Translational Immunology
TRANSLATIONAL AUTOIMMUNITY, VOL. 2

Translational Immunology

TRANSLATIONAL AUTOIMMUNITY, VOL. 2

Treatment of Autoimmune Diseases

Edited by

NIMA REZAEI

*Professor, Department of Immunology, School of Medicine;
Head, Research Center for Immunodeficiencies, Children's Medical Center,
Tehran University of Medical Sciences; Founding President,
Universal Scientific Education and Research Network (USERN),
Tehran, Iran*

Editorial Assistant

NILOUFAR YAZDANPANAH

*Managing Director, Network of Immunity in Infection,
Malignancy and Autoimmunity (NIIMA),
Universal Scientific Education and Research Network, (USERN); and School of Medicine,
Tehran University of Medical Sciences,
Tehran, Iran*

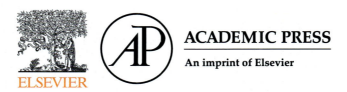

Academic Press is an imprint of Elsevier
125 London Wall, London EC2Y 5AS, United Kingdom
525 B Street, Suite 1650, San Diego, CA 92101, United States
50 Hampshire Street, 5th Floor, Cambridge, MA 02139, United States
The Boulevard, Langford Lane, Kidlington, Oxford OX5 1GB, United Kingdom

Copyright © 2022 Elsevier Inc. All rights reserved.

No part of this publication may be reproduced or transmitted in any form or by any means, electronic or mechanical, including photocopying, recording, or any information storage and retrieval system, without permission in writing from the publisher. Details on how to seek permission, further information about the Publisher's permissions policies and our arrangements with organizations such as the Copyright Clearance Center and the Copyright Licensing Agency, can be found at our website: www.elsevier.com/permissions.

This book and the individual contributions contained in it are protected under copyright by the Publisher (other than as may be noted herein).

Notices

Knowledge and best practice in this field are constantly changing. As new research and experience broaden our understanding, changes in research methods, professional practices, or medical treatment may become necessary.

Practitioners and researchers must always rely on their own experience and knowledge in evaluating and using any information, methods, compounds, or experiments described herein. In using such information or methods they should be mindful of their own safety and the safety of others, including parties for whom they have a professional responsibility.

To the fullest extent of the law, neither the Publisher nor the authors, contributors, or editors, assume any liability for any injury and/or damage to persons or property as a matter of products liability, negligence or otherwise, or from any use or operation of any methods, products, instructions, or ideas contained in the material herein.

Library of Congress Cataloging-in-Publication Data
A catalog record for this book is available from the Library of Congress

British Library Cataloguing-in-Publication Data
A catalogue record for this book is available from the British Library

ISBN: 978-0-12-824390-9

For information on all Academic Press publications
visit our website at https://www.elsevier.com/books-and-journals

Publisher: Stacy Masucci
Acquisitions Editor: Linda Versteeg-Buschman
Editorial Project Manager: Billie Jean Fernandez
Production Project Manager: Omer Mukthar
Cover Designer: Christian J. Bilbow

Typeset by STRAIVE, India

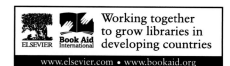

Dedication

This book would not have been possible without the continuous encouragement of my family. I dedicate the book to my daughters, Ariana and Arnika, in the hope that we learn enough from today to make a brighter future for the next generation.

Contents

Contributors xi
Preface xv
Series editor biography xvii
Acknowledgment xix
Abbreviations xxi

1. Introduction on therapeutic opportunities for autoimmunity

Nima Rezaei and Niloufar Yazdanpanah

1 Introduction 2
2 From the very first known treatment to the recent developments in therapeutic strategies 2
3 Conclusion 8
References 8

2. Innate lymphoid cells as therapeutic targets in autoimmune diseases

Prince Amoah Barnie, Xia Lin, and Su Zhaoliang

1 Introduction 13
2 The biology of innate lymphoid cells 15
3 Properties and functions of ILCs 18
4 ILC in autoimmune diseases 19
5 ILCs as immunoregulators in autoimmune diseases 26
6 ILC as a potential therapeutic target in autoimmune diseases 27
7 Future perspectives 29
8 Conclusion 29
References 29

3. B regulatory cells in patients with autoimmune diseases: Pathogenic significance and therapeutic potential

Athanasios Mavropoulos, Efterpi Zafiriou, Efthymios Dardiotis, Lazaros I. Sakkas, and Dimitrios P. Bogdanos

1 Introduction 38
2 Identification of Breg cells 38

3 Functional properties 39
4 B regulatory cells and autoimmunity: Pathogenic significance 43
5 Therapeutic potential 44
6 Conclusion 46
References 46

4. Regulatory T cells in autoimmunity and potential therapeutic targets

Ankur Kumar Jindal, Aaqib Zaffar Banday, and Rahul Tyagi

1 Introduction 56
2 Discovery of Treg cells 56
3 Development and activation of Treg cells 56
4 FoxP3—The transcriptional master regulator of Treg cells 58
5 Phenotype of Treg cells 58
6 Treg/T cell subtypes with regulatory function 60
7 Protocols for estimation of Treg cells in the peripheral blood 62
8 Isolation of Treg cells for therapeutic purposes 63
9 Tissue-resident Treg cells 63
10 Clinical and translational significance of Treg cells 64
11 Regulatory T cells (Tregs) as potential therapeutic targets 72
12 Conclusion 75
References 75

5. Application of IL-6 antagonists in autoimmune disorders

Tiago Borges, Arsénio Barbosa, and Sérgio Silva

1 Introduction 83
2 Signaling 85
3 Roles of IL-6 86
4 IL-6 in ADs and autoimmune-related disorders 89

viii   Contents

5 Laboratory clues 92
6 IL-6 blockade 94
7 Conclusion 103
References 104

6. The search for monomer-interaction-based alternative TNF-α therapies

Mark Farrugia and Byron Baron

1 Introduction 115
2 TNF-α in relation to stages in life 119
3 Structure of TNF-α 121
4 TNF-α therapies 124
5 Conclusion 127
References 127

7. Generation of thymic cells from pluripotent stem cells for basic research and cell therapy

Stephan Ramos and Holger A. Russ

1 Introduction 136
2 Thymus organogenesis 136
3 Thymus function 137
4 Common thymic disorders 137
5 Human pluripotent stem cells to TECs: A new frontier 138
6 Mimicking development in vitro to generate hPSC-derived anterior foregut endoderm 139
7 Generating thymic epithelial progenitor cells in vitro 139
8 hPSC-derived thymic epithelial cells 141
9 In vitro coculture systems to model thymic function 142
10 Conclusion 144
References 145

8. The NLRP3 inflammasome pathway in autoimmune diseases: a chronotherapeutic perspective?

Cécilia Bellengier, Hélène Duez, and Benoit Pourcet

1 Introduction 150
2 The NLRP3 inflammasome 151
3 NLRP3 and autoimmune diseases 154

4 The clock and autoimmune diseases 163
5 NLRP3 as a chronotherapeutic target for autoimmune diseases treatment 166
6 Conclusion 168
References 169

9. Plasmocyte depletion in autoimmune diseases

Nathalie Sturm and Bertrand Huard

1 Introduction 179
2 The plasmocyte 180
3 New drugs targeting the humoral immunity 183
4 Drugs in the pipeline 185
5 Autoimmune diseases that may benefit from plasmocyte targeting 187
6 Conclusion 188
References 189

10. Biological aging and autoimmunity

Mustafa Erinç Sitar

1 Introduction 193
2 Immunosenescence 194
3 Immune and autoimmune theories of aging 195
4 Autoimmune diseases, cancer, and their relations with aging 196
5 Conclusion 200
References 200

11. Efficacy and safety of immune checkpoint inhibitors and cytokine therapy in autoimmune diseases

Reyhaneh Sabourian, Seyedeh Zohreh Mirjalili, and Nima Rezaei

1 Introduction 206
2 Immunogenicity of mAbs and its effect on efficacy and safety 206
3 Inflammatory cytokine inhibition in autoimmune diseases 207
4 ICIs in autoimmune disease 231
5 Conclusion 234
References 235

12. Nutritional implications for the pathophysiology and treatment of autoimmune disorders

Catherine J. Andersen and Julia M. Greco

1 Introduction 244
2 Body composition and metabolic health 244
3 Dietary patterns 246
4 Macronutrients 249
5 Micronutrients 252
6 Additional non-nutrient dietary factors 254
7 Conclusion 255
References 256

13. Dysbiosis and probiotic applications in autoimmune diseases

Larissa Vedovato Vilela de Salis, Luísa Sales Martins,
Guilherme Siqueira Pardo Rodrigues, and
Gislane Lelis Vilela de Oliveira

1 Introduction 270
2 Dysbiosis in autoimmune diseases 271
3 Dysbiosis in autoimmune diabetes 272
4 Dysbiosis in autoimmune thyroid diseases 273
5 Dysbiosis in rheumatoid arthritis 275
6 Dysbiosis in systemic lupus erythematosus 277
7 Dysbiosis in Sjögren's syndrome 278
8 Probiotic applications in autoimmune diseases 279
9 Probiotics in autoimmune diabetes 280
10 Probiotics in autoimmune thyroid diseases 283
11 Probiotics in rheumatoid arthritis 284
12 Probiotics in systemic lupus erythematous 285
13 Probiotics in Sjögren's syndrome 286
14 Conclusion 287
References 287

14. Precision medicine to manage chronic immune-related conditions

David S. Gibson, Phil Egan, Guangran Guo, Catriona Kelly,
Paula McClean, Victoria McGilligan, Roisin McAllister,
Kyle B. Matchett, Chloe A. Martin, Elaine K. Murray,
Coral R. Lapsley, Taranjit Singh Rai, and Anthony J. Bjourson

1 Introduction 296
2 Immunosenescence 296
3 Diabetes mellitus 299
4 Atherosclerotic cardiovascular disease 300

5 Musculoskeletal conditions and arthritis 303
6 Mental health conditions 306
7 Cancer 308
8 Conclusion 310
References 311

15. New advanced therapy medicinal products in treatment of autoimmune diseases

Shahrbanoo Jahangir, Sareh Zeydabadinejad, Zhila Izadi,
Mahdi Habibi-Anbouhi, and Ensiyeh Hajizadeh-Saffar

1 Introduction 320
2 Autoimmune disorders 322
3 Conclusion 352
References 353

16. Targeting autoimmune disorders through metal nanoformulation in overcoming the fences of conventional treatment approaches

Krishna Yadav, Madhulika Pradhan, Deependra Singh,
and Manju Rawat Singh

1 Introduction 362
2 Nanotechnology and nanomaterials 365
3 Targeting of metal nanoparticles for autoimmune conditions 377
4 Safety concern of metallic nanoparticles 385
5 Conclusion 386
References 387

17. Immunomodulatory effects of parasites on autoimmunity

Amir Abdoli, Alireza Badirzadeh, Nazanin Mojtabavi,
Ahmadreza Meamar, and Reza Falak

1 Introduction 396
2 Mechanism of action in helminth therapy 397
3 Application and protective roles of helminth therapy 399
4 Current challenges in helminth therapy 402
5 Animal models for helminth therapy 402
6 Immunomodulatory roles of parasites on inflammatory or autoimmune diseases 413
7 Leishmaniasis and autoimmune disorders 414

x   Contents

8 *Toxoplasmosis* and autoimmune disorders   415
9 Conclusion   416
References   416

18. Prediction of autoimmune diseases: From bench to bedside

Álvaro J. Vivas and Gabriel J. Tobón

1 Introduction   425
2 Using genetics to estimate the risk of developing AIDs   427
3 Epigenetics to predict AIDs   430
4 Using antibodies and serum biomarkers to predict AIDs   432
5 Perspectives   440
6 Prevention   441
7 Conclusion   445
References   445

Index   451

Contributors

Amir Abdoli Zoonosis Research Center; Department of Parasitology and Mycology, Jahrom University of Medical Sciences, Jahrom, Iran

Catherine J. Andersen Department of Biology, Fairfield University, Fairfield; Department of Nutritional Sciences, University of Connecticut, Storrs, CT, United States

Alireza Badirzadeh Department of Parasitology and Mycology, School of Medicine, Iran University of Medical Sciences, Tehran, Iran

Aaqib Zaffar Banday Allergy and Immunology Unit, Department of Pediatrics, Advanced Pediatric Centre, Postgraduate Institute of Medical Education and Research, Chandigarh, India

Arsénio Barbosa Department of Internal Medicine, University Hospital Center of São João, Porto, Portugal

Prince Amoah Barnie The Central Laboratory, The Fourth Affiliated Hospital of Jiangsu University; International Genome Center, Jiangsu University, Zhenjiang, China; Department of Biomedical Sciences, School of Allied Health Sciences, University of Cape Coast, Cape Coast, Ghana

Byron Baron Centre for Molecular Medicine and Biobanking, University of Malta, Msida, Malta

Cécilia Bellengier Univ. Lille, U1011 – EGID; Inserm, U1011; CHU Lille; Institut Pasteur de Lille, Lille, France

Anthony J. Bjourson Northern Ireland Centre for Stratified Medicine, Ulster University, Londonderry, United Kingdom

Dimitrios P. Bogdanos Department of Rheumatology and Clinical Immunology, Faculty of Medicine, School of Health Sciences, University of Thessaly, Larissa, Greece

Tiago Borges Department of Internal Medicine, Trofa Saúde Private Hospital, Vila Nova de Gaia, Portugal

Efthymios Dardiotis Department of Neurology, Faculty of Medicine, School of Health Sciences, University of Thessaly, Larissa, Greece

Hélène Duez Univ. Lille, U1011 – EGID; Inserm, U1011; CHU Lille; Institut Pasteur de Lille, Lille, France

Phil Egan Northern Ireland Centre for Stratified Medicine, Ulster University, Londonderry, United Kingdom

Reza Falak Department of Immunology, School of Medicine; Immunology Research Center, Iran University of Medical Sciences, Tehran, Iran

Mark Farrugia Centre for Molecular Medicine and Biobanking, University of Malta, Msida, Malta

David S. Gibson Northern Ireland Centre for Stratified Medicine, Ulster University, Londonderry, United Kingdom

Julia M. Greco Department of Biology, Fairfield University, Fairfield, CT, United States

Guangran Guo Northern Ireland Centre for Stratified Medicine, Ulster University, Londonderry, United Kingdom

Mahdi Habibi-Anbouhi National Cell Bank of Iran, Pasteur Institute of Iran, Tehran, Iran

Ensiyeh Hajizadeh-Saffar Advanced Therapy Medicinal Product Technology Development Center (ATMP-TDC); Department of Regenerative Medicine; Department of Diabetes, Obesity, and Metabolism, Cell Science Research Center, Royan Institute for Stem Cell Biology and Technology, Tehran, Iran

Bertrand Huard TIMC-IMAG Laboratory, CNRS UMR5525, University Grenoble-Alpes, La Tronche, France

Zhila Izadi Pharmaceutical Sciences Research Center, Health Institute, Kermanshah University of Medical Sciences, Kermanshah, Iran

Shahrbanoo Jahangir Department of Stem Cells and Developmental Biology; Advanced Therapy Medicinal Product Technology Development Center (ATMP-TDC), Cell Science Research Center, Royan Institute for Stem Cell Biology and Technology, Tehran, Iran

Ankur Kumar Jindal Allergy and Immunology Unit, Department of Pediatrics, Advanced Pediatric Centre, Postgraduate Institute of Medical Education and Research, Chandigarh, India

Catriona Kelly Northern Ireland Centre for Stratified Medicine, Ulster University, Londonderry, United Kingdom

Coral R. Lapsley Northern Ireland Centre for Stratified Medicine, Ulster University, Londonderry, United Kingdom

Xia Lin International Genome Center, Jiangsu University, Zhenjiang, China

Chloe A. Martin Northern Ireland Centre for Stratified Medicine, Ulster University, Londonderry, United Kingdom

Luísa Sales Martins Microbiology Program, Institute of Biosciences, Humanities and Exact Sciences (IBILCE), São Paulo State University (UNESP), São Paulo, Brazil

Kyle B. Matchett Northern Ireland Centre for Stratified Medicine, Ulster University, Londonderry, United Kingdom

Athanasios Mavropoulos Department of Rheumatology and Clinical Immunology, Faculty of Medicine, School of Health Sciences, University of Thessaly, Larissa, Greece

Roisin McAllister Northern Ireland Centre for Stratified Medicine, Ulster University, Londonderry, United Kingdom

Paula McClean Northern Ireland Centre for Stratified Medicine, Ulster University, Londonderry, United Kingdom

Victoria McGilligan Northern Ireland Centre for Stratified Medicine, Ulster University, Londonderry, United Kingdom

Ahmadreza Meamar Department of Parasitology and Mycology, School of Medicine, Iran University of Medical Sciences, Tehran, Iran

Seyedeh Zohreh Mirjalili Department of Drug and Food Control, Faculty of Pharmacy, Tehran University of Medical Sciences; Network of Immunity in Infection, Malignancy and Autoimmunity (NIIMA), Universal Scientific Education and Research Network (USERN), Tehran, Iran

Nazanin Mojtabavi Department of Immunology, School of Medicine; Immunology Research Center, Iran University of Medical Sciences, Tehran, Iran

Elaine K. Murray Northern Ireland Centre for Stratified Medicine, Ulster University, Londonderry, United Kingdom

Gislane Lelis Vilela de Oliveira Microbiology Program, Institute of Biosciences, Humanities and Exact Sciences (IBILCE); Department of Food Engineering and Technology, Institute of Biosciences, Humanities and Exact Sciences, São Paulo State University (UNESP), São Paulo, Brazil

Benoit Pourcet Univ. Lille, U1011 – EGID; Inserm, U1011; CHU Lille; Institut Pasteur de Lille, Lille, France

Madhulika Pradhan Rungta College of Pharmaceutical Sciences and Research, Bhilai, Chhattisgarh, India

Taranjit Singh Rai Northern Ireland Centre for Stratified Medicine, Ulster University, Londonderry, United Kingdom

Stephan Ramos Barbara Davis Center for Diabetes, Department of Pediatrics, School of Medicine, University of Colorado Anschutz Medical Campus, Aurora, CO, United States

Nima Rezaei Research Center for Immunodeficiencies, Children's Medical Center; Department of Immunology, School of Medicine, Tehran University of Medical Sciences; Network of Immunity in Infection, Malignancy and Autoimmunity (NIIMA), Universal Scientific Education and Research Network (USERN), Tehran, Iran

Guilherme Siqueira Pardo Rodrigues Department of Pediatrics, Hospital from School of Medicine from Botucatu (HCFMB), São Paulo State University (UNESP), Botucatu, Brazil

Holger A. Russ Barbara Davis Center for Diabetes, Department of Pediatrics, School of Medicine, University of Colorado Anschutz Medical Campus, Aurora, CO, United States

Reyhaneh Sabourian Department of Drug and Food Control, Faculty of Pharmacy, Tehran University of Medical Sciences; Network of Immunity in Infection, Malignancy and Autoimmunity (NIIMA), Universal Scientific Education and Research Network (USERN), Tehran, Iran

Lazaros I. Sakkas Department of Rheumatology and Clinical Immunology, Faculty of Medicine, School of Health Sciences, University of Thessaly, Larissa, Greece

Larissa Vedovato Vilela de Salis Microbiology Program, Institute of Biosciences, Humanities and Exact Sciences (IBILCE), São Paulo State University (UNESP), São Paulo, Brazil

Sérgio Silva Department of Internal Medicine, Trofa Saúde Private Hospital, Vila Nova de Gaia, Portugal

Deependra Singh University Institute of Pharmacy, Pt. Ravishankar Shukla University, Raipur, Chhattisgarh, India

Manju Rawat Singh University Institute of Pharmacy, Pt. Ravishankar Shukla University, Raipur, Chhattisgarh, India

Mustafa Erinç Sitar Faculty of Medicine, Department of Clinical Biochemistry, Maltepe University; Maltepe University Experimental Animals Application and Research Center, Istanbul, Turkey

Nathalie Sturm Department of Pathology, University Hospital, Grenoble; TIMC-IMAG Laboratory, CNRS UMR5525, University Grenoble-Alpes, La Tronche, France

Gabriel J. Tobón Universidad Icesi, CIRAT: Centro de Investigación en Reumatología,

Autoinmunidad y Medicina Traslacional, Cali, Colombia

Rahul Tyagi Allergy and Immunology Unit, Department of Pediatrics, Advanced Pediatric Centre, Postgraduate Institute of Medical Education and Research, Chandigarh, India

Álvaro J. Vivas Universidad Icesi, Facultad de Ciencias de la Salud, Calle 18 No. 122 -135; Universidad Icesi, CIRAT: Centro de Investigación en Reumatología, Autoinmunidad y Medicina Traslacional, Cali, Colombia

Krishna Yadav University Institute of Pharmacy, Pt. Ravishankar Shukla University, Raipur, Chhattisgarh, India

Niloufar Yazdanpanah Research Center for Immunodeficiencies, Children's Medical Center, Tehran University of Medical Sciences; Network of Immunity in Infection, Malignancy and Autoimmunity (NIIMA), Universal Scientific Education and Research Network (USERN), Tehran, Iran

Efterpi Zafiriou Department of Dermatology, Faculty of Medicine, School of Health Sciences, University of Thessaly, Larissa, Greece

Sareh Zeydabadinejad Cellular and Molecular Endocrine Research Center, Research Institute for Endocrine Sciences, Shahid Beheshti University of Medical Sciences, Tehran, Iran

Su Zhaoliang The Central Laboratory, The Fourth Affiliated Hospital of Jiangsu University; International Genome Center, Jiangsu University, Zhenjiang, China

Preface

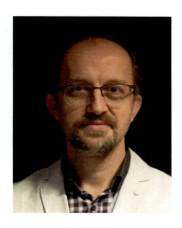

The scientific world has witnessed remarkable developments in the field of immunology during recent decades. The novel discovery of genes related to different immune-mediated diseases has enhanced our knowledge about the immune system and its interactions with other systems in the human body and has also enlightened the different aspects of its complexity that lead to promoting diagnostic strategies, designing more efficient therapeutic agents, and reducing the potential morbidities and mortality. Due to the broad spectrum of immune-mediated diseases, from immunodeficiency to hypersensitivity and autoimmune diseases, immune system diseases collectively contribute to a considerable prevalence, although every single immune-mediated disease represents a low prevalence.

The concern of applying the latest research findings has long been with scientists. Translational research is recognized as a potential tool to utilize scientific findings in clinical settings and patient care. Considering the wide spectrum of diseases related to the immune system, besides their huge burden on individuals, healthcare settings, families, and society, identifying promising alternative diagnostic and therapeutic strategies through translational studies is of interest.

The *Translational Immunology* Book series is a major new suite of books in immunology, which covers both basic and clinical immunology. This series seeks to discuss and provide foundational content from bench to bedside in immunology. The series is intended to discuss recent immunological findings and translate them into clinical practice. The first volumes of the book series are specifically devoted to autoimmune diseases.

Translational Autoimmunity: Treatment of Autoimmune Diseases is a comprehensive guide that attempts to cover the latest data on all the current therapeutic measures and promising future treatments. Despite the notable progress in animal studies concerning finding new targets and treatment strategies, the advancement in clinical practice is not as what was expected. The complexity of the human body and innate differences with animal models besides the existing impediments to conducting large-scale human studies are the main reasons for this issue, which potentially highlights the importance of translational studies. This book starts with recapitulating all the current and potential future therapeutic options in Chapter 1, which briefly discusses therapeutic measures and introduces alternative treatments for future autoimmunity medicines. Considering immune cells as important components in the etiopathology of autoimmune diseases, Chapters 2, 3, and 4 focus on innate lymphoid cells, B-regulatory cells, and T-regulatory cells, respectively. Meanwhile, the role of immune mediators in the initiation and progress of autoimmune diseases is inevitable. Therefore, Chapter 5 is devoted to interleukin 6 as a therapeutic target and Chapter 6 is about targeting the tumor necrosis factor, as the two pivotal immune mediators in autoimmune reactions. Chapter 7 dives deep into cell therapy research, thymic cell generation in particular. Moreover, considering the growing interest in the role of NLRP3 inflammasome in immune-mediated diseases, Chapter 8 discusses the potentials of targeting the NLRP3 pathway. Concerning the importance of antibodies and antibody-producing cells, targeting plasmocytes are explored in Chapter 9. Furthermore, Chapter 10 discusses the association between biological aging and autoimmunity. To evaluate the currently available treatments and highlight the existing challenges, Chapter 11 takes a focused view on the efficacy and safety of biologic agents. With regard to the growing body of evidence on the role of nutrition and diet on human health by itself and by modulating the microbiota, Chapters 12 and 13 are devoted to the nutritional implications in the management of autoimmune diseases and the therapeutic targeting of microbiota, respectively. With the progress of genetic studies and the emergence of the concept of personalized medicine, Chapter 14 goes into details about the application of precision medicine in autoimmune diseases. In addition, advanced therapy medicinal products (ATMPs), which are novel treatments based on genes, cells, and tissues, and the application of nanotechnology in the treatment of autoimmune diseases are discussed is Chapters 15 and 16, respectively. Finally, as often stated about various types of diseases, prevention is better than cure. Hence, prediction of autoimmune diseases might help diagnose patients either before the onset of the disease or at the early stages of the disease, which in turn leads to a better prognosis and lower disease burden. The topic of prediction in autoimmune diseases is explored in Chapter 17.

The *Translational Immunology* Book series is the outcome of the invaluable contributions of scientists and clinicians from well-known universities/institutes worldwide. I hereby appreciate and acknowledge the expertise of all contributors for generously devoting their time and considerable effort in preparing their respective chapters. I also express my gratitude to Elsevier for providing me with the opportunity to publish this book. Finally, I hope this translational book will be comprehensible, cogent, and of special value to researchers and clinicians who wish to extend their knowledge on immunology.

Nima Rezaei

Series editor biography

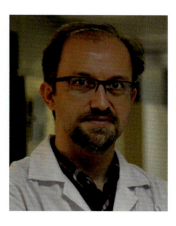

Professor Nima Rezaei obtained his medical degree (MD) from Tehran University of Medical Sciences and subsequently obtained an MSc in molecular and genetic medicine and a PhD in clinical immunology and human genetics from the University of Sheffield, United Kingdom. He also spent a short-term fellowship of Pediatric Clinical Immunology and Bone Marrow Transplantation in the Newcastle General Hospital. Rezaei is now the Full Professor of Immunology and Vice Dean of International Affairs, School of Medicine, Tehran University of Medical Sciences, and the Cofounder and Head of the Research Center for Immunodeficiencies. He is also the founding President of Universal Scientific Education and Research Network (USERN). Prof. Rezaei has already been the Director of more than 50 research projects and has designed and participated in several international collaborative projects. Prof. Rezaei is an editorial assistant or board member for more than 30 international journals. He has edited more than 30 international books, has presented more than 500 lectures/posters in congresses/meetings, and has published more than 1000 scientific papers in international journals.

Acknowledgment

I express my gratitude to the editorial assistant of this book, Dr. Niloufar Yazdanpanah. Without a doubt, this book would not have been completed without her contribution.

Nima Rezaei

Abbreviations

1,25(OH)$_2$D$_3$	1,25-dihydroxy vitamin D$_3$	AOSD	adult-onset Still's disease
25(OH)D$_3$	25-hydroxy vitamin D$_3$	APCs	antigen-presenting cells
A20/Tnfaip3	tumor necrosis factor, alpha-induced protein 3	APECED	autoimmune polyendocrinopathy-candidiasis-ectodermal dystrophy
A23187	calcium ionophore	aPLs	antiphospholipid antibodies
AAV	adeno-associated virus	APPs	acute-phase proteins
AAV	ANCA-associated vasculitis	APRIL	a proliferation-inducing ligand
aCLs	anticardiolipin antibodies	APS	antiphospholipid syndrome
ACPAs	anticitrullinated protein antibodies	APS-1	autoimmune polyendocrine syndrome type 1
ACS	acute coronary syndrome	AS	ankylosing spondylitis
ACTH	adrenocorticotropic hormone	ASC	apoptosis-associated speck-like protein containing a CARD domain
ADABs	antibody-binding fragments		
ADABs	antidrug antibodies	ASD	autism spectrum disorder
ADAM10/17	metalloproteinase domain-containing proteins 10 and 17	ATMPs	advanced therapy medicinal products
ADAMTS13	a disintegrin and metalloproteinase with a thrombospondin type 1 motif, member 13	ATP	adenosine triphosphate
		AUC	area under the curve
		AUC	area under the ROC curve
ADCC	antibody-dependent cellular cytotoxicity	Aβ$_{1-42}$	β-amyloid peptide (1-42)
		B19V	parvovirus B19
AD-MSCs	adipose-derived mesenchymal stem cells	BAFF	B-cell activation factor from the TNF superfamily
ADs	autoimmune diseases	BAs	bile acids
AEs	adverse effects	BASDAI	Bath Ankylosing Spondylitis Disease Activity Index
AFEs	anterior foregut endoderm cells		
AFG	anterior foregut	BASFI	Bath Ankylosing Spondylitis Functional Index
AFG	autologous fat grafting		
AIA	arthritis induced by adjuvant	BBI	Bowman-Birk inhibitor
AIDS	acquired immunodeficiency syndrome	BC4d	B-cell-bound C4d
		BCG	Bacillus Calmette-Guérin
AIDs	autoimmune diseases	BCMA	B-cell maturation antigen
AIM2	absent in melanoma 2	BCR	B-cell receptor
AIRE	autoimmune regulator	BMAL1	brain and muscle ARNT-like 1
AIT	autoimmune thyroiditis	BMI	body mass index
AITD	autoimmune thyroid disease	BM-MSCs	bone marrow-derived mesenchymal stem cells
Akt	AKT serine/threonine kinase		
ALPS	autoimmune lymphoproliferative syndrome	BMP4	bone morphogenic protein 4
		BRCC3	Lys-63-specific deubiquitinase BRCC36
ALT	alanine transaminase		
ANAs	antinuclear antibodies	Breg	B regulatory
ANCAs	antineutrophil cytoplasm antibodies	Breg	regulatory B cell
		BS	Behçet's syndrome
ANCAs	antineutrophil cytoplasmic autoantibodies	BSF	B-cell stimulatory factor
		BSF-2	B-cell stimulatory factor-2
Anti-CarPs	anti-carbamylated protein antibodies	BTD	breakthrough therapy designation

xxi

CA	curculigoside A	CXCL	C-X-C motif chemokine ligand
CAI	Clinical Activity Index	CYC	cyclophosphamide
CAMs	cell-adhesion molecules	D2	type 2 iodothyronine deiodinase
CAPS	cryopyrin-associated periodic syndrome	DAMPs	damage-associated molecular patterns
CAR T cells	chimeric antigen receptor T cells	DAS-28	disease activity score in 28 joints
CAR	chimeric antigen receptor	DAS28-CRP	disease activity score-28 for
CARMIL2	capping protein regulator and myosin 1 linker 2		rheumatoid arthritis with C-reactive protein
cATMPs	combined ATMPs	DCreg	regulatory dendritic cell
CB	HSCs cord blood-derived HSCs	DCs	dendritic cells
CB-CAPs	cell-bound complement activation products	DEPTOR	DEP domain-containing mTOR-interacting protein
CCL	C-C motif chemokine ligand	DEs	definitive endoderm cells
CCP	cyclic citrullinated peptide	DFNB	dinitrofluorobenzene
CCR	C-C chemokine receptor	DHA	docosahexaenoic acid
CD	cluster of differentiation	diC8	1,2-dioctanoylglycerol
CD	Crohn's disease	DM	diabetes mellitus
CDAI	CD Activity Index	DMARDs	disease-modifying antirheumatic
CDC	complement-dependent cytotoxicity	DMOAD	drugs disease-modifying osteoarthritis
cDMARD	conventional disease-modifying antirheumatic drug		drug
CDSs	coding sequences	DNA	deoxyribonucleic acid
CeD	celiac disease	DNBS	dinitrobenzene sulfonic acid
CFA	complete Freund's adjuvant	DNTs	double-negative T cells
CFU-M	megakaryocytic colony-forming cells	DOCK8	dedicator of cytokinesis 8
cGAS	cyclic GMP-AMP synthase	DPT-1	diabetes prevention trial-type1
CIA	collagen-induced arthritis	dsDNA	double-stranded DNA
CITR	collaborative islet transplant registry	DSS	dextran sodium
CL	cutaneous leishmaniasis	DSS	dextran sodium sulfate
CLICs	chloride intracellular channels	DSS	dextran sulfate sodium
CLOCK	circadian locomotor output cycles kaput	EAE	experimental autoimmune encephalomyelitis
CLP	common lymphoid progenitor	EAT	experimental autoimmune thyroiditis
CLRs	C-lectin receptors	EBMT	European Society for Bone Marrow
CLZ	clazakizumab		Transplantation
C_{max}	maximum plasma concentration	EBV	Epstein-Barr virus
CMV	cytomegalovirus	EC4d	erythrocyte-bound C4d
CNS	central nervous system	ECL	electrochemiluminescence
CNTF	ciliary neurotrophic factor	EDSS	Expanded Disability Status Scale
COX-2	cyclooxygenase 2	EGF	epidermal growth factor
CRDs	cysteine-rich domains	eNOS	endothelial nitric oxide synthase
CRP	C-reactive protein	EPA	eicosapentaenoic acid
CRY	cryptochrome	ER	endoplasmic reticulum
cs	conventional synthetic	ERKs	extracellular signal-regulated kinases
CSF	cerebrospinal fluid	ESPs	excretory/secretory products
CT-1	cardiotropin 1	ESR	erythrocyte sedimentation rate
cTECs	cortical thymic epithelial cells	EU	European Union
CTLA	cytotoxic T-lymphocyte antigen	EULAR	European League against
CVD	cardiovascular disease		Rheumatism
CVID	common variable immunodeficiency	EVOO	extra virgin olive oil
		EYA1	eyes absent homolog 1

Abbreviations

Fc	fragment crystallizable
FDA	Food and Drug Administration
FDRs	first-degree relatives
FEZF2	fasciculation and elongation protein zeta 2
FGF10	fibroblast growth factor 10
FGF8	fibroblast growth factor
FMO3	flavin-dependent monooxygenase
FOXN1	forkhead box N1
FoxP3	forkhead box P3
FSS	Fatigue Severity Scale
fTreg	follicular regulatory T cell
FVC	forced vital capacity
GAD-65	glutamic acid decarboxylase
GADAs	glutamic acid decarboxylase antibodies
GC	germinal center
GCA	giant cell arteritis
GCM2	glial cells missing transcription factor 2
GD	Graves' disease
GFAP	glial fibrillary acidic protein
GFD	gluten-free diet
GFP	green fluorescence protein
GGT	gamma-glutamyl transferase
GH	growth hormone
GI	gastrointestinal
GM-CSF	granulocyte-macrophage colony-stimulating factor
GMP	good manufacturing practice
GO	Graves' ophthalmopathy
GO	Graves' orbitopathy
GPA	granulomatosis with polyangiitis
GRSs	genetic risk scores
GSDMD	Gasdermin D
GTF2i	general transcription factor IIi
GTMPs	gene therapy medicinal products
GWASs	genome-wide association studies
HbA1c	glycated hemoglobin
HCV	hepatitis C virus
hEMPs	human embryonic mesoderm progenitors
HFLS	human fibroblast-like synoviocytes
HIF-1α	hypoxia-inducible factor-1α
hiPSCs	human induced pluripotent stem cells
HIV	human immunodeficiency virus
HLA	human leukocyte antigen
HMGB1	high-mobility group box-1
HMW Ag	high-molecular-weight antigen
HOMA-B	homeostatic model assessment of B-cell function
HOXA3	homeobox A3
HPA axis	hypothalamic pituitary adrenal axis
HPA	hypothalamus-pituitary-adrenal
HPGF	hybridoma/plasmacytoma growth factor
hPSCs	human pluripotent stem cells
hsCRP	high-sensitivity C-reactive protein
Hs-CRP	high-sensitivity C-reactive protein
HSCs	hematopoietic stem cells
HSCT	hematopoietic stem cell transplantation
HSF	hepatocyte-stimulating factor
HSP	Henoch-Schönlein purpura
HSP90	heat shock protein 90
Hsp90	heat shock protein 90
HSPGs	heparan sulfate proteoglycans
HT	Hashimoto's thyroiditis
hUC-MSC	human umbilical cord-derived MSC
IA	intra-articular
IA-2A	islet tyrosine phosphatase 2 antibodies
IAAs	insulin autoantibodies
IAPP	islet amyloid polypeptide precursor
IBD	inflammatory bowel disease
IBD	inflammatory bowel disorder
ICAM-1	intercellular adhesion molecule 1
ICAs	islet cell antibodies
IDO	immunosuppressant indoleamine dioxygenase
IFA	indirect fluorescent antibody
IFNs	interferons
IFN-γ	interferon gamma
IgG	Immunoglobulin G
IIF	indirect immunofluorescence
IKBKB	inhibitor of nuclear factor kappa B kinase subunit beta
IL	interleukin
IL-6R	IL-6 receptor
ILC	innate lymphoid cell
iNKTs	invariant natural killer T cells
iNOS	inducible nitric oxide synthase
IPEX	immune dysregulation, polyendocrinopathy, enteropathy X-linked
IRF1	interferon regulatory factor 1
IRF3	interferon regulatory factor 3
IRF6	interferon-regulatory factor 5 (IRF5) locus
IUGR	intrauterine growth retardation
IV	intravenous
IVIg	intravenous immunoglobulin
JAKs	Janus kinases
JIA	juvenile idiopathic arthritis
JIA	juvenile inflammatory arthritis

Abbreviations

JNK	c-Jun N-terminal kinase
KD	Kawasaki disease
KGF	keratinocyte growth factor, also known as fibroblast growth factor 7
KLRG1	killer-cell lectin-like receptor 1
KO	gene knockout model
LAG-3	lymphocyte activation gene-3
LBP	LPS-binding protein
LCD	low-carbohydrate diet
LDL	low-density cholesterol
LDL	low-density lipoprotein
LFTs	liver function tests
LH	luteinizing hormone
LIF	leukemia inhibitory factor
LPCs	lymphoid progenitor cells
LPS	lipopolysaccharide
LRBA	LPS-responsive and beige-like anchor
LRR	leucine-rich repeat
LT4	levothyroxine
LVL	levilimab
LXRs	liver X receptors
MAAA	multiplex assays with algorithmic analyses
mAbs	monoclonal antibodies
MAPK	mitogen-activated protein kinase
MAS	macrophage activation syndrome
MAS	multiplex assay technologies
MAVS	mitochondrial antiviral-signaling protein
MBP	myelin basic protein
MCP	metacarpophalangeal
MCS	mental component summary
M-CSF	macrophage colony-stimulating factor
MDP	muramyl dipeptide
MetS	metabolic syndrome
MGI-2A	macrophage granulocyte inducer type 2
MHCs	major histocompatibility complexes
miR	microRNA
miRNAs	micro RNAs
MMF	mycophenolate mofetil
MMP	matrix metallopeptidase
MPO	myeloperoxidase
MR	mineralocorticoid receptor
mRNA	messenger RNA
MS	multiple sclerosis
MSCs	mesenchymal stem cells
mt	mitochondrial
mTECs	medullary thymic epithelial cells
mTOR	mammalian target of rapamycin
MTX	methotrexate
MyD88	myeloid differentiation primary response 88

MyoD	myoblast determination protein 1
NADPH	nicotinamide adenine dinucleotide phosphate
NB-UVB	narrowband ultraviolet B
NEK7	NIMA-related kinase 7
NETs	neutrophil extracellular traps
NF-IL6	nuclear factor for controlling IL-6 expression (C/EBPβ)
NF-κB	nuclear factor kappa B
NF-κB	nuclear factor kappa-light-chain-enhancer of activated B cells
NF-κB	nuclear factor-κB
NHL	non-Hodgkin's lymphoma
NHS	Nurses' Health Study
NK cells	natural killer cells
NK	natural killer
NKT	natural killer T
NLRP3	NLR family pyrin domain containing 3
NLRP3	nucleotide-binding, LRR and PYD domain-containing protein 3
NLRs	NOD-like receptors
NMO	neuromyelitis optica
NO	nitric oxide
NOD mice	nonobese diabetic mice
NOD	nonobese diabetic
NOD	nonobese diabetic mice
NOD	nucleotide-binding and oligomerization domain
NOD	nucleotide-binding domain
NOD2	nucleotide-binding oligomerization domain containing 2
NOX	NADPH oxidase
NPD	neuropsychiatric disorder
NRLP	nucleotide-binding and oligomerization domain-like receptor, leucine-rich repeat, and pyrin domain-containing
NSAIDs	nonsteroidal anti-inflammatory drugs
NSTEMI	non-ST wave-elevated myocardial infarction
nTreg	natural Treg
OA	osteoarthritis
OKZ	olokizumab
OM	oncostatin M
OVA	ovalbumin
ox-LDL	oxidized low-density lipoprotein
oxPTM-INS-Ab	antibodies specific to oxidative PTM-insulin
P2rx7	P2X purinoceptor 7
p53	tumor protein 53
PAMPs	pathogen-associated molecular patterns

Abbreviations

PAN	polyarteritis nodosa	RTOCs	reaggregated thymic organotypic cultures
PAP	prostatic acid phosphatase	SAA	serum amyloid A
PAX1	paired box 1	SASP	senescence-associated secretory phenotype
PBMCs	peripheral blood mononuclear cells		
PC4d	platelet-bound C4d	SA-β-gal	senescence-associated β-galactosidase
PD	pharmacodynamics		
PD-1	programmed cell death protein 1	SC	subcutaneous
PDC	proportion of follow-up days covered	SCFAs	short-chain fatty acids
		SCOT	scleroderma cyclophosphamide or transplantation
pDCs	plasmacytoid dendritic cells		
PDGF	platelet-derived growth factor	SCTMPs	somatic cell therapy medicinal products
PER	period		
PGE2	prostaglandin E_2	Se	selenium
PGF2α	prostaglandin F2α	SeMet	selenomethionine
PGI2	prostacyclin	SF-36	36-item short form health survey
PI3K	phosphatidylinositol-4,5-bisphosphate 3-kinase	SFB	segmented filamentous bacteria
		sgp130Fc	soluble gp130
PIAS	protein inhibitors of activated STATs	SHH	sonic hedgehog
		sIL-6R	soluble form of IL-6R
PJIA	polyarticular juvenile idiopathic arthritis	SIX1/4	sine oculis homeobox homolog 1
		SJIA	systemic juvenile idiopathic arthritis
PK	pharmacokinetics		
PLAD	pre-ligand-binding assembly domain	SLAM-R	systemic lupus activity measure
		SLE	systematic lupus erythematosus
Platr4	pluripotency-associated transcript 4	SLE	systemic lupus erythematosus
		SLE	systemic lupus erythematous
PMA	phorbol myristate acetate	SLEDAI	SLE Disease Activity Index
PMG	physcion-8-O-β-D-monoglucoside	SLEDAI	Systemic Lupus Erythematous Disease Activity Index
PMR	polymyalgia rheumatica		
PP	pharyngeal pouch	SMYD2	SET and MYND domain-containing protein 2
PR	palindromic rheumatism		
PRRs	pattern recognition receptors	SNPs	single nucleotide polymorphisms
PsA	psoriatic arthritis	SNPs	single nucleotides polymorphisms
PSCs	pluripotent stem cells	SOCS3	suppressor of cytokine signaling 3
PTMs	post-translational modifications	SpA	spondyloarthritis/ankylosing spondylitis
PTU	propylthiouracil		
PUFAs	polyunsaturated fatty acids	SPT	skin prick test
PV	plasma viscosity	SRK	sirukumab
PYCARD	PYD and CARD domain containing	SRL	sarilumab
qPCR	quantitative polymerase chain reaction	SS	Sjögren's syndrome
		SSc	systemic sclerosis
RA	rheumatoid arthritis	STAT3	signal transducer and activator of transcription 3
RANKL	receptor activator of NF-$\kappa\beta$ ligand		
RCT	randomized controlled trial	STEMI	ST wave-elevated myocardial infarction
ReA	reactive arthritis		
RF	rheumatoid factor	STHs	soil-transmitted helminths
RIG-1	retinoid acid-inducible gene I	STING	stimulator of interferon genes
RLRs	(RIG-1)-like receptors	STL	satralizumab
ROR	receptor tyrosine kinase-like orphan receptor	sTNF-α	soluble TNF-α
		STOCs	stem cell-derived thymic organoids
ROS	reactive oxygen species	STZ	streptozotocin
RPM	revolution per minute	T1D	type 1 diabetes
RS3PE	remitting seronegative symmetrical synovitis with pitting edema	T1DM	type 1 diabetes mellitus

Abbreviations

T2D	type 2 diabetes	TPOAbs	thyroid peroxidase antibodies
TA	takayasu arteritis	TPP	third pharyngeal pouch
TAA	tumor-associated antigen	Treg cell	regulatory T cell
TACE	tumor necrosis factor-alpha converting enzyme	Treg	regulatory T cell
		Treg	T regulatory
TACE; ADAM17	matrix metalloproteinase TNF-α-converting enzyme	Tregs	regulatory T cells
		TRIF	Toll-like receptor adaptor molecule
TACI	transmembrane activator, calcium modulator, and cyclophilin ligand interactor	TSH	thyroid-stimulating hormone
		TSHR	thyrotropin receptor
		TSLP	thymic stromal lymphopoietin
TBK1	TANK-binding kinase 1	TSO	*Trichuris suis* ova
TBX1	T-box transcription factor 1	TWIK2	two-pore domain weak inwardly rectifying K + channel 2
TCRs	T-cell receptors	
TCZ	tocilizumab	TXNIP	thioredoxin-interacting protein
TECs	thymic epithelial cells	UA	unstable angina
TEPs	thymic epithelial progenitor cells	UC	ulcerative colitis
TEPs	tissue-engineered products	UCB	umbilical cord blood
TG	thyroglobulin	UC-MSCs	umbilical cord-derived MSCs
TgAb	thyroglobulin antibody	ULN	upper limit of normal range
TGF	transforming growth factor	uPAR	urokinase-type plasminogen activator receptor
TGF-β	transforming growth factor-β	
TGF-β1	transforming growth factor-β1	UPLC-MS	ultra-performance liquid chromatography-mass spectrometry
Th1	T-helper 1	
Th1	T-helper type 1	
Th17	T-helper 17	USA	United States of America
Th17/1	T-helper 17/1	UTR	untranslated region
Th2	T-helper 2	vAFE	ventral anterior foregut endoderm
THD	TNF homology domain	VAFG	ventral anterior foregut
TLRs	Toll-like receptors	VAT	visceral adipose tissue
TMAO	trimethylamine *N*-oxide	VBR	vobarilzumab
tmTNF-α	transmembrane TNF-α	VCAM-1	vascular cell-adhesion molecule 1
TNBS	trinitrobenzene sulfonic acid	Vd	volume of distribution at steady state
TNF	tumor necrosis factor	
TNFi	TNF-α inhibitor	VEGF	vascular endothelial growth factor
TNFR	tumor necrosis factor receptor	VL	visceral leishmaniasis
TNFR1	tumor necrosis factor receptor 1	WHO	World Health Organization
TNFSF	tumor necrosis factor superfamily	WNT3a	wingless family member 3a
TNF-α	tumor necrosis factor alpha	WNT5b	wingless family member 5b
TNF-α	tumor necrosis factor-α	ZnT8	zinc transporter 8 antibodies
tol-DCs	tolerogenic dendritic cells	ZnT8A	zinc transporter 8 autoantibody
TPO	thyroid peroxidase	ZT	Zeitgeber time

CHAPTER

1

Introduction on therapeutic opportunities for autoimmunity

Nima Rezaei[a,b,c,*] and Niloufar Yazdanpanah[a,c]

[a]Research Center for Immunodeficiencies, Children's Medical Center, Tehran University of Medical Sciences, Tehran, Iran [b]Department of Immunology, School of Medicine, Tehran University of Medical Sciences, Tehran, Iran [c]Network of Immunity in Infection, Malignancy and Autoimmunity (NIIMA), Universal Scientific Education and Research Network (USERN), Tehran, Iran

*Corresponding author

Abstract

Autoimmune diseases have induced a huge burden on individuals, families, economy, and the healthcare system. Considering their wide spectrum of manifestations and systemic involvement in some of the cases, different complications are associated with these diseases. On the other hand, since most of the current treatments systematically target the immune system, patients might experience a variety of adverse effects. Despite the progress in finding new targets and treatment strategies in animal studies, the development of treatments in clinical application is not seen to the same extent. One important explanation regarding this issue is the difference between the animal and human physiological systems. Moreover, the genetic and epigenetic differences between individuals potentially result in different disease manifestations even with the same underlying pathology besides different spectra of response to treatment. Therefore, finding proper treatment for autoimmune diseases by conducting translational studies that facilitate the application of current evidence from laboratory, animal studies, and preclinical findings in clinical practice is of interest. In this chapter, a brief review of currently available treatments for autoimmune diseases and existing challenges in this field are provided.

Keywords

Immunology, Immunity, Autoimmunity, Treatment, Translational studies

1 Introduction

Affecting about 5% of the population [1], a considerable burden of society and healthcare service is attributed to autoimmune diseases. In spite of the efforts and time devoted to the discovery of an appropriate treatment for autoimmune diseases, multiple challenges exist in the treatment of these patients. For instance, unexpected side effects, several remissions or disease flare after the period of taking the treatment, and complications resulting from the nonselectivity of therapeutic agents are of the major foresaid challenges.

Considering the recent attempts in understanding the pathophysiology and multifactorial etiology of autoimmunity, it might be expected to witness a great progress in the discovery of novel promising therapeutic approaches. Meanwhile, regardless of how deep is the current knowledge about underlying mechanisms of autoimmunity, many challenges exist in linking the laboratory and preclinical findings to clinical benefits. In this chapter, current therapeutic strategies as well as challenges in the field of drug discovery are discussed.

2 From the very first known treatment to the recent developments in therapeutic strategies

The first rationale for the treatment of autoimmune diseases has been based on suppressing the immune system. In spite of the variety of side effects and complications resulting from the nonselectivity of the immune suppression, this approach is still the gold standard in the treatment and control of autoimmune diseases [2]. The most noticeable side effect of the nonselective immunosuppressive drugs is inducing an increased vulnerability to infections and emergence of malignancies that might progress to life-threatening conditions since they disturb nonrelevant pathways and cell functions. Meanwhile, as in other types of diseases, conservative therapies with the aim of reducing the symptoms of the patients had had their role in the management of autoimmune patients [3]. In the following sections, different therapeutic agents involved in the management of autoimmune diseases are briefly discussed.

2.1 Corticosteroids

Glucocorticoid therapy was primarily suggested in the 1950s by Philip Hench and his colleagues [4]. Undoubtedly, it was a milestone in the management of autoimmune reactions in autoinflammatory and rheumatoid diseases. In addition, these immunosuppressant antiinflammatory agents are favorable in transplant rejection, allergic reactions, ambulatory care service, and as a part of chemotherapy process in oncology [5]. Although several side effects have been reported for corticosteroids due to their systemic effects, they are still part of treatment strategies concerning their fast mechanism of action that potentially covers the gap between the administration of other therapeutic agents and the start of their effects [6–9]. Furthermore, these drugs are beneficial in the maintenance therapy as well [6, 8]. Considering the vast spectrum of corticosteroids' targets and different mechanisms of action, long-term and high-dose administration is associated with serious side effects. For instance, psychiatric complications, gastric problems, osteoporotic fractures, adrenal suppression, metabolic problems and undesired weight gain, hypertension, and cardiovascular complications as well as increased susceptibility to infections due to the global suppression of the immune system [5, 10]. Since all the cells possess the same glucocorticoid receptors, their modulatory effects on inflammation and their metabolic effects are inseparable. To reduce these adverse effects and optimize the use of corticosteroids, different aspects of corticosteroid therapy have been investigated. One important finding might be the optimal pattern of administration as it has been revealed that administration with an alternate-day pattern potentially decreases the adverse effects and autoantibodies' level compared to daily administration [11, 12]. It has been reported that local (inhaled or topical corticosteroids) administration potentially reduces the systemic side effects. However, local prescription of corticosteroids is accompanied with different side effects as well. Although the local side effects are not as dangerous as the systemic complications, the presence of these side effects could potentially decrease the patients' compliance with the treatment that could result in detrimental consequences [13] such as the flare-up of the disease and prednisolone withdrawal symptoms in the case of the abrupt stop in taking the drug. That being so, regardless of all the benefits of the corticosteroids that make them an important part of the management strategies of autoimmune diseases, there are still considerable challenges remained to be solved.

2.2 Disease-modifying antirheumatic drugs

Disease-modifying antirheumatic drugs (DMARDs) are therapeutic agents that modulate or suppress the immune system. DMARDs are classified into conventional such as methotrexate, sulfasalazine, and hydroxychloroquine, and biological consists of monoclonal antibodies and the antagonist of different factors in the immune system [14]. In contrast to the nonspecific targeting of corticosteroids, biological DMARDs target a specific pathway or component of the immune system. Hence, the adverse effects related to this group of drugs might be less serious and observed at lower rates. However, they are not completely safe since a number of side effects have been reported for DMARDs. Gastrointestinal problems, increased risk of infection, hepatotoxicity, bone marrow suppression, and hypersensitivity reactions are demonstrated as side effects in patients treated with conventional DMARDs [15, 16]. While these effects have been reported in most of the conventional DMARDs administration, hydroxychloroquine has represented milder complications such as allergic reactions and diarrhea [17, 18]. On the other hand, ophthalmological complications (drug-induced retinopathy or maculopathy) have been reported as rare but serious side effects exclusively for hydroxychloroquine prescription [19]. The most remarkable and common undesirable effect of biological DMARDs is predisposing individuals to different infections, while a spectrum of different rare adverse effects has been reported as well [14, 20].

2.3 Targeting the different immune components

Moreover, the medical society has witnessed developments in the treatment of autoimmune diseases by discovering promising alternative targets. Since both the innate and adaptive immune systems are involved in autoimmunity, a broad spectrum of medications has been approved and indicated for specific conditions. B cells, T cells, T regulatory (Treg) cells, complement pathways, costimulatory molecules and receptors, Toll-like receptors (TLRs), cytokines, immunoglobulins, JAK enzymes, and tolerance mechanisms have been the target of different treatment strategies so far [2, 3, 21, 22].

As a comprehensive concept, immunotherapy is a therapeutic method having the manipulated components of the immune system as its tools. Monoclonal antibodies, receptor fusion proteins, cytokines, and immune cells are functional tools in immunotherapy [21]. Although many of these tools have shown promising results in animal models, their efficacy for human cases has faced several challenges. The complexity of the human immune system, the issue of applying the animal and laboratory finding to the human system, and the crucial matter of preoccupation with safety in human immunotherapy studies are some of the most prominent obstacles in this field [21, 23, 24]. The dynamic progressive route of scientific discoveries results in finding novel targets for immunotherapy in autoimmune diseases. For instance, investigating the diversity and unique functional pathways of antigen-presenting cells (APCs), discovery of the cytokine alteration in the immune environment action sites, and the immune cells' interaction with the resident cells in different tissues led to the conceptualization of plasticity in the differentiation process of T cells into various subtypes [25–28]. Therefore, these kinds of findings might reveal potential novel treatment targets such as T helper 17 (Th17) cells and inducible Treg (iTreg) cells [27, 28].

2.4 Targeting cytokines

Due to the wide spectrum of biological effects of cytokines, they have attracted special attention as treatment targets. Inhibition of proinflammatory cytokines either by special monoclonal antibodies or by soluble receptors, interfering in the pathways related to the function of cytokines, and impairing the function of the cytokines' receptors by both monoclonal antibodies and receptor antagonists are the strategies applied to tackle autoimmune diseases by means of cytokines [29–33]. Furthermore, provoking the immune system to produce autoantibodies against cytokines by novel methods of anticytokine vaccination [34, 35] and the introduction of cytokine traps that have represented promising results in vitro and in vivo [36, 37] are other potential treatment strategies targeting cytokines. On the other hand, administration of antiinflammatory cytokines such as TGF-β, IFN-β, IL-4, and IL-10 to attenuate the autoimmune responses might be beneficial as well [33]. In addition to immune mediators, infiltration of immune cells plays a significant role in the induction of chronic inflammation. Hence, targeting the related pathways' components such as chemokines and adhesion molecules might be beneficial for the management of chronic conditions in autoimmune diseases [38–41].

2.5 Targeting immune cells

OKT3 (Ortho Kung 3) or muromonab, a CD3-recognizing antibody, was the first monoclonal antibody of murine origin [42]. Furthermore, rituximab, an anti-CD20 antibody, one of the successful applied targeted B cell therapies in autoimmune patients highlighted the possible efficacy of the therapeutic agents targeting immune cells as promising groups of medications for autoimmune diseases [43]. Rituximab selectively targets CD20$^+$ cells such as pre-B cells and B cells through different mechanisms, while it does not affect bone marrow stem cells and evolved plasma cells. This is counted as one of the best aspects of rituximab whereas some of the B- and T-cell targeting agents function nonselectively, which in turn enhances the risk of developing cancer and opportunistic infection [44]. However, assessment of the balance between risks and benefits has always remained a challenge [45]. An example in the field of immunotherapy for autoimmune diseases might be the application of alemtuzumab, an anti-CD52 antibody that nonselectively inhibits B cells, T cells, natural killer (NK) cells, and monocytes, in multiple sclerosis patients. Promising impressive results have been observed in the related trials; however, due to its broad spectrum of effects on different immune cells, different deleterious side effects have been reported for it. Progressive multifocal leukoencephalopathy and even other autoimmune conditions such as idiopathic thrombocytopenic purpura (ITP) are of the mentioned unwanted adverse effects [46, 47].

Besides the aforementioned therapeutic agents that mostly inhibit the function of immune cells, immune-related receptors, proinflammatory cytokines, and leukocyte infiltration, some agents do not inhibit or negate a function, but modulate, convert, or induce a function. For instance, stimulation or induction of regulatory immune cells, altering the antigen recognition process, and conversion of the immune responses to protective ones.

2.6 Vaccination

In 1911, by demonstrating how hay fever potentially resolved after a patient's inoculation with the related antigen, the first antigen-specific immunotherapy (SIT) was suggested [48]. Considering the concept of inducing antigen-specific Treg cells to target the underlying pathological mechanisms of autoimmunity rather than treating the symptoms of the diseases, therapeutic vaccination for autoimmune diseases emerged [49, 50]. Antigen-presenting cells (APCs) facing the stimulating antigens in a proinflammatory environment (in the presence of proinflammatory cytokines and innate immunity receptors) potentially results in the progress of the immune response through the Th1 and Th2 mediated pathways that might induce autoreactive immune cells [51, 52]. Meanwhile, encounter of APCs with antigens in a nonproinflammatory environment stabilizes these cells and leads to induction of regulatory cells and responses as they confront T cells in the periphery in a noninflammatory state [49, 51]. Deletion and anergy processes have been suggested as the main action mechanism of APCs (e.g., dendritic cells or DCs) [53, 54]. However, how administration of a peptide component of one antigen could stop the immune response against another antigen still remained a challenge. Bystander suppression has been suggested as an explanation for this observation [55, 56]. To further elucidate the action mechanism of this method of immunotherapy in autoimmune diseases, it has been observed that frequent exposure of the APCs with the synthetic antigen results in the production of IL-10 secreting regulatory cells. It has been demonstrated that these regulatory cells originate from naïve T cells without the expression of *FOXP3*, but with approximately equivalent regulatory potency as $CD4^+$ $CD25^+$ Treg cells [57, 58]. An antigen potent to bind MHC molecules and simulate the characteristics of naturally processed antigens to be capable of inducing tolerance in the involved immune cells might be a proper option to develop autoimmune therapeutic vaccination. In addition, the proposed antigen might be nonstimulating for the innate immune system so that an appropriate environment is provided to result in the induction of regulatory immune responses [49]. To avoid the local inflammation and facilitate the APCs to arrive in the peripheral lymphoid tissues, the designed antigen must be soluble [49, 59]. It is worth mentioning that DCs can be used either as cellular vaccines after ex vivo manipulations or can be the target of in vivo peptide delivery system [60, 61]. Although promising results have been achieved for the application of antigen-specific immunotherapy in animal studies, translation of these results to clinical studies and usage is still the main challenge in this field.

Oral tolerance has been known as a physiologic route to reduce inflammation and autoimmune reactions. The advantage of oral tolerance is its potential specificity for defined antigens and rare chance of toxicity that is due to its administration route that resembles a physiologic process [62]. Whether the antigen fed is in low or high dose, it could lead to the emergence of Treg cells or the stimulation of clonal anergy/clonal deletion, respectively [62, 63]. Furthermore, there are different factors affecting the initiation and maintenance of the oral tolerance including the administrated dosage of the antigen and the characteristics of it, age and gender of the patient, and the variation in genetic background of patients [64]. Considering the integration of these complex factors besides the difference between the human and animal physiologic systems, further investigations are necessary to translate the current finding regarding the efficacy of oral tolerance, which is mostly from animal and preclinical studies, to clinical practice in humans [64, 65].

2.7 Gene therapy

Gene therapy, defined as a novel therapeutic strategy in which the impaired genes are inactivated or substituted in the targeted cells, could offer a treatment opportunity for autoimmune diseases [66]. The existing records of the efficacy of gene therapy in attenuating the autoimmune reactions and complications in animal models have attracted considerable attention whether this method is applicable in humans as well [67]. Meanwhile, with the introduction of appropriate vectors for gene delivery, the investigations regarding gene therapy in autoimmune diseases have been strengthened [68]. Adjustment of the activation and function of autoreactive immune cells, expression level and the function of immune systems' immunomodulatory molecules, and immune tolerance are of the focused fields in animal models for the improvement of gene therapy strategies [68]. In spite of the recent advancements in gene therapy studies, there are few approved clinical trials with limited number of participants due to the safety and efficacy concerns, since there are major differences between animal and human physiologic systems [68, 69].

2.8 Cell therapy

Cell therapy, which is the method of reconfiguration of the immune system to the naïve and self-tolerant nonautoreactive cells, holds great promises in the treatment of autoimmune diseases [70]. Although it has been established to combat malignancies, recent promising reports concerning the application of this method on severe forms of autoimmune diseases, and in cases with poor or no response to targeted therapies [71]. The initial translational study that has constructed the basic concept of the application of HSCT in autoimmunity using murine model was conducted by Ikehara et al. in 1985 [72]. They have suggested the bone marrow as the root of autoimmune diseases and claimed that bone marrow transplantation could be beneficial in reconfiguration of the immune system while thymus transplantation might not be effective [72]. Hematopoietic stem cell transplantation (HSCT), regulatory T cell therapy, and mesenchymal stromal cell therapy are different cells employed in methods of cell therapy. The integration of different processes, such as restriction of the autoreactive B cells and T cells besides impeding the aging process in the remained normal cell repertoires, maintaining the immune system's defense potency against environmental treats by saving memory cells, and reinstating the regulatory process of the immune system, results in the effectiveness of the cell therapy in autoimmune diseases [71].

2.9 Microbiota manipulation and probiotic application

Drastically developing data on the association of microbiota and the immune system function has highlighted the potentials of the application of microbiota manipulation for the treatment of autoimmune diseases [73]. Some of the resident normal flora bacteria in the gut and airways trigger the formation of T helper 17 (Th17) cells by affecting the normal response of dendritic cells, which Th17 is one of the pivotal components of the autoimmune reactions in some autoimmune diseases [74, 75]. However, the microbiota perform antiinflammatory roles by facilitating the Treg responses by means of secreting substances such as polysaccharide A or short-chain fatty acids [75, 76]. Several approaches have been established for the modulation of microbiota for therapeutic purposes. For instance, antimicrobial interventions, fecal transplantation, prebiotics diets, and the administration of selective bacterial candidates [77]. Furthermore, dietary treatments, with the goal of microbiota change, could be a promising alternative treatment due to its reasonable economical costs, feasibility, and noninvasiveness [78].

2.10 Immunometabolism

The mutual connection between the immune system and the metabolism, as the two most vital components of survival, is detectable in health and disease. To go into further detail, the inflammatory processes are responsible for the physiopathology of metabolic syndromes [79]. Meanwhile, the metabolic processes determine the proliferation, differentiation, and function of the immune cells [79, 80]. The observations concerning the fat tissue's secretion of TNF-α in a murine model of obesity [81] in addition to the widely accepted notion that malnutrition leads to immunosuppression [82] have strengthened the link between metabolic alteration and immune system function. Indeed, each type of the immune cells represents specific metabolic characteristics in different steps of their life span and they acquire specific features and undergo reprogramming as they enter different tissues [79, 83]. With regard to these observations, modification of the function of immune cells by manipulating their microenvironment of the infiltrated tissue or their origin tissue, which in turn results in the metabolic reprogramming of these cells, has opened new chapters in investigating new treatment methods for autoimmune diseases. Since this method could potentially target specific components of the immune system according to their distinct metabolic features, it could be a favorable alternative to systemic immunosuppression. It is worth mentioning that some of the immune cells' metabolic pathways have already been targeted in the classic treatment. For instance, methotrexate potentially affects the JAK-STAT pathway as one of its action mechanisms [84]. However, specifically targeting immunometabolic targets to optimize the treatment results and reduce the undesired adverse effects of conventional medications requires further research.

3 Conclusion

As reviewed throughout this chapter, there are different treatment strategies established for the management of autoimmune diseases during the recent decades, however, no definite long-lasting treatment is available so far. In spite of the considerable progress in the animal studies aiming to elucidate the etiopathogenesis and contributing factors to the initiation and progress of autoimmune diseases, the advancement in clinical practice is not to that extent. This inequivalent progress is due to the difference between animal and human systems besides the restrictions in conducting human studies with large number of participants. Hence, the importance of translational studies in the attempt to apply the laboratory, preclinical, and animal studies finding in clinical practice is highlighted once more.

References

[1] D.L. Jacobson, et al., Epidemiology and estimated population burden of selected autoimmune diseases in the United States, Clin. Immunol. Immunopathol. 84 (3) (1997) 223–243.

[2] M.D. Rosenblum, et al., Treating human autoimmunity: current practice and future prospects, Sci. Transl. Med. 4 (125) (2012) 125sr1.

[3] S. Chandrashekara, The treatment strategies of autoimmune disease may need a different approach from conventional protocol: a review, Indian J. Pharmacol. 44 (6) (2012) 665–671.

[4] C.M. Burns, The history of cortisone discovery and development, Rheum. Dis. Clin. North Am. 42 (1) (2016) 1–14. vii.

[5] E. Sarnes, et al., Incidence and US costs of corticosteroid-associated adverse events: a systematic literature review, Clin. Ther. 33 (10) (2011) 1413–1432.

[6] B. Hellmich, et al., 2018 update of the EULAR recommendations for the management of large vessel vasculitis, Ann. Rheum. Dis. 79 (1) (2020) 19.

[7] A. Fanouriakis, et al., 2019 update of the EULAR recommendations for the management of systemic lupus erythematosus, Ann. Rheum. Dis. 78 (6) (2019) 736.

[8] C. Mukhtyar, et al., EULAR recommendations for the management of primary small and medium vessel vasculitis, Ann. Rheum. Dis. 68 (3) (2009) 310.

[9] J.S. Smolen, et al., EULAR recommendations for the management of rheumatoid arthritis with synthetic and biological disease-modifying antirheumatic drugs: 2019 update, Ann. Rheum. Dis. 79 (6) (2020) 685.

[10] A.K. McDonough, J.R. Curtis, K.G. Saag, The epidemiology of glucocorticoid-associated adverse events, Curr. Opin. Rheumatol. 20 (2) (2008) 131–137.

[11] G.M. Chaia-Semerena, et al., The effects of alternate-day corticosteroids in autoimmune disease patients, Autoimmune Dis. 2020 (2020), 8719284.

[12] M. Suda, et al., Safety and efficacy of alternate-day corticosteroid treatment as adjunctive therapy for rheumatoid arthritis: a comparative study, Clin. Rheumatol. 37 (8) (2018) 2027–2034.

[13] N.J. Roland, R.K. Bhalla, J. Earis, The local side effects of inhaled corticosteroids: current understanding and review of the literature, Chest 126 (1) (2004) 213–219.

[14] O. Benjamin, S.L. Lappin, Disease modifying anti-rheumatic drugs (DMARD), in: StatPearls, StatPearls Publishing, 2019 (Internet).

[15] W. Wang, H. Zhou, L. Liu, Side effects of methotrexate therapy for rheumatoid arthritis: a systematic review, Eur. J. Med. Chem. 158 (2018) 502–516.

[16] W. Katchamart, et al., Efficacy and toxicity of methotrexate (MTX) monotherapy versus MTX combination therapy with non-biological disease-modifying antirheumatic drugs in rheumatoid arthritis: a systematic review and meta-analysis, Ann. Rheum. Dis. 68 (7) (2009) 1105–1112.

[17] A. Srinivasa, S. Tosounidou, C. Gordon, Increased incidence of gastrointestinal side effects in patients taking hydroxychloroquine: a brand-related issue? J. Rheumatol. 44 (3) (2017) 398.

[18] A.N. Sharma, N.A. Mesinkovska, T. Paravar, Characterizing the adverse dermatologic effects of hydroxychloroquine: a systematic review, J. Am. Acad. Dermatol. 83 (2020) 563–578.

[19] R.B. Melles, M.F. Marmor, The risk of toxic retinopathy in patients on long-term hydroxychloroquine therapy, JAMA Ophthalmol. 132 (12) (2014) 1453–1460.

[20] T.T. Hansel, et al., The safety and side effects of monoclonal antibodies, Nat. Rev. Drug Discov. 9 (4) (2010) 325–338.

[21] M. Feldmann, L. Steinman, Design of effective immunotherapy for human autoimmunity, Nature 435 (7042) (2005) 612–619.

[22] F.J. Barrat, R.L. Coffman, Development of TLR inhibitors for the treatment of autoimmune diseases, Immunol. Rev. 223 (1) (2008) 271–283.

[23] B.O. Roep, M. Atkinson, M. von Herrath, Satisfaction (not) guaranteed: re-evaluating the use of animal models of type 1 diabetes, Nat. Rev. Immunol. 4 (12) (2004) 989–997.

[24] R.S. Blumberg, et al., Unraveling the autoimmune translational research process layer by layer, Nat. Med. 18 (1) (2012) 35–41.

[25] J.J. O'Shea, C.A. Hunter, R.N. Germain, T cell heterogeneity: firmly fixed, predominantly plastic or merely malleable? Nat. Immunol. 9 (5) (2008) 450–453.

[26] M. Veldhoen, et al., Transforming growth factor-beta 'reprograms' the differentiation of T helper 2 cells and promotes an interleukin 9-producing subset, Nat. Immunol. 9 (12) (2008) 1341–1346.

[27] W. Chen, et al., Conversion of peripheral CD4+CD25- naive T cells to CD4+CD25+ regulatory T cells by TGF-beta induction of transcription factor Foxp3, J. Exp. Med. 198 (12) (2003) 1875–1886.

[28] L.E. Harrington, et al., Interleukin 17–producing CD4+ effector T cells develop via a lineage distinct from the T helper type 1 and 2 lineages, Nat. Immunol. 6 (11) (2005) 1123–1132.

[29] M. Cargill, et al., A large-scale genetic association study confirms IL12B and leads to the identification of IL23R as psoriasis-risk genes, Am. J. Hum. Genet. 80 (2) (2007) 273–290.

[30] R.H. Duerr, et al., A genome-wide association study identifies IL23R as an inflammatory bowel disease gene, Science 314 (5804) (2006) 1461–1463.

[31] E. Lubberts, et al., Treatment with a neutralizing anti-murine interleukin-17 antibody after the onset of collagen-induced arthritis reduces joint inflammation, cartilage destruction, and bone erosion, Arthritis Rheum. 50 (2) (2004) 650–659.

[32] M. Pesu, et al., Therapeutic targeting of Janus kinases, Immunol. Rev. 223 (2008) 132–142.

[33] L. Adorini, Cytokine-based immunointervention in the treatment of autoimmune diseases, Clin. Exp. Immunol. 132 (2) (2003) 185–192.

[34] L. Semerano, E. Assier, M.-C. Boissier, Anti-cytokine vaccination: a new biotherapy of autoimmunity? Autoimmun. Rev. 11 (11) (2012) 785–786.

[35] L. Delavallée, et al., Vaccination with cytokines in autoimmune diseases, Ann. Med. 40 (5) (2008) 343–351.

[36] A.N. Economides, et al., Cytokine traps: multi-component, high-affinity blockers of cytokine action, Nat. Med. 9 (1) (2003) 47–52.

[37] C.R. Zamecnik, et al., An injectable cytokine trap for local treatment of autoimmune disease, Biomaterials 230 (2020) 119626.

[38] R. Bonecchi, et al., Differential expression of chemokine receptors and chemotactic responsiveness of type 1 T helper cells (Th1s) and Th2s, J. Exp. Med. 187 (1) (1998) 129–134.

[39] N. Godessart, Chemokine receptors: attractive targets for drug discovery, Ann. N. Y. Acad. Sci. 1051 (2005) 647–657.

[40] R.W. McMurray, Adhesion molecules in autoimmune disease, Semin. Arthritis Rheum. 25 (4) (1996) 215–233.

[41] N. Oppenheimer-Marks, P.E. Lipsky, Adhesion molecules as targets for the treatment of autoimmune diseases, Clin. Immunol. Immunopathol. 79 (3) (1996) 203–210.

[42] P. Kung, et al., Monoclonal antibodies defining distinctive human T cell surface antigens, Science 206 (4416) (1979) 347–349.

[43] V. Strand, R. Kimberly, J.D. Isaacs, Biologic therapies in rheumatology: lessons learned, future directions, Nat. Rev. Drug Discov. 6 (1) (2007) 75–92.

[44] C. Balagué, S.L. Kunkel, N. Godessart, Understanding autoimmune disease: new targets for drug discovery, Drug Discov. Today 14 (19–20) (2009) 926–934.

[45] M. Yasunaga, Antibody therapeutics and immunoregulation in cancer and autoimmune disease, Semin. Cancer Biol. 64 (2020) 1–12.

[46] C.L. Hirst, et al., Campath 1-H treatment in patients with aggressive relapsing remitting multiple sclerosis, J. Neurol. 255 (2) (2008) 231–238.

1. Introduction on therapeutic opportunities for autoimmunity

[47] L.H. Calabrese, E.S. Molloy, Progressive multifocal leucoencephalopathy in the rheumatic diseases: assessing the risks of biological immunosuppressive therapies, Ann. Rheum. Dis. 67 (Suppl. 3) (2008) iii64–5.

[48] L. Noon, Prophylactic inoculation against hay fever, Lancet 177 (4580) (1911) 1572–1573.

[49] M. Larché, D.C. Wraith, Peptide-based therapeutic vaccines for allergic and autoimmune diseases, Nat. Med. 11 (4) (2005) S69–S76.

[50] I. Van Brussel, et al., Tolerogenic dendritic cell vaccines to treat autoimmune diseases: can the unattainable dream turn into reality? Autoimmun. Rev. 13 (2) (2014) 138–150.

[51] H. Jonuleit, et al., Induction of interleukin 10–producing, nonproliferating CD4+ T cells with regulatory properties by repetitive stimulation with allogeneic immature human dendritic cells, J. Exp. Med. 192 (9) (2000) 1213–1222.

[52] S.M. Anderton, et al., Influence of a dominant cryptic epitope on autoimmune T cell tolerance, Nat. Immunol. 3 (2) (2002) 175–181.

[53] D.C. Wraith, Therapeutic peptide vaccines for treatment of autoimmune diseases, Immunol. Lett. 122 (2) (2009) 134–136.

[54] R.P. Anderson, B. Jabri, Vaccine against autoimmune disease: antigen-specific immunotherapy, Curr. Opin. Immunol. 25 (3) (2013) 410–417.

[55] A.M. Faria, H.L. Weiner, Oral tolerance: mechanisms and therapeutic applications, Adv. Immunol. 73 (1999) 153–264.

[56] H.L. Weiner, Oral tolerance: immune mechanisms and treatment of autoimmune diseases, Immunol. Today 18 (7) (1997) 335–343.

[57] P.L. Vieira, et al., IL-10-secreting regulatory T cells do not express Foxp3 but have comparable regulatory function to naturally occurring CD4+CD25+ regulatory T cells, J. Immunol. 172 (10) (2004) 5986–5993.

[58] K.S. Nicolson, et al., Antigen-induced IL-10+ regulatory T cells are independent of CD25+ regulatory cells for their growth, differentiation, and function, J. Immunol. 176 (9) (2006) 5329–5337.

[59] B. Metzler, et al., Kinetics of peptide uptake and tissue distribution following a single intranasal dose of peptide, Immunol. Invest. 29 (1) (2000) 61–70.

[60] C.M. Hilkens, J.D. Isaacs, A.W. Thomson, Development of dendritic cell-based immunotherapy for autoimmunity, Int. Rev. Immunol. 29 (2) (2010) 156–183.

[61] C.C. Gross, H. Wiendl, Dendritic cell vaccination in autoimmune disease, Curr. Opin. Rheumatol. 25 (2) (2013) 268–274.

[62] H.L. Weiner, et al., Oral tolerance, Immunol. Rev. 241 (1) (2011) 241–259.

[63] A.M.C. Faria, H.L. Weiner, Oral tolerance, Immunol. Rev. 206 (1) (2005) 232–259.

[64] L. Mayer, L. Shao, Therapeutic potential of oral tolerance, Nat. Rev. Immunol. 4 (6) (2004) 407–419.

[65] T. Sricharunrat, P. Pumirat, P. Leaungwutiwong, Oral tolerance: recent advances on mechanisms and potential applications, Asian Pac. J. Allergy Immunol. 36 (4) (2018) 207–216.

[66] C.E. Dunbar, et al., Gene therapy comes of age, Science 359 (6372) (2018), eaan4672.

[67] E. Sloane, et al., Anti-inflammatory cytokine gene therapy decreases sensory and motor dysfunction in experimental multiple sclerosis: MOG-EAE behavioral and anatomical symptom treatment with cytokine gene therapy, Brain Behav. Immun. 23 (1) (2009) 92–100.

[68] S.A. Shu, et al., Gene therapy for autoimmune disease, Clin. Rev. Allergy Immunol. 49 (2) (2015) 163–176.

[69] P.S. Leung, et al., Gene therapy in autoimmune diseases: challenges and opportunities, Autoimmun. Rev. 9 (3) (2010) 170–174.

[70] T. Alexander, et al., Hematopoietic stem cell therapy for autoimmune diseases—clinical experience and mechanisms, J. Autoimmun. 92 (2018) 35–46.

[71] F. Dazzi, et al., Cell therapy for autoimmune diseases, Arthritis Res. Ther. 9 (2) (2007) 1–9.

[72] S. Ikehara, et al., Rationale for bone marrow transplantation in the treatment of autoimmune diseases, Proc. Natl. Acad. Sci. U. S. A. 82 (8) (1985) 2483–2487.

[73] G. Fitzgibbon, K.H.G. Mills, The microbiota and immune-mediated diseases: opportunities for therapeutic intervention, Eur. J. Immunol. 50 (3) (2020) 326–337.

[74] I.I. Ivanov, et al., Induction of intestinal Th17 cells by segmented filamentous bacteria, Cell 139 (3) (2009) 485–498.

[75] Y. Belkaid, T.W. Hand, Role of the microbiota in immunity and inflammation, Cell 157 (1) (2014) 121–141.

[76] M. Kim, et al., Microbial metabolites, short-chain fatty acids, restrain tissue bacterial load, chronic inflammation, and associated cancer in the colon of mice, Eur. J. Immunol. 48 (7) (2018) 1235–1247.

[77] B. Balakrishnan, V. Taneja, Microbial modulation of the gut microbiome for treating autoimmune diseases, Expert Rev. Gastroenterol. Hepatol. 12 (10) (2018) 985–996.

[78] J.L. Richards, et al., Dietary metabolites and the gut microbiota: an alternative approach to control inflammatory and autoimmune diseases, Clin. Transl. Immunol. 5 (5) (2016), e82.

[79] L. Makowski, M. Chaib, J.C. Rathmell, Immunometabolism: from basic mechanisms to translation, Immunol. Rev. 295 (1) (2020) 5–14.

[80] M. Galgani, S. Bruzzaniti, G. Matarese, Immunometabolism and autoimmunity, Curr. Opin. Immunol. 67 (2020) 10–17.

[81] G.S. Hotamisligil, N.S. Shargill, B.M. Spiegelman, Adipose expression of tumor necrosis factor-alpha: direct role in obesity-linked insulin resistance, Science 259 (5091) (1993) 87–91.

[82] M.K. Ibrahim, et al., Impact of childhood malnutrition on host defense and infection, Clin. Microbiol. Rev. 30 (4) (2017) 919–971.

[83] C. Stathopoulou, D. Nikoleri, G. Bertsias, Immunometabolism: an overview and therapeutic prospects in autoimmune diseases, Immunotherapy 11 (9) (2019) 813–829.

[84] S. Thomas, et al., Methotrexate is a JAK/STAT pathway inhibitor, PLoS One 10 (7) (2015), e0130078.

CHAPTER

2

Innate lymphoid cells as therapeutic targets in autoimmune diseases

Prince Amoah Barnie[a,b,c], Xia Lin[b], and Su Zhaoliang[a,b,]*

[a]The Central Laboratory, The Fourth Affiliated Hospital of Jiangsu University, Zhenjiang, China
[b]International Genome Center, Jiangsu University, Zhenjiang, China [c]Department of Biomedical Sciences, School of Allied Health Sciences, University of Cape Coast, Cape Coast, Ghana
*Corresponding author

Abstract

The recent identification of a complex group of innate lymphocyte cells, now collectively termed innate lymphoid cells (ILCs), has been implicated in the pathogenesis of inflammatory disorders. Basically, three classes of ILCs have been described according to how they function and develop as well as the type of cytokines they produce and how the interactions between innate and adaptive immune cells are influenced during inflammatory disorders. Data from clinical and experimental animal models suggest that ILCs modulate various autoimmune diseases. The ILCs play this role possibly through their ability to produce cytokines, which influence the activities of important cells, particularly the effector CD4[+] cells. Due to their identified functions in the pathogenesis of autoimmune diseases, researchers have proposed that they may be viable therapeutic targets. This review outlines the biology and functions of ILCs in autoimmune diseases and attempts to further identify their potential as therapeutic targets.

Keywords

ILC, Autoimmune diseases, Inflammatory bowel disease, IBD, Multiple sclerosis, MS, Systemic lupus erythematosus, SLE

1 Introduction

Innate lymphoid cells (ILCs) represent a group of recently identified innate immune cells, which play important roles in innate and adaptive immunity [1]. They were previously identified and associated with mucosal immunity [2] but more functions have been discovered. Their recent discovery attracted considerable attention and led to the initiation of different

Translational Autoimmunity, Vol. 2
https://doi.org/10.1016/B978-0-12-824390-9.00020-7

Copyright © 2022 Elsevier Inc. All rights reserved.

research activities to better characterize their roles. They have been reported to share many phenotypic and functional characteristics with CD4$^+$ and CD8$^+$ T cells [3]. The roles of some innate and adaptive immune cells and their interplay have received much attention lately. Our understanding of the important roles of ILCs in autoimmune diseases has increased due to the recent investigations. It is interesting to note that more innate cells, particularly ILCs, have been added to the list of immune cells that play vital roles in autoimmune diseases such as inflammatory bowel disease (IBD) [4], psoriasis [5], rheumatoid arthritis (RA) [6], atopic dermatitis (AD) [7], systemic lupus erythematosus (SLE) [8], and multiple sclerosis (MS) [9]. The quest of the researchers in this field to obtain knowledge and further understand the roles of ILCs in autoimmune diseases is gradually making progress, however, there is more to be explored. Research activities have provided enough evidence to support the speculation that ILCs can act in response to microbiota through communication with both epithelial cells and intestinal mononuclear phagocytes via cytokine signaling [10]. However, little information is known about how the functions of cytokines from ILCs and their effects on other cells in the pathogenesis of autoimmune diseases can be targeted for therapeutic aims. As a group of cells related to the development, ILCs are involved in providing immunity and tissue development as well as remodeling [11]. Notably, ILCs are innate immune cells that are commonly distributed in lymphoid and nonlymphoid tissues. They are known to be enriched at mucosal and barrier surfaces and are rapid and potent in cytokine production, which participates in a variety of immune responses [12, 13]. These ILCs are emerging as important effectors of innate immunity and have been found to play a central role in tissue remodeling. Three main features are known to define the ILC family: the lack of recombination activating gene (RAG)-dependent rearranged antigen receptors; absence of markers typical of myeloid and dendritic cells (DCs); and the morphology of their lymphoid origin. The ILC populations exhibit a typical illustration of natural killer (NK) cells and lymphoid tissue-inducer (LTi) cells. Immunologically, NK cells have been found to mediate early immune responses against viruses (pathogens) and cancer cells [14]. LTi cells are essential for the formation of lymph nodes during embryogenesis and also for the formation of secondary lymphoid tissues [15]. Despite the functional differences between NK cells and LTi cells, they are developmentally related because both cell types require common cytokine receptor γ-chain (γc; also known as IL-2Rγ) and the transcriptional repressor inhibitor of DNA binding 2 (ID2) for their development. Based on recent findings, ILC populations have been shown to demonstrate significant effector functions against microorganisms as well as contribution to tissue repair during the early stages of immune responses. Actually, ILCs lack the expression of antigen-specific receptors and do not directly mediate antigen-specific responses as compared with T helper (Th) subsets [16, 17]. Instead, they act as central organizers of immune responses by coordinating signals from the epithelium, the microbiota, pathogens, and other immune cells via the expression of an array of cytokines, cytokine receptors, and eicosanoid receptors [18, 19]. In autoimmune diseases, ILC's signature cytokines influence the pathophysiology of autoimmune diseases such as IBD and psoriasis. This chapter reviews the biology and diverse role of ILCs in autoimmune diseases and discusses how ILCs contribute to the pathogenesis of various autoimmune diseases. A clear understanding of the role of these cells in the pathogenesis of various autoimmune diseases could offer new treatment strategies targeting autoimmune diseases.

2 The biology of innate lymphoid cells

Several distinct members of ILCs have been identified recently and many different names have been used to characterize these newly identified ILC subsets because there is no systematic naming protocol [11]. This has generated many confusing arguments. ILCs have been identified in blood [20], thymus [21], tonsils [22], gut [23], liver [24], skin [25], lungs [26], bone marrow [27], and uterus [28]. All ILCs share three main characteristics: (i) the absence of somatically rearranged antigen receptors, (ii) a lack of myeloid and dendritic cell phenotypic markers, and (iii) their lymphoid morphology [29]. ILC subsets mirror the cytokine and transcriptional profile of CD4[+] T helper cell subsets [30]. Therefore, it was proposed that ILCs should be categorized into three groups based on cytokines that they produce and transcription factors that regulate their development and effector functions [11]. The three groups are group 1 (ILC1s), group 2 (ILC2s), and group 3 (ILC3s) innate lymphoid cells [31]. The ILC1s express the transcription factor T-box that is expressed in T cells (T-bet) and produce IFN-γ. This makes them the main contributors to cell-mediated immune responses to bacteria and protozoan parasites [10, 32, 33]. Likewise, ILC2s promote type 2 immune responses that protect against helminthic infection, cause allergic inflammation, mediate tissue repair, and maintain metabolic homeostasis by the expression of GATA3, type 2 cytokines such as IL-4, IL-5, IL-9, and IL-13, as well as the growth factor amphiregulin (Areg) and met-enkephalin peptides [34–37]. On the other hand, ILC3s express retinoid-related orphan receptor γt (RORγt) and produce IL-17A, IL-22, and lymphotoxin [38–40]. Notably, ILC3s are the most heterogeneous ILC population and can be further divided into two main groups: lymphoid tissue-inducer cells (LTi) and LTi-like C–C chemokine receptor type 6 (CCR6)–expressing ILC3s that are responsible for the development of lymphoid structures and intestinal inflammation while the T-bet[+] natural cytotoxicity receptor NCR[+] and NCR[−] ILC3s function to promote tissue homeostasis, antibacterial immunity, and autoimmune inflammation [40–42]. However, with the increased understanding of the development and function of ILCs, researchers recently proposed to reclassify ILCs into five subsets, namely NK cells, ILC1s, ILC2s, ILC3s, and lymphoid tissue-inducer (LTi) cells, which was approved by the International Union of Immunological Societies (IUIS). These ILCs have been documented to regulate immunity, inflammation, and tissue homeostasis by producing cytokines, integrating environmental signals as well as interacting with many other immune cells such as MDSCs, macrophages, and DCs [13, 16, 17].

2.1 ILC1

Cytotoxicity, macrophage activation, immunity to viruses, immunological aspects of cancer, and chronic inflammation are some of the functions mediated by ILC1 cells [13]. Actually, ILC1s are known to respond to IL-12, and are dependent on the transcription factor T-bet (encoded by the *Tbx21* gene), and produce effector cytokines, such as interferon (IFN)-γ and tumor necrosis factor (TNF) [10, 33]. Usually, the differentiation of ILC1s from common lymphoid progenitor (CLP) to a resident in the bone marrows requires eomesodermin (Eomes), T-bet, IL-15, and IL-7. The ILC1s can be divided into at least three subsets based on the difference in the expression of their products and requirements for their regulation. The first subset includes conventional NK cells, which require eomesodermin and IL-15, but not IL-7 or T-bet, for their development from NKps [33]. Likewise, the second subset of ILC1s or CD103[+] intraepithelial ILC1s develop from an as yet unknown precursor in a process that requires T-bet, NFIL3, and Id2, but not IL-15 and eomes expression [33]. The third identified subset is known to develop from CHILPs in a T-bet- and IL-15-dependent manner, but not dependent on IL-7 and does not express eomes [10, 33].

2.2 ILC2

The identification of lymphoid-like producing IL-13 and IL-5 cells was first reported in IL-25-treated Rag2[−/−] mice (which are unable to produce mature T or B cells). Those non-B/non-T (NBNT) cells were identified to be MHC class II high, CD11 null, and Lin—cells that were able to maximize type 2 immune responses upon treatment with IL-25 [43]. CD117, CD127 (IL-7Rα), inducible T cell costimulator (ICOS), CRTH2 (CD294), IL-1R, ST2, IL-17RB, NK1.1 (CD161), and CCR6 are the main surface markers and cytokines produced by ILC2s. More importantly, ILC2 has been identified to play vital roles in anthelminthic response [44] and the development of allergy-related inflammations such as asthma, atopic dermatitis, and chronic rhinosinusitis [45, 46]. Zhu et al. demonstrated that transcription factors GATA-3 and retinoic acid receptor-related orphan receptor-α (RORα) are responsible for the generation of ILC2, which are dependent on and can be maintained based on the growth factor independent 1 transcriptional repressor (Gfi-1) [47] and possibly on other yet to be identified conditions. In response to stimulation, it has been found that ILC2 cells produce effector cytokines via alarming cytokines, which are described as master stimulants of ILC2 activation. Examples of these master stimulants of ILC2 activation are IL-25, IL-33, and TSLP [48]. Basically, two distinct subtypes: nILC2 cells and iILC2 cells are known. The nILC2 cells represent the tissue-resident ST2[+] ILC2 cells that primarily respond to IL-33 and are present in steady-state. The iILC2 cells represent IL25-induced ST2[−] IL-17RB[+] ILC2 cells and they are undetectable in steady-state but can be rapidly elicited by IL-25 or infections [49]. ILC2s reside in both human and murine skin and are solely activated by TSLP vis-a-vis being responsible for promoting inflammation of the skin upon activation [50]. Tumor necrosis factor (TNF) superfamily cytokine TL1A (TNFSF15) promotes ILC2 to produce IL-13 ex vivo. In addition, the expansion of ILC2 is costimulated by TL1A through their highly expressed TNF-receptor superfamily member DR3 (TNFRSF25), which is independent of the IL-25 or IL-33 stimulation pathways [51]. The deregulated ILC2 functions are due to their lack of co-stimulation by TL1A and the disruption of the stimulation of ILC2. This results in reduced T cell accumulation and response in T-cell-dependent allergic models, which was suggested to be potentially beneficial for ILC2-related allergies such as allergic asthma [52].

2.3 ILC3

The ILC3s differ from the other two ILC groups owing to their ability to take part in intestinal homeostasis and lymphoid tissue development together with the provision of immunity against extracellular bacteria and chronic inflammation [44]. ILC3s require transcription factor RORγt for development and function [53], characterized by the production of IL-17A, IL-22, and granulocyte-macrophage colony-stimulating factor (GM-CSF) [54].

Significantly, various subsets of RORγt$^+$ group 3 ILCs have been reported both in humans and mice [55]. Accordingly, ILC3 in both mice and humans has been characterized using CD3$^-$Tcrab$^-$Tcrγδ$^-$CD11b$^-$Cd19$^-$CD45$^+$ CD127$^+$ Ckit$^+$ RORγt$^+$ IL-23R$^+$. Currently, the ILC3 community categorizes them into three major groups (LTi cells, NCR$^-$ILC3s, and NCR$^+$ ILC3s). However, these three major groups do not represent final states and vary in their expression of various cell surface markers upon exposure to different microenvironments with specific stimuli. More research is highly recommended in this area to understand how different stimuli lead to the expression of other cell surface markers on ILC3s. The LTi, one of the subgroups of ILC3s, was first found in developing lymph nodes, strictly dependent on RORγt for development and expresses high levels of CC6, which is essential in the formation of lymphoid tissue during organogenesis [56].

Two other subgroups of ILC3s that depend on GATA-3 and RORγt for their expressions are NCR$^+$ILC3 and NCR$^-$ILC3. ILC3s can switch from NCR$^-$ phenotype to NCR$^+$ phenotype when the microenvironment contains IL-1β and IL-23. This is termed phenotype switching and has been reported in recent studies [57]. ILC3s require RORγt for both development and function unlike ILC2s, which require RORγt only for development. This is one of the main differences observed between ILC2s and ILC3s. One other documented function of GATA-3 is its ability to regulate NCR$^+$ILC3 as well as NK cells of their crucial role in IL-22 production by these cells [58]. The activating NKp46 orNKp44 receptors are also expressed by NCR$^+$ILC3 [59]. Phenotypically, there is a distinguishing chemokine receptor expression in LTi but not NCR$^+$ILC3, theCCR6. The LTi and NCR$^-$ILC3 also produce IL-17, which is a cytokine associated with Th17 and granulocyte-macrophage colony-stimulating factor (GM-CSF) and contributes to proinflammatory responses [60]. These NCR$^-$ILC3 are able to produce interferon-gamma (IFN-γ) in addition to IL-22 and IL-17 [61]. Elevated ILC3 numbers have been reported in many autoimmune diseases including how their elevated levels influence the pathogenesis of these diseases [17]. Typically, in psoriasis, elevated levels of ILC3 have been observed in both skin and blood. It was also found that the elevated levels of ILC3s either producing IL-22 or IL-17A contribute to the pathogenesis of psoriatic disease [62] Table 1.

TABLE 1   Characteristics of innate lymphoid cells.

ILC subsets	Surface markers	Transcription factors	Modulators	Effector mediators
NK	NCR, NKG2D, KLRG1, CD122	T-bet, Eomes, NFIL3	NKG2D, KIRs	Perforins, IFN-γ, granzymes,
ILC1	CD122, CD160, CD103, CD39, NCR, NK1.1, TRAIL, CD200R.	T-bet, Eomes, NFIL3	IL-18, IL-12	TNF, IFN-γ
ILC2	CD127, ST2, ICOS, MHC-II, Sca-1	Bcl11b, GATA3, TCF-1, RORα	TSLP, IL-22, IL-33, IL-25	IL-4, IL-5, IL-9, IL-13
ILC3	NCR, IL23R, MHC-II, RANKL, CD49d	RORγt, T-bet	IL-1β, IL-7	IL-17, IL-22, TNF-α, GM-CSF
LTi	IL-23R, RANKL, CCRG, CD117, CD127, MHC-II	RORγt	EBI2	CCR6, IL-17, IL-22, TNF, lymphotoxin

2. Innate lymphoid cells as therapeutic targets

3 Properties and functions of ILCs

ILCs are found in both lymphoid and nonlymphoid tissues. All ILCs express CD45 and IL-7Rα and share a common lymphoid cell precursor with T and B cells but are lineage negative (lin⁻), lacking antigen receptors and other cell surface markers that define T cells, B cells, and myeloid cells. The functions of ILCs are numerous. Principally, ILCs orchestrate pathogen attacks, mediate homeostasis and participate in autoimmune pathologies via crosstalk with other immune cells. The tissue-resident ILCs execute important effector functions that make them key regulators in tissue homeostasis, repair, remodeling, microbial defense, and anti-tumor immunity [63, 64]. ILCs have been identified as antigen-presenting cells. ILC2s and ILC3s have the ability to process and present foreign antigens (Ags) via major histocompatibility complex class II (MHC-II), and to induce cognate $CD4^+$ T cell responses [65].

3.1 ILCs play protective immune functions

ILCs are involved in diverse immune responses such as participating in attacking and clearing pathogens from the immune system. The presence of increased populations of ILC at barrier surfaces such as the skin and other vital organs, which are prevalent sites of pathogen entry, enables ILCs to perform protective immune functions. The epithelial cells and myeloid cells communicate effectively to sense infection and/or tissue damage and produce cytokines and alarmins, which in turn facilitate the rapid activation of distinct ILCs' populations [66]. ILCs respond to these activations by producing cytokines in different ways. ILC1 are activated by IL-12, IL-15, and IL-18 [67], while IL-25, IL-33, and TSLP activate ILC2 [68] and IL-1 and IL-23 stimulate ILC3 [69]. What however remains unknown is whether the cytokines produced by the three groups of ILC work together to achieve immune protective functions. In other words, without activating a group of ILC, the other groups, if activated, cannot function to provide immune protection (Fig. 1).

3.2 ILCs in homeostasis

ILCs are present in all tissues, but they are particularly enriched in mucosal surfaces and barriers surfaces [70]. ILCs are also present in nonbarrier tissues, such as the meninges and the liver, where they maintain tissue homeostasis [71, 72]. ILCs mediate the maintenance of tissue homeostasis in different organs. This is principally achieved through crosstalk between myeloid immune cells [73] and T cells [74]. ILCs also crosstalk with the resident cells of the tissue by sensing the cytokines present in the microenvironments and subsequent production of signature cytokines, which in turn regulate innate immunity and homeostasis of hemato-poietic and nonhematopoietic cells in the tissues [75]. Ignacio et al. reported that ILC3s maintain homeostasis in lymph nodes in mice by inhibiting the recruitment of B and T cells. They failed to provide direct mechanistic pathways connecting ILC3 to B and T cells recruitment [75]. ILC3s contribute to the control of intestinal homeostasis by two main mechanisms. First, ILC3s directly sense diet-derived retinoic acid and AhR-ligands; and second, by responding with the production of IL-22. This enforces the integrity of the epithelial barrier by inducing mucus production, fucosylation, and antimicrobial peptide production. Again, sensing of intestinal commensals by macrophages induces the secretion of IL-1β, which triggers GM-CSF

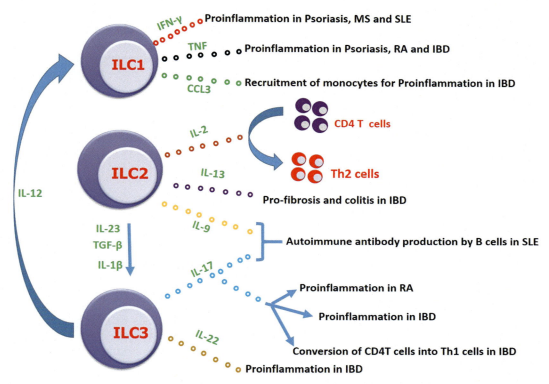

FIG. 1 Pathogenic roles of ILC in autoimmune diseases: ILCs play different functions in the pathogenesis of different autoimmune diseases. ILC1, ILC2, and ILC3 express surface receptors and mediators, which influence the activities of other cells in disease pathogenesis.

production by ILC3s that instructs intestinal phagocytes to produce regulatory molecules such as retinoic acid and IL-10 to expand regulatory T cells, thereby inducing oral tolerance [76, 77].

3.3 ILCs in disease pathology

Abnormal populations and dysregulation of ILCs are instrumental factors in the development of different diseases such as inflammatory diseases, autoimmune diseases, and cancers. Over the years, it has become clear that when the activities of ILCs are not well regulated, they contribute to chronic inflammation, tissue damage, autoimmunity, metabolic diseases, and cancer [16].

4 ILC in autoimmune diseases

Knowing the anatomical locations of ILCs and their ability to rapidly secrete immunoregulatory cytokines, it is important to outline how they crosstalk with other innate and adaptive immune cells during autoimmune diseases. This is because ILCs are proving to be important in the regulation of immune responses as well as promoting or ameliorating inflammation in autoimmunity. ILCs are known to respond to environmental stress in infections, allergy, and autoimmunity by producing cytokines that target stromal and epithelial cells, which potentially lead to the disease pathology [78]. ILCs' functions vary depending on their phenotype. Typically, ILC1s secrete type I cytokines, which promote inflammation in a variety of autoimmune diseases. Moreover, ILC2s play important roles in the induction of fibrosis in different tissues and organs in various autoimmune diseases. In addition, IL-17 and IL-22 derived from ILC3s can promote or inhibit local inflammation in autoimmune diseases. ILCs play a role in the initiation and exacerbation of autoimmune responses through the amplification of the IL-23/IL-17 cytokine axis [79, 80].

4.1 ILC in psoriasis

Psoriasis is a common immune-mediated inflammatory disease that affects the skin and joints [81]. The immunopathogenesis of psoriasis is based on a combination of genetic susceptibility and environmental risk factors triggering pathogenic crosstalk between innate and adaptive immune cells [82]. The IL-23/IL-17A pathway plays a key role in the pathogenesis of psoriasis. Until recently, it was believed that T cells were the only group of cells responsible for the production of cytokines such as IL-17 known to play crucial roles in the pathogenesis of psoriasis. The discovery of the ILCs provided insight into other sources of IL-17 production. ILCs are involved in early effector cytokine-mediated responses during infections in peripheral tissues. ILCs also play an important role in chronic inflammatory skin diseases, including psoriasis [83]. Pantelyushin et al. were the first to provide evidence about the involvement of IL-17 and IL-22-producing ILCs in the pathogenesis of psoriasis. They identified that IL-17F, IL-17A, and IL-22-producing RoRγt$^+$ innate lymphocytes and γδ T cells were the primary inducers of imiquimod-induced psoriasis-like skin inflammation in mice [84]. This study stimulated further research work about the functional roles of ILC subsets in the pathophysiology of psoriasis. In 2014, Villanova et al. characterized the ILCs in PBMC and human skin biopsies from healthy individuals and patients with psoriasis. They identified increased populations of IL-17A- and IL-22-producing cells in the skin and blood of psoriasis patients, which were CD3-negative innate lymphocytes. After immunophenotyping, the human ILC subsets showed a statistically significant increase in the frequency of circulating NKp44$^+$ILC3 in the blood of psoriasis patients compared with healthy individuals. More than 50% of circulating NKp44$^+$ILC3 expressed cutaneous lymphocyte associated antigens, which indicates their potential for skin homing. Analysis of skin tissues revealed a significantly increased proportion of total ILCs in the skin compared with the blood. Moreover, the frequency of NKp44$^+$ILC3 was significantly increased in nonlesional psoriatic skin compared with normal skin [5]. Villanova et al. concluded that the increase in the frequency of NKp44$^+$ILC3 subset in noninflamed skin tissue of psoriasis patients indicates that they are potentially major innate contributors of IL-17 and IL-22 production in skin homeostasis and inflammatory pathology [5]. Increased populations of NCR$^+$ ILC3 in psoriatic skin lesions compared to healthy skin have been reported through other studies as well [85]. The authors reported increased frequency of NCR$^+$ILC3 in psoriatic skin without lesions, which suggests that the altered populations of ILCs in the skin can potentially be an initiating factor for the development of psoriasis. It has now become clear that ILC3s accumulate in psoriatic skin but the mechanisms that mediate this accumulation remain unclear. In this regard, Keren et al. determined whether human ILC3 (CD3$^-$ RORγt$^+$ NKp44$^+$ cells) could induce psoriatic lesions in healthy human skin in vivo. This study provided the first functional evidence that ILC3s' populations increase in human psoriatic skin and can initiate the development of the human psoriatic phenotype independent of Th17 cells. In addition, they found that ILCs promote T cell activation in the pathophysiology of psoriasis [86]. Future research should focus on identifying the expression levels of cytokine receptors on ILC3s and the levels of different cytokines promoting different ILC subsets in psoriasis that will help clarify the functional roles of ILCs in psoriasis.

4.2 ILC in autoimmune cardiac diseases

4.2.1 *ILC in rheumatic heart diseases*

Rheumatic heart disease (RHD) is an autoimmune disease that is mediated by both humoral and cellular immune responses that follow an untreated *Streptococcus pyogenes* infection [87]. The autoimmune reactions are the hallmark of disease pathogenesis. Both cross-reactive antibodies and T cells play important roles in the cross-recognition between streptococcal antigens and human proteins leading to inflammation and autoimmunity [88]. Activation of T lymphocytes in the presence of antigen-presenting cells such as macrophages and DCs has been reported to be involved in the pathogenesis of inflammation in RHD [89]. Currently, the role of ILCs in the pathogenesis of RHD remains unknown. Researchers are encouraged to delve into this direction to unravel how the diverse ILC groups function during the pathogenesis of RHD.

4.2.2 *ILC in autoimmune myocarditis*

Myocarditis is the inflammation of the myocardium (muscle tissues of the heart). After a pathological cardiac-specific inflammatory process, it may progress to chronic damage and dilated cardiomyopathy [90]. It results from an autoimmune process. The development of autoimmune myocarditis arises from different predisposing factors such as viral infection, systemic/local preexisting autoimmune condition, HLA gene variations, molecular mimicry, exposure of cryptic antigens, and deficient thymic training or Treg induction. During the pathogenesis of autoimmune myocarditis, there is a recruitment of various immune cells in the heart [91], which orchestrate a sustained attack toward myocardial tissues. We have previously described and reported direct interplays between cardiac fibroblast, dendritic, macrophages, and CD4 T cells in the pathogenesis of myocarditis [92]. Available evidence concerning the role of ILCs in the pathogenesis of myocarditis was limited until recent publication by Bracamonte-Baran et al. [93]. The authors observed an increased proportion of the ILC2 population in the heart of patients with chronic ischemic cardiomyopathy and myocarditis, in contrast to a predominantly undifferentiated ILC profile in healthy human hearts. They also identified elevated proportions of ILC2 in murine models of myocarditis and myocardial infarctions. These together led to the conclusion that the heart's ILCs are a quiescent and phenotypically undifferentiated population, which develop ILC type 2 features during inflammatory processes such as ischemia and autoimmunity in cardiac tissues [93]. Recently, other researchers have identified ILC2s to play pathogenic roles in pericarditis [94]. There is no study currently available, which has assessed the populations on ILC1 and ILC3 in myocarditis. We argue that because GM-CSF, which mediates autoimmunity, is produced from ILC3 and activates Th17 to function in promoting experimental autoimmune myocarditis (EAM), ILC3 could possibly play pathogenic roles indirectly in myocarditis and should be further explored.

4.3 ILC in inflammatory bowel disease

Inflammatory bowel disease (IBD), chronic inflammation of the gastrointestinal tract, consists of ulcerative colitis (UC) and Crohn's disease (CD). IBD is attributed to dysregulated immune responses. There is more to be unraveled about the pathogenesis of IBD, however, it is believed that the intestinal epithelium shows an increased permeability, which permits enhanced immune responses against the commensal microbiota [95]. IBD is driven by aberrant T cell responses to the intestinal microbiota. Over the years, the roles of CD4$^+$ T cells in the pathogenesis of IBD became the research focus in this field. The IBD-relevant cytokines were believed to be produced exclusively by Th1 and Th17 cells until researchers reported potent IL-17A and IL-22 responses in mice lacking T cells and B cells. These IL-23 responsive IL-22 producing innate mucosal immune cells are now termed ILCs. Interestingly, ILC1s, ILC2s, and ILC3s have all been implicated in IBD [96, 97]. Understanding how pathogenic ILCs emerge and function inhuman IBD could give novel insights in finding better therapeutic strategies for IBD patients. It is important to note that under normal functioning of the colon and ileum, the intestinal lamina propria has increased levels of IL-22-producing ILC3 subsets, however, the ILC composition and cytokine profile within the colon and ileum in IBD is markedly altered [98]. The altered cytokine profile in the intestines of patients with CD or UC leads to elevated IL-17-producing ILC3s and IFN-γ producing ILC1s in the intestines of CD patients, while IL-17 and type 2 cytokines are elevated in UC patients [98]. It is interesting to note that ILC1s accumulate in inflamed intestinal tissues resected from CD patients whereas the frequencies of NCR$^+$ILC3s decrease [10]. Other researchers have reported increased populations of IL-12- and IL-15-responsive intraepithelial CD103$^+$NKp46$^+$ILC1 and lamina propria NKp46$^+$ILC1 in CD patients [99]. Based on their findings and considering prior reports, the authors concluded that ILC1 cells might have a pathogenic role in the ileum [99]. The accumulation of ILC1 translates into increased levels of IFN-γ, which promotes neutrophil migration, and activation of lymphocytes, macrophages, and endothelial cells. Furthermore, the IFN-γ affects tight junctions' function that leads to impairments in the epithelial barrier, which is an important defense mechanism against pathogens in the intestine. Researchers have provided evidence to support the notion regarding the involvement of ILC2 in the pathogenesis of IBD. They have identified abundant IL-13 producing CD3$^-$KIR$^+$ cells in fibrotic areas of the intestine in CD patients and these fibrotic lesions had higher levels of IL-13, IL-13Rα2, and collagen expression than nonfibrotic lesions. It can therefore be concluded that ILC2s might contribute to intestinal fibrosis via IL-13 production in the gut [100]. ILC3s are known to play a dual role in IBD pathology. While an increased population of IL-17-producing NCR$^-$ILC3s was found in both the ileum and colon of CD patients [101], ILC3s expressed IFN-γ and IL-17 and antibodies against these cytokines potentially ameliorated IBD. This confirmed the pathogenic role of IL-17 where it is known to help in the recruitment of other immune cells. These findings point to the fact that IL-17 does not play a pathogenic role in CD as reported in the pathogenesis of other autoimmune diseases such as ankylosing spondylitis and psoriasis. These stimulated arguments that IL-17 can have both protective and disease-causing roles depending on the disease context and possible competition between Th1 and Th17. In all ILCs contribute to intestinal inflammation through production of cytokine such as IL17A and IFN-γ, recruitment of other inflammatory cells and organization of the inflammatory tissue during the pathogenesis of IBD.

4.4 ILC in systemic lupus erythematosus

Systemic lupus erythematosus (SLE) is an autoimmune disease, which affects the skin, joints, kidneys, brain, and other organs. SLE is characterized by various degrees of immune system dysfunctions, including immune complex depositions, pathogenic autoantibody production, and immune cells infiltration, which together lead to inflammation and damage within targeted organs. Considering the recent discovery of ILCs and their inflammatory mediators, innate immunity is emerging as a key player in disease pathology. Researchers have highlighted the importance of innate lymphoid cells through their signature cytokines molecule in promoting and potentiating the immunopathology of SLE. In SLE, different cytokines are overexpressed and contribute to the pathogenesis of the disease. Alterations in the frequency and function of ILCs have been implicated in the pathophysiology of SLE and other systemic autoimmune diseases. In 2019, Chu et al. analyzed the subsets of ILCs in PBMC of SLE patients and correlated their frequencies with clinical serologic markers, IL-4, IL-33, and IFN-γ. They reported a significant elevation of ILC1 percentage in SLE active group. ILC2 population was decreased significantly in both remission and active groups while ILC3 was decreased significantly in active group. The authors, therefore, speculated that ILCs generally could have both protective and pathogenic roles in SLE [102]. Düster et al. investigated the role of ILC2s in the MRL/MpJ-Fas^{lpr} (MRL-lpr) mouse model for severe organ manifestation of systemic lupus erythematosus (SLE). The authors reported that the progression of lupus nephritis is accompanied by a reduction of ILC2 population in the inflamed renal tissue and again the cytokine production of kidney-residing ILC2s was suppressed by IFN-γ. Most importantly, restoration of ILC2 numbers by IL-33-mediated expansion ameliorated lupus nephritis and prevented mortality in MRL-*lpr* mice. Based on their findings, they concluded that the development of SLE-like kidney inflammation results in the downregulation of the renal ILC2 response and proposed further that an ILC2-expanding therapy may be a promising therapeutic option for autoimmune diseases [103].

In 2019, Blokland et al. assessed the frequency and phenotype of circulating ILCs in SLE and their relationship to the IFN signature. They identified increased ILC1 frequencies in peripheral blood of patients with SLE as compared with healthy controls and correlate with disease activity. However, they found no differences between the frequency of ILC2s or ILC3s in patients with SLE and the healthy controls. The authors concluded that type I IFN signature is related to Fas expression and frequencies of circulating ILC2s and ILC3s in patients with SLE and may possibly influence ILC balance [104]. We recommend more studies to increase our understanding of how ILC populations can be manipulated together with other possible unidentified roles of ILC and how they could be good candidates for future therapeutic approaches.

4.5 ILC in multiple sclerosis

Multiple sclerosis (MS) is a chronic inflammatory, autoimmune, demyelinating and degenerative disease of the central nervous system (CNS) resulting in axonal loss with consequential clinical impairments [105]. The interplay between innate and adaptive immunity is important in multiple sclerosis. This complex disease involves interplay between many different immune cells involved in its pathogenesis. Recently an important immunological site, which influences the pathogenesis of MS is the meninges, has been identified [106]. The meninges composing of three layers, the outermost dura mater, the arachnoid mater, and the pia mater surrounds the brain and spinal cord and lies outside of the blood–brain barrier (BBB). Aggregation of innate immune cells in the meningeal space has been documented in MS [107]. The meninges functions as immune border sites where immune surveillance of the CNS occurs. ILC3s together with ILC2 and ILC1 are normally present in the meninges and CNS [108]. ILC1s and ILC3s are implicated in promoting severe EAE [109]. The proportions of ILC3 increase in number after disease induction. When activated ILC3 produces IFNγ, IL-17, GM-CSF, and other cytokines that have been linked to EAE pathogenesis [109]. The authors identified group 3 ILCs, (ILC3s–CD45$^+$ Lin-IL-7Ra$^+$RORct$^+$) as are normal residents of the meninges and exhibit disease-induced accumulation and activation in EAE. They proposed that CD45$^+$ Lin-IL-7Ra$^+$RORct$^+$ ILC3s in the meninges, and to a lesser extent in the CNS, play a major and essential role in these disease-promoting events of EAE. Again the group adoptively transferred encephalitogenic Th17 cells to $Rorc^{-/-}$ mice, lacking both ILC3s. They found that the ability to generate Th17 responses is not sufficient to induce disease indicating that ILC3s are also required to initiate EAE [109].

In 2016, Gross et al. assessed the patterns of distinct lesion in MS patients and for the first time showed that distinct T helper cell and helper-like ILC subsets are associated with preferential cerebral or spinal lesion development in humans [110]. In clarifying the potential role of ILCs in the early stages of MS, Degn et al. in 2016 analyzed the proportions and phenotype of ILCs in the cerebrospinal fluid (CSF) of patients experiencing their first or second demyelinating event. They found significant proportions of LTi subset of the ILCs, which suggests their accumulation in the CNS over time leads to the development of the ectopic lymphoid follicles, a hallmark of MS disease [111]. The role of natural killer cells, a subset of ILC1 cells in the pathogenesis of MS remains unexplored. Over the past years, it was unclear whether they exert a beneficial or detrimental role. It is gradually becoming acceptable that NK cells play beneficial roles. In MS, most studies report a deficiency of NK cytolytic activity in peripheral blood and IFN-β appears to induce a slight decrease of total circulating NK cells in MS patients [112]. NK cell depletion exacerbated EAE disease activity in rodents and could therefore be a potential therapeutic target in MS. Many researchers found that IFN-β therapy resulted in elevated populations of immunoregulatory NK cell subset CD56^{bright} coupled with a decrease of the cytotoxic CD56^{dim}NK cells in the periphery [113, 114].

4.6 ILC in diabetes

4.6.1 *ILC in type 1 diabetes*

Type 1 Diabetes (T1D) is an autoimmune disease driven by autoreactive T cells that results in the destruction of pancreatic islet insulin-producing beta cells and hyperglycemia [115].

The pathogenesis of T1D involves various arms of the innate immune systems. Two types of T1D are described; the aggressive type of T1D that is a T cell-driven autoimmune disease, and the T cell-independent type of T1D, which is largely mediated by innate immune effectors [116]. Studies of the pathogenesis of T1D have largely focused on the analysis of diabetogenic T cells and their control by Treg cells and several clinical trials in humans are targeting this cell type [117, 118]. Currently, there is little data on the role of innate immune cells specifically, ILCs in the pathogenesis of T1D. There is increasing evidence that innate cells play critical roles in T1D onset [119]. Many observations support a protective role of these cells following their triggering upon the microbial infections early phase of the disease [120]. Researchers have speculated that the activation of these innate immune cells in the pancreas through continued β-cell death may promote their pathogenic functions [121]. One group of innate lymphoid cells, which has been implicated in T1D are the natural killer cells. The specific role of NK cells remains unclear but it was reported that $CD56^{dim}CD16^{pos}$ NKs are reduced at onset of T1D [122]. This accounts for the reported diminished responses to IL-2 and IL-15 and lipopolysaccharide (LPS), cytotoxicity and defective IFN-γ secretion [123]. There should be more investigations to identify the unique roles of the other ILC groups in the pathogenesis of T1D. It is believed that increasing the knowledge of regulatory mechanisms in T1D by innate lymphoid cells would open up to promising therapeutic approaches.

4.6.2 *ILC in type 2 diabetes*

Type 2 diabetes is a chronic condition, which results from the body's inability to effectively use the insulin produced by the pancreas to enter blood sugar into cells to produce sufficient energy [124]. This leads to high blood glucose levels, which subsequently elicit an inflammatory response as a result of the immune response to high blood glucose levels and the presence of inflammatory mediators from immune cells [125]. Interestingly, increasing studies report an emerging role of innate lymphoid cells in the development of type 2 diabetes. These researchers have provided convincing data regarding the role of ILCs in T2D. it has been reported that ILCs promote inflammation and insulin resistance [126, 127]. Dalmas et al. researched resident immune cells in the pancreatic islets and possibly identify their roles in the pathogenesis of T2D. The authors found increased frequencies and cell numbers of ILC2, dendritic cells, and NK cells. They further discovered ILC2 as the primary immune subset expressing IL-33-receptor T1/ST2 within islets. This provided evidence for the first time that there is immunometabolic crosstalk between islet-derived IL-33, ILC2, and myeloid cells contributes to the maintenance of insulin secretion [128]. In 2019, Liu et al. employed FCM to assess the populations of ILC1 in the PBMC and adipose tissues from T2D patients to identify the relationship between ILC and glucose homeostasis. They reported elevated populations of circulating and adipose ILC1. The authors concluded that type 1 innate lymphoid cells are associated with type 2 diabetes [127]. It has become convincingly clear that group 2 innate lymphoid cells are associated with chronic inflammation and dysregulated metabolic homeostasis in T2D, while ILC1 facilitates T2D.

4.7 ILC in rheumatoid arthritis

Rheumatoid arthritis (RA) is an autoimmune disease characterized by joint inflammation [129]. Both innate and adaptive mechanisms closely interplay to promote chronic joint inflammation. Although the pathogenesis remains unclear, RA is characterized by the infiltration of immune cells in the synovial tissue promoting the production of autoantibodies and contributing to the persistent joint damage [130]. There is limited research detailing the roles of ILC in the pathogenesis of RA. It has been hypothesized that ILCs stimulate other immune cells such as macrophages and fibroblast-like synoviocytes (FLS) to produce proinflammatory cytokines, such as TNF-α, IL-1β, IL-6, IL-15, and IL-23, which are involved in the pathogenesis of RA [131]. In 2015, Leijten et al. characterized ILC classes and subsets in the peripheral blood (PB) of healthy controls and in the synovial fluid of rheumatoid arthritis patients. They reported elevated populations of all classes of ILCs in rheumatoid arthritis [132]. These results were consistent with a study conducted in 2002, which reported a subset of NK cells to be elevated in peripheral blood and synovial fluid from patients with inflammatory arthritis [133]. Characterized by early lymph node (LN) activation in the pathogenesis of RA, Javier Rodriguez-Carrio et al. used FCM to analyze the frequency and distribution of ILCs in LN biopsies obtained during the earliest phases of RA. They reported ILC distribution changes within the LN compartments before the onset of symptoms as well as the early phase of RA. They also identified that individuals who are prone to RA, produce RA-specific autoantibodies and subsequently display features of systemic autoimmunity associated with RA, thereby suggesting a role for ILCs during RA development [134]. To further unravel the roles of ILCs in the pathogenesis of RA, Al-Mossawi et al. attempted to identify and characterize ILCs in the joints of patients with inflammatory arthritis. They found that ILC populations (type 1 and type 3) are present in the synovial fluid and synovial tissue of inflamed RA joints. They reported that these cells have the ability to secrete enormous levels of cytokines, which are important components of inflammatory status. Moreover, they discovered that ILC1 and ILC3 play a role in antigen presentation through HLADR expression [135]. There are inconsistent findings of the roles of ILC2 in RA, while Hirota et al. reported years ago that GM-CSF-producing ILC2s had a pathogenic role in the development of arthritis [136], another recent publication argues that ILC2s have a protective role in RA [137].

In 2019, Takaki-Kuwahara et al. investigated the ILCs' function in the development of RA using a mouse model of collagen-induced arthritis (CIA). In this research, they used fluorescence-activated cell sorting and quantitative PCR to identify and purified the ILC subsets in the joints, peripheral blood (PB), local lymph nodes (LNs) and to assess the expression levels of representative cytokines. They analyzed their data by correlating the frequencies of each ILC subset in synovial fluid of RA patients. They reported increased populations of CCR6$^+$ILC3s in the total proportion of ILCs in the joints with active inflammation compared to the controls. Again CCR6$^+$ILC3s from mice with arthritis expressed significantly higher levels of IL-17A and IL-22 cytokines [6].

5 ILCs as immunoregulators in autoimmune diseases

ILC plays important function in regulation of immune responses. Similar to T regulatory cells, ILCs inhibit both innate and adaptive immune cells. Known to promote inflammatory immune responses, recent studies provide evidence that populations of ILCs inhibit immune responses through a variety of mechanisms. ILCs contribute to shaping the type and intensity of the immune response by producing cytokines and other mediators, and via cell-cell interactions [138]. Their ability to modulate immune responses remains an important function of ILCs. ILCs inhibit inflammatory immune responses and mouse studies demonstrate their potential to directly limit T cell responses in transplantation, autoimmunity, and host defense [65]. ILC1s mediate several autoimmune diseases through their secreted mediators such as IFN-γ, TNF-α, and CCL3 resulting from their activation by IL-12 and IL-15 produced from stromal cells [139]. Several studies defined a regulatory role for cNK cells in controlling T-cell-dependent immune responses by direct cytotoxic activity toward CD4$^+$ and CD8$^+$ T cells [140]. ILC2 produces IL4, IL-5, IL-9, and IL-13 after been activated by IL-25, IL-33, and TSLP from stromal cells and perform different functions in various autoimmune diseases. Typically, IL-9 enhances the generation of autoimmune antibodies and therefore serves to worsen the pathologic condition of systemic lupus erythematosus [140], while IL-13 plays a crucial role in the induction of fibrosis in systemic sclerosis [141] and in the pathogenesis of inflammatory bowel diseases [142]. ILC3s are also emerging as key orchestrators and regulators of adaptive immune responses. They have the capacity to modulate a broad variety of specialized adaptive immune responses through cell-cell interactions via additional nonclassical costimulatory and co-inhibitory molecules [143]. ILC3 are endowed with a broad array of accessory co-activating and co-inhibitory molecules that mediate further modulation and tuning of adaptive immune cell function. ILC3s are associated with the secretion of effector cytokines and these soluble mediators can modulate the functions of immune cells and nonimmune cells during the pathogenesis of autoimmune diseases. It is reported that ILC3-associated CD30L and OX40L are responsible for the modulation of T memory cell through cognate interactions with CD30/OX40L [143] and also promote inflammatory effector T cell responses in autoimmune diseases. In addition, ILC3 have been reported to express co-inhibitory and immune checkpoint molecules such as PD1 and PDL1, further suggesting their immunoregulatory functions [144].

6 ILC as a potential therapeutic target in autoimmune diseases

Current pharmacological treatments used in autoimmune diseases are not effective, can produce significant side effects and their efficacy is speculated to diminish over time. In fact, the majority of patients with autoimmune diseases do not show a satisfactory response to these therapies. As a result, there is an urgent need to introduce alternatives for specific targeted therapies, which could significantly improve the care and disease management for autoimmune patients. Most targeted therapies have been directed at altering T cell function in the pathogenesis of autoimmune diseases. The recent understanding that ILCs can exert profound influences on T cell polarization and effector functions could lead to extensive research on finding new therapeutic strategies targeting immunological pathways involved in autoimmune diseases. Researchers speculate that due to the multiple roles of ILCs in autoimmune diseases, they represent an attractive therapeutic target. Excessive accumulation and/or activation of specific ILC populations have been related to the pathogenesis of a number of diseases such as inflammatory bowel disease, psoriasis, and asthma. Possible therapeutic strategies have been proposed with the goal of preventing ILCs' activation by the blockade of activation and/or survival signals, interference with intracellular signaling pathways that lead to dysregulation of ILC populations, and the neutralization of effector pathogenic cytokines that they produce, or inhibition of ILC recruitment to target organs.

6.1 Blocking the activation and/or survival signals of ILC

Several cytokines serve as signals responsible for activating ILCs either to increase their populations or reduce their populations, thereby influencing the pathogenesis of autoimmune diseases. Typically, IL-23 potently stimulates IL-17A and IL-22 production by pathogenic ILC3 and also triggers the production of IFN-γ and TNF-α by ILC1 in IBD patients [4]. Some other cytokines mediating IL-23-induced cytokine production include IL-1, IL-6, IL-15, IL-18, and TL1A [145, 146]. IL-7 also augments pathogenic cytokine production by ILC3. Increased levels of these cytokines are reported in the gut of patients with IBD [147]. Blocking these cytokines reduces effector cytokine production and attenuates ILC dependent mechanisms in autoimmune pathology of Crohn's disease [148] and IBD [149]. There is evidence of increased numbers of ILCs in patients with active MS. Treatment with daclizumab, an antibody against IL-2 receptor (CD25), substantially diminishes the number of circulating ILCs and inhibits atrophy of brain structures in direct contact with the meninges by 38%–60% [150].

6.2 Inhibiting intracellular signaling pathways leads to dysregulation of ILC populations

Intracellular signaling pathways are initiated by cytokines, which their receptors are on the cells. Evidence suggests that experimental targeting of these subsets leading to decreased ILC counts and disease alleviation. Most cytokine receptors signal through Janus kinase (JAK) and STAT pathways. Specifically inhibiting JAK/STAT signaling suppresses effector cytokine production by ILCs [151]. STAT3 inhibition is expected to suppress the activation of ILCs mediated by IL-23 and IL-6, limiting the pathogenic potential of ILCs in the gut involvement as in some other diseases [152].

6.3 Neutralization of the effector pathogenic cytokines that they produce

Targeting the ability of ILC3s to produce GM-CSF is proposed to be an alternative treatment option in some autoimmune diseases [153]. Cytokines such as IL-23, IL-17, and IL-22 can serve as unique therapeutic targets because the dysregulation of either IL-17 or IL-22, however, has been linked to autoimmune diseases such as psoriasis, RA, and IBD [154]. IL-23/IL-17 axis overactivation and IL-17 overexpression are reported in CD and psoriasis. Therefore, blocking IL-17 could be beneficial and may provide a novel therapeutic target in the treatment of IBD patients. Therapies designed to target IL-23, IL-6, and JAK signaling, in addition to suppressing ILCs also influence other cells such as Th17 cells, which are crucial in the progression of the pathogenesis of a group of autoimmune diseases. Targeted therapy against IL-17 has been very successful in the treatment of RA and have been reviewed extensively [155]. Furthermore, IL-9 and IL-17 are important cytokines secreted by ILC2s and ILC3s, respectively. IL-9 promotes the production of autoantibodies and increases the severity of lupus nephritis. The authors used anti-IL-9 and anti-IL-17 antibodies to neutralize IL-9 and IL-17 in vivo, they observed significantly decreased autoantibody levels and relief of symptoms of lupus nephritis [156].

6.4 Inhibition of ILC recruitment to target organs

ILCs trafficking in the pathogenesis of autoimmune disease remains a critical aspect in identifying therapeutic targets for autoimmune diseases. Altered local populations can additionally result from the migration of ILCs within an organ or from/to distal organs. IL-17- and IL-22-producing ILC3s expand in the peripheral blood, gut, synovial fluid, and bone marrow of RA patients. These cells express elevated levels of gut-homing integrin α4β7 compared with healthy controls, indicating the possibility that gut-derived ILC3s emigrate from the intestine to α4β7 ligand-expressing synovial tissue, promoting local joint inflammation by producing IL-17 and IL-22. Based on this, it was recorded that ILC3s travel from the gut to extra-intestinal synovial tissues in the pathogenesis of RA [157]. Therefore, researchers anticipate that blockade of the ILC trafficking or trafficking pathway would prevent the recruitment of ILC precursors to organs, which could serve as a new therapeutic opportunity. Drugs targeting inflammatory ILCs trafficking into organs may be very helpful because as they inhibit an important part of disease pathogenesis.

7 Future perspectives

A better and precise understanding of the roles of ILC types in autoimmune diseases or exploring a way to control them will facilitate the opportunity to manipulate their functions to develop new interventions and therapeutic strategies. More research is recommended to explore the regulatory pathways in various autoimmune diseases, which will help to design effective strategies for treating autoimmune diseases.

8 Conclusion

ILCs are the latest discovered group of innate immune cells known to modulate the pathogenesis of autoimmune diseases. Recent studies have investigated ILCs in various autoimmune diseases. The interesting discovery of their various roles, especially identifying them as major drivers of autoimmune diseases, could potentially lead to the discovery of novel therapeutic strategies to combat these diseases. This chapter has provided possible mechanistic roles of ILC and their potential as therapeutic targets in various autoimmune diseases.

References

[1] I. Kortekaas Krohn, et al., Emerging roles of innate lymphoid cells in inflammatory diseases: clinical implications, Allergy 73 (4) (2018) 837–850.

[2] J.P. Di Santo, An IL-1β-dependent switch in innate mucosal immunity? Immunity 32 (6) (2010) 734–736.

[3] A. Kurioka, P. Klenerman, C.B. Willberg, Innate-like CD 8+ T-cells and NK cells: converging functions and phenotypes, Immunology 154 (4) (2018) 547–556.

[4] A.R. Moschen, H. Tilg, T. Raine, IL-12, IL-23 and IL-17 in IBD: immunobiology and therapeutic targeting, Nat. Rev. Gastroenterol. Hepatol. 16 (3) (2019) 185–196.

[5] F. Villanova, et al., Characterization of innate lymphoid cells in human skin and blood demonstrates increase of NKp44+ ILC3 in psoriasis, J. Investig. Dermatol. 134 (4) (2014) 984–991.

[6] A. Takaki-Kuwahara, et al., CCR6+ group 3 innate lymphoid cells accumulate in inflamed joints in rheumatoid arthritis and produce Th17 cytokines, Arthritis Res. Ther. 21 (1) (2019) 1–9.

[7] M. Salimi, et al., A role for IL-25 and IL-33–driven type-2 innate lymphoid cells in atopic dermatitis, J. Exp. Med. 210 (13) (2013) 2939–2950.

[8] C. Guo, et al., Innate lymphoid cell disturbance with increase in ILC1 in systemic lupus erythematosus, Clin. Immunol. 202 (2019) 49–58.

[9] F. Roan, et al., CD4+ group 1 innate lymphoid cells (ILC) form a functionally distinct ILC subset that is increased in systemic sclerosis, J. Immunol. 196 (5) (2016) 2051–2062.

[10] J.H. Bernink, et al., Human type 1 innate lymphoid cells accumulate in inflamed mucosal tissues, Nat. Immunol. 14 (3) (2013) 221.

[11] H. Spits, et al., Innate lymphoid cells—a proposal for uniform nomenclature, Nat. Rev. Immunol. 13 (2) (2013) 145–149.

[12] E.D.T. Wojno, D. Artis, Emerging concepts and future challenges in innate lymphoid cell biology, J. Exp. Med. 213 (11) (2016) 2229–2248.

[13] D. Artis, H. Spits, The biology of innate lymphoid cells, Nature 517 (7534) (2015) 293–301.

[14] C.A. Vosshenrich, J.P. Di Santo, Developmental programming of natural killer and innate lymphoid cells, Curr. Opin. Immunol. 25 (2) (2013) 130–138.

[15] R.E. Mebius, Organogenesis of lymphoid tissues, Nat. Rev. Immunol. 3 (4) (2003) 292–303.

[16] A.N. McKenzie, H. Spits, G. Eberl, Innate lymphoid cells in inflammation and immunity, Immunity 41 (3) (2014) 366–374.

[17] A. Diefenbach, M. Colonna, S. Koyasu, Development, differentiation, and diversity of innate lymphoid cells, Immunity 41 (3) (2014) 354–365.

[18] G. Eberl, M. Colonna, J.P. Di Santo, A.N. McKenzie, Innate lymphoid cells: a new paradigm in immunology, Science 348 (6237) (2015), aaa6566.

[19] C. Pearson, H.H. Uhlig, F. Powrie, Lymphoid microenvironments and innate lymphoid cells in the gut, Trends Immunol. 33 (6) (2012) 289–296.

[20] J. Mjösberg, L. Mazzurana, ILC-poiesis: making tissue ILCs from blood, Immunity 46 (3) (2017) 344–346.

[21] T. Cupedo, ILC2: at home in the thymus, Eur. J. Immunol. 48 (9) (2018) 1441–1444.

[22] A. Eken, et al., ILC3 deficiency and generalized ILC abnormalities in DOCK8-deficient patients, Allergy 75 (4) (2020) 921–932.

[23] M.H. Kim, E.J. Taparowsky, C.H. Kim, Retinoic acid differentially regulates the migration of innate lymphoid cell subsets to the gut, Immunity 43 (1) (2015) 107–119.

[24] H.C. Jeffery, et al., Human intrahepatic ILC2 are IL-13positive amphiregulinpositive and their frequency correlates with model of end stage liver disease score, PLoS One 12 (12) (2017), e0188649.

[25] B.S. Kim, Innate lymphoid cells in the skin, J. Investig. Dermatol. 135 (3) (2015) 673–678.

[26] K.C. De Grove, et al., Characterization and quantification of innate lymphoid cell subsets in human lung, PloS One 11 (1) (2016), e0145961.

[27] Q. Yang, et al., TCF-1 upregulation identifies early innate lymphoid progenitors in the bone marrow, Nat. Immunol. 16 (10) (2015) 1044–1050.

[28] E. Montaldo, et al., Unique Eomes+ NK cell subsets are present in uterus and decidua during early pregnancy, Front. Immunol. 6 (2016) 646.

[29] S. Amarnath, Protocols for innate lymphoid cell phenotypic and functional characterization: an overview, in: Innate Lymphoid Cells, Springer, 2020, pp. 1–6.

[30] M. Colonna, Innate lymphoid cells: diversity, plasticity, and unique functions in immunity, Immunity 48 (6) (2018) 1104–1117.

[31] F. Annunziato, C. Romagnani, S. Romagnani, The 3 major types of innate and adaptive cell-mediated effector immunity, J. Allergy Clin. Immunol. 135 (3) (2015) 626–635.

[32] G. Sciumé, et al., Distinct requirements for T-bet in gut innate lymphoid cells, J. Exp. Med. 209 (13) (2012) 2331–2338.

[33] C.S. Klose, et al., Differentiation of type 1 ILCs from a common progenitor to all helper-like innate lymphoid cell lineages, Cell 157 (2) (2014) 340–356.

[34] K. Moro, et al., Innate production of TH2 cytokines by adipose tissue-associated c-Kit+ Sca-1+ lymphoid cells, Nature 463 (7280) (2010) 540–544.

[35] J.I. Odegaard, A. Chawla, The immune system as a sensor of the metabolic state, Immunity 38 (4) (2013) 644–654.

[36] D.R. Neill, et al., Nuocytes represent a new innate effector leukocyte that mediates type-2 immunity, Nature 464 (7293) (2010) 1367–1370.

[37] A.E. Price, et al., Systemically dispersed innate IL-13–expressing cells in type 2 immunity, Proc. Natl. Acad. Sci. U. S. A. 107 (25) (2010) 11489–11494.

[38] R.E. Mebius, P. Rennert, I.L. Weissman, Developing lymph nodes collect CD4+ CD3− LTβ+ cells that can differentiate to APC, NK cells, and follicular cells but not T or B cells, Immunity 7 (4) (1997) 493–504.

[39] N. Satoh-Takayama, et al., Microbial flora drives interleukin 22 production in intestinal NKp46+ cells that provide innate mucosal immune defense, Immunity 29 (6) (2008) 958–970.

[40] S. Sawa, et al., Lineage relationship analysis of RORγt+ innate lymphoid cells, Science 330 (6004) (2010) 665–669.

[41] G.F. Sonnenberg, L.A. Monticelli, M.M. Elloso, L.A. Fouser, D. Artis, CD4+ lymphoid tissue-inducer cells promote innate immunity in the gut, Immunity 34 (1) (2011) 122–134.

[42] L.C. Rankin, et al., The transcription factor T-bet is essential for the development of NKp46+ innate lymphocytes via the notch pathway, Nat. Immunol. 14 (4) (2013) 389–395.

[43] M.M. Fort, et al., IL-25 induces IL-4, IL-5, and IL-13 and Th2-associated pathologies in vivo, Immunity 15 (6) (2001) 985–995.

[44] J.A. Walker, J.L. Barlow, A.N. McKenzie, Innate lymphoid cells—how did we miss them? Nat. Rev. Immunol. 13 (2) (2013) 75.

[45] P. Licona-Limón, L.K. Kim, N.W. Palm, R.A. Flavell, TH2, allergy and group 2 innate lymphoid cells, Nat. Immunol. 14 (6) (2013) 536–542.

[46] Y.-J. Chang, et al., Innate lymphoid cells mediate influenza-induced airway hyper-reactivity independently of adaptive immunity, Nat. Immunol. 12 (7) (2011) 631–638.

[47] J. Zhu, T helper 2 (Th2) cell differentiation, type 2 innate lymphoid cell (ILC2) development and regulation of interleukin-4 (IL-4) and IL-13 production, Cytokine 75 (1) (2015) 14–24.

[48] Y. Huang, W.E. Paul, Inflammatory group 2 innate lymphoid cells, Int. Immunol. 28 (1) (2015) 23–28.

[49] K. Juelke, C. Romagnani, Differentiation of human innate lymphoid cells (ILCs), Curr. Opin. Immunol. 38 (2016) 75–85.

[50] B.S. Kim, et al., TSLP elicits IL-33–independent innate lymphoid cell responses to promote skin inflammation, Sci. Transl. Med. 5 (170) (2013) 170ra16.

[51] X. Yu, et al., TNF superfamily member TL1A elicits type 2 innate lymphoid cells at mucosal barriers, Mucosal Immunol. 7 (3) (2014) 730–740.

[52] J.L. Barlow, A.N. McKenzie, Type-2 innate lymphoid cells in human allergic disease, Curr. Opin. Allergy Clin. Immunol. 14 (5) (2014) 397.

[53] Y. Tanriver, A. Diefenbach, Transcription factors controlling development and function of innate lymphoid cells, Int. Immunol. 26 (3) (2014) 119–128.

[54] F. Melo-Gonzalez, M.R. Hepworth, Functional and phenotypic heterogeneity of group 3 innate lymphoid cells, Immunology 150 (3) (2017) 265–275.

[55] S. Cording, J. Medvedovic, M. Cherrier, G. Eberl, Development and regulation of RORγt+ innate lymphoid cells, FEBS Lett. 588 (22) (2014) 4176–4181.

[56] G. Eberl, S. Marmon, M.-J. Sunshine, P.D. Rennert, Y. Choi, D.R. Littman, An essential function for the nuclear receptor RORγt in the generation of fetal lymphoid tissue inducer cells, Nat. Immunol. 5 (1) (2004) 64.

[57] B. Zeng, S. Shi, G. Ashworth, C. Dong, J. Liu, F. Xing, ILC3 function as a double-edged sword in inflammatory bowel diseases, Cell Death Dis. 10 (4) (2019) 1–12.

[58] C. Seillet, et al., Nfil3 is required for the development of all innate lymphoid cell subsets, J. Exp. Med. 211 (9) (2014) 1733–1740.

[59] A. Moretta, et al., Activating receptors and coreceptors involved in human natural killer cell-mediated cytolysis, Annu. Rev. Immunol. 19 (1) (2001) 197–223.

[60] G.F. Sonnenberg, D. Artis, Innate lymphoid cells in the initiation, regulation and resolution of inflammation, Nat. Med. 21 (7) (2015) 698.

[61] L.A. Mielke, et al., Retinoic acid expression associates with enhanced IL-22 production by γδ T cells and innate lymphoid cells and attenuation of intestinal inflammation, J. Exp. Med. 210 (6) (2013) 1117–1124.

[62] B. Dyring-Andersen, et al., Increased number and frequency of group 3 innate lymphoid cells in nonlesional psoriatic skin, Br. J. Dermatol. 170 (3) (2014) 609–616.

[63] A. Soriani, H. Stabile, A. Gismondi, A. Santoni, G. Bernardini, Chemokine regulation of innate lymphoid cell tissue distribution and function, Cytokine Growth Factor Rev. 42 (2018) 47–55.

[64] C.S. Klose, D. Artis, Innate lymphoid cells control signaling circuits to regulate tissue-specific immunity, Cell Res. 30 (2020) 1–17.

[65] G.F. Sonnenberg, M.R. Hepworth, Functional interactions between innate lymphoid cells and adaptive immunity, Nat. Rev. Immunol. 19 (10) (2019) 599–613.

[66] A. Mortha, K. Burrows, Cytokine networks between innate lymphoid cells and myeloid cells, Front. Immunol. 9 (2018) 191.

[67] N. Oka, et al., IL-12 regulates the expansion, phenotype, and function of murine NK cells activated by IL-15 and IL-18, Cancer Immunol. Immunother. 69 (2020) 1699–1712.

[68] A. Camelo, et al., IL-33, IL-25, and TSLP induce a distinct phenotypic and activation profile in human type 2 innate lymphoid cells, Blood Adv. 1 (10) (2017) 577–589.

[69] J.W. McGinty, J. von Moltke, A three course menu for ILC and bystander T cell activation, Curr. Opin. Immunol. 62 (2020) 15–21.

[70] F. Almeida, G. Belz, Innate lymphoid cells: models of plasticity for immune homeostasis and rapid responsiveness in protection, Mucosal Immunol. 9 (5) (2016) 1103–1112.

[71] C.H. Kim, S. Hashimoto-Hill, M. Kim, Migration and tissue tropism of innate lymphoid cells, Trends Immunol. 37 (1) (2016) 68–79.

[72] F. Karagiannis, C. Wilhelm, Innate lymphoid cells—key immune integrators of overall body homeostasis, Semin. Immunopathol. 40 (4) (2018) 319–330. Springer.

[73] N. Branzk, K. Gronke, A. Diefenbach, Innate lymphoid cells, mediators of tissue homeostasis, adaptation and disease tolerance, Immunol. Rev. 286 (1) (2018) 86–101.

[74] J. von Moltke, R.M. Locksley, ILC-2 it: type 2 immunity and group 2 innate lymphoid cells in homeostasis, Curr. Opin. Immunol. 31 (2014) 58–65.

[75] A. Ignacio, C.N.S. Breda, N.O.S. Camara, Innate lymphoid cells in tissue homeostasis and diseases, World J. Hepatol. 9 (23) (2017) 979.

[76] Y. Goto, et al., Innate lymphoid cells regulate intestinal epithelial cell glycosylation, Science 345 (6202) (2014) 1248.

[77] A. Mortha, et al., Microbiota-dependent crosstalk between macrophages and ILC3 promotes intestinal homeostasis, Science 343 (6178) (2014) 1477.

[78] F. Flores-Borja, et al., Crosstalk between innate lymphoid cells and other immune cells in the tumor microenvironment, J. Immunol. Res. 2016 (2016) 1–14.

[79] S.L. Gaffen, R. Jain, A.V. Garg, D.J. Cua, IL-23-IL-17 immune axis: discovery, mechanistic understanding, and clinical testing, Nat. Rev. Immunol. 14 (9) (2014) 585.

[80] M.P. Schön, L. Erpenbeck, The interleukin-23/interleukin-17 axis links adaptive and innate immunity in psoriasis, Front. Immunol. 9 (2018) 1323.

[81] S.P. Raychaudhuri, A cutting edge overview: psoriatic disease, Clin Rev Allergy Immunol 44 (2) (2013) 109–113.

[82] M.A. Lowes, C.B. Russell, D.A. Martin, J.E. Towne, J.G. Krueger, The IL-23/T17 pathogenic axis in psoriasis is amplified by keratinocyte responses, Trends Immunol. 34 (4) (2013) 174–181.

[83] L.M. Mora-Velandia, et al., A human Lin− CD123+ CD127low population endowed with ILC features and migratory capabilities contributes to immunopathological hallmarks of psoriasis, Front. Immunol. 8 (2017) 176.

[84] S. Pantelyushin, et al., Rorγt+ innate lymphocytes and γδ T cells initiate psoriasiform plaque formation in mice, J. Clin. Invest. 122 (6) (2012) 2252–2256.

[85] M.B. Teunissen, et al., Composition of innate lymphoid cell subsets in the human skin: enrichment of NCR+ ILC3 in lesional skin and blood of psoriasis patients, J. Investig. Dermatol. 134 (9) (2014) 2351–2360.

[86] A. Keren, et al., Innate lymphoid cells 3 induce psoriasis in xenotransplanted healthy human skin, J. Allergy Clin. Immunol. 142 (1) (2018) 305–308. e6.

[87] L. Guilherme, J. Kalil, Rheumatic fever and rheumatic heart disease: cellular mechanisms leading autoimmune reactivity and disease, J. Clin. Immunol. 30 (1) (2010) 17–23.

[88] L. Guilherme, K. Köhler, J. Kalil, Rheumatic heart disease: mediation by complex immune events, Adv. Clin. Chem. 53 (2) (2011) 31–50.

[89] M. Shiba, et al., Presence of increased inflammatory infiltrates accompanied by activated dendritic cells in the left atrium in rheumatic heart disease, PloS one 13 (9) (2018), e0203756.

[90] Z. Kaya, P. Raczek, N.R. Rose, Myocarditis and dilated cardiomyopathy, in: The Autoimmune Diseases, Elsevier, 2020, pp. 1269–1284.

[91] B. Chen, N.G. Frangogiannis, Immune cells in repair of the infarcted myocardium, Microcirculation 24 (1) (2017) e12305.

[92] P.A. Barnie, X. Lin, Y. Liu, H. Xu, Z. Su, IL-17 producing innate lymphoid cells 3 (ILC3) but not Th17 cells might be the potential danger factor for preeclampsia and other pregnancy associated diseases, Int. J. Clin. Exp. Pathol. 8 (9) (2015) 11100.

[93] W. Bracamonte-Baran, et al., Non-cytotoxic cardiac innate lymphoid cells are a resident and quiescent type 2-commited population, Front. Immunol. 10 (2019) 634.

[94] H.S. Choi, et al., Innate Lymphoid Cells Play a Pathogenic Role in Pericarditis, Cell Rep. 30 (9) (2020) 2989–3003. e6.

[95] R. Okumura, K. Takeda, Maintenance of intestinal homeostasis by mucosal barriers, Inflamm. Regen. 38 (1) (2018) 1–8.

[96] M. Forkel, J. Mjösberg, Dysregulation of group 3 innate lymphoid cells in the pathogenesis of inflammatory bowel disease, Curr. Allergy Asthma Rep. 16 (10) (2016) 73.

[97] S.H. Lee, J.E. Kwon, M.-L. Cho, Immunological pathogenesis of inflammatory bowel disease, Intest. Res. 16 (1) (2018) 26.

[98] A. Geremia, et al., IL-23–responsive innate lymphoid cells are increased in inflammatory bowel disease, J. Exp. Med. 208 (6) (2011) 1127–1133.

[99] A. Fuchs, et al., Intraepithelial type 1 innate lymphoid cells are a unique subset of IL-12-and IL-15-responsive IFN-γ-producing cells, Immunity 38 (4) (2013) 769–781.

[100] J.R. Bailey, et al., IL-13 promotes collagen accumulation in Crohn's disease fibrosis by down-regulation of fibroblast MMP synthesis: a role for innate lymphoid cells? PloS one 7 (12) (2012) e52332.

[101] J. Li, A.L. Doty, A. Iqbal, S.C. Glover, The differential frequency of Lineage− CRTH2− CD45+ NKp44− CD117− CD127+ ILC subset in the inflamed terminal ileum of patients with Crohn's disease, Cell. Immunol. 304 (2016) 63–68.

[102] H. Chu, et al., AB0049B Changes of Innate Lymphoid Cells in Peripheral Blood of Patients With Primary SJöGREN'S Syndrome and its Correlations with Clinical Markers, BMJ Publishing Group Ltd, 2019.

[103] M. Düster, M. Becker, A.C. Gnirck, M. Wunderlich, U. Panzer, J.E. Turner, T cell-derived IFN-γ downregulates protective group 2 innate lymphoid cells in murine lupus erythematosus, Eur. J. Immunol. 48 (8) (2018) 1364–1375.

[104] S.L. Blokland, et al., Increased expression of Fas on group 2 and 3 innate lymphoid cells is associated with an interferon signature in systemic lupus erythematosus and Sjögren's syndrome, Rheumatology 58 (10) (2019) 1740–1745.

[105] L.K. Peterson, R.S. Fujinami, Inflammation, demyelination, neurodegeneration and neuroprotection in the pathogenesis of multiple sclerosis, J. Neuroimmunol. 184 (1–2) (2007) 37–44.

[106] R.J. Bevan, et al., Meningeal inflammation and cortical demyelination in acute multiple sclerosis, Ann. Neurol. 84 (6) (2018) 829–842.

[107] L. Van Kaer, J.L. Postoak, C. Wang, G. Yang, L. Wu, Innate, innate-like and adaptive lymphocytes in the pathogenesis of MS and EAE, Cell. Mol. Immunol. 16 (6) (2019) 531–539.

[108] S. Romero-Suárez, et al., The central nervous system contains ILC1s that differ from NK cells in the response to inflammation, Front. Immunol. 10 (2019) 2337.

[109] J.K. Hatfield, M.A. Brown, Group 3 innate lymphoid cells accumulate and exhibit disease-induced activation in the meninges in EAE, Cell. Immunol. 297 (2) (2015) 69–79.

[110] C.C. Gross, et al., Alemtuzumab treatment alters circulating innate immune cells in multiple sclerosis, Neurol. Neuroimmunol. Neuroinflamm. 3 (6) (2016) 1–9.

[111] M. Degn, et al., Increased prevalence of lymphoid tissue inducer cells in the cerebrospinal fluid of patients with early multiple sclerosis, Mult. Scler. J. 22 (8) (2016) 1013–1020.

[112] T.A. Johnson, et al., Reduction of the peripheral blood CD56bright NK lymphocyte subset in FTY720-treated multiple sclerosis patients, J. Immunol. 187 (1) (2011) 570–579.

[113] A.A. Vandenbark, et al., Interferon-beta-1a treatment increases CD56bright natural killer cells and CD4+ CD25+ Foxp3 expression in subjects with multiple sclerosis, J. Neuroimmunol. 215 (1–2) (2009) 125–128.

[114] J. Martinez-Rodriguez, A. Saez-Borderias, E. Munteis, N. Romo, J. Roquer, M. Lopez-Botet, Natural killer receptors distribution in multiple sclerosis: relation to clinical course and interferon-beta therapy, Clin. Immunol. 137 (1) (2010) 41–50.

[115] J. Ozougwu, K. Obimba, C. Belonwu, C. Unakalamba, The pathogenesis and pathophysiology of type 1 and type 2 diabetes mellitus, J. Physiol. Pathophysiol. 4 (4) (2013) 46–57.

[116] M. Clark, C.J. Kroger, R.M. Tisch, Type 1 diabetes: a chronic anti-self-inflammatory response, Front. Immunol. 8 (2017) 1898.

[117] H. Yu, et al., Intestinal type 1 regulatory T cells migrate to periphery to suppress diabetogenic T cells and prevent diabetes development, Proc. Natl. Acad. Sci. U. S. A. 114 (39) (2017) 10443–10448.

[118] B.O. Roep, M. Peakman, Diabetogenic T lymphocytes in human type 1 diabetes, Curr. Opin. Immunol. 23 (6) (2011) 746–753.

[119] A. Lehuen, J. Diana, P. Zaccone, A. Cooke, Immune cell crosstalk in type 1 diabetes, Nat. Rev. Immunol. 10 (7) (2010) 501–513.

[120] J. Diana, L. Gahzarian, Y. Simoni, A. Lehuen, Innate immunity in type 1 diabetes, Discov. Med. 11 (61) (2011) 513–520.

[121] W. Quan, E.K. Jo, M.S. Lee, Role of pancreatic β-cell death and inflammation in diabetes, Diabetes. Obes. Metab. 15 (s3) (2013) 141–151.

[122] M. Hussain, L. Alviggi, B. Millward, R. Leslie, D. Pyke, D. Vergani, Evidence that the reduced number of natural killer cells in type 1 (insulin-dependent) diabetes may be genetically determined, Diabetologia 30 (12) (1987) 907–911.

[123] C. Fraker, A.L. Bayer, The expanding role of natural killer cells in type 1 diabetes and immunotherapy, Curr. Diab. Rep. 16 (11) (2016) 109.

[124] S. Chatterjee, K. Khunti, M.J. Davies, Type 2 diabetes, Lancet 389 (10085) (2017) 2239–2251.

[125] M.Y. Donath, J. Størling, K. Maedler, T. Mandrup-Poulsen, Inflammatory mediators and islet β-cell failure: a link between type 1 and type 2 diabetes, J. Mol. Med. 81 (8) (2003) 455–470.

[126] L. Galle-Treger, et al., Costimulation of type-2 innate lymphoid cells by GITR promotes effector function and ameliorates type 2 diabetes, Nat. Commun. 10 (1) (2019) 1–14.

[127] F. Liu, et al., Type 1 innate lymphoid cells are associated with type 2 diabetes, Diabetes Metab. 45 (4) (2019) 341–346.

[128] E. Dalmas, et al., Interleukin-33-activated islet-resident innate lymphoid cells promote insulin secretion through myeloid cell retinoic acid production, Immunity 47 (5) (2017) 928–942. e7.

[129] I.B. McInnes, G. Schett, Pathogenetic insights from the treatment of rheumatoid arthritis, Lancet 389 (10086) (2017) 2328–2337.

[130] G.S. Firestein, I.B. McInnes, Immunopathogenesis of rheumatoid arthritis, Immunity 46 (2) (2017) 183–196.

[131] J. Zhu, et al., Interleukin-22 secreted by NKp44+ natural killer cells promotes proliferation of fibroblast-like synoviocytes in rheumatoid arthritis, Medicine 94 (52) (2015) 1–10.

[132] E.F. Leijten, et al., Brief report: enrichment of activated group 3 innate lymphoid cells in psoriatic arthritis synovial fluid, Arthritis Rheumatol. 67 (10) (2015) 2673–2678.

[133] N. Dalbeth, M.F. Callan, A subset of natural killer cells is greatly expanded within inflamed joints, Arthritis Rheum. 46 (7) (2002) 1763–1772.

[134] J. Rodríguez-Carrio, et al., Altered innate lymphoid cells subsets in human lymph node biopsies during the at risk and earliest phase of rheumatoid arthritis, Arthritis Rheumatol. 69 (2016) 70–76.

[135] M. Al-Mossawi, J. De Wit, B. Kendrick, R. Gundle, P. Bowness, A1. 1 Identification and Phenotyping of Innate Lymphoid Cells Present in the Diseased Joints of Patients with Spondyloarthritis, Rheumatoid Arthritis and Psoriatic Arthritis, BMJ Publishing Group Ltd, 2015.

[136] K. Hirota, et al., Autoimmune Th17 cells induced synovial stromal and innate lymphoid cell secretion of the cytokine GM-CSF to initiate and augment autoimmune arthritis, Immunity 48 (6) (2018) 1220–1232. e5.

[137] W. Fang, Y. Zhang, Z. Chen, Innate lymphoid cells in inflammatory arthritis, Arthritis Res. Ther. 22 (1) (2020) 25.

[138] S.Q. Crome, P.S. Ohashi, Immunoregulatory functions of innate lymphoid cells, J. Immunother. Cancer 6 (1) (2018) 1–4.

[139] S. Li, D. Yang, T. Peng, Y. Wu, Z. Tian, B. Ni, Innate lymphoid cell-derived cytokines in autoimmune diseases, J. Autoimmun. 83 (2017) 62–72.

[140] N. von Burg, G. Turchinovich, D. Finke, Maintenance of immune homeostasis through ILC/T cell interactions, Front. Immunol. 6 (2015) 416.

[141] S. O'Reilly, Role of interleukin-13 in fibrosis, particularly systemic sclerosis, Biofactors 39 (6) (2013) 593–596.

[142] G. Latella, J. Di Gregorio, V. Flati, F. Rieder, I.C. Lawrance, Mechanisms of initiation and progression of intestinal fibrosis in IBD, Scand. J. Gastroenterol. 50 (1) (2015) 53–65.

[143] R.G. Domingues, M.R. Hepworth, Immunoregulatory sensory circuits in group 3 innate lymphoid cell (ILC3) function and tissue homeostasis, Front. Immunol. 11 (2020) 116.

[144] F.R. Mariotti, L. Quatrini, E. Munari, P. Vacca, L. Moretta, Innate lymphoid cells: expression of PD-1 and other checkpoints in normal and pathological conditions, Front. Immunol. 10 (2019) 910.

[145] A. Geremia, P. Biancheri, P. Allan, G.R. Corazza, A. Di Sabatino, Innate and adaptive immunity in inflammatory bowel disease, Autoimmun. Rev. 13 (1) (2014) 3–10.

[146] J. Ermann, T. Staton, J.N. Glickman, R. de Waal Malefyt, L.H. Glimcher, Nod/Ripk2 signaling in dendritic cells activates IL-17A–secreting innate lymphoid cells and drives colitis in T-bet−/−. Rag2−/−(TRUC) mice, Proc. Natl. Acad. Sci. U. S. A. 111 (25) (2014) E2559–E2566.

[147] G. Monteleone, D. Fina, R. Caruso, F. Pallone, New mediators of immunity and inflammation in inflammatory bowel disease, Curr. Opin. Gastroenterol. 22 (4) (2006) 361–364.

[148] H. Ito, et al., A pilot randomized trial of a human anti-interleukin-6 receptor monoclonal antibody in active Crohn's disease, Gastroenterology 126 (4) (2004) 989–996.

[149] M. Coccia, et al., IL-1β mediates chronic intestinal inflammation by promoting the accumulation of IL-17A secreting innate lymphoid cells and CD4+ Th17 cells, J. Exp. Med. 209 (9) (2012) 1595–1609.

[150] J.S. Perry, et al., Inhibition of LTi cell development by CD25 blockade is associated with decreased intrathecal inflammation in multiple sclerosis, Sci. Transl. Med. 4 (145) (2012) 145ra106.

[151] H. Stabile, et al., JAK/STAT signaling in regulation of innate lymphoid cells: the gods before the guardians, Immunol. Rev. 286 (1) (2018) 148–159.

[152] J.J. O'Shea, D.M. Schwartz, A.V. Villarino, M. Gadina, I.B. McInnes, A. Laurence, The JAK-STAT pathway: impact on human disease and therapeutic intervention, Annu. Rev. Med. 66 (2015) 311–328.

[153] C. Pearson, et al., ILC3 GM-CSF production and mobilisation orchestrate acute intestinal inflammation, Elife 5 (2016), e10066.

[154] W. Ouyang, J.K. Kolls, Y. Zheng, The biological functions of T helper 17 cell effector cytokines in inflammation, Immunity 28 (4) (2008) 454–467.

[155] S. Kunwar, K. Dahal, S. Sharma, Anti-IL-17 therapy in treatment of rheumatoid arthritis: a systematic literature review and meta-analysis of randomized controlled trials, Rheumatol. Int. 36 (8) (2016) 1065–1075.

[156] J. Yang, Q. Li, X. Yang, M. Li, Interleukin-9 is associated with elevated anti-double-stranded DNA antibodies in lupus-prone mice, Mol. Med. 21 (1) (2015) 364–370.

[157] F. Ciccia, et al., Potential involvement of IL-9 and Th9 cells in the pathogenesis of rheumatoid arthritis, Rheumatology 54 (12) (2015) 2264–2272.

CHAPTER

3

B regulatory cells in patients with autoimmune diseases: Pathogenic significance and therapeutic potential

Athanasios Mavropoulos[a], Efterpi Zafiriou[b], Efthymios Dardiotis[c], Lazaros I. Sakkas[a,†], and Dimitrios P. Bogdanos[a,,†]*

[a]Department of Rheumatology and Clinical Immunology, Faculty of Medicine, School of Health Sciences, University of Thessaly, Larissa, Greece [b]Department of Dermatology, Faculty of Medicine, School of Health Sciences, University of Thessaly, Larissa, Greece [c]Department of Neurology, Faculty of Medicine, School of Health Sciences, University of Thessaly, Larissa, Greece
*Corresponding author

Abstract

Regulatory B cells (Breg cells) emerge as critical immunoregulators in autoimmune disease as they inhibit T helper 1 (Th1) and T helper 17 (Th17) cells. Although there are several phenotypic B cell subsets with immuno-suppressing functions, the best-characterized subset is the Interleukin (IL)-10-producing B cell subset. IL-10-producing Breg cells are reduced in several autoimmune diseases and restored during the disease remission. Furthermore, they exhibited an inverse correlation with Th1 and Th17 cells in psoriasis and psoriatic arthritis, insinuating possible therapeutic importance in human autoimmune diseases in vivo. Focusing on promising data such as that demonstrating that fusion of granulocyte monocyte-colony stimulating factor (GM-CSF) with IL-15 (GIFT15 fusokine) induces Breg cells and suppresses experimental autoimmune encephalomyelitis may underline a new strategy of Breg cell expansion for B cell-based therapies for organ- and nonorgan specific human autoimmune diseases.

Keywords

Breg cell, Regulatory B cell, Autoimmune disease, Multiple sclerosis, Psoriatic arthritis, Psoriasis, Rheumatoid arthritis, Systemic sclerosis

[†] Shared last authorship.

1 Introduction

B regulatory cell (Breg cells) is a term given to designate a class of B cells with suppressive properties capable of regulating inflammation in certain pathological conditions. The ability of splenic B cells to suppress delayed-type hypersensitivity (DTH) responses has been first described in guinea pigs [1, 2]. However, it was until much later in the mid-1990s when Janeway and his group reported the existence of immunosuppressive B cells in the experimental autoimmune encephalitis (EAE) mouse model of multiple sclerosis (MS) [3]. Bregs were subsequently described as key immune regulators in murine models of collagen-induced arthritis and colitis [4–6]. In humans, B cell subsets with established regulatory capacity that contribute to the maintenance of immune tolerance and the suppression of inflammatory responses have been described in different clinical settings, including autoimmunity, malignancies, and infections [7].

2 Identification of Breg cells

Up to date, any B cell subset that exerts immune regulatory functions can be termed as regulatory, since neither a specific phenotypic marker has been documented, nor a consensus on its classification has been reached. Despite the fact that certain signaling molecules such as Galphaq (Gαq) have been identified to be involved in B cell suppressive functions [8], none of them yet proved the existence of a lineage commitment Breg-specific transcription factor, equivalent to Foxp3 in T regulatory cells (Tregs). Likewise, while some studies have reported B cell-specific Foxp3 expression, whether Foxp3 can be used as a potential marker for Breg cells remained inconclusive [9–11].

Furthermore, whether Breg cells acquire their suppressive function upon inflammatory environmental conditions remains to be fully clarified. Interleukin (IL)-1β, IL-6, and GM-CSF when combined with IL-15 are capable of inducing the differentiation of murine Breg cells [12, 13]. In addition, bacterial lipopolysaccharide (LPS) and CpG rich DNA components can activate and expand Breg cells through Toll-like receptor (TLR) signaling pathways, a method routinely used to propagate both murine and human Breg cells in vitro [14, 15].

The currently supported notion is that Breg cell subsets might arise from a common progenitor and that all B cells even the more mature memory B and plasma cells, can differentiate into Bregs following appropriate stimulation with TLR ligands, CD40 ligand, and B cell receptor (BCR) cross-linking [16, 17]. Moreover, the cytokines IL-21 [18] and IL-35 [19] are also crucial for Breg cell development and maintenance.

In human peripheral blood mononuclear cells (PBMCs), several Breg cell phenotypes have been identified spanning from immature B cell subsets up to fully differentiated plasmablasts. These include transitional B cells ($CD19^+CD24^{hi}CD38^{hi}$), memory B cells ($CD19^+CD24^{hi}CD27^+$), $CD19^+CD5^+CD1d^{hi}$ B cells, T cell immunoglobulin and mucin domain 1 $CD19^+$ B cells (TIM-1^+ B cells), programmed death-ligand 1 $CD19^+$ B cells (PD-L1^+ B cells), plasmablasts ($CD19^+CD27^{int}CD38^+$), $CD19^+CD39^{hi}$ cells, and B regulatory 1 (Br1) cells ($CD19^+CD25^+CD71^+CD73^-$) [20–27].

3 Functional properties

Breg cells exert suppressive functions on different cell types, including T cells, dendritic cells (DCs), and monocytes [28] (Fig. 1). Several studies have provided strong evidence that B cells can influence Tregs dynamics and function, through the induction of Foxp3 expression

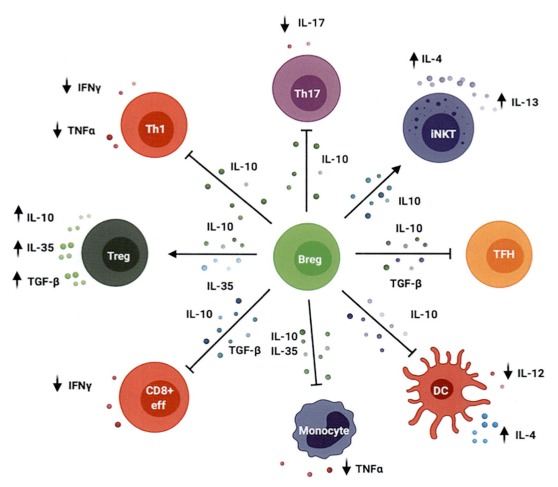

FIG. 1 Effect of B regulatory cells on various cell subsets. B regulatory cells (Breg) exert either an inductor or an inhibitory effect on various immune cells via the induction of cytokines. *Treg*, T regulatory cells; *Th1*, T helper; *Th17*, T helper 17; *TFH*, T follicular helper; *DC*, dendritic cell; *eff*, effector.

by several mechanisms including B cell production of IL-10 and TGF-β [29–32]. Foxp3[+] Tregs are also required for IL-33 mediated expansion of Bregs [33, 34]. Breg cells are generally highly immunosuppressive and can diminish both effector Th1 and Th17 CD4[+] cell responses [35, 36]. IL-10 producing Breg cells are the most widely studied Breg cells in collagen-induced arthritis (CIA) and experimental autoimmune encephalitis (EAE) models [37]. Mice lacking endogenous IL-10-producing Breg cells exhibit an increased frequency of Th1/Th17, decreased numbers of Tregs [29], and exacerbation of CIA [5]. On the other hand, the adoptive transfer of Breg cells suppresses inflammatory responses and CD4[+] T cell activation. For instance, adoptive transfer of CD11b[+] B subset to experimental autoimmune hepatitis (EAH) model mice suppressed CD4[+] T cell proliferation and IFNγ/TNF-α production and ameliorated disease manifestations [38].

The role of B cells in autoimmune diseases has been further studied by their depletion using anti-CD20 monoclonal antibody (mAb), which targets B cells from the pre-B cell to memory stages. For example, in the EAE model, B cell depletion using an anti-CD20 mAb during the early phase of the disease exacerbated the disease [39]. In contrast, depletion of B cells during the late phase of the EAE reduced the severity and alleviated disease symptoms. It is thought that IL-10-producing Breg cells are the early responders at the onset of the inflammatory response and that anti-CD20-mediated depletion is effective in established EAE disease because it depletes the antigen-presenting B cell subsets.

Breg cells can also regulate the cellular immune response via other suppressor cytokines such as IL-35 [40]. In addition, certain contact-dependent and receptor-mediated mechanisms of inhibition have also been reported via programmed death-ligand 1 (PD-L1), Fas ligand (FasL), and glucocorticoid-induced TNFR-related ligand (GITRL) expression [19, 41, 42].

3.1 IL-10 producing Breg cells

Thus far, IL-10 production remains the best hallmark of Breg cells, namely, IL-10[+] B cells (B10 cells) [17]. B10 cells represent a distinct subset of B cells that reflects a unique functional program (IL-10-competency in vivo and IL-10 production following a 5-h stimulation with phorbol 12-myristate 13-acetate (PMA) and ionomycin ex vivo) [43]. B10 cells are detected within subsets bearing phenotypic markers for transitional B cells [20, 22, 44], memory B cells [21, 22], germinal center B cells [45], and plasmablasts [46].

The majority of IL-10[+] B cells in blood are found within the subsets of CD19[+]CD24[hi]CD27[+] (memory) or CD19[+]CD24[hi]CD38hi (transitional) subpopulations [21, 22]. A study that examined B10 cells across the entire age range of normal human development, showed that up to 30% of B cells are competent to produce IL-10 during childhood [47]. Most adult B10 cells were CD27[+] and ~50% were CD24[hi]CD27[+], whereas only 12% of B10 cells in children were CD24[hi]CD27[+]. On the other hand, 32% of B10 cells in children were CD24[hi]CD38[hi], compared to only 8% of adult B10 cells that were CD24[hi]CD38[hi] [47]. Interestingly, the CD19[+]CD24[hi]CD27[+] B cell subset includes not only IL-10-competent B10 cells but also B10 pro cells which are capable of IL-10 production in the absence of specific in vitro stimulation [21, 48].

Ding et al. successively demonstrated in mice that Tim-1 is predominantly expressed on B rather than T cells and that 70% of IL-10-producing B cells are Tim-1 positive [49]. Tim-1 is essential for the induction and maintenance of IL-10 in Breg cells and their regulation of tissue inflammation [50]. Moreover, Tim-1 is the primary receptor responsible for Breg cell induction by apoptotic cells (ACs) [51]. In human B cells, up to 60% of IL-10 producing transitional and 30% of memory B cells can also co-express the Tim-1 [52]. Sorted Tim-1$^+$ B cells from healthy individuals strongly suppressed the expression of proinflammatory cytokines such as IFN-γ, TNF-α, and IL-17 by CD4$^+$ T cells, compared to Tim-1$^-$ B cells [52]. Furthermore, IgG4 has been implicated in B cell regulatory function, and IgG4-expressing B cells are detected within the IL-10$^+$ B cell subset in humans [26].

3.2 IL-35-producing Breg cells

IL-10-independent Breg cell properties have also been reported [53]. IL-35 is a critical antiinflammatory cytokine that plays an important role in various autoimmune diseases, however, the suppressive activities of IL-35 remain poorly understood [54, 55]. IL-35 is a heterodimer composed of IL-12p35 and Ebi3 subunits. The IL-12p35 subunit is shared with IL-12 (IL-12p35/IL-12p40) cytokine that promotes inflammatory responses. Recently, Dambuza et al. showed that the IL-12p35 subunit has immunoregulatory functions inducing the expansion of IL-10- and IL-35-producing B cells and ameliorating autoimmune uveitis in mice by antagonizing pathogenic Th17 responses [56].

Most of the information concerning IL-35 producing Breg cells has been obtained in murine autoimmune disease models thus far. Mice with deficiencies in both TLR2 and TLR4 restricted to B cells developed a chronic EAE after immunization with the encephalitogenic peptide from myelin oligodendrocyte glycoprotein [16]. Shen et al. have reported that mice bearing a targeted B cell deletion of TLR4 developed severe EAE, which emphasize the critical role for B-cell-mediated suppression [40]. Interestingly, naïve B cells were capable of IL-10 production upon activation by lipopolysaccharide (LPS) but costimulation with LPS and anti-CD40 switched off IL-10 production and produced IL-35. About the same time, Wang et al. reported the existence of a unique IL-35-producing Breg (IL-35$^+$ Breg) subpopulation that conferred protection from experimental autoimmune uveitis (EAU) [19]. Treatment of mice with IL-35 conferred protection from uveitis, whereas mice lacking IL-35 or defective in IL-35-signaling produced fewer Breg cells and developed severe uveitis. IL-35-producing B cells (i35-Breg) have been subsequently proposed as a new mediator of regulatory B cell functions especially in the central nervous system (CNS)-related autoimmune diseases [57].

3.3 TGF-β producing Breg cells

TGF-β is one of the fundamental regulatory cytokines that direct the generation of Tregs and tolerogenic DCs [58, 59]. Studies in murine models have shown that B cells can express high levels of TGF-β1 and dampen the Th1 mediated immunity. More specifically, LPS-activated B cells can express high levels of TGF-β and upon transfer into nonobese diabetic (NOD) mice prevent spontaneous Th1 immunity and disease progression by downregulating T cell responses and controlling the function of antigen-presenting cells (APCs) [14]. B cell-derived TGF-β can also induce anergy in CD8$^+$ T cells and can constrain Th1 and Th17 responses in EAE by downregulating the function of DCs [60, 61]. TGF-β-producing B cells are CD5$^+$ and co-localize with CD4$^+$Foxp3$^+$ T cells in lymph nodes of tolerant mice in a murine model of allergic airway disease [62]. Through induction of Tregs and upregulation of Foxp3 expression in CD4$^+$CD25$^-$ T cells, TGF-β-producing Breg subsets can also promote transplantation tolerance [63]. Recently, TGFβin conjunction with IL-10 has been shown to suppress metabolism in murine and human B cells and ameliorate systemic lupus erythematosus (SLE) [64].

3.4 Granzyme B expressing Breg cells

Granzyme B (GrB) is a protease localized in the cytotoxic granules of T cells and NK cells that mediates commitment to T cell apoptosis and suppression of proliferation [65]. GrB secretion was also noted in B cells having a significant role in the initiation of early antiviral immune responses, regulation of autoimmune responses, and cancer immunosurveillance [66]. B cells have been detected adjacent to IL-21-secreting Tregs that contribute to the maintenance of immune tolerance of tumor antigens. These B cells expressed high levels of GrB and inhibited Tcell proliferation by a GrB-dependent degradation of the Tcell receptor (TCR) ζ-chain [67]. Other studies have also reported GrB expression by subsets of B cells capable of decreasing T cell proliferation [68, 69]. GrB-producing Bregs were found to be significantly decreased and functionally impaired in patients with rheumatoid arthritis (RA) [70]. These cells exhibited low levels of IL-21 receptor expression, and impaired suppressive action on Th1 and Th17 cells while they were negatively correlated with RA disease activity.

3.5 Receptor-mediated inhibitory mechanisms

In an elegant study, Ray et al. showed that B cell depletion with anti-CD20mAb resulted in the rapid onset of EAE and colitis, accompanied by a significant reduction of Tregs [42]. They found that B cell expression of GITRL, but not IL-10, induced Treg proliferation, suggesting that B cells, via expression of GITRL, play an essential role in Treg homeostasis by maintaining their numbers above a threshold required for the prevention of autoimmunity.

Programmed death-ligand 1 (PD-L1), is another critical suppressive molecule, constitutively expressed on B lymphocytes, DCs, and monocytes [71]. Guan et al. found higher PD-L1 expression on Breg cells in breast cancer patients and showed a significant correlation between CD19$^+$CD24$^+$CD38$^+$PD-L1$^+$ Breg cells and CD19$^+$CD24$^+$CD38$^+$ Breg cells [41]. Notably, the Breg cell expression of PD-L1 was positively correlated with Tregs. Khan et al. also elegantly showed that PD-L1hi B cells play a critical role in regulating humoral immunity mediated by CD4$^+$CXCR5$^+$PD-1$^+$ follicular helper T cells, and can suppress inflammation [72].

The expression of PD-L1 is often induced following cell surface receptor ligation and/or stimulation with the Th1-associated cytokine, IFN-γ [73]. Its receptor, the programmed death-1 (PD-1), is upregulated in activated T cells and B cells [74]. PD-1 is an inhibitory costimulatory molecule whose expression on T cells and interaction with the ligand on APCs induces T cell anergy and exhaustion [75]. PD-1 also affects T cell function directly by downregulating cytokine production (IFN-γ, TNFα, and IL-2) and cell proliferation [76]. The PD-1/PD-L1 signaling pathway plays a crucial role in dampening T cell immune responses and has been attributed as a critical regulator for maintaining peripheral tolerance through the conversion of human Th1 cells into Treg cells [73].

Besides PD-L1, other death-inducing ligands such as TRAIL and Fas ligand are also found to be expressed by B cells and regulatory subsets such as $CD19^+CD5^+CD1d^{hi}$ cells [77, 78]. FasL expression in $CD5^+CD1d^{hi}$ B cells rapidly increased after TLR4 ligation but not after anti-CD40 or CpG and anti-CD40 stimulation [77]. The FasL/Fas pathway has been extensively studied as a mechanism of killing overactive $CD4^+$ T cells and other immune cell subsets.

4 B regulatory cells and autoimmunity: Pathogenic significance

4.1 Rheumatoid arthritis and systemic sclerosis as models of autoimmune rheumatic diseases

In RA, Breg subsets are decreased and functionally impaired, particularly in RA-associated lung fibrosis [79, 80]. More specifically, the frequencies of both transitional ($CD19^+CD24^{hi}CD38^{hi}$) and memory ($CD19^+CD24^{hi}CD27^+$) Bregs cells were found to be decreased in patients with RA [36, 48, 81, 82]. Their IL-10-producing function was also diminished and their proportions inversely correlated with disease activity [81]. The impairment in $CD19^+CD24^{hi}CD27^+$ B10 cells was partially attributed to the decreased expression of CD27 induced by the upregulated CD70 expression on $CD19^+$ B cells and $CD4^+$ T cells [48]. $CD19^+CD27^+IL-10^+$ cells in RA patients were functionally defective in suppressing IFN-γ production by $CD4^+$ T cells [82]. IL-21 greatly increased $IL-10^+$ Breg cells within the $CD19^+CD27^+$ and $CD19^+CD27^-$ cellular compartments.

Circulating $CD19^+TIM1^+IL10^+$ B cells, $CD19^+CD5^+CD1d^+IL10^+$ B cells, and $CD4^+CD25^+Foxp3^+$ T cells were also reported to be reduced in patients with RA [83]. Deficits in peripheral $CD19^+Foxp3^+$ and $CD19^+TGFβ^+$ Breg cell populations have also been described in RA patients with interstitial lung disease (ILD) [10]. Patients with ILD had a considerably lower percentage of $CD19^+TGFβ^+$ Breg cells compared to RA patients without ILD and there was also a negative association between $CD19^+Foxp3^+$ Bregs and disease severity scores [10]. $CD19^+CD5^+CD1d^{hi}$ B cells were also decreased in RA patients and negatively correlated with disease activity score (DAS28), whereas $CD19^+CD5^+GrB^+$ B cells were significantly higher in RA [84]. However, another study reported that GrB-producing Breg cells were significantly decreased in RA concomitant with lower levels of IL-21 receptor and negatively correlated with disease activity and recovered during disease remission [70]. $PD-L1^+$ Bregs are also significantly decreased in RA patients and increased after efficacious treatment [25].

Similar to RA, significant memory and transitional Breg cell depletion accompanied by diminished IL-10-producing ability was first reported by Mavropoulos et al. in patients with systemic sclerosis (SSc) and especially in those with associated ILD diagnosis [80]. B10 cells were also markedly diminished and inversely correlated with T cell IL-17 and IFN-γ production [85]. Furthermore, B cells from SSc patients exhibited impaired p38 MAPK and STAT-3 activation upon stimulation with BCR and TLR9, which are two fundamental signals for optimal IL-10 production by B cells [80, 86]. Others also found significantly lower B cell IL-10 production in SSc but no difference in IL-6 production [87]. The decreased Breg cells were negatively associated with autoantibody production [88]. In addition, transitional $TIM-1^+IL-10^+$ B cells were significantly decreased in SSc and were functionally defective as $TIM-1^+$ B cells failed to suppress $CD4^+$ T cell activation [52].

4.2 Psoriasis as a paradigm of inflammatory skin disease

Psoriasis is an inflammatory cutaneous disorder characterized by epidermal thickening and extensive Th1 and Th17 cell infiltration. About 30% of psoriasis patients develop an inflammatory arthritic disorder, psoriatic arthritis (PsA) [89]. In both psoriasis and PsA, IL-10$^+$ Breg cells were found to be decreased and inversely correlated with Th1 and Th17 cells and the severity of psoriasis. Thus, an antiinflammatory potential of Breg cells was insinuated in a clinical setting, extending previous observations from experimental animal models of psoriasis [90]. Similar findings were also obtained for CD19$^+$CD24^{hi}CD38^{hi} B cells in a cohort of psoriasis vulgaris patients who had not received any immunosuppressant in a period of 6 months [91].

4.3 Multiple sclerosis as a model of autoimmune neurological disorder

Several B cell subpopulations have displayed regulatory capacities and antiinflammatory cytokine expression in response to stimuli in vitro, as well as in thein the experimental autoimmune encephalomyelitis (EAE), animal model of multiple sclerosis (MS). However, the functional role of Breg cells in MS has not been fully elucidated in vivo [92, 93]. Hence, although the general notion in patients with MS is that Breg subsets are numerically decreased [94, 95], some studies have reported that Breg cells remain unaltered or even increase during the course of the disease [96, 97]. Regardless of their proportions, Breg cell function was consistently found to be impaired in MS patients, with defects in both IL-10 production and suppressive capacity of B cells [98–100]. Furthermore, the proportion of naïve Breg cells during MS relapse is reduced, leading to an increased memory/naïve cell ratio [94]. Whether this reduction is the cause or the consequence of relapsing MS remains to be clarified. However, a recent study found that the reduced peripheral blood Breg cell levels were not associated with the Expanded Disability Status Scale (EDSS) score in MS [101].

5 Therapeutic potential

5.1 In vivo maintenance/expansion of B regulatory cells following standard therapy

5.1.1 Restoration of Breg cells in RA: The experience with the anti-CD20 mAb (rituximab)

B cells play an important role in the development of RA through the secretion of autoantibodies, such as rheumatoid factor (RF) and anticyclic citrullinated peptide antibodies (anti-CCP) [102, 103]. The importance of Breg cells in RA is highlighted in patients receiving treatment with the B cell-depleting monoclonal antibody (mAb), rituximab (RTX), which targets the B lymphocyte cell surface marker, CD20 [104]. B cell depletion using RTX has been effective for the treatment of RA; however, its clinical efficacy varies through different reports. Although the B cell depletion rate is almost 100%, clinical response is observed in only 60%–70% of patients [105, 106]. Following the withdrawal of RTX treatment, B cell levels recover within 6–20 months.

Interestingly, the efficacy of RTX was subsequently shown to derive in part from the expansion of rare Breg cell populations, and disease suppression was directly related to the secretion of the antiinflammatory cytokine, IL-10, by Breg cells [107–110]. B cell repopulation following RTX administration occurred after a mean of 8 months and was dependent on the formation of naïve B cells, which showed an increased expression of CD38 and CD5 [111]. During repopulation, increased numbers of circulating immature $CD19^+ IgD^+ CD38^{hi} CD10lowCD24^{hi}$ B cells were identified [111]. RTX spared Breg cell subsets and these represent the first population to develop from the bone marrow following B cell depletion, thus becoming a dominant B cell population [42]. IL-10-producing B cells and their association with responsiveness to RTX have been also described in other autoimmune disorders such as primary Sjögren's syndrome and myasthenia gravis [112, 113].

5.1.2 *Restoration of Breg cells in psoriasis and psoriatic arthritis: The experience with apremilast*

Evidence that rituximab also depletes regulatory B cells comes from reports that it can lead to severe exacerbation of colitis as well as the onset of colitis and psoriasis soon after the start of the treatment [114–117].

The phosphodiesterase 4 inhibitor, apremilast, increases cyclic adenosine monophosphate levels and suppresses tumor necrosis alpha (TNF-α) production [118]. Apremilast has been approved for the treatment of moderate to severe psoriasis and PsA. Apremilast can expand IL-10-producing Breg cells in vivo in both psoriasis and PsA patients [119]. Furthermore, the apremilast-induced increase of Breg cells was strongly associated with a reduction of Th1 cells, IFNγ-producing NKT cells, and IL-17-producing NKT cells.

5.1.3 *Restoration of Breg cells in multiple sclerosis: The experience from anti-CD52mAb (alemtuzumab)*

In MS, anti-CD20 mAbs (rituximab, ocrelizumab, and ofatumumab) demonstrated clinical efficacy in both relapsing-remitting (RR) and primary-progressive (PP) MS in phase III clinical trials providing evidence that B cells have a pathogenic role in MS [120]. However, B cell depletion therapy had also deleterious effects in some patients with MS [121, 122]. Following depletion, naïve and immature B cells are primarily reconstituted, and B cells producing antiinflammatory cytokines increase [110, 123, 124].

Depletion of CD52 expressing T cells, B cells, and monocytes by the anti-CD52mAb (alemtuzumab) also resulted in impressive and durable suppression of disease activity in mouse models of MS and in RRMS patients [125, 126]. The effects of such treatment were accompanied by markedly decreased absolute numbers of Th1 and Th17 cells, which remained below baseline level in complete responders [127]. Some studies have provided information on the composition of repopulating B cell pool following alemtuzumab administration. Heidt et al. described a transient increase in transitional B cells and long-lasting predominance of naïve B cells following alemtuzumab administration [128]. In accordance with this evidence, Kim et al. found decreased proportions of $CD19^+ CD24^{hi} CD38^{hi}$ and $CD19^+ PD-L1^{hi}$ Breg subsets during relapse compared to remission and healthy controls. Meanwhile, following alemtuzumab administration there was a shift in the distribution of B cells toward naïve phenotype and $CD19^+ CD24^{hi} CD38^{hi}$ Breg cells percentages were restored [129]. The frequency of $CD19^+ PD-L1^{hi}$ cells also significantly increased up to 12 months following treatment.

Besides alemtuzumab, dimethyl fumarate and fingolimod treatment have been shown to influence B cell subsets and favor the induction of Breg cells, in particular circulating $CD24^{hi}CD38^{hi}$ cells [130–132].

5.2 Alternative protocols for expansion of B regulatory cells

In recent years, a new family of engineered fusion cytokines has been developed for cell-based immune modulation in order to treat cancer or autoimmune diseases [133]. For instance, the combination of GM-CSF and IL-15 as a fusokine (GIFT15) induced Breg cells that suppressed EAE, suggesting the involvement of cytokines in the development or expansion of Bregcells [13]. Likewise, a fusion of GM-CSF with IL-21 could initiate hypersignaling through the IL-21Rα chain with immune-modulating effects in vivo [134].

Deng et al. in an extensive review outlined how to reprogram B cells into regulatory cells with engineered fusokines [135]. The novel fusion cytokine GIFT15 is successfully able to reprogram naïve B cells to become inducible Breg cells (iBregs). The phenotype, function, and immune suppressive properties of iBregs are similar to the naturally occurring subsets.

Intriguingly, they also explored the possibility of converting B cells from peripheral blood of patients with MS to iBreg by GIFT15. Indeed, a population of IL-10-producing GIFT15-iBregs was reprogrammed from peripheral blood naïve B cells in the circulation of MS patients after 6 days of GIFT15 treatment [135]. The authors showed that the ex vivo manipulation of autologous naïve B cells from peripheral blood of patients is an entirely feasible procedure in MS. The successful generation of human iBregs with GIFT15 provides the rationale for developing personalized GIFT15-iBregs-based adoptive therapy for MS patients.

6 Conclusion

Interventions, aiming to drug-induced or direct expansion of Breg cells could in principle be effective in the induction of remission and maintenance of tolerance in several autoimmune conditions. While the use of these agents in vivo may be limited by other immune stimulatory parameters, these approaches are promising in creating platforms for B cell-based therapies with reinfusion of ex vivo expanded autologous Breg cells. Further studies expanding our knowledge on Breg functions will ensure that these cells will be efficiently expanded with beneficial therapeutic outcomes.

References

[1] S.I. Katz, D. Parker, J.L. Turk, B-cell suppression of delayed hypersensitivity reactions, Nature 251 (5475) (1974) 550–551.

[2] R. Neta, S.B. Salvin, Specific suppression of delayed hypersensitivity: the possible presence of a suppressor B cell in the regulation of delayed hypersensitivity, J. Immunol. 113 (6) (1974) 1716–1725.

[3] S.D. Wolf, B.N. Dittel, F. Hardardottir, C.A. Janeway Jr., Experimental autoimmune encephalomyelitis induction in genetically B cell-deficient mice, J. Exp. Med. 184 (6) (1996) 2271–2278.

[4] S. Fillatreau, C.H. Sweenie, M.J. McGeachy, D. Gray, S.M. Anderton, B cells regulate autoimmunity by provision of IL-10, Nat. Immunol. 3 (10) (2002) 944–950.

[5] C. Mauri, D. Gray, N. Mushtaq, M. Londei, Prevention of arthritis by interleukin 10-producing B cells, J. Exp. Med. 197 (4) (2003) 489–501.

[6] A. Mizoguchi, E. Mizoguchi, H. Takedatsu, R.S. Blumberg, A.K. Bhan, Chronic intestinal inflammatory condition generates IL-10-producing regulatory B cell subset characterized by CD1d upregulation, Immunity 16 (2) (2002) 219–230.

[7] C. Mauri, M. Menon, Human regulatory B cells in health and disease: therapeutic potential, J. Clin. Invest. 127 (3) (2017) 772–779.

[8] Y. He, X. Yuan, Y. Li, C. Zhong, Y. Liu, H. Qian, J. Xuan, L. Duan, G. Shi, Loss of Galphaq impairs regulatory B-cell function, Arthritis Res. Ther. 20 (1) (2018) 186.

[9] J. Noh, W.S. Choi, G. Noh, J.H. Lee, Presence of Foxp3-expressing CD19(+)CD5(+) B cells in human peripheral blood mononuclear cells: human CD19(+)CD5(+)Foxp3(+) regulatory B cell (Breg), Immune Netw. 10 (6) (2010) 247–249.

[10] Y. Guo, X. Zhang, M. Qin, X. Wang, Changes in peripheral CD19(+)Foxp3(+) and CD19(+)TGFbeta(+) regulatory B cell populations in rheumatoid arthritis patients with interstitial lung disease, J. Thorac. Dis. 7 (3) (2015) 471–477.

[11] Z. Vadasz, E. Toubi, FoxP3 expression in macrophages, cancer, and B cells-is it real? Clin. Rev. Allergy Immunol. 52 (3) (2017) 364–372.

[12] E.C. Rosser, K. Oleinika, S. Tonon, R. Doyle, A. Bosma, N.A. Carter, K.A. Harris, S.A. Jones, N. Klein, C. Mauri, Regulatory B cells are induced by gut microbiota-driven interleukin-1beta and interleukin-6 production, Nat. Med. 20 (11) (2014) 1334–1339.

[13] M. Rafei, J. Hsieh, S. Zehntner, M. Li, K. Forner, E. Birman, M.N. Boivin, Y.K. Young, C. Perreault, J. Galipeau, A granulocyte-macrophage colony-stimulating factor and interleukin-15 fusokine induces a regulatory B cell population with immune suppressive properties, Nat. Med. 15 (9) (2009) 1038–1045.

[14] J. Tian, D. Zekzer, L. Hanssen, Y. Lu, A. Olcott, D.L. Kaufman, Lipopolysaccharide-activated B cells downregulate Th1 immunity and prevent autoimmune diabetes in nonobese diabetic mice, J. Immunol. 167 (2) (2001) 1081–1089.

[15] K. Yanaba, J.D. Bouaziz, T. Matsushita, T. Tsubata, T.F. Tedder, The development and function of regulatory B cells expressing IL-10 (B10 cells) requires antigen receptor diversity and TLR signals, J. Immunol. 182 (12) (2009) 7459–7472.

[16] V. Lampropoulou, K. Hoehlig, T. Roch, P. Neves, E. Calderon Gomez, C.H. Sweenie, Y. Hao, A.A. Freitas, U. Steinhoff, S.M. Anderton, S. Fillatreau, TLR-activated B cells suppress T cell-mediated autoimmunity, J. Immunol. 180 (7) (2008) 4763–4773.

[17] I. Kalampokis, A. Yoshizaki, T.F. Tedder, IL-10-producing regulatory B cells (B10 cells) in autoimmune disease, Arthritis Res. Ther. 15 (Suppl. 1) (2013), S1.

[18] A. Yoshizaki, T. Miyagaki, D.J. DiLillo, T. Matsushita, M. Horikawa, E.I. Kountikov, R. Spolski, J.C. Poe, W.J. Leonard, T.F. Tedder, Regulatory B cells control T-cell autoimmunity through IL-21-dependent cognate interactions, Nature 491 (7423) (2012) 264–268.

[19] R.X. Wang, C.R. Yu, I.M. Dambuza, R.M. Mahdi, M.B. Dolinska, Y.V. Sergeev, P.T. Wingfield, S.H. Kim, C.E. Egwuagu, Interleukin-35 induces regulatory B cells that suppress autoimmune disease, Nat. Med. 20 (6) (2014) 633–641.

[20] P.A. Blair, L.Y. Norena, F. Flores-Borja, D.J. Rawlings, D.A. Isenberg, M.R. Ehrenstein, C. Mauri, CD19(+) CD24(hi)CD38(hi) B cells exhibit regulatory capacity in healthy individuals but are functionally impaired in systemic lupus erythematosus patients, Immunity 32 (1) (2010) 129–140.

[21] Y. Iwata, T. Matsushita, M. Horikawa, D.J. Dilillo, K. Yanaba, G.M. Venturi, P.M. Szabolcs, S.H. Bernstein, C.M. Magro, A.D. Williams, R.P. Hall, E.W.S. Clair, T.F. Tedder, Characterization of a rare IL-10-competent B-cell subset in humans that parallels mouse regulatory B10 cells, Blood 117 (2) (2011) 530–541.

[22] A. Khoder, A. Sarvaria, A. Alsuliman, C. Chew, T. Sekine, N. Cooper, S. Mielke, H. de Lavallade, M. Muftuoglu, I. Fernandez Curbelo, E. Liu, P.A. Muraro, A. Alousi, K. Stringaris, S. Parmar, N. Shah, H. Shaim, E. Yvon, J. Molldrem, R. Rouce, R. Champlin, I. McNiece, C. Mauri, E.J. Shpall, K. Rezvani, Regulatory B cells are enriched within the IgM memory and transitional subsets in healthy donors but are deficient in chronic GVHD, Blood 124 (13) (2014) 2034–2045.

[23] M. Matsumoto, A. Baba, T. Yokota, H. Nishikawa, Y. Ohkawa, H. Kayama, A. Kallies, S.L. Nutt, S. Sakaguchi, K. Takeda, T. Kurosaki, Y. Baba, Interleukin-10-producing plasmablasts exert regulatory function in autoimmune inflammation, Immunity 41 (6) (2014) 1040–1051.

[24] Y. Zhang, X. Zhang, Y. Xia, X. Jia, H. Li, Y. Zhang, Z. Shao, N. Xin, M. Guo, J. Chen, S. Zheng, Y. Wang, L. Fu, C. Xiao, D. Geng, Y. Liu, G. Cui, R. Dong, X. Huang, T. Yu, CD19+ Tim-1+ B cells are decreased and negatively correlated with disease severity in Myasthenia Gravis patients, Immunol. Res. 64 (5–6) (2016) 1216–1224.

3. Bregs and autoimmune diseases

[25] E.R. Zacca, L.I. Onofrio, C.D.V. Acosta, P.V. Ferrero, S.M. Alonso, M.C. Ramello, E. Mussano, L. Onetti, I.I. Cadile, M.I. Stancich, M.C. Taboada Bonfanti, C.L. Montes, E.V. Acosta Rodriguez, A. Gruppi, PD-L1(+) regulatory B cells are significantly decreased in rheumatoid arthritis patients and increase after successful treatment, Front. Immunol. 9 (2018) 2241.

[26] W. van de Veen, B. Stanic, G. Yaman, M. Wawrzyniak, S. Sollner, D.G. Akdis, B. Ruckert, C.A. Akdis, M. Akdis, IgG4 production is confined to human IL-10-producing regulatory B cells that suppress antigen-specific immune responses, J. Allergy Clin. Immunol. 131 (4) (2013) 1204–1212.

[27] F. Figueiro, L. Muller, S. Funk, E.K. Jackson, A.M. Battastini, T.L. Whiteside, Phenotypic and functional characteristics of CD39(high) human regulatory B cells (Breg), Oncoimmunology 5 (2) (2016), e1082703.

[28] E.C. Rosser, P.A. Blair, C. Mauri, Cellular targets of regulatory B cell-mediated suppression, Mol. Immunol. 62 (2) (2014) 296–304.

[29] N.A. Carter, E.C. Rosser, C. Mauri, Interleukin-10 produced by B cells is crucial for the suppression of Th17/ Th1 responses, induction of T regulatory type 1 cells and reduction of collagen-induced arthritis, Arthritis Res. Ther. 14 (1) (2012), R32.

[30] J.S. Ellis, H. Braley-Mullen, Mechanisms by which B cells and regulatory T cells influence development of murine organ-specific autoimmune diseases, J. Clin. Med. 6 (2) (2017) 13.

[31] S. Shah, L. Qiao, Resting B cells expand a CD4+CD25+Foxp3+ Treg population via TGF-beta3, Eur. J. Immunol. 38 (9) (2008) 2488–2498.

[32] M. Tarique, H. Naz, S.V. Kurra, C. Saini, R.A. Naqvi, R. Rai, M. Suhail, N. Khanna, D.N. Rao, A. Sharma, Interleukin-10 producing regulatory B cells transformed CD4(+)CD25(−) into Tregs and enhanced regulatory T cells function in human leprosy, Front. Immunol. 9 (2018) 1636.

[33] S. Sattler, G.S. Ling, D. Xu, L. Hussaarts, A. Romaine, H. Zhao, L. Fossati-Jimack, T. Malik, H.T. Cook, M. Botto, Y.L. Lau, H.H. Smits, F.Y. Liew, F.P. Huang, IL-10-producing regulatory B cells induced by IL-33 (Breg(IL-33)) effectively attenuate mucosal inflammatory responses in the gut, J. Autoimmun. 50 (2014) 107–122.

[34] J. Zhu, Y. Xu, C. Zhu, J. Zhao, X. Meng, S. Chen, T. Wang, X. Li, L. Zhang, C. Lu, H. Liu, X. Sun, IL-33 induces both regulatory B cells and regulatory T cells in dextran sulfate sodium-induced colitis, Int. Immunopharmacol. 46 (2017) 38–47.

[35] J.D. Bouaziz, H. Le Buanec, A. Saussine, A. Bensussan, M. Bagot, IL-10 producing regulatory B cells in mice and humans: state of the art, Curr. Mol. Med. 12 (5) (2012) 519–527.

[36] F. Flores-Borja, A. Bosma, D. Ng, V. Reddy, M.R. Ehrenstein, D.A. Isenberg, C. Mauri, CD19+CD24hiCD38hi B cells maintain regulatory T cells while limiting TH1 and TH17 differentiation, Sci. Transl. Med. 5 (173) (2013), 173ra23.

[37] T. Matsushita, M. Horikawa, Y. Iwata, T.F. Tedder, Regulatory B cells (B10 cells) and regulatory T cells have independent roles in controlling experimental autoimmune encephalomyelitis initiation and late-phase immunopathogenesis, J. Immunol. 185 (4) (2010) 2240–2252.

[38] X. Liu, X. Jiang, R. Liu, L. Wang, T. Qian, Y. Zheng, Y. Deng, E. Huang, F. Xu, J.Y. Wang, Y. Chu, B cells expressing CD11b effectively inhibit CD4+ T-cell responses and ameliorate experimental autoimmune hepatitis in mice, Hepatology 62 (5) (2015) 1563–1575.

[39] T. Matsushita, K. Yanaba, J.D. Bouaziz, M. Fujimoto, T.F. Tedder, Regulatory B cells inhibit EAE initiation in mice while other B cells promote disease progression, J. Clin. Invest. 118 (10) (2008) 3420–3430.

[40] P. Shen, T. Roch, V. Lampropoulou, R.A. O'Connor, U. Stervbo, E. Hilgenberg, S. Ries, V.D. Dang, Y. Jaimes, C. Daridon, R. Li, L. Jouneau, P. Boudinot, S. Wilantri, I. Sakwa, Y. Miyazaki, M.D. Leech, R.C. McPherson, S. Wirtz, M. Neurath, K. Hoehlig, E. Meinl, A. Grutzkau, J.R. Grun, K. Horn, A.A. Kuhl, T. Dorner, A. Bar-Or, S.H.E. Kaufmann, S.M. Anderton, S. Fillatreau, IL-35-producing B cells are critical regulators of immunity during autoimmune and infectious diseases, Nature 507 (7492) (2014) 366–370.

[41] H. Guan, Y. Wan, J. Lan, Q. Wang, Z. Wang, Y. Li, J. Zheng, X. Zhang, Z. Wang, Y. Shen, F. Xie, PD-L1 is a critical mediator of regulatory B cells and T cells in invasive breast cancer, Sci. Rep. 6 (2016) 35651.

[42] A. Ray, S. Basu, C.B. Williams, N.H. Salzman, B.N. Dittel, A novel IL-10-independent regulatory role for B cells in suppressing autoimmunity by maintenance of regulatory T cells via GITR ligand, J. Immunol. 188 (7) (2012) 3188–3198.

[43] J.M. Lykken, K.M. Candando, T.F. Tedder, Regulatory B10 cell development and function, Int. Immunol. 27 (10) (2015) 471–477.

[44] Q. Simon, J.O. Pers, D. Cornec, L. Le Pottier, R.A. Mageed, S. Hillion, In-depth characterization of CD24(high) CD38(high) transitional human B cells reveals different regulatory profiles, J. Allergy Clin. Immunol. 137 (5) (2016) 1577–1584. e10.

[45] W. Lin, D. Cerny, E. Chua, K. Duan, J.T. Yi, N.B. Shadan, J. Lum, M. Maho-Vaillant, F. Zolezzi, S.C. Wong, A. Larbi, K. Fink, P. Musette, M. Poidinger, S. Calbo, Human regulatory B cells combine phenotypic and genetic hallmarks with a distinct differentiation fate, J. Immunol. 193 (5) (2014) 2258–2266.

[46] A. de Masson, J.D. Bouaziz, H. Le Buanec, M. Robin, A. O'Meara, N. Parquet, M. Rybojad, E. Hau, J.B. Monfort, M. Branchtein, D. Michonneau, V. Dessirier, F. Sicre de Fontbrune, A. Bergeron, R. Itzykson, N. Dhedin, D. Bengoufa, R. Peffault de Latour, A. Xhaard, M. Bagot, A. Bensussan, G. Socie, CD24(hi)CD27(+) and plasmablast-like regulatory B cells in human chronic graft-versus-host disease, Blood 125 (11) (2015) 1830–1839.

[47] I. Kalampokis, G.M. Venturi, J.C. Poe, J.A. Dvergsten, J.W. Sleasman, T.F. Tedder, The regulatory B cell compartment expands transiently during childhood and is contracted in children with autoimmunity, Arthritis Rheumatol. 69 (1) (2017) 225–238.

[48] L. Shi, F. Hu, L. Zhu, C. Xu, H. Zhu, Y. Li, H. Liu, C. Li, N. Liu, L. Xu, R. Mu, Z. Li, CD70-mediated CD27 expression downregulation contributed to the regulatory B10 cell impairment in rheumatoid arthritis, Mol. Immunol. 119 (2020) 92–100.

[49] Q. Ding, M. Yeung, G. Camirand, Q. Zeng, H. Akiba, H. Yagita, G. Chalasani, M.H. Sayegh, N. Najafian, D.M. Rothstein, Regulatory B cells are identified by expression of TIM-1 and can be induced through TIM-1 ligation to promote tolerance in mice, J. Clin. Invest. 121 (9) (2011) 3645–3656.

[50] S. Xiao, C.R. Brooks, R.A. Sobel, V.K. Kuchroo, Tim-1 is essential for induction and maintenance of IL-10 in regulatory B cells and their regulation of tissue inflammation, J. Immunol. 194 (4) (2015) 1602–1608.

[51] M.Y. Yeung, Q. Ding, C.R. Brooks, S. Xiao, C.J. Workman, D.A. Vignali, T. Ueno, R.F. Padera, V.K. Kuchroo, N. Najafian, D.M. Rothstein, TIM-1 signaling is required for maintenance and induction of regulatory B cells, Am. J. Transplant. 15 (4) (2015) 942–953.

[52] O. Aravena, A. Ferrier, M. Menon, C. Mauri, J.C. Aguillon, L. Soto, D. Catalan, TIM-1 defines a human regulatory B cell population that is altered in frequency and function in systemic sclerosis patients, Arthritis Res. Ther. 19 (1) (2017) 8.

[53] A. Ray, L. Wang, B.N. Dittel, IL-10-independent regulatory B-cell subsets and mechanisms of action, Int. Immunol. 27 (10) (2015) 531–536.

[54] L.I. Sakkas, A. Mavropoulos, C. Perricone, D.P. Bogdanos, IL-35: a new immunomodulator in autoimmune rheumatic diseases, Immunol. Res. 66 (3) (2018) 305–312.

[55] M. Bettini, A.H. Castellaw, G.P. Lennon, A.R. Burton, D.A. Vignali, Prevention of autoimmune diabetes by ectopic pancreatic beta-cell expression of interleukin-35, Diabetes 61 (6) (2012) 1519–1526.

[56] I.M. Dambuza, C. He, J.K. Choi, C.R. Yu, R. Wang, M.J. Mattapallil, P.T. Wingfield, R.R. Caspi, C.E. Egwuagu, IL-12p35 induces expansion of IL-10 and IL-35-expressing regulatory B cells and ameliorates autoimmune disease, Nat. Commun. 8 (1) (2017) 719.

[57] C.E. Egwuagu, C.R. Yu, L. Sun, R. Wang, Interleukin 35: critical regulator of immunity and lymphocyte-mediated diseases, Cytokine Growth Factor Rev. 26 (5) (2015) 587–593.

[58] W. Chen, W. Jin, N. Hardegen, K.J. Lei, L. Li, N. Marinos, G. McGrady, S.M. Wahl, Conversion of peripheral CD4+CD25− naive T cells to CD4+CD25+ regulatory T cells by TGF-beta induction of transcription factor Foxp3, J. Exp. Med. 198 (12) (2003) 1875–1886.

[59] Q. Lan, X. Zhou, H. Fan, M. Chen, J. Wang, B. Ryffel, D. Brand, R. Ramalingam, P.R. Kiela, D.A. Horwitz, Z. Liu, S.G. Zheng, Polyclonal CD4+Foxp3+ Treg cells induce TGFbeta-dependent tolerogenic dendritic cells that suppress the murine lupus-like syndrome, J. Mol. Cell Biol. 4 (6) (2012) 409–419.

[60] V.V. Parekh, D.V. Prasad, P.P. Banerjee, B.N. Joshi, A. Kumar, G.C. Mishra, B cells activated by lipopolysaccharide, but not by anti-Ig and anti-CD40 antibody, induce anergy in CD8+ T cells: role of TGF-beta 1, J. Immunol. 170 (12) (2003) 5897–5911.

[61] K. Bjarnadottir, M. Benkhoucha, D. Merkler, M.S. Weber, N.L. Payne, C.C.A. Bernard, N. Molnarfi, P.H. Lalive, B cell-derived transforming growth factor-beta1 expression limits the induction phase of autoimmune neuroinflammation, Sci. Rep. 6 (2016) 34594.

[62] P. Natarajan, A. Singh, J.T. McNamara, E.R. Secor Jr., L.A. Guernsey, R.S. Thrall, C.M. Schramm, Regulatory B cells from hilar lymph nodes of tolerant mice in a murine model of allergic airway disease are CD5+, express TGF-beta, and co-localize with CD4+Foxp3+ T cells, Mucosal Immunol. 5 (6) (2012) 691–701.

[63] K.M. Lee, R.T. Stott, G. Zhao, J. SooHoo, W. Xiong, M.M. Lian, L. Fitzgerald, S. Shi, E. Akrawi, J. Lei, S. Deng, H. Yeh, J.F. Markmann, J.I. Kim, TGF-beta-producing regulatory B cells induce regulatory T cells and promote transplantation tolerance, Eur. J. Immunol. 44 (6) (2014) 1728–1736.

[64] T. Komai, M. Inoue, T. Okamura, K. Morita, Y. Iwaski, S. Sumitomo, H. Shoda, K. Yamamoto, K. Fujio, Transforming growth factor-beta and interleukin-10 synergistically regulate humoral immunity via modulating metabolic signals, Front. Immunol. 9 (2018) 1364.

[65] S. Hoves, J.A. Trapani, I. Voskoboinik, The battlefield of perforin/granzyme cell death pathways, J. Leukoc. Biol. 87 (2) (2010) 237–243.

[66] M. Hagn, B. Jahrsdorfer, Why do human B cells secrete granzyme B? Insights into a novel B-cell differentiation pathway, Oncoimmunology 1 (8) (2012) 1368–1375.

[67] S. Lindner, K. Dahlke, K. Sontheimer, M. Hagn, C. Kaltenmeier, T.F. Barth, T. Beyer, F. Reister, D. Fabricius, R. Lotfi, O. Lunov, G.U. Nienhaus, T. Simmet, R. Kreienberg, P. Moller, H. Schrezenmeier, B. Jahrsdorfer, Interleukin 21-induced granzyme B-expressing B cells infiltrate tumors and regulate T cells, Cancer Res. 73 (8) (2013) 2468–2479.

[68] Q. Zeng, Y.H. Ng, T. Singh, K. Jiang, K.A. Sheriff, R. Ippolito, S. Zahalka, Q. Li, P. Randhawa, R.A. Hoffman, B. Ramaswami, F.E. Lund, G. Chalasani, B cells mediate chronic allograft rejection independently of antibody production, J. Clin. Invest. 124 (3) (2014) 1052–1056.

[69] M. Chesneau, L. Michel, E. Dugast, A. Chenouard, D. Baron, A. Pallier, J. Durand, F. Braza, P. Guerif, D.A. Laplaud, J.P. Soulillou, M. Giral, N. Degauque, E. Chiffoleau, S. Brouard, Tolerant kidney transplant patients produce B cells with regulatory properties, J. Am. Soc. Nephrol. 26 (10) (2015) 2588–2598.

[70] L. Xu, X. Liu, H. Liu, L. Zhu, H. Zhu, J. Zhang, L. Ren, P. Wang, F. Hu, Y. Su, Impairment of granzyme B-producing regulatory B cells correlates with exacerbated rheumatoid arthritis, Front. Immunol. 8 (2017) 768.

[71] Z.Y. Huang, P. Xu, J.H. Li, C.H. Zeng, H.F. Song, H. Chen, Y.B. Zhu, Y.Y. Song, H.L. Lu, C.P. Shen, X.G. Zhang, M.Y. Wu, X.F. Wang, Clinical significance of dynamics of programmed death ligand-1 expression on circulating CD14(+) monocytes and CD19(+) B cells with the progression of hepatitis B virus infection, Viral Immunol. 30 (3) (2017) 224–231.

[72] A.R. Khan, E. Hams, A. Floudas, T. Sparwasser, C.T. Weaver, P.G. Fallon, PD-L1hi B cells are critical regulators of humoral immunity, Nat. Commun. 6 (2015) 5997.

[73] S. Amarnath, C.W. Mangus, J.C. Wang, F. Wei, A. He, V. Kapoor, J.E. Foley, P.R. Massey, T.C. Felizardo, J.L. Riley, B.L. Levine, C.H. June, J.A. Medin, D.H. Fowler, The PDL1-PD1 axis converts human TH1 cells into regulatory T cells, Sci. Transl. Med. 3 (111) (2011), 111ra120.

[74] Z.Z. Yang, D.M. Grote, S.C. Ziesmer, B. Xiu, A.J. Novak, S.M. Ansell, PD-1 expression defines two distinct T-cell sub-populations in follicular lymphoma that differentially impact patient survival, Blood Cancer J. 5 (2015), e281.

[75] M.T. Zdrenghea, S.L. Johnston, Role of PD-L1/PD-1 in the immune response to respiratory viral infections, Microbes Infect. 14 (6) (2012) 495–499.

[76] L.M. Francisco, P.T. Sage, A.H. Sharpe, The PD-1 pathway in tolerance and autoimmunity, Immunol. Rev. 236 (2010) 219–242.

[77] K. Wang, L. Tao, J. Su, Y. Zhang, B. Zou, Y. Wang, M. Zou, N. Chen, L. Lei, X. Li, TLR4 supports the expansion of FasL(+)CD5(+)CD1d(hi) regulatory B cells, which decreases in contact hypersensitivity, Mol. Immunol. 87 (2017) 188–199.

[78] T.J. Kemp, J.M. Moore, T.S. Griffith, Human B cells express functional TRAIL/Apo-2 ligand after CpG-containing oligodeoxynucleotide stimulation, J. Immunol. 173 (2) (2004) 892–899.

[79] L.I. Sakkas, D. Daoussis, A. Mavropoulos, S.N. Liossis, D.P. Bogdanos, Regulatory B cells: new players in inflammatory and autoimmune rheumatic diseases, Semin. Arthritis Rheum. 48 (6) (2019) 1133–1141.

[80] A. Mavropoulos, T. Simopoulou, A. Varna, C. Liaskos, C.G. Katsiari, D.P. Bogdanos, L.I. Sakkas, Breg cells are numerically decreased and functionally impaired in patients with systemic sclerosis, Arthritis Rheumatol. 68 (2) (2016) 494–504.

[81] C.I. Daien, S. Gailhac, T. Mura, R. Audo, B. Combe, M. Hahne, J. Morel, Regulatory B10 cells are decreased in patients with rheumatoid arthritis and are inversely correlated with disease activity, Arthritis Rheumatol. 66 (8) (2014) 2037–2046.

[82] Z. Banko, J. Pozsgay, T. Gati, B. Rojkovich, I. Ujfalussy, G. Sarmay, Regulatory B cells in rheumatoid arthritis: alterations in patients receiving anti-TNF therapy, Clin. Immunol. 184 (2017) 63–69.

[83] L. Ma, B. Liu, Z. Jiang, Y. Jiang, Reduced numbers of regulatory B cells are negatively correlated with disease activity in patients with new-onset rheumatoid arthritis, Clin. Rheumatol. 33 (2) (2014) 187–195.

[84] D. Cui, L. Zhang, J. Chen, M. Zhu, L. Hou, B. Chen, B. Shen, Changes in regulatory B cells and their relationship with rheumatoid arthritis disease activity, Clin. Exp. Med. 15 (3) (2015) 285–292.

[85] A. Mavropoulos, C. Liaskos, T. Simopoulou, D.P. Bogdanos, L.I. Sakkas, IL-10-producing regulatory B cells (B10 cells), IL-17+ T cells and autoantibodies in systemic sclerosis, Clin. Immunol. 184 (2017) 26–32.

[86] F. Mion, S. Tonon, B. Toffoletto, D. Cesselli, C.E. Pucillo, G. Vitale, IL-10 production by B cells is differentially regulated by immune-mediated and infectious stimuli and requires p38 activation, Mol. Immunol. 62 (2) (2014) 266–276.

[87] L. Soto, A. Ferrier, O. Aravena, E. Fonseca, J. Berendsen, A. Biere, D. Bueno, V. Ramos, J.C. Aguillon, D. Catalan, Systemic sclerosis patients present alterations in the expression of molecules involved in B-cell regulation, Front. Immunol. 6 (2015) 496.

[88] T. Matsushita, Y. Hamaguchi, M. Hasegawa, K. Takehara, M. Fujimoto, Decreased levels of regulatory B cells in patients with systemic sclerosis: association with autoantibody production and disease activity, Rheumatology (Oxford) 55 (2) (2016) 263–267.

[89] L.I. Sakkas, D.P. Bogdanos, Are psoriasis and psoriatic arthritis the same disease? The IL-23/IL-17 axis data, Autoimmun. Rev. 16 (1) (2017) 10–15.

[90] K. Yanaba, M. Kamata, N. Ishiura, S. Shibata, Y. Asano, Y. Tada, M. Sugaya, T. Kadono, T.F. Tedder, S. Sato, Regulatory B cells suppress imiquimod-induced, psoriasis-like skin inflammation, J. Leukoc. Biol. 94 (4) (2013) 563–573.

[91] M. Hayashi, K. Yanaba, Y. Umezawa, Y. Yoshihara, S. Kikuchi, Y. Ishiuji, H. Saeki, H. Nakagawa, IL-10-producing regulatory B cells are decreased in patients with psoriasis, J. Dermatol. Sci. 81 (2) (2016) 93–100.

[92] G.K. Vasileiadis, E. Dardiotis, A. Mavropoulos, Z. Tsouris, V. Tsimourtou, D.P. Bogdanos, L.I. Sakkas, G.M. Hadjigeorgiou, Regulatory B and T lymphocytes in multiple sclerosis: friends or foes? Auto Immun. Highlights 9 (1) (2018) 9.

[93] E. Staun-Ram, A. Miller, Effector and regulatory B cells in multiple sclerosis, Clin. Immunol. 184 (2017) 11–25.

[94] S. Knippenberg, E. Peelen, J. Smolders, M. Thewissen, P. Menheere, J.W. Cohen Tervaert, R. Hupperts, J. Damoiseaux, Reduction in IL-10 producing B cells (Breg) in multiple sclerosis is accompanied by a reduced naive/memory Breg ratio during a relapse but not in remission, J. Neuroimmunol. 239 (1–2) (2011) 80–86.

[95] F. Piancone, M. Saresella, I. Marventano, F. La Rosa, M. Zoppis, S. Agostini, R. Longhi, D. Caputo, L. Mendozzi, M. Rovaris, M. Clerici, B lymphocytes in multiple sclerosis: Bregs and BTLA/CD272 expressing-CD19+ lymphocytes modulate disease severity, Sci. Rep. 6 (2016) 29699.

[96] L. Michel, M. Chesneau, P. Manceau, A. Genty, A. Garcia, M. Salou, A. Elong Ngono, A. Pallier, M. Jacq-Foucher, F. Lefrere, S. Wiertlewski, J.P. Soulillou, N. Degauque, D.A. Laplaud, S. Brouard, Unaltered regulatory B-cell frequency and function in patients with multiple sclerosis, Clin. Immunol. 155 (2) (2014) 198–208.

[97] C. de Andres, M. Tejera-Alhambra, B. Alonso, L. Valor, R. Teijeiro, R. Ramos-Medina, D. Mateos, F. Faure, S. Sanchez-Ramon, New regulatory CD19(+)CD25(+) B-cell subset in clinically isolated syndrome and multiple sclerosis relapse. Changes after glucocorticoids, J. Neuroimmunol. 270 (1–2) (2014) 37–44.

[98] M. Hirotani, M. Niino, T. Fukazawa, S. Kikuchi, I. Yabe, S. Hamada, Y. Tajima, H. Sasaki, Decreased IL-10 production mediated by Toll-like receptor 9 in B cells in multiple sclerosis, J. Neuroimmunol. 221 (1–2) (2010) 95–100.

[99] T. Kinnunen, N. Chamberlain, H. Morbach, T. Cantaert, M. Lynch, P. Preston-Hurlburt, K.C. Herold, D.A. Hafler, K.C. O'Connor, E. Meffre, Specific peripheral B cell tolerance defects in patients with multiple sclerosis, J. Clin. Invest. 123 (6) (2013) 2737–2741.

[100] Y. Okada, H. Ochi, C. Fujii, Y. Hashi, M. Hamatani, S. Ashida, K. Kawamura, H. Kusaka, S. Matsumoto, M. Nakagawa, T. Mizuno, R. Takahashi, T. Kondo, Signaling via Toll-like receptor 4 and CD40 in B cells plays a regulatory role in the pathogenesis of multiple sclerosis through interleukin-10 production, J. Autoimmun. 88 (2018) 103–113.

[101] S. Guo, Q. Chen, X. Liang, M. Mu, J. He, Q. Fang, C. Song, D. Sang, Reduced peripheral blood regulatory B cell levels are not associated with the Expanded Disability Status Scale score in multiple sclerosis, J. Int. Med. Res. 46 (9) (2018) 3970–3978.

[102] L.I. Sakkas, D.P. Bogdanos, C. Katsiari, C.D. Platsoucas, Anti-citrullinated peptides as autoantigens in rheumatoid arthritis-relevance to treatment, Autoimmun. Rev. 13 (11) (2014) 1114–1120.

[103] S. Modi, M. Soejima, M.C. Levesque, The effect of targeted rheumatoid arthritis therapies on anti-citrullinated protein autoantibody levels and B cell responses, Clin. Exp. Immunol. 173 (1) (2013) 8–17.

[104] J.C. Edwards, L. Szczepanski, J. Szechinski, A. Filipowicz-Sosnowska, P. Emery, D.R. Close, R.M. Stevens, T. Shaw, Efficacy of B-cell-targeted therapy with rituximab in patients with rheumatoid arthritis, N. Engl. J. Med. 350 (25) (2004) 2572–2581.

[105] A. Rubbert-Roth, P.P. Tak, C. Zerbini, J.L. Tremblay, L. Carreno, G. Armstrong, N. Collinson, T.M. Shaw, M.T. Investigators, Efficacy and safety of various repeat treatment dosing regimens of rituximab in patients with active rheumatoid arthritis: results of a Phase III randomized study (MIRROR), Rheumatology (Oxford) 49 (9) (2010) 1683–1693.

[106] B. Haraoui, M. Bokarewa, I. Kallmeyer, V.P. Bykerk, R. Investigators, Safety and effectiveness of rituximab in patients with rheumatoid arthritis following an inadequate response to 1 prior tumor necrosis factor inhibitor: the RESET Trial, J. Rheumatol. 38 (12) (2011) 2548–2556.

[107] J.D. Bouaziz, K. Yanaba, G.M. Venturi, Y. Wang, R.M. Tisch, J.C. Poe, T.F. Tedder, Therapeutic B cell depletion impairs adaptive and autoreactive CD4+ T cell activation in mice, Proc. Natl. Acad. Sci. U. S. A. 104 (52) (2007) 20878–20883.

[108] J.O. Pers, C. Daridon, B. Bendaoud, V. Devauchelle, C. Berthou, A. Saraux, P. Youinou, B-cell depletion and repopulation in autoimmune diseases, Clin. Rev. Allergy Immunol. 34 (1) (2008) 50–55.

[109] K. Hofmann, A.K. Clauder, R.A. Manz, Targeting B cells and plasma cells in autoimmune diseases, Front. Immunol. 9 (2018) 835.

[110] P. Roll, A. Palanichamy, C. Kneitz, T. Dorner, H.P. Tony, Regeneration of B cell subsets after transient B cell depletion using anti-CD20 antibodies in rheumatoid arthritis, Arthritis Rheum. 54 (8) (2006) 2377–2386.

[111] M.J. Leandro, G. Cambridge, M.R. Ehrenstein, J.C. Edwards, Reconstitution of peripheral blood B cells after depletion with rituximab in patients with rheumatoid arthritis, Arthritis Rheum. 54 (2) (2006) 613–620.

[112] W.H. Abdulahad, J.M. Meijer, F.G. Kroese, P.M. Meiners, A. Vissink, F.K. Spijkervet, C.G. Kallenberg, H. Bootsma, B cell reconstitution and T helper cell balance after rituximab treatment of active primary Sjögren's syndrome: a double-blind, placebo-controlled study, Arthritis Rheum. 63 (4) (2011) 1116–1123.

[113] F. Sun, S.S. Ladha, L. Yang, Q. Liu, S.X. Shi, N. Su, R. Bomprezzi, F.D. Shi, Interleukin-10 producing-B cells and their association with responsiveness to rituximab in myasthenia gravis, Muscle Nerve 49 (4) (2014) 487–494.

[114] S. Dass, E.M. Vital, P. Emery, Development of psoriasis after B cell depletion with rituximab, Arthritis Rheum. 56 (8) (2007) 2715–2718.

[115] F. Mielke, J. Schneider-Obermeyer, T. Dorner, Onset of psoriasis with psoriatic arthropathy during rituximab treatment of non-Hodgkin lymphoma, Ann. Rheum. Dis. 67 (7) (2008) 1056–1057.

[116] M. Goetz, R. Atreya, M. Ghalibafian, P.R. Galle, M.F. Neurath, Exacerbation of ulcerative colitis after rituximab salvage therapy, Inflamm. Bowel Dis. 13 (11) (2007) 1365–1368.

[117] D. El Fassi, C.H. Nielsen, J. Kjeldsen, O. Clemmensen, L. Hegedus, Ulcerative colitis following B lymphocyte depletion with rituximab in a patient with Graves' disease, Gut 57 (5) (2008) 714–715.

[118] P. Schafer, Apremilast mechanism of action and application to psoriasis and psoriatic arthritis, Biochem. Pharmacol. 83 (12) (2012) 1583–1590.

[119] A. Mavropoulos, E. Zafiriou, T. Simopoulou, A.G. Brotis, C. Liaskos, A. Roussaki-Schulze, C.G. Katsiari, D.P. Bogdanos, L.I. Sakkas, Apremilast increases IL-10-producing regulatory B cells and decreases proinflammatory T cells and innate cells in psoriatic arthritis and psoriasis, Rheumatology (Oxford) 58 (12) (2019) 2240–2250.

[120] S.L. Hauser, A. Bar-Or, G. Comi, G. Giovannoni, H.P. Hartung, B. Hemmer, F. Lublin, X. Montalban, K.W. Rammohan, K. Selmaj, A. Traboulsee, J.S. Wolinsky, D.L. Arnold, G. Klingelschmitt, D. Masterman, P. Fontoura, S. Belachew, P. Chin, N. Mairon, H. Garren, L. Kappos, I. Opera, O.I.C. Investigators, Ocrelizumab versus interferon beta-1a in relapsing multiple sclerosis, N. Engl. J. Med. 376 (3) (2017) 221–234.

[121] L. Benedetti, D. Franciotta, T. Vigo, M. Grandis, E. Fiorina, E. Ghiglione, L. Roccatagliata, G.L. Mancardi, A. Uccelli, A. Schenone, Relapses after treatment with rituximab in a patient with multiple sclerosis and anti myelin-associated glycoprotein polyneuropathy, Arch. Neurol. 64 (10) (2007) 1531–1533.

[122] R. Milo, Therapeutic strategies targeting B-cells in multiple sclerosis, Autoimmun. Rev. 15 (7) (2016) 714–718.

[123] M. Duddy, M. Niino, F. Adatia, S. Hebert, M. Freedman, H. Atkins, H.J. Kim, A. Bar-Or, Distinct effector cytokine profiles of memory and naive human B cell subsets and implication in multiple sclerosis, J. Immunol. 178 (10) (2007) 6092–6099.

[124] J.J. Sabatino Jr., S.S. Zamvil, S.L. Hauser, B-cell therapies in multiple sclerosis, Cold Spring Harb. Perspect. Med. 9 (2) (2019) a032037.

[125] M. Simon, R. Ipek, G.A. Homola, D.M. Rovituso, A. Schampel, C. Kleinschnitz, S. Kuerten, Anti-CD52 antibody treatment depletes B cell aggregates in the central nervous system in a mouse model of multiple sclerosis, J. Neuroinflammation 15 (1) (2018) 225.

[126] J.R. Evan, S.B. Bozkurt, N.C. Thomas, F. Bagnato, Alemtuzumab for the treatment of multiple sclerosis, Expert Opin. Biol. Ther. 18 (3) (2018) 323–334.

[127] K. Akgun, J. Blankenburg, M. Marggraf, R. Haase, T. Ziemssen, Event-driven Immunoprofiling predicts return of disease activity in alemtuzumab-treated multiple sclerosis, Front. Immunol. 11 (2020) 56.

[128] S. Heidt, J. Hester, S. Shankar, P.J. Friend, K.J. Wood, B cell repopulation after alemtuzumab induction-transient increase in transitional B cells and long-term dominance of naive B cells, Am. J. Transplant. 12 (7) (2012) 1784–1792.

[129] Y. Kim, G. Kim, H.J. Shin, J.W. Hyun, S.H. Kim, E. Lee, H.J. Kim, Restoration of regulatory B cell deficiency following alemtuzumab therapy in patients with relapsing multiple sclerosis, J. Neuroinflammation 15 (1) (2018) 300.

[130] S. Blumenfeld-Kan, E. Staun-Ram, A. Miller, Fingolimod reduces CXCR4-mediated B cell migration and induces regulatory B cells-mediated anti-inflammatory immune repertoire, Mult. Scler. Relat. Disord. 34 (2019) 29–37.

[131] S.K. Lundy, Q. Wu, Q. Wang, C.A. Dowling, S.H. Taitano, G. Mao, Y. Mao-Draayer, Dimethyl fumarate treatment of relapsing-remitting multiple sclerosis influences B-cell subsets, Neurol. Neuroimmunol. Neuroinflamm. 3 (2) (2016), e211.

[132] S. Medina, N. Villarrubia, S. Sainz de la Maza, J. Lifante, L. Costa-Frossard, E. Roldan, C. Picon, J.C. Alvarez-Cermeno, L.M. Villar, Optimal response to dimethyl fumarate associates in MS with a shift from an inflammatory to a tolerogenic blood cell profile, Mult. Scler. 24 (10) (2018) 1317–1327.

[133] S. Ng, J. Galipeau, Concise review: engineering the fusion of cytokines for the modulation of immune cellular responses in cancer and autoimmune disorders, Stem Cells Transl. Med. 4 (1) (2015) 66–73.

[134] P. Williams, M. Rafei, M. Bouchentouf, J. Raven, S. Yuan, J. Cuerquis, K.A. Forner, E. Birman, J. Galipeau, A fusion of GMCSF and IL-21 initiates hypersignaling through the IL-21Ralpha chain with immune activating and tumoricidal effects in vivo, Mol. Ther. 18 (7) (2010) 1293–1301.

[135] J. Deng, J. Galipeau, Reprogramming of B cells into regulatory cells with engineered fusokines, Infect. Disord. Drug Targets 12 (3) (2012) 248–254.

CHAPTER

4

Regulatory T cells in autoimmunity and potential therapeutic targets

Ankur Kumar Jindal*, Aaqib Zaffar Banday, and Rahul Tyagi

**Allergy and Immunology Unit, Department of Pediatrics, Advanced Pediatric Centre,
Postgraduate Institute of Medical Education and Research, Chandigarh, India
*Corresponding author**

Abstract

Regulatory T cells (Treg cells) are a subset of T cells that have an important role in maintaining immune homeostasis in the body. Germline mutations in *FOXP3* gene, the transcriptional master regulator for Treg cells, resulting in diminished number and function of Treg cells leading to immune dysregulation polyendocrinopathy enteropathy X-linked (IPEX) syndrome. This syndrome is characterized by the presence of autoantibodies (such as antiislet cell, antiinsulin, antiglutamic acid decarboxylase, antithyroglobulin, antithyroid peroxidase, antienterocyte, antivillin, antiharmonin, antismooth muscle, and antimicrosomal antibodies) and autoimmune manifestations. Acquired abnormalities in the number or function of Treg cells may play a crucial role in the development of autoimmune diseases such as systemic lupus erythematous, type 1 diabetes mellitus, and rheumatoid arthritis and have been the focus of intense research over the last decade or so. Additionally, Treg cell therapy is an upcoming area of investigation in therapeutics of several autoimmune manifestations. Ovalbumin-specific Treg cells have already been shown to be efficacious and well tolerated in patients with refractory Crohn's disease and type 1 diabetes mellitus. Here in, we review the basics of the development and function of Treg cells with a detailed overview of the pathogenic role of these cells in autoimmune and primary immunodeficiency diseases. In addition, we provide an overview of the therapeutic potentials of Treg cells in the management of various autoimmune diseases.

Keywords

Autoimmunity, Diabetes, Immune deficiency, Inflammatory bowel disease, IPEX syndrome, Kawasaki disease, Multiple sclerosis, Regulatory T cell, Rheumatoid arthritis, SLE

1 Introduction

Regulatory T cells (Treg cells) are an important subset of T cells that have a very important role of maintaining the immune homeostasis in the body. These cells are generated either in the thymus or in the periphery. There are several different subsets of Treg cells that are distinguished from each other by cell surface markers. Each one of these cells has a specialized and unique function in maintaining immune homeostasis. An abnormality in the number or function of Treg cells (either inherited or acquired) may lead to severe and life-threatening autoimmune diseases such as systemic lupus erythematosus (SLE), type 1 diabetes mellitus (T1DM), rheumatoid arthritis, and immune dysregulation polyendocrinopathy enteropathy X-linked (IPEX) syndrome. In this chapter, the basics of the development and function of Treg cells with a detailed overview of the pathogenic role of these cells in autoimmune and primary immunodeficiency diseases are discussed. In addition, an overview of therapeutic potentials of Treg cells in the management of various autoimmune diseases is provided.

2 Discovery of Treg cells

Experiments that led to the discovery of Treg cells were carried out almost half a century ago. It was observed that T cells not only generate immune responses but also suppress it [1, 2]. Literature in the early 1970s labeled these T cells as "suppressor T cells" [3, 4]. However, the term regulatory T cells was also used at the same time depicting the counterbalance between the T cell subtypes [5] Research into this specialized subgroup, suppressor T cells typified them to be $CD4^+CD25^+$ [6]. In the early 2000s, Forkhead box P3 *(FOXP3)* gene was found out to be transcriptional master regulator for Treg cells [7–9]. This was preceded by the identification of *Foxp3* as the defective gene in scurfy mice and that mutations in the same gene were responsible for causing the scurfy mice equivalent disorder in humans, the IPEX syndrome [10–13]. Decrease in the proportion of $CD4^+CD25^+FoxP3^+$ T cells (Treg cells) suggested the immune 'dysregulation/autoimmunity' seen in this genetic disorder [14]. Indeed, discovery of Treg cells has ushered us into a new era of research into immune dysregulation and its implications in autoimmune diseases. The discovery of Treg cells is probably the most interesting story in the field of autoimmunity [15].

3 Development and activation of Treg cells

Treg cells are derived from common lymphoid progenitor (CLP) cells in the bone marrow followed by their migration to the thymus via the bloodstream. Cellular development occurs in specialized microenvironments. These cells target the autoreactive T cells that have escaped the negative selection process in the thymus. During the development of CLPs in the thymus, double-negative cells ($CD4^-CD8^-$) emerge that subsequently are converted to double-positive cells ($CD4^+CD8^+$) following a sequence of events. The polarization of Treg cell subsets has been considered an instructive selection via self-reactive thymocytes. This selection requires stimulation of $CD25^{high}$ Treg precursors by IL-2 or IL-15, which in turn express the FoxP3. In vivo animal studies have shown that models deficient in IL-2/IL-2R

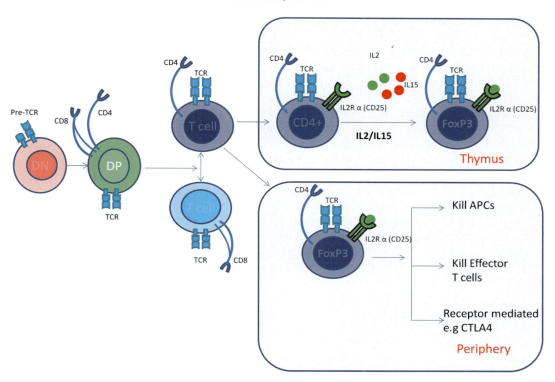

FIG. 1 Illustration of the developmental trajectory of Treg Cells in the thymus and in the periphery. TCR: T cell receptor; APC: antigen-presenting cells.

interaction lead to lethal autoimmunity similar to the phenotype of FoxP3 deficiency [7]. This interaction between IL-2 and IL-2R is reported to affect the thymic Treg cells. Animal studies expressing green fluorescence protein (GFP) under the influence of *Foxp3* locus revealed that the majority of FoxP3 expression is limited to CD4$^+$T cells [16]. Moreover, along with CD25^{high} cells, a few CD25$^{low/lacking}$ cells also express FoxP3 [16]. The steps of development of Treg cells have been illustrated in Fig. 1.

Treg cells are generated either in the thymus or in the periphery. As described earlier, thymic Treg cells develop from immature thymocytes due to high-affinity interactions with self-antigens. In contrast, peripheral Treg cells develop from naïve thymic immigrants in the presence of cytokines such as transforming growth factor-β1(TGF-β1). TGF-β1 activates downstream molecules and specific transcription factors including Smad2 and Smad3 [17]. Smad2/3 double knock-out mouse model developed fatal inflammatory consequences along with high proportions of IFN-γ and reduced Treg cells expressing FoxP3 [17]. Peripheral Treg cells that develop from escaped naïve T cells are induced to express FoxP3. These cells in contact-dependent and independent manners may either kill antigen-presenting cells (APCs) and effector T cells or act on APCs by receptor-mediated inactivation.

4 FoxP3—The transcriptional master regulator of Treg cells

FoxP3 is a 431 amino acid-long protein encoded by the *FOXP3* gene comprising of 12 exons (located on the X chromosome at q11.3–13.3) [18]. *FOXP3* gene is a member of a large family of 44 genes that encode for forkhead box/winged-helix transcription factors, named after *forkhead* gene in *Drosophila melanogaster* [19]. The name *forkhead* was used because mutations in this gene, cloned in the late 1980s, led to head shape abnormalities in the fruit fly [20]. The term winged-helix is derived from the crystal structure of the DNA-binding domain of these transcription factors that consists of about 100-odd amino acids with high sequence homology [21]. The *FOXP* subfamily is unique from most other *FOX* subfamilies as it has a DNA-binding domain located at C-terminus (rather than N-terminus) and can bind to two molecules of DNA by protein dimerization through domain-swapping [22, 23]. This could confer a greater ability of transcriptional regulation to this subfamily [24].

Among the FoxP subfamily, FoxP3 dimers are the most stable which additionally highlights its role as a transcriptional regulator. The hinge-loop region of FoxP3 contains the hydrophobic aromatic amino acid, phenylalanine, at position 373 that increases the dimer stability as compared to other subfamily members that contain polar tyrosine residue at the corresponding amino acid position [25]. In addition to its capability to form homodimers, FoxP3 can form multiprotein complexes that can regulate both gene activation and repression. More than 350 associated proteins have already been identified that include other transcription factors such as IKZF1, NFAT, and GATA-3 [26]. This complex networking of various proteins with FoxP3 is required for Treg cell development and functioning. Epigenetic modifications, microRNAs, and transcription factors such as FoxO1, FoxO3, and c-Rel have in turn been implicated in regulating the expression of *FOXP3* gene in Treg cells [27].

5 Phenotype of Treg cells

There are several canonical markers expressed on Treg cells that distinguish these cells from other T lymphocytes. FoxP3 is a definite marker for screening of functional Treg cells (commonly labeled as $CD4^+CD25^+FoxP3^+$ Treg cells). However, few studies have shown that IL-7 receptor or CD127 gets downregulated in $CD4^+FoxP3^+$ cells [28]. Therefore, a combination of $CD4^+CD25^+CD127^-$ cell surface markers may also represent Treg cells [28]. Several other markers have also been characterized for the specific screening of Treg cells. CD25 is a crucial marker for the suppressive Treg cells as has been studied in thymectomized mice. Moreover, strong presence of CD45RO has been observed in the $CD25^{high}$ regulatory cells, unlike naïve T cells that express CD45RA. The function of $CD4^+CD25^{high}$ cells has appeared critical in maintaining self-tolerance and regulating the fate of autoreactive T cells. Though the above-mentioned markers are sufficient for immunophenotyping of Treg cells, but to understand and interlink Treg cell functions, various other markers involved in the activation, maintenance, and inhibition of Treg cells are also important (Table 1). In vitro and in vivo studies have revealed the role of a few inhibitory molecules governing the suppressive function of Treg cells such as Ox40 and 4-1BB, especially applicable to tumor immunity. In contrast to the function of Ox-40 and 4-1BB, the neuropilin-1 receptor potentiates the Treg cell function in vitro and may act at inflammatory sites in vivo [29].

Various markers of Treg cells have been described in Table 1 and Fig. 2.

TABLE 1 Intracellular and extracellular markers of T regulatory cells.

Marker	Cellular location	Function
FoxP3	Intracellular	Master regulator of T regulatory cells
CD127	Extracellular	Negative regulator of T regulatory cells
CD4	Extracellular	T helper cell marker
CD25	Extracellular	Expressed on activated Treg Cells
CTLA-4 (CD152)	Extracellular	Transmits an inhibitory signal to T cells. Expressed in high levels in Treg cells
Neuropilin-1 (CD304)	Extracellular	Required for the stability of Treg cells
Glycoprotein A repetitions predominant (GARP)	Extracellular	Serves as a receptor for latent TGF-β in the surface of activated Tregs (CD4+, CD25+, FoxP3+ cells)
CD39	Extracellular	Activated Treg cells. Implicated in the suppressive function of Treg cells. Stronger stability and function under inflammatory conditions
LAG3 (CD223)	Extracellular	Maintenance of active Treg cell subsets
Latency-associated peptide (LAP)	Extracellular	Immunosuppressive TGFbeta-mediated function
Ox40 (CD134)	Extracellular	Reduce the FoxP3 expression leading to abrogation of Treg mediated suppression
4-1BB	Extracellular	Inhibit Treg cells by blocking IL-9 production

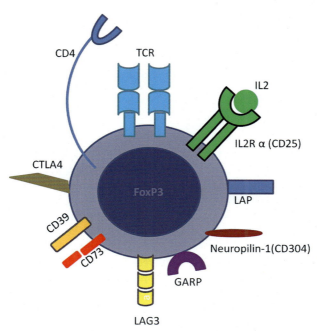

FIG. 2 Phenotype of T regulatory cells.

6 Treg/T cell subtypes with regulatory function

6.1 Follicular Treg cells

Follicular regulatory T cells (fTreg) are a subset of FoxP3$^+$ Treg cells that resemble follicular T helper cells in their expression of certain cell surface markers (CXCR5, ICOS) and transcriptional regulator Bcl6 [30]. These cells are able to access B cell follicles thereby regulating B cell responses, development of germinal centers, and appear to have a crucial role in the protection against the development of autoimmunity, allergies, or even malignancies [30, 31]. Quantitative alterations, predominantly an increase, in the circulating fTreg cells have been reported in many autoimmune disorders such as systemic lupus erythematosus, primary Sjögren syndrome, rheumatoid arthritis, and ankylosing spondylitis [32]. These contrasting findings need to be interpreted with caution as a majority of the circulating fTregs in humans are CD45RA positive whereas most of the tissue fTregs are negative for CD45RA [33].

6.2 FoxP3 expressing invariant NKT cells

In 2010, Monteiro et al. identified a population of regulatory invariant natural killer T cells (iNKT) in mice with immunosuppressive properties. These cells express FoxP3, CD25, and cytotoxic T-lymphocyte-associated protein 4 (CTLA4) (similar to Treg cells) and promyelocytic leukemia zinc finger protein (PLZF) characteristic of iNKT cells [34]. Subsequently, human iNKT cells were shown to express FoxP3 and acquire immunosuppressive properties in presence of TGF-β and sirolimus. It was postulated that sirolimus resulted in a positive selection of FoxP3 expressing iNKT cells among other iNKT subsets facilitating their recognition [35]. Additionally, iNKT cell clones have been demonstrated to express FoxP3 upon stimulation with anti-CD3 and PMA-ionomycin [36]. The role of the FoxP3 expressing iNKT cells in human autoimmune diseases is largely unknown [37]. As sirolimus has been speculated to positively select these immunosuppressive cells, future research in this area may have implications in the management of autoimmune diseases.

6.3 FoxP3$^+$ γδT cells

Similar to FoxP3$^+$ iNKT cells, FoxP3$^+$ γδT cells were discovered just more than a decade ago [38, 39]. In humans, these cells with nontransient FoxP3 expression and a specific phenotype (elevated CTLA-4 expression) were derived from CD25 negative helper T cells using antigenic stimulation (TGF-β1 and IL-15) [38]. The capability of these cells to suppress T cell proliferation was also validated subsequently [38, 40] Li et al. showed γδT cells, CD27$^+$CD45RA$^-$γδT cells, and Vδ1 cells to negatively correlate with disease activity in systemic lupus erythematosus although it was noted that only CD27$^+$CD45RA$^-$Vδ1 cells expressed FoxP3 [40]. The data on the correlation of this specific subset of FoxP3$^+$ γδT cells with disease activity was, however, unavailable. Further research is required to elucidate the role of these cells in autoimmune diseases. Recently, vitamin C was shown to facilitate the generation of regulatory FoxP3$^+$ γδT cells via alteration of DNA methylation pattern of various genes [41]. Although, vitamin C has been said to have immunomodulatory effects [42] more data are required to elucidate the clinical significance of this observation.

6.4 Double-negative regulatory T cells

An increasing number of studies are demonstrating the double-negative T (DNT) cells ($TCR\alpha\beta^+CD4^-CD8^-$) to have an effective immune regulatory function. These cells suppress $CD4^+$ T cell proliferation and modulate $CD4^+$ T cell function. Suppression of mTOR mediated signaling is among the several important mechanisms elucidated till date for the function of DN Treg cells [43]. Hyperactivity of mTOR signaling in DNT cells has been implicated to be a key pathogenic mechanism underlying the pathogenesis of autoimmune lymphoproliferative syndrome (ALPS) [44]. However, contrary to the previous thought, recent data may reflect the elevated peripheral blood percentage or tissue infiltration by DNT cells to be a secondary regulatory homeostatic response rather than the primary pathogenic mechanism. Increased rate of DNT cell apoptosis on administration of sirolimus in patients with ALPS could then be explained by its effect on the abnormally proliferating $CD4^+$ T cells that could potentially result in abatement of regulatory homeostatic cascades resulting in DNT cell proliferation. The efficacy of sirolimus in monogenic illnesses presenting with an ALPS-like phenotype that has normal DNT cells [45] favors the concept that elevated mTOR activity in $CD4^+$ T cells rather than the DNTs may be the primary disease-causing mechanism.

6.5 Th3 cells

Th3 cells are a subset of induced Treg cells that have been reported to be maintained in an inverse relationship with the proinflammatory Th17 cells. A transitional phenotype has also been described that expresses characteristics of both Treg cells (FoxP3) and Th17 cells (RORγt and RORα) [46]. These cells that are believed to be $CD4^+CD25^-FoxP3^-$ latency-associated peptide (LAP)$^+$ were discovered about three decades ago and play a vital role in maintaining tolerance to ingested antigens [47]. LAP is a membrane-bound propeptide that binds to TGF-β and Helios has been suggested to be a marker of $CD4^+LAP^+$ Tregs [48]. There is a paucity of data with regard to the role of these Treg cells in the pathogenesis of autoimmune diseases.

6.6 Tr1 cells

Among the various subsets of Treg cells, Tr1 cells are by far the earliest to be identified (in the late 1980s) [49]. These induced $CD4^+$ T cells are characterized by production of IL-10, TGF-β, IFN-γ, and IL-5, in vivo suppressive capabilities, expression of (at least on a subset of Tr1 cells) LAG-3 (lymphocyte activation gene-3) and CD49b (an integrin), and lack of a stable expression of FoxP3 and CD25 [49, 50]. Decreased Tr1 cells have been documented in patients with a variety of autoimmune diseases including multiple sclerosis, psoriasis, rheumatoid arthritis, type 1 diabetes mellitus, Graves' disease, and Hashimoto's thyroiditis [51]. Infusion of ovalbumin-specific Tr1 cells has already been employed in patients with refractory Crohn's disease with promising results [52]. However, long-term data regarding the safety (including bystander immune effects) and outcome are lacking. Extensive research is required in the future regarding Tr1 cell therapy in autoimmune diseases.

4. Regulatory T cells in autoimmunity and potential therapeutic targets

7 Protocols for estimation of Treg cells in the peripheral blood

Treg cells may be assessed using distinct extracellular markers [positive (CD3, CD4, CD25) and negative (CD127)] and by assessing the intracellular transcription factor FoxP3. CD3 identifies T cell receptors, CD4 identifies T helper cell subsets, and CD25 identifies activated cells whereas low/null CD127 expression identifies Treg cells. A combination of CD3, CD4, CD25, and CD127 requires a surface staining protocol. However, a combination of CD3, CD4, CD25, and FoxP3 requires surface as well as intracellular staining protocols. Intracellular staining is performed using additional steps of fixation and permeabilization followed by intracellular staining. Fixation retains targeted proteins at their original cellular locations and permeabilization is required to transport the intracellular antibodies through the plasma membrane for binding to the target protein.

7.1 Surface staining protocol ($CD4^+CD25^+CD127^{-/low}$)

1. Microfuge the monoclonal antibodies (mAbs) reagent vials before experiments.
2. Add pretitered mAbs in the $100\,\mu L$ volume of cells.
3. Mix the cell-mAb cocktail by vortexing for nearly 3s or pipetting up and down 10 times.
4. Incubate the cell-mAb cocktail for 30min.
5. Wash the cells by adding wash buffer.
6. Centrifuge tubes for 10min at 1100 revolution per minute (rpm).
7. Decant the tubes for discarding the supernatant.
8. The tube now is ready to be acquired in flow cytometry.

7.2 Intracellular staining protocol ($CD4^+CD25^+FoxP3^+$)

1. Surface staining protocol until point-7 would be applicable for intracellular staining.
2. Fixation/permeabilization: Add $1\,\mu L$ of Fix/Perm buffer for tubes.
3. Vortex the mixture for 3s or pipetting up-down for 10 times.
4. Incubate the mixture for 45min at ambient temperature/as per the manufacturer's protocol.
5. Centrifuge the tubes for 8min a 4°C and decant the supernatant.
6. Blocking: Add blocking reagent as per instruction.
7. Vortex the mixture for 3s or pipetting up-down for 10 times.
8. Incubate the mixture for 15min.
9. Intracellular staining: microfuge the mAbs.
10. Add fluorescently labeled mAbs to the mixture.
11. Vortex the mixture for 3s or pipetting up-down for 10 times.
12. Incubate the cell-mAb cocktail for 30min.
13. Wash the cells by adding wash buffer and decant the supernatant.
14. Add $200\,\mu L$ fixative (1%) and vortex the mixture for 3s or pipetting up-down for 10 times.
15. Keep the tubes in dark at 4°C until acquiring flow cytometry.

16. Gating strategy.
    (i) Identification of $CD3^+CD4^+$ T helper subsets.
    (ii) Identification of activated T cell subsets through $CD4^+CD25^+$.
    (iii) Displaying CD25 versus $CD127^-$ or $FoxP3^+$ would be the Treg cell populations.

8 Isolation of Treg cells for therapeutic purposes

Umbilical cord blood (UCB) [53], peripheral blood [54], or thymus [55] may be used to isolate the Treg cells either by depletion of $CD8^+$ and/or $CD19^+$ cells followed by enrichment of $CD25^+$ cells. For this procedure magnetic associated cell sorter (MACS) from Miltenyi Biotec is preferred. However, the purified fraction has been reported to have approximately 80% of $FoxP3^+$ cells [56]. Alternatively, Treg cells may also be purified by sorting of cells based on extracellular markers ($CD4^+$, $CD25^+$, $FoxP3^+$, or CD127, $CD45RA^+$) with enhanced purified fraction [57]. The $CD4^+CD25^+CD127^-$ based sorting results in a highly purified (>99%) fraction of Tregs. However, to obtain epigenetically stable and Th17 conversion resistant cells another gating for $CD45RA^+$ has also been performed [58]. Another strategy to obtain higher number of Tregs is expansion with anti-CD3/CD28-coated beads in the presence of IL2. Rapamycin is used as suppressor of mammalian target of rapamycin (mTOR) protein kinase, which results in the inhibition of T effector cells. It also favors upregulation of FoxP3 expressing T cells by blocking AkT–mTOR-SMAD3 pathway [59]. Mathew et al. developed rapamycin, IL2, and TGF-β-dependent Treg expansion protocol [60].

9 Tissue-resident Treg cells

In addition to the two main subtypes of Treg cells, i.e., central Treg cells (that are primarily located in lymphoid tissues and express homing molecules such as CD62L and CCR7) and effector Treg cells (that are primarily located outside lymphoid tissue and downregulate homing molecules and upregulate activation receptors), there is another specialized group of Treg cells that are primarily located in extra lymphoid tissues (known as tissue-resident Treg cells). Tissue-resident Tregs may have tissue-specific expression of molecules and a unique phenotype and function. These cells have been reported to be present in the skin, intestine, adipose tissue, muscle, and central nervous system (CNS) [61, 62] and have a crucial role in maintaining the local tissue homeostasis.

Visceral adipose tissue (VAT) Tregs are specialized cells critical for insulin sensitivity in the adipose tissues. Studies suggest a higher proportion (up to 50%) of $CD4^+$ FoxP3 expressing Treg cells in the visceral fat. Phenotypically VAT-Tregs have shown differential expression of various markers, e.g., higher levels of CD25, CTLA-4, FoxP3, and reduced levels of CCL5 and CXCR3 [63]. VAT-Tregs were found to be reduced in obese people and led to an insulin-resistant state. Animal studies have shown that adipose tissue depleted of tissue-resident Treg cells delays the onset of age-associated insulin resistance but does not affect the obesity-associated insulin resistance.

Intestine is reported to have at least three different subsets of Treg cells: (a) $GATA3^+Helios^+(Nrp1^+)$ (b) retinoic acid receptor-related orphan receptor γt (RORγt) expressing $RORγt^+Helios^-$ and, (c) $RORγt^-Nrp1^-(Helios^-)$ subsets. Intestine-specific Tregs express a variety of proteins concerned with tissue repair [64]. Another higher proportion (20%–30%) of resident Treg cells populate in the human skin. Cutaneous Tregs share less TCRβ sequences than conventional Tregs. These tissue-resident Treg cells have several unique phenotypic characteristics and have an important role to play in the pathogenesis of autoimmune cutaneous diseases such as psoriasis [65].

10 Clinical and translational significance of Treg cells

Treg cells have an important function of maintaining immune homeostasis and this is particularly achieved by inhibiting the function of effector T cells. An abnormality in the number or function of Treg cells may lead to an overactive and aberrant immune response and may predispose individuals to develop autoimmune and autoinflammatory complications. Herein, the role of Treg cells in the pathogenesis of autoimmune diseases is reviewed.

10.1 Systemic lupus erythematosus (SLE)

SLE is the prototypic autoimmune disease characterized clinically by multisystem involvement and the presence of autoantibodies. Treg cells have been reported to have an important role in the pathogenesis of SLE. Studies have shown that patients with active SLE have a significantly lower proportion of Treg cells as compared to patients with inactive disease and healthy controls. Treg cells had an inverse correlation with the SLE disease activity index (SLEDAI) [66–68]. However, several authors have reported no significant difference in peripheral blood Treg cells in patients with SLE. A recent meta-analysis published in 2018 critically analyzed various subsets of Treg cells in patients with SLE [69]. Pooled analysis of 44 different studies showed that the definition of Treg cells (depending on the status of CD127, CD25, and FoxP3 expression) was variably used in different studies. When Treg cells were compared in patients with SLE as compared to healthy controls (irrespective of the definition used to label Treg cells), there was no difference in Treg cells between the two groups. On subgroup analysis, it was observed that in studies where CD25 positivity (CD25$^+$ or CD25^{high}) was used as a marker to define Treg cells, these cells were found to be reduced in patients with SLE as compared to controls. Similarly, when CD127 negativity was used as a marker to define Treg cells, a significant difference was observed between patients with SLE and controls. However, in studies that used FoxP3 positivity as a marker for Treg cells (irrespective of the status of CD25 or CD127), no significant difference was observed between patients and controls. Rather a few studies in the latter case showed higher Treg cells in patients with SLE as compared to controls [69]. When Treg cells were compared between patients with active and inactive disease (irrespective of the criteria to define Treg cells), these cells were found to be reduced in patients with active disease.

Few animal studies have suggested the role of Treg cells in the pathogenesis of SLE. Humrich et al. studied Treg cells in the NZBxNZW- F(1) mouse model of lupus and showed a reduced poll of Treg cells in the lymphoid organs and an imbalance of conventional T cells and Treg cells [70]. It was also observed that these Treg cells were functionally active and were capable of controlling the conventional T cells. Exogenous administration of IL-2 led to a proliferation of Treg cells and restored the balance between conventional T cells and Treg cells [70]. These data support the therapeutic efficacy of the use of IL-2 in patients with SLE to restore the homeostasis of immune system and control the disease.

Pathogenic role of Treg cells in patients with SLE is also suggested by studies that have used sirolimus, a potential inhibitor of the mammalian target of rapamycin (mTOR), for the management of this disease. mTOR pathway is a potential inhibitor of Treg cell proliferation and inhibition of mTOR pathway using sirolimus has been shown to increase the proportion of Treg cells and clinical improvement in patients with SLE [71–73].

Similarly, the immunomodulatory effect of 25-hydroxyvitamin D or vitamin D has also been assessed in patients with SLE. Vitamin D supplementation has been reported to increase the Treg cells and decrease the Th17 cells in patients with active SLE and has been found to improve the disease activity as well [74–79].

10.2 Type 1 diabetes mellitus (T1DM)

T1DM is a chronic autoimmune condition characterized by the destruction of pancreatic β-cells primarily mediated by T and B cells. In vivo nonobese diabetic (NOD) mouse model has revealed the crucial role of Treg cell in the pathogenesis of DM and suggested Treg cell-based therapeutic strategies or adoptive transfer approaches. Moreover, the susceptible loci (*IL2RA, IL2, PTPN2, CTLA4*, and *IL10*) identified through genome-wide association studies (GWASs) are known to influence Treg cell function. Based on these observations, $CD4^+CD127^{low/-}CD25^+$ polyclonal Treg cell-based therapies have been tried in phase I (NCT01210664) clinical trial.

10.3 Common variable immunodeficiency (CVID)

CVID is clinically characterized by the presence of recurrent sinopulmonary infections, lymphadenopathy, lymphoproliferation, and autoimmunity. It is known to be in association with hypogammaglobulinemia and B cell differentiation defects. A quarter of CVID cases also suffer from autoimmune manifestations [80]. Autoimmune cytopenias are the most frequent autoimmune condition in CVID. Few studies have reported the role of Treg cells in the pathogenesis of CVID [81–85]. Moreover, specific clinical manifestations including autoimmunity and splenomegaly have been associated with a markedly reduced number of Treg cells (Table 2). Recent studies indicate a higher proportion of monogenic defects in CVID especially in patients who have early-onset disease with autoimmune and autoinflammatory complications. Haploinsufficiency of CTLA-4 and deficiency of lipopolysaccharide (LPS)-responsive and beige-like anchor protein (LRBA) are the common monogenic causes of CVID and have been reported to have a reduction in the proportion and function of Treg cells [86]. CTLA-4 and LRBA proteins exert similar effects on Treg cells.

10.4 IPEX syndrome

As mentioned previously, IPEX syndrome is the human equivalent of *scurfy* in mice. Experiments following the landmark discovery of male *scurfy* in 1949 and the exceptional female *scurfy* in 1950 resulted in the elucidation of sex-linked inheritance in mice [87, 88].

TABLE 2 A review of studies showing the role of Treg cells in the pathogenesis of common variable immunodeficiency (CVID).

S. No	Author, year, and country	Clinical condition	Analysis	Markers	Outcome
1	López-Herrera et al. 2019, Mexico [81]	CVID patients with autoimmune diseases	Autoimmune manifestation and Treg cell association	CD4$^+$CD25$^+$CD127^{low} and CD4$^+$CD25$^+$FoxP3$^+$	Study reported autoimmune (AI) manifestations in 39%. AI included Autoimmune thrombocytopenia (31%), Vitiligo (6%), systemic lupus erythematosus (3%), and multiple sclerosis (1%). CVID cases with AI had a reduced proportion of Tregs (Both CD127- and FoxP3$^+$) AI group also had expanded CD21^{low} B cell populations
2	Melo et al. 2009, Brazil [82]	CVID	Treg cells proportion and immune activation	CD4$^+$CD25^{high}FOXP3 T cells for Tregs and CD38$^+$ and HLA-DR$^+$ as activation markers	Significantly lowered proportion of CD4$^+$CD25^{high}FOXP3$^+$ Tregs No significant correlation between Treg and immune activation was found
3	Fevang et al. 2007, Norway [83]	CVID patients with splenomegaly	Association of Tregs and chronic inflammation	CD4$^+$CD25^{high}FOXP3$^+$	The lowered proportion of Tregs accompanied by reduced mRNA expression. CVID cases with splenomegaly had even lower Tregs Negative correlation of Treg to inflammatory markers
4	Yesillik et al. 2019, USA [84]	CVID	To evaluate CD4$^+$ Treg and CD8$^+$ Treg cells in CVID patients	nCD4$^+$ Treg (CD4$^+$CD127^{low} CD25^{high}FoxP3$^+$)	Various Tregs (nTreg/iTregs) were reduced CD8$^+$ CD25high CD183$^+$ FoxP3$^+$ Tregs were also reduced
5	Arandi et al. 2013, Iran [85]	CVID patients with autoimmunity	Treg cells	CD4$^+$CD25^{high}FOXP3$^+$	Markedly reduced Tregs in CVID cases with autoimmunity and diminished iTreg markers cytotoxic T-lymphocyte-associated protein 4 (CTLA4) and Glucocorticoid-induced tumor necrosis factor receptor (TNFR) (GITR) were found to have lowered expression on Treg cells

Similar clinical phenotype in humans was first reported in 1982 when Powell et al. described an X-linked syndrome with recurrent infections and a myriad of autoimmune manifestations including enteropathy, immune hemolytic anemia, type I diabetes mellitus, and autoimmune thyroiditis. Out of the eight patients described, the fatal outcome in infancy or early childhood was noted in six. In addition, 11 other male children in the kindred had already succumbed due to a similar illness [89]. Over the years, IPEX syndrome has emerged as one of the most notable monogenic multisystem autoimmune disorders with more than 300 mutation-proven cases reported till date [90]. Qualitative defects in Treg cells (with or without quantitative defects) are the central pathogenic mechanism in IPEX syndrome. Although patients with IPEX syndrome may have normal proportion of Treg cells, overall, the proportion of Treg cells has been shown to be lower as compared to healthy controls. Very rarely, high Treg proportions have been reported in patients with IPEX syndrome which may be a reflection of Treg cell dysfunction [91]. Functional analyses of Treg cells have suggested decreased suppressive function and even conversion of these cells from suppressive to a proinflammatory phenotype [92, 93]. Qualitative defects in Treg cells in IPEX syndrome result in aberrant effector T cell distribution and amassing of self-reactive B cells [94, 95]. These immunologic abnormalities result in multisystem autoimmunity often in the presence of a variety of autoantibodies such as antiislet cells, antiinsulin, antiglutamic acid decarboxylase, antithyroglobulin, antithyroid peroxidase, antienterocyte, antivillin, antiharmonin, antismooth muscle, and antimicrosomal antibodies [90].

Long-term, often a combination, immunosuppressive therapy with or without hematopoietic stem cell transplantation (HSCT) is the most common treatment protocol employed in patients with IPEX. Corticosteroids, sirolimus, and calcineurin inhibitors, which are among the most common agents used, seem to show the maximum clinical benefit [91, 96]. Although HSCT is the only therapy that can prove to be curative and recent studies have shown promising results, data definitively asserting the superiority of early HSCT over chronic immunosuppressive therapy are lacking. Additionally, (poly)endocrinopathy may persist post HSCT [90, 91, 96, 97].

10.5 Other inborn errors of immunity with Treg dysfunction

In addition to IPEX, many other inborn errors of immunity have been known to be associated with Treg cell abnormalities. Notably, these include mutations in *DOCK8*, *IKBKB*, *STAT5B* (autosomal recessive form), *IL2RA* (CD25), *IL2RB* (CD122), *CTLA4*, *LRBA*, *DEF6*, *STAT3* (autosomal dominant gain of function form), *BACH2*, *CD70*, and *CARMIL2* [98]. Together with *FOXP3*, these gene defects may be collectively grouped under the umbrella term "Tregopathies" [99]. These genetic defects may have IPEX-like clinical presentation and/or multiple autoimmune manifestations along with Treg cell abnormalities and are summarized below:

10.5.1 *DOCK8 deficiency*

DOCK8 (dedicator of cytokinesis 8) deficiency is a combined inborn error of immunity that usually presents with cutaneous viral and bacterial infections, recurrent sinopulmonary infections, and atopic manifestations. These patients may also develop autoimmune manifestations such as cytopenias, vasculitis, endocrinopathy, and systemic lupus erythematosus

[100]. In 2014, Janssen et al. described the presence of a multitude of autoantibodies (in variable titres) in 22 patients with *DOCK8* deficiency. Additionally, they demonstrated decreased proportion of Treg cells with impaired suppressive capabilities [101]. Subsequently, Alroqi et al. described few patients with *DOCK8* deficiency who had IPEX-like clinical manifestations with the presence of chronic diarrhea, eczematous rash, and Treg cell dysfunction [102]. A number of mechanisms have been postulated to explain Treg dysfunction in *DOCK8* deficiency which includes the impaired formation of the immunological synapse (via aberrancies in remodeling of actin cytoskeleton), impaired STAT3/5 activation, and impaired IL-2 signaling [102, 103].

10.5.2 IκBKβ deficiency

Mutations in *IKBKB* gene (which encodes for inhibitor of nuclear factor-kappa B kinase subunit beta (IκBKβ)) result in combined immunodeficiency that usually present in infancy with persistent oral thrush, disseminated Bacillus Calmette–Guérin (BCG) disease, viral infections, and bacterial sepsis commonly caused by Gram-negative organisms [104–107]. These patients also have low to absent peripheral Treg cells; [104, 105] however, autoimmune manifestations have not been reported. Profound immunodeficiency (resembling severe combined immune deficiency (SCID)) affecting the adaptive and innate immunity in these patients resulting in early death [106, 107] before the development of autoimmune manifestations may be the likely explanation. Secondly, only homozygous nonsense or frameshift mutations have been reported; hypomorphic missense or compound heterozygous mutations, which may result in autoimmune manifestations (as in the case of hypomorphic SCID) have not been reported till date.

10.5.3 CD25 deficiency

In 1997, even before the first mutation-proven case of IPEX syndrome was published, Sharfe et al. reported a mutation-proven case of CD25/IL2RA (Interleukin 2 Receptor Subunit Alpha) deficiency. This child had been symptomatic since the age of 6 months with cytomegalovirus (CMV) pneumonitis and esophageal/oropharyngeal candidiasis. However, data on autoimmune manifestations and Tregs were unavailable [108]. The second patient was reported 10 years later by Caudy et al. with an IPEX syndrome-like clinical presentation (with the following autoimmune manifestations—enteropathy, hemolytic anemia, neutropenia, and hypothyroidism). The proportion of FoxP3$^+$ cells was normal; however, IL-10 expression was markedly reduced [109]. Goudy et al. reported the third patient in 2013 who, similar to the second case, also had IPEX-like clinical presentation, absence of CD25 expression on CD4$^+$ T cells, and normal proportion of Treg cells [110]. The autoimmune manifestations are seen in CD25 deficiency, hence, appear to be the result of dysfunctional Treg cells.

10.5.4 CD122 deficiency

In 2001, an infant with CD122/IL2RB (Interleukin 2 Receptor Subunit Beta) deficiency was reported with a T$^-$B$^+$NK$^-$ SCID-like phenotype. Although no mutation in *IL2RB* gene was reported, there was a markedly reduced expression of IL-2Rβ on flow cytometry, western blot, and northern blot analysis [111]. In 2019, a total of 10 mutation-proven cases of *CD122* deficiency were reported for the first time [112]. In contrast to *CD25* deficiency, these patients had marked reductions in Treg cell population. A number of autoimmune manifestations have been reported in these patients including direct Coombs test positive hemolytic anemia, lymphocytic infiltration of lungs, skin, and other organs, autoimmune thyroid disease, enteropathy, elevated antineutrophil cytoplasmic antibodies (ANCA) titres with/without vasculitis, elevated antinuclear antibody (ANA) and antismooth muscle antibody titres. Additionally, these patients develop florid CMV or Epstein–Barr virus (EBV) disease [112].

10.5.5 *CARMIL2 deficiency*

CARMIL2 (capping protein regulator and myosin 1 linker 2) deficiency manifests as cutaneous viral infections (such as human papillomavirus, molluscum contagiosum, and herpesviruses), noninfectious dermatitis, and EBV positive smooth muscle tumors [113]. Among the various immunologic abnormalities seen in patients with CARMIL2 deficiency, profound reduction in the Treg cell population has been reported [113]. Autoimmune manifestations have occasionally been reported in patients with CARAMIL deficiency and have been attributed to defective CD28-mediated costimulatory signaling [113].

10.6 Rheumatoid arthritis (RA)

RA is a systemic autoimmune disease characterized by the presence of inflammatory and destructive arthritis. Pathogenesis of RA is not clear. However, it is believed to be due to an abnormality in the adaptive arm of the immune system with the role of both B and T cells. T helper cells have been found to play an important role in causing cartilage damage in patients with RA [114]. However, there have been conflicting observations with regard to the number and proportion of circulating Treg cells in patients with RA and their role in the pathogenesis of this disease. While few studies have shown that Treg cells are decreased in patients with RA as compared to control [115–117] others have shown these cells to be normal or increased [118, 119]. Contrary to the belief, most studies have consistently shown that Treg cells are increased in the synovium of patients with RA as compared to the synovium of healthy controls and the peripheral blood of patients with RA [116–118]. This observation is quite intriguing and questions the role of Treg cells in the pathogenesis of RA. One may ask that despite the presence of excess Treg cells in the synovium, why are these cells unable to control the local inflammation? There may be several explanations for excess of Treg cells in the synovium of inflamed joints. One, FoxP3 may transiently be expressed on conventional T cells especially during inflammation and it may be speculated that excess of apparently looking Treg cells in synovium is actually T helper cells that have transiently acquired FoxP3 expression. Second, Treg cells have a property of plasticity and may assume the role of effector T cells and lose the ability of suppressive function under inflammatory conditions. Walter et al. studied the $CD4^+CD45RO^+CD25^+CD127^{low}$ T cells (memory Treg cells) in the peripheral blood and synovial fluid of patients with RA and carried out the in vitro activation of healthy $CD4^+CD45RO^+CD25^+CD127^{low}$ T cells (memory Treg cells) by activated monocytes using anti-CD3 monoclonal antibodies. It was observed that memory Treg cells and activated monocytes were higher in synovial fluid as compared to peripheral blood. On activating the memory Treg cells using monocytes, there was increased percentage of IL-17, IFN-γ, and TNF-α positive Treg cells as well as the IL-10 positive Treg cells. Despite excess cytokine expression, these cells maintained their suppressive phenotype. Therefore, it appears that excess Treg cells maintain their suppressive phenotype in the inflamed environment of synovium and uncontrolled inflammation could be related to the effector T cell population that becomes resistant to suppressive actions of Treg cells [120]. However, it has also been observed that there may be differences in the in vitro properties of Treg cells as was seen in the experiments by Walter et al. and in vivo properties of Treg cells seen in the real-life environment of the synovium, which is under control of several other factors [121]. It is possible that in vivo, the Treg cells are ineffective in suppressing the activity of antigen-presenting cells, and because of the plasticity, there is loss of function [121]. It has also been observed that inflamed synovium abnormally phosphorylate FoxP3 resulting in the abnormal suppressive effects of Treg cells [122]. Nie et al. observed specific dephosphorylation at Ser418 position of the C-terminal DNA-binding domain of FoxP3 transcription factor by enzyme protein phosphatase 1 (PPT1). The enzyme was found to be induced in the synovium niche in the presence of tumor necrosis factor α (TNF-α), which ultimately resulted in the reduction of Treg function. Indeed, treatment with TNF-α antibody restored the Treg cell functions [122, 123].

A recent study by Avdeeva et al. published in 2020 evaluated the peripheral blood Treg cells and their activation markers in patients with untreated RA and patients who received methotrexate. It was observed that Treg cell number, proportion, and activation markers were reduced in patients with untreated RA. These abnormalities were found to be correlated with antibody levels and the severity of the disease. On initiating treatment with methotrexate, these abnormalities tend to get better.

Although there have been several published reports on the role of Treg cells in the pathogenesis of RA, the results of these studies are variable. Based on these studies, it may be hypothesized that Treg cells have a role in the pathogenesis of RA. However, whether they control effector T cells in the synovium or these Treg cells change their phenotype in the synovium to a stronger proinflammatory phenotype is a question that needs to be answered by doing more studies.

10.7 Inflammatory bowel disease (IBD)

Treg cells are crucial for maintaining gut homeostasis and preventing an immune response against commensal flora and dietary antigens. Similar to RA, it has been observed that Treg cells are reduced in the peripheral blood of patients with IBD while these cells are increased in the intestinal tissue [124–129]. However, it is not known that how Treg cells function in the intestinal tissue of patients with IBD. It may be hypothesized that effector T cells may become resistant to the inhibitory action of Treg cells in the inflammatory milieu of the intestine or Treg cells have lost their ability to cause suppression. Treg cells may also be irreversibly converted to the Th17 phenotype [130–132]. Intact TGF-β signaling is required for optimal functioning of Treg cells and inhibition of effector T cells. However, this signaling is inhibited by the upregulation of an inflammatory molecule Smad-7 in the inflamed bowel [133, 134]. Anti-Smad7 antisense oligonucleotide has been found to reverse this inhibition of TGF-β signaling [135].

A recent study by Zhou et al. published in 2019 studied the role of group 3 innate lymphoid cells (ILC3) in supporting the intestinal development of Treg cells via the production of IL-2 [136]. It was observed that MyD88- and Nod2-dependent microbial sensing by macrophages leads to production of IL-1β that further stimulates the production of IL-2 by ILC3. This IL-2 is crucial for survival of Treg cells in the intestine and maintains immunologic homeostasis. In patients with IBD, there may be an impaired ILC3 derived IL-2 production leading to impaired Treg cells and inflammation. This may suggest a therapeutic role of low-dose IL-2 in these patients to control the aberrant inflammation.

Although the potential role of Treg cells in the pathogenesis of IBD, similar to its role in RA, remains speculative, there have been few studies that have assessed the role of Treg cells as potential therapeutic targets in IBD [52]. Canavan et al. demonstrated that $CD4^+CD25^+CD127^{low}CD45RA^+$ Treg cells isolated from patients with Crohn's disease had stable *FOXP3*locus and did not convert to Th17 phenotype in vitro when compared with $CD4^+CD25^+CD127^{low}CD45RA^-$ Treg cells. $CD4^+CD25^+CD127^{low}CD45RA^+$ Treg cells express α4β7 integrin, CD62L, and CCR7, and preferentially tend to accumulate in the small intestine and inhibit the lymphocytes in lamina propria and mesenteric lymph nodes [58]. Thus, $CD4^+CD25^+CD127^{low}CD45RA^+$ Treg cells isolated from patients with Crohn's disease may be the most appropriate cell lines for autologous Treg therapy.

10.8 Multiple sclerosis (MS)

MS has genetically been associated with CTLA-4 and CD25 along with the reduced expression of Treg master regulator FoxP3 as well as IL-10 [137]. Primate studies have shown that the diminished Il-10 levels in active MS cases are restored in inactive stages. The acute stage population of $CD4^+CD25^+$ Tregs was also found to be reduced in MS [138]. Adoptive transfer of Treg cells could be a potential therapy in the management of MS [139].

10.9 Kawasaki disease (KD)

Kawasaki Disease (KD) is a medium vessel vasculitis and the most common cause of acquired heart diseases in children in the developed world. Etiology of KD remains obscure, although clinical and epidemiological features suggest a possible infectious, genetic, and immunological insult. Seasonal change and wind flow have also been associated with KD epidemics. The acute stage in KD leads to alterations in innate and adaptive immune responses. Studies have reported the association of altered Treg cells in KD [140, 141] along with an elevated proportion of antagonistic Th17 cells, cytokines including IL-17, IL-6, and IL-23, and transcription factors including (IL-17A/F, ROR-γt), in the acute phase of KD [141]. These studies report a marked imbalance in the Th17/Treg cell homeostasis in KD. One study on 187 patients with KD analyzed the plasma levels of Th17 cells and Treg-associated cytokines before giving intravenous immunoglobulin, on 3rd day after giving IVIg, and 21 days after giving IVIg. Compared to the febrile control group, a marked increase in IL-17A and IL6 was found in the KD cases. IVIg treatment resulted in elevated proportions of $FoxP3^+$ Treg cells and reduced plasma IL-17A and IL6 levels even at day 21 [142]. Given the proinflammatory nature of Th17 cells and inflammatory conditions in KD, treatment strategies to enhance Treg cells would be of paramount importance [143]. An association between Treg cells abnormalities, IVIg resistant KD, and coronary artery abnormalities have also been reported [144]. Though the mechanism of action of IVIg in KD is not completely understood, recognizing the heavy constant region (Fc) of IgG by Treg cells may be responsible for its immunomodulatory action [145].

4. Regulatory T cells in autoimmunity and potential therapeutic targets

11 Regulatory T cells (Tregs) as potential therapeutic targets

Tregs have a crucial role in suppressing and controlling the function of various effector cells in humans. These effectors cells include T effector cells, neutrophils, monocytes, macrophages, NK cells, and B cells. There are several mechanisms for suppression of these effector cells by Tregs. A few of these include the use of various cytokines such as IL-10, IL-35, and TGF-β and release of perforin and granzymes (direct inhibition), and expression of surface molecules such as CD39/CD73 that depletes ATP from microenvironment and by virtue of high expression of CD25 on Tregs that depletes IL-2 in the microenvironment (indirect inhibition). IL-2 is an important cytokine for survival of various effector cells. In addition, there are several cell-specific mechanisms for suppression of the action of individual effector cells (e.g., increased expression of CD163 (hemoglobin scavenger receptor) and CD206 (mannose scavenger receptor) on monocytes thereby leading to antiinflammatory M2 macrophage phenotype and decreased expression of chemokines such as CXCL1 and CXCL2 on neutrophils thereby leading to decreased tissue infiltration). Several of these effector cells such as monocytes and neutrophils when co-cultured with Tregs produce antiinflammatory cytokines [146].

As several of these effector cells are central to the pathogenesis of autoimmune diseases such as SLE, type 1 DM, pemphigus, and autoimmune manifestations in the context of primary immunodeficiency diseases (e.g., CVID), role of Tregs is now being explored as immunomodulators to controls aberrant immune response and thereby suppressing the autoimmunity [52, 57, 147].

Desreumaux et al. from France evaluated the safety and efficacy of Ovalbumin-specific Treg cells in 20 patients with refractory Crohn's disease in a phase I/IIa, open-label multicentric trial. Infusions of Tregs were well tolerated in most patients and were found to have dose-related efficacy in patients with refractory Crohn's disease activity (assessed using Crohn's Disease Activity Index) (Table 3).

The therapeutic implication of Treg cells in patients with type 1 diabetes mellitus was assessed in two non-randomized trials published in 2014 (Trzonkowska et al.) and 2015 (Bluestone et al.). Trzonkowska et al. [149] showed that polyclonal Tregs cell infusions were safe in children with type 1 DM and were effective in most patients when compared with patients who did not receive Treg infusions. Many children who received Treg infusions were in disease remission and had higher C-peptide levels for at least 1 year following infusions. Bluestone et al. [57] studied the role of ex vivo-expanded autologous $CD4^+CD127^{low/-}CD25^+$ polyclonal Tregs in adult patients with type 1 DM in an open-label, interventional phase I clinical trial. It was observed that one-fourth of all infused Tregs were still present 1 year after infusions while C-peptide was present even 2 years after infusions of Treg cells. However, the clinical efficacy was not assessed in this study (Table 3).

IL-2 is a critical molecule required for the proliferation of Treg cells and even a small concentration of IL-2 can potentially cause proliferation of Treg cells, because of higher expression of IL-2 receptors on these cells. Low-dose IL-2 has been tried therapeutically in autoimmune diseases that are associated with abnormal Treg cell compartments such as SLE, T1DM, and vasculitis. Saadoun et al. studied low-dose IL-2 in 10 patients with hepatitis C virus (HCV) induced vasculitis [151]. It was observed that low-dose IL-2 lead to the proliferation of $CD4^+CD25^{high}FoxP3^+$ Tregs in 10/10and clinical improvement in 8/10 patients. No patient showed a flare of vasculitis and HCV viremia following initiation of treatment.

TABLE 3 Review of studies that have evaluated the clinical implications of Treg cell therapy in autoimmune diseases.

S. no.	Author, year and country	Disease studied	Number of patients	Type of study	Intervention	Results and conclusions
1	Saadoun et al., 2011, France [148]	Hepatitis C virus (HCV) induced vasculitis	10	Prospective open-label, phase1—phase 2a study	one course of IL-2 (1.5 million IU per day) for 5 days, followed by three 5-day courses of 3 million IU per day at weeks 3, 6,9	Proliferation of $CD4^+CD25^{high}FOXP3^+$ Tregs in all and clinical improvement in 8/10 patients. No patient showed flare of vasculitis and HCV viremia following initiation of treatment
2	Desreumaux et al., 2012, France [52]	Refractory Crohn's disease	20	Open-label,single injection, escalating-dose, phase 1/2a clinical study	Ovalbumin-specific Treg cells	Ovalbumin-specific Treg cells were well tolerated and had dose-related efficacy in patients with refractory Crohn's disease assessed using Crohn's Disease Activity Index
3	Hartemann et al., 2013, France [148]	Adults with type 1 diabetes	24	Randomized phase 1/phase 2 study *Four groups*: • Placebo • IL2 (0·33 MIU/day) for 5 days • IL2 (1 MIU/day) for 5 days • IL2 (3 MIU/day) for 5 days	Low-dose IL-2	IL-2 induced a dose-dependent increase in Treg cells which was significantly higher than placebo at all doses. IL-2 therapy was well tolerated in most patients
4	Trzonkowska et al., 2014, Poland [149]	Children with type 1 diabetes	12	Nonrandomized trial	Polyclonal Tregs	No serious adverse events At 1-year, 66% of patients were into remission Insulin doses were significantly less and fasting C-peptide levels were significantly higher in Treg treated group as compared to the not-treated group at 4 months and 1 year. Additional Treg infusions provided beneficial effects but the effect was less when compared to first infusion Treg untreated patients continued to remain insulin-dependent and had lower C-peptide levels

Continued

TABLE 3 Review of studies that have evaluated the clinical implications of Treg cell therapy in autoimmune diseases—cont'd

S. no.	Author, year and country	Disease studied	Number of patients	Type of study	Intervention	Results and conclusions
5	Bluestone et al., 2015, United States [57]	Adults with type 1 diabetes	14	Open-label, interventional phase I clinical trial	Ex vivo-expanded autologous $CD4^+CD127lo/-CD25^+$ polyclonal Tregs	25% of adoptively transferred Tregs were present in the circulation even 1 year after infusion and in several patients, C-peptides were present even after 2 years after infusion. Tregs retained a broad phenotype and infusions were well tolerated
6	Dall'Era et al., 2019, United States [150]	1 patient with active cutaneous lupus	1	–	Autologous adoptive Treg cells	Treg cells appeared transiently in circulation and disappeared in 4 weeks followed by an increased concentration of Treg cells in diseased skin tissue. It was accompanied by suppression of IFN-γ pathway and augmentation of IL-17 pathway. No significant clinical recovery

Hartemann et al. studied the safety of IL-2 and increase in Treg cells in response to IL-2 in adult patients with type 2 DM [148]. IL-2 was used in three different doses and was found to be well tolerated. Dose-dependent increase in Treg cells was observed and the response was significantly higher at all doses as compared to placebo. Dall'Era et al. studied the role of IL-2 on cutaneous lupus in one single patient [150]. This study was supposed to be carried out on several patients with cutaneous lupus using dose escalation of Treg cells. However, because of issues with recruitment, only a single patient could be studied. It was observed that after infusing Treg cells, there was a transient appearance of these cells in the periphery followed by a persistent rise in affected skin tissue. In addition, the T cells in skin tissue showed a transition from IFN-γ producing cells to IL-17 producing cells. There was no demonstrable clinical effect.

There have been recent attempts on creating special subsets of Treg cells by modifying one or more of the surface receptors. This is based on the plasticity of Treg cells and as a result of this property, Treg cells fail to work in an inflammatory environment or may sometimes be counter-productive in such situations. These modified Treg cells are therapeutically more active than natural Treg cells. One such cell was created by Chen et al. by reducing the CD126 expression ($CD162^{low/-}$ Treg cells). These cells were found to be more effective in treating colitis and collagen-induced arthritis as compared to $CD126^{high}$ natural Treg cells [152].

In the last few years, several studies have been carried out on the role of Treg cells in autoimmune diseases. While most studies have assessed the safety of the use of Treg cells as a therapeutic modality and have found it to be safe in most patients, there are preliminary data on their clinical efficacy as well. With the available information, it may be too premature to make a judgment about the future prospects of Treg cells as potential therapeutic targets in autoimmune diseases. However, we are likely to get more published literature on the clinical effects of these cells in several autoimmune diseases. At present, there are several ongoing clinical trials on Treg cells in patients with autoimmune diseases including SLE, psoriasis, type 1 DM, inflammatory bowel disease, and Sjögren's syndrome [146, 153]. The results of these trials are still awaited.

12 Conclusion

To conclude, Treg cells appear to have an important role in several autoimmune diseases such as SLE, DM, RA, IBD, KD, IPEX syndrome, and autoimmune manifestations seen in patients with several primary immunodeficiency diseases. However, the pathogenic role of these cells needs to be further explored in the context of autoimmune diseases. Last few years have witnessed several trials on the therapeutic efficacy of Treg cells in several autoimmune diseases. Currently, there are several ongoing trials in this field. Based on the results of these trials, Treg cells may be a potential therapeutic option in several autoimmune manifestations in the next few years.

References

[1] Y. Nishizuka, T. Sakakura, Thymus and reproduction: sex-linked dysgenesis of the gonad after neonatal thymectomy in mice, Science 166 (3906) (1969) 753–755.

4. Regulatory T cells in autoimmunity and potential therapeutic targets

[2] R.K. Gershon, K. Kondo, Cell interactions in the induction of tolerance: the role of thymic lymphocytes, Immunology 18 (5) (1970) 723–737.

[3] R.K. Gershon, P. Cohen, R. Hencin, S.A. Liebhaber, Suppressor T cells, J. Immunol. 108 (3) (1972) 586–590.

[4] M.J. Taussig, Demonstration of suppressor T cells in a population of 'educated' T cells, Nature 248 (5445) (1974) 236–238.

[5] P.J. Baker, N.D. Reed, P.W. Stashak, D.F. Amsbaugh, B. Prescott, Regulation of the antibody response to type III pneumococcal polysaccharide, J. Exp. Med. 137 (6) (1973) 1431–1441.

[6] S. Sakaguchi, N. Sakaguchi, M. Asano, M. Itoh, M. Toda, Immunologic self-tolerance maintained by activated T cells expressing IL-2 receptor alpha-chains (CD25). Breakdown of a single mechanism of self-tolerance causes various autoimmune diseases, J. Immunol. 155 (3) (1995) 1151–1164.

[7] J.D. Fontenot, M.A. Gavin, A.Y. Rudensky, Foxp3 programs the development and function of CD4+CD25+ regulatory T cells, Nat. Immunol. 4 (4) (2003) 330–336.

[8] R. Khattri, T. Cox, S.A. Yasayko, F. Ramsdell, An essential role for Scurfin in CD4+CD25+ T regulatory cells, Nat. Immunol. 4 (4) (2003) 337–342.

[9] S. Hori, Control of regulatory T cell development by the transcription factor Foxp3, Science 299 (5609) (2003) 1057–1061.

[10] T.A. Chatila, F. Blaeser, N. Ho, H.M. Lederman, C. Voulgaropoulos, C. Helms, et al., JM2, encoding a fork head–related protein, is mutated in X-linked autoimmunity–allergic disregulation syndrome, J. Clin. Invest. 106 (12) (2000) R75–R81.

[11] R.S. Wildin, F. Ramsdell, J. Peake, F. Faravelli, J.L. Casanova, N. Buist, et al., X-linked neonatal diabetes mellitus, enteropathy and endocrinopathy syndrome is the human equivalent of mouse scurfy, Nat. Genet. 27 (1) (2001) 18–20.

[12] C.L. Bennett, J. Christie, F. Ramsdell, M.E. Brunkow, P.J. Ferguson, L. Whitesell, et al., The immune dysregulation, polyendocrinopathy, enteropathy, X-linked syndrome (IPEX) is caused by mutations of FOXP3, Nat. Genet. 27 (1) (2001) 20–21.

[13] M.E. Brunkow, E.W. Jeffery, K.A. Hjerrild, B. Paeper, L.B. Clark, S.A. Yasayko, et al., Disruption of a new forkhead/winged-helix protein, scurfin, results in the fatal lymphoproliferative disorder of the scurfy mouse, Nat. Genet. 27 (1) (2001) 68–73.

[14] K. Lahl, C. Loddenkemper, C. Drouin, J. Freyer, J. Arnason, G. Eberl, et al., Selective depletion of Foxp3+ regulatory T cells induces a scurfy-like disease, J. Exp. Med. 204 (1) (2007) 57–63.

[15] S. Sakaguchi, K. Wing, M. Miyara, Regulatory T cells—a brief history and perspective, Eur. J. Immunol. 37 (S1) (2007) S116–S123.

[16] J.D. Fontenot, J.P. Rasmussen, M.A. Gavin, A.Y. Rudensky, A function for interleukin 2 in Foxp3-expressing regulatory T cells, Nat. Immunol. 6 (11) (2005) 1142–1151.

[17] T. Takimoto, Y. Wakabayashi, T. Sekiya, N. Inoue, R. Morita, K. Ichiyama, et al., Smad2 and Smad3 are redundantly essential for the TGF-beta-mediated regulation of regulatory T plasticity and Th1 development, J. Immunol. 185 (2) (2010) 842–855.

[18] R. Bacchetta, F. Barzaghi, M.G. Roncarolo, From IPEX syndrome to *FOXP3* mutation: a lesson on immune dysregulation: IPEX syndrome and *FOXP3*, Ann. N. Y. Acad. Sci. 1417 (1) (2018) 5–22.

[19] M.L. Golson, K.H. Kaestner, Fox transcription factors: from development to disease, Development 143 (24) (2016) 4558–4570.

[20] D. Weigel, G. Jürgens, F. Küttner, E. Seifert, H. Jäckle, The homeotic gene fork head encodes a nuclear protein and is expressed in the terminal regions of the Drosophila embryo, Cell 57 (4) (1989) 645–658.

[21] S. Hannenhalli, K.H. Kaestner, The evolution of fox genes and their role in development and disease, Nat. Rev. Genet. 10 (4) (2009) 233–240.

[22] J.C. Stroud, Y. Wu, D.L. Bates, A. Han, K. Nowick, S. Paabo, et al., Structure of the forkhead domain of FOXP2 bound to DNA, Structure 14 (1) (2006) 159–166.

[23] H.S. Bandukwala, Y. Wu, M. Feuerer, Y. Chen, B. Barboza, S. Ghosh, et al., Structure of a domain-swapped FOXP3 dimer on DNA and its function in regulatory T cells, Immunity 34 (4) (2011) 479–491.

[24] B.C. Jackson, C. Carpenter, D.W. Nebert, V. Vasiliou, Update of human and mouse forkhead box (FOX) gene families, Hum. Genomics 4 (5) (2010). Available from https://humgenomics.biomedcentral.com/articles/10.1186/1479-7364-4-5-345.

[25] K. Perumal, H.W. Dirr, S. Fanucchi, A single amino acid in the hinge loop region of the FOXP Forkhead domain is significant for dimerisation, Protein J. 34 (2) (2015) 111–121.

[26] D. Rudra, P. deRoos, A. Chaudhry, R.E. Niec, A. Arvey, R.M. Samstein, et al., Transcription factor Foxp3 and its protein partners form a complex regulatory network, Nat. Immunol. 13 (10) (2012) 1010–1019.

[27] A. Colamatteo, F. Carbone, S. Bruzzaniti, M. Galgani, C. Fusco, G.T. Maniscalco, et al., Molecular mechanisms controlling Foxp3 expression in health and autoimmunity: from epigenetic to post-translational regulation, Front. Immunol. 10 (2020). Available from: https://www.frontiersin.org/article/10.3389/fimmu.2019.03136/full.

[28] W. Liu, A.L. Putnam, Z. Xu-Yu, G.L. Szot, M.R. Lee, S. Zhu, et al., CD127 expression inversely correlates with FoxP3 and suppressive function of human CD4+ T reg cells, J. Exp. Med. 203 (7) (2006) 1701–1711.

[29] G.M. Delgoffe, S.R. Woo, M.E. Turnis, D.M. Gravano, C. Guy, A.E. Overacre, et al., Stability and function of regulatory T cells is maintained by a neuropilin-1-semaphorin-4a axis, Nature 501 (7466) (2013) 252–256.

[30] P.T. Sage, A.H. Sharpe, T follicular regulatory cells, Immunol. Rev. 271 (1) (2016) 246–259.

[31] R.L. Clement, J. Daccache, M.T. Mohammed, A. Diallo, B.R. Blazar, V.K. Kuchroo, et al., Follicular regulatory T cells control humoral and allergic immunity by restraining early B cell responses, Nat. Immunol. 20 (10) (2019) 1360–1371.

[32] J. Deng, Y. Wei, V.R. Fonseca, L. Graca, D. Yu, T follicular helper cells and T follicular regulatory cells in rheumatic diseases, Nat. Rev. Rheumatol. 15 (8) (2019) 475–490.

[33] V.R. Fonseca, F. Ribeiro, L. Graca, T follicular regulatory (Tfr) cells: dissecting the complexity of Tfr-cell compartments, Immunol. Rev. 288 (1) (2019) 112–127.

[34] M. Monteiro, C.F. Almeida, M. Caridade, J. Ribot, J. Duarte, A. Agua-Doce, et al., Identification of regulatory Foxp3 + invariant NKT cells induced by TGF-β, J. Immunol. 185 (4) (2010) 2157–2163.

[35] L. Moreira-Teixeira, M. Resende, O. Devergne, J.P. Herbeuval, O. Hermine, E. Schneider, et al., Rapamycin combined with TGF-β converts human invariant NKT cells into suppressive Foxp3 + regulatory cells, J. Immunol. 188 (2) (2012) 624–631.

[36] P. Engelmann, K. Farkas, J. Kis, G. Richman, Z. Zhang, C.W. Liew, et al., Characterization of human invariant natural killer T cells expressing FoxP3, Int. Immunol. 23 (8) (2011) 473–484.

[37] H.M. Buechel, M.H. Stradner, L.M. D'Cruz, Stages versus subsets: invariant natural killer T cell lineage differentiation, Cytokine 72 (2) (2015) 204–209.

[38] R. Casetti, C. Agrati, M. Wallace, A. Sacchi, F. Martini, A. Martino, et al., Cutting edge: TGF-β1 and IL-15 induce FOXP3 + γδ regulatory T cells in the presence of antigen stimulation, J. Immunol. 183 (6) (2009) 3574–3577.

[39] N. Kang, L. Tang, X. Li, D. Wu, W. Li, X. Chen, et al., Identification and characterization of Foxp3+ γδ T cells in mouse and human, Immunol. Lett. 125 (2) (2009) 105–113.

[40] X. Li, N. Kang, X. Zhang, X. Dong, W. Wei, L. Cui, et al., Generation of human regulatory γδ T cells by TCRγδ stimulation in the presence of TGF-β and their involvement in the pathogenesis of systemic lupus erythematosus, J. Immunol. 186 (12) (2011) 6693–6700.

[41] L. Kouakanou, C. Peters, Q. Sun, S. Floess, J. Bhat, J. Huehn, et al., Vitamin C supports conversion of human γδ T cells into FOXP3-expressing regulatory cells by epigenetic regulation, Sci. Rep. 10 (1) (2020). Available from http://www.nature.com/articles/s41598-020-63572-w.

[42] S. Mousavi, S. Bereswill, M.M. Heimesaat, Immunomodulatory and antimicrobial effects of vitamin C, Eur. J. Microbiol. Immunol. (Bp) 9 (3) (2019) 73–79.

[43] T. Haug, M. Aigner, M.M. Peuser, C.D. Strobl, K. Hildner, D. Mougiakakos, et al., Human double-negative regulatory T-cells induce a metabolic and functional switch in effector T-cells by suppressing mTOR activity, Front. Immunol. 10 (2019). Available from https://www.frontiersin.org/article/10.3389/fimmu.2019.00883/full.

[44] S. Völkl, A. Rensing-Ehl, A. Allgäuer, E. Schreiner, M.R. Lorenz, J. Rohr, et al., Hyperactive mTOR pathway promotes lymphoproliferation and abnormal differentiation in autoimmune lymphoproliferative syndrome, Blood 128 (2) (2016) 227–238.

[45] A.Z. Banday, A.K. Jindal, R. Tyagi, S. Singh, P.K. Patra, Y. Kumar, et al., Refractory autoimmune cytopenia in a young boy with a novel LRBA mutation successfully managed with sirolimus, J. Clin. Immunol. (2020). Epub ahead of print: 2020 Sep 10; available from: http://link.springer.com/10.1007/s10875-020-00835-1.

[46] R.A. Peterson, Regulatory T-cells: diverse phenotypes integral to immune homeostasis and suppression, Toxicol. Pathol. 40 (2) (2012) 186–204.

[47] H.L. Weiner, A.P. da Cunha, F. Quintana, H. Wu, Oral tolerance: basic mechanisms and applications of oral tolerance, Immunol. Rev. 241 (1) (2011) 241–259.

[48] E. Elkord, M.A. Al Samid, B. Chaudhary, Helios, and not FoxP3, is the marker of activated Tregs expressing GARP/LAP, Oncotarget 6 (24) (2015) 20026–20036.

4. Regulatory T cells in autoimmunity and potential therapeutic targets

[49] M.G. Roncarolo, S. Gregori, R. Bacchetta, M. Battaglia, N. Gagliani, The biology of T regulatory type 1 cells and their therapeutic application in immune-mediated disease, Immunity 49 (6) (2018) 1004–1019.

[50] H. Zeng, R. Zhang, B. Jin, L. Chen, Type 1 regulatory T cells: a new mechanism of peripheral immune tolerance, Cell. Mol. Immunol. 12 (5) (2015) 566–571.

[51] X. Jia, T. Zhai, B. Wang, Q. Yao, Q. Li, K. Mu, et al., Decreased number and impaired function of type 1 regulatory T cells in autoimmune diseases, J. Cell. Physiol. 234 (8) (2019) 12442–12450.

[52] P. Desreumaux, A. Foussat, M. Allez, L. Beaugerie, X. Hébuterne, Y. Bouhnik, et al., Safety and efficacy of antigen-specific regulatory T-cell therapy for patients with refractory Crohn's disease, Gastroenterology 143 (5) (2012) 1207–1217.e2.

[53] N. Safinia, T. Vaikunthanathan, H. Fraser, S. Thirkell, K. Lowe, L. Blackmore, et al., Successful expansion of functional and stable regulatory T cells for immunotherapy in liver transplantation, Oncotarget 7 (7) (2016) 7563–7577.

[54] C.G. Brunstein, J.S. Miller, Q. Cao, D.H. McKenna, K.L. Hippen, J. Curtsinger, et al., Infusion of ex vivo expanded T regulatory cells in adults transplanted with umbilical cord blood: safety profile and detection kinetics, Blood 117 (3) (2011) 1061–1070.

[55] I.E. Dijke, R.E. Hoeppli, T. Ellis, J. Pearcey, Q. Huang, A.N. McMurchy, et al., Discarded human thymus is a novel source of stable and long-lived therapeutic regulatory T cells, Am. J. Transplant. 16 (1) (2016) 58–71.

[56] M. Di Ianni, B. Del Papa, T. Zei, R.I. Ostini, D. Cecchini, M.G. Cantelmi, et al., T regulatory cell separation for clinical application, Transfus. Apher. Sci. 47 (2) (2012) 213–216.

[57] J.A. Bluestone, J.H. Buckner, M. Fitch, S.E. Gitelman, S. Gupta, M.K. Hellerstein, et al., Type 1 diabetes immunotherapy using polyclonal regulatory T cells, Sci. Transl. Med. 7 (315) (2015) 315ra189.

[58] J.B. Canavan, C. Scottà, A. Vossenkämper, R. Goldberg, M.J. Elder, I. Shoval, et al., Developing in vitro expanded CD45RA+ regulatory T cells as an adoptive cell therapy for Crohn's disease, Gut 65 (4) (2016) 584–594.

[59] A.W. Thomson, H.R. Turnquist, G. Raimondi, Immunoregulatory functions of mTOR inhibition, Nat. Rev. Immunol. 9 (5) (2009) 324–337.

[60] J.M. Mathew, J. H-Voss, A. LeFever, I. Konieczna, C. Stratton, J. He, et al., A phase I clinical trial with ex vivo expanded recipient regulatory T cells in living donor kidney transplants, Sci. Rep. 8 (1) (2018) 7428.

[61] A. Sharma, D. Rudra, Emerging functions of regulatory T cells in tissue homeostasis, Front. Immunol. 9 (2018) 883.

[62] J. Lu, H. Meng, A. Zhang, J. Yang, X. Zhang, Phenotype and function of tissue-resident unconventional Foxp3-expressing CD4(+) regulatory T cells, Cell. Immunol. 297 (1) (2015) 53–59.

[63] M. Feuerer, L. Herrero, D. Cipolletta, A. Naaz, J. Wong, A. Nayer, et al., Lean, but not obese, fat is enriched for a unique population of regulatory T cells that affect metabolic parameters, Nat. Med. 15 (8) (2009) 930–939.

[64] C. Schiering, T. Krausgruber, A. Chomka, A. Fröhlich, K. Adelmann, E.A. Wohlfert, et al., The alarmin IL-33 promotes regulatory T-cell function in the intestine, Nature 513 (7519) (2014) 564–568.

[65] R. Sanchez Rodriguez, M.L. Pauli, I.M. Neuhaus, S.S. Yu, S.T. Arron, H.W. Harris, et al., Memory regulatory T cells reside in human skin, J. Clin. Invest. 124 (3) (2014) 1027–1036.

[66] J.C. Crispin, A. Martínez, J. Alcocer-Varela, Quantification of regulatory T cells in patients with systemic lupus erythematosus, J. Autoimmun. 21 (3) (2003) 273–276.

[67] M. Habibagahi, Z. Habibagahi, M. Jaberipour, A. Aghdashi, Quantification of regulatory T cells in peripheral blood of patients with systemic lupus erythematosus, Rheumatol. Int. 31 (9) (2011) 1219–1225.

[68] M. Żabińska, M. Krajewska, K. Kościelska-Kasprzak, K. Jakuszko, D. Bartoszek, M. Myszka, et al., CD4(+) CD25(+)CD127(−) and CD4(+)CD25(+)Foxp3(+) regulatory T cell subsets in mediating autoimmune reactivity in systemic lupus erythematosus patients, Arch. Immunol. Ther. Exp. (Warsz.) 64 (5) (2016) 399–407.

[69] S.X. Zhang, X.W. Ma, Y.F. Li, N.L. Lai, Z.H. Huang, K. Fan, et al., The proportion of regulatory T cells in patients with systemic lupus erythematosus: a meta-analysis, J. Immunol. Res. 2018 (2018), 7103219.

[70] J.Y. Humrich, H. Morbach, R. Undeutsch, P. Enghard, S. Rosenberger, O. Weigert, et al., Homeostatic imbalance of regulatory and effector T cells due to IL-2 deprivation amplifies murine lupus, Proc. Natl. Acad. Sci. U. S. A. 107 (1) (2010) 204–209.

[71] L. Ji, W. Xie, Z. Zhang, Efficacy and safety of sirolimus in patients with systemic lupus erythematosus: a systematic review and meta-analysis, Semin. Arthritis Rheum. 50 (5) (2020) 1073–1080.

[72] Z.W. Lai, R. Kelly, T. Winans, I. Marchena, A. Shadakshari, J. Yu, et al., Sirolimus in patients with clinically active systemic lupus erythematosus resistant to, or intolerant of, conventional medications: a single-arm, open-label, phase 1/2 trial, Lancet 391 (10126) (2018) 1186–1196.

[73] L. Peng, C. Wu, R. Hong, Y. Sun, J. Qian, J. Zhao, et al., Clinical efficacy and safety of sirolimus in systemic lupus erythematosus: a real-world study and meta-analysis, Ther. Adv. Musculoskelet. Dis. 12 (2020), 1759720X20953336.

[74] B. Terrier, N. Derian, Y. Schoindre, W. Chaara, G. Geri, N. Zahr, et al., Restoration of regulatory and effector T cell balance and B cell homeostasis in systemic lupus erythematosus patients through vitamin D supplementation, Arthritis Res. Ther. 14 (5) (2012) R221.

[75] A. Marinho, C. Carvalho, D. Boleixa, A. Bettencourt, B. Leal, J. Guimarães, et al., Vitamin D supplementation effects on FoxP3 expression in T cells and FoxP3+/IL-17A ratio and clinical course in systemic lupus erythematosus patients: a study in a Portuguese cohort, Immunol. Res. 65 (1) (2017) 197–206.

[76] S.A. Fisher, M. Rahimzadeh, C. Brierley, B. Gration, C. Doree, C.E. Kimber, et al., The role of vitamin D in increasing circulating T regulatory cell numbers and modulating T regulatory cell phenotypes in patients with inflammatory disease or in healthy volunteers: a systematic review, PLoS One 14 (9) (2019), e0222313.

[77] J.R. Mora, M. Iwata, U.H. von Andrian, Vitamin effects on the immune system: vitamins A and D take centre stage, Nat. Rev. Immunol. 8 (9) (2008) 685–698.

[78] I. Ben-Zvi, C. Aranow, M. Mackay, A. Stanevsky, D.L. Kamen, L.M. Marinescu, et al., The impact of vitamin D on dendritic cell function in patients with systemic lupus erythematosus, PLoS One 5 (2) (2010), e9193.

[79] L.E. Jeffery, F. Burke, M. Mura, Y. Zheng, O.S. Qureshi, M. Hewison, et al., J. Immunol, 1,25-Dihydroxyvitamin D3 and IL-2 combine to inhibit T cell production of inflammatory cytokines and promote development of regulatory T cells expressing CTLA-4 and FoxP3, 183 (9) (2009) 5458–5467.

[80] K. Warnatz, R.E. Voll, Pathogenesis of autoimmunity in common variable immunodeficiency, Front. Immunol. 3 (2012) 210.

[81] G. López-Herrera, N.H. Segura-Méndez, P. O'Farril-Romanillos, M.E. Nuñez-Nuñez, M.C. Zarate-Hernández, D. Mogica-Martínez, et al., Low percentages of regulatory T cells in common variable immunodeficiency (CVID) patients with autoimmune diseases and its association with increased numbers of CD4+CD45RO+ T and CD21^{low} B cells, Allergol. Immunopathol. (Madr) 47 (5) (2019) 457–466.

[82] K.M. Melo, K.I. Carvalho, F.R. Bruno, L.C. Ndhlovu, W.M. Ballan, D.F. Nixon, et al., A decreased frequency of regulatory T cells in patients with common variable immunodeficiency, PLoS One 4 (7) (2009), e6269.

[83] B. Fevang, A. Yndestad, W.J. Sandberg, A.M. Holm, F. Müller, P. Aukrust, et al., Low numbers of regulatory T cells in common variable immunodeficiency: association with chronic inflammation in vivo, Clin. Exp. Immunol. 147 (3) (2007) 521–525.

[84] S. Yesillik, S. Agrawal, S.V. Gollapudi, S. Gupta, Phenotypic analysis of CD4+ Treg, CD8+ Treg, and Breg cells in adult common variable immunodeficiency patients, Int. Arch. Allergy Immunol. 180 (2) (2019) 150–158.

[85] N. Arandi, A. Mirshafiey, H. Abolhassani, M. Jeddi-Tehrani, R. Edalat, B. Sadeghi, et al., Frequency and expression of inhibitory markers of CD4(+) CD25(+) FOXP3(+) regulatory T cells in patients with common variable immunodeficiency, Scand. J. Immunol. 77 (5) (2013) 405–412.

[86] T.Z. Hou, N. Verma, J. Wanders, A. Kennedy, B. Soskic, D. Janman, et al., Identifying functional defects in patients with immune dysregulation due to LRBA and CTLA-4 mutations, Blood 129 (11) (2017) 1458–1468.

[87] W.L. Russell, L.B. Russell, J.S. Gower, Exceptional inheritance of a sex-linked gene in the mouse explained on the basis that the X/O sex-chromosome constitution is female, Proc. Natl. Acad. Sc.i U. S. A. 45 (4) (1959) 554–560.

[88] W.J. Welshons, L.B. Russell, The Y-chromosome as the bearer of male determining factors in the mouse, Proc. Natl. Acad. Sci. U. S. A. 45 (4) (1959) 560–566.

[89] B.R. Powell, N.R.M. Buist, P. Stenzel, An X-linked syndrome of diarrhea, polyendocrinopathy, and fatal infection in infancy, J. Pediatr. 100 (5) (1982) 731–737.

[90] M. Jamee, M. Zaki-Dizaji, B. Lo, H. Abolhassani, F. Aghamahdi, M. Mosavian, et al., Clinical, immunological, and genetic features in patients with immune dysregulation, polyendocrinopathy, enteropathy, X-linked (IPEX) and IPEX-like syndrome, J. Allergy Clin. Immunol. Pract. 8 (8) (2020) 2747–2760.e7.

[91] E. Gambineri, S. Ciullini Mannurita, D. Hagin, M. Vignoli, S. Anover-Sombke, S. DeBoer, et al., Clinical, immunological, and molecular heterogeneity of 173 patients with the phenotype of immune dysregulation, polyendocrinopathy, enteropathy, X-linked (IPEX) syndrome, Front. Immunol. 9 (2018) 2411.

[92] R. Bacchetta, Defective regulatory and effector T cell functions in patients with FOXP3 mutations, J. Clin. Invest. 116 (6) (2006) 1713–1722.

[93] L. Passerini, S. Olek, S. Di Nunzio, F. Barzaghi, S. Hambleton, M. Abinun, et al., Forkhead box protein 3 (FOXP3) mutations lead to increased TH17 cell numbers and regulatory T-cell instability, J. Allergy Clin. Immunol. 128 (6) (2011) 1376–1379.e1.

4. Regulatory T cells in autoimmunity and potential therapeutic targets

[94] F.R. Santoni de Sio, L. Passerini, S. Restelli, M.M. Valente, A. Pramov, M.E. Maccari, et al., Role of human forkhead box P3 in early thymic maturation and peripheral T-cell homeostasis, J. Allergy Clin. Immunol. 142 (6) (2018) 1909–1921.e9.

[95] T. Kinnunen, N. Chamberlain, H. Morbach, J. Choi, S. Kim, J. Craft, et al., Accumulation of peripheral autoreactive B cells in the absence of functional human regulatory T cells, Blood 121 (9) (2013) 1595–1603.

[96] F. Barzaghi, L.C. Amaya Hernandez, B. Neven, S. Ricci, Z.Y. Kucuk, J.J. Bleesing, et al., Long-term follow-up of IPEX syndrome patients after different therapeutic strategies: an international multicenter retrospective study, J. Allergy Clin. Immunol. 141 (3) (2018) 1036–1049.e5.

[97] J.H. Park, K.H. Lee, B. Jeon, H.D. Ochs, J.S. Lee, H.Y. Gee, et al., Immune dysregulation, polyendocrinopathy, enteropathy, X-linked (IPEX) syndrome: a systematic review, Autoimmun. Rev. 19 (6) (2020) 102526.

[98] S.G. Tangye, W. Al-Herz, A. Bousfiha, T. Chatila, C. Cunningham-Rundles, A. Etzioni, et al., Human inborn errors of immunity: 2019 update on the classification from the international union of immunological societies expert committee, J. Clin. Immunol. 40 (1) (2020) 24–64.

[99] A.M. Cepika, Y. Sato, J.M.-H. Liu, M.J. Uyeda, R. Bacchetta, M.G. Roncarolo, Tregopathies: monogenic diseases resulting in regulatory T-cell deficiency, J. Allergy Clin. Immunol. 142 (6) (2018) 1679–1695.

[100] C.M. Biggs, S. Keles, T.A. Chatila, DOCK8 deficiency: insights into pathophysiology, clinical features and management, Clin. Immunol. 181 (2017) 75–82.

[101] E. Janssen, H. Morbach, S. Ullas, J.M. Bannock, C. Massad, L. Menard, et al., Dedicator of cytokinesis 8–deficient patients have a breakdown in peripheral B-cell tolerance and defective regulatory T cells, J. Allergy Clin. Immunol. 134 (6) (2014) 1365–1374.

[102] F.J. Alroqi, L.-M. Charbonnier, S. Keles, F. Ghandour, P. Mouawad, R. Sabouneh, et al., DOCK8 deficiency presenting as an IPEX-like disorder, J. Clin. Immunol. 37 (8) (2017) 811–819.

[103] E. Janssen, S. Kumari, M. Tohme, S. Ullas, V. Barrera, J.M.J. Tas, et al., DOCK8 enforces immunological tolerance by promoting IL-2 signaling and immune synapse formation in Tregs, JCI Insight 2 (19) (2017). Available from https://insight.jci.org/articles/view/94298.

[104] U. Pannicke, B. Baumann, S. Fuchs, P. Henneke, A. Rensing-Ehl, M. Rizzi, et al., Deficiency of innate and acquired immunity caused by an *IKBKB* mutation, N. Engl. J. Med. 369 (26) (2013) 2504–2514.

[105] T. Mousallem, J. Yang, T.J. Urban, H. Wang, M. Adeli, R.E. Parrott, et al., A nonsense mutation in IKBKB causes combined immunodeficiency, Blood 124 (13) (2014) 2046–2050.

[106] Z. Alsum, M.S. AlZahrani, H. Al-Mousa, N. Alkhamis, A.A. Alsalemi, H.E. Shamseldin, et al., Multiple family members with delayed cord separtion and combined immunodeficiency with novel mutation in IKBKB, Front. Pediatr. 8 (2020). Available from https://www.frontiersin.org/article/10.3389/fped.2020.00009/full.

[107] G.D.E. Cuvelier, T.S. Rubin, A. Junker, R. Sinha, A.M. Rosenberg, D.A. Wall, et al., Clinical presentation, immunologic features, and hematopoietic stem cell transplant outcomes for IKBKB immune deficiency, Clin. Immunol. 205 (2019) 138–147.

[108] N. Sharfe, H.K. Dadi, M. Shahar, C.M. Roifman, Human immune disorder arising from mutation of the chain of the interleukin-2 receptor, Proc. Natl. Acad. Sci. U. S. A. 94 (7) (1997) 3168–3171.

[109] A.A. Caudy, S.T. Reddy, T. Chatila, J.P. Atkinson, J.W. Verbsky, CD25 deficiency causes an immune dysregulation, polyendocrinopathy, enteropathy, X-linked–like syndrome, and defective IL-10 expression from CD4 lymphocytes, J. Allergy Clin. Immunol. 119 (2) (2007) 482–487.

[110] K. Goudy, D. Aydin, F. Barzaghi, E. Gambineri, M. Vignoli, S.C. Mannurita, et al., Human IL2RA null mutation mediates immunodeficiency with lymphoproliferation and autoimmunity, Clin. Immunol. 146 (3) (2013) 248–261.

[111] K.C. Gilmour, H. Fujii, T. Cranston, E.G. Davies, C. Kinnon, H.B. Gaspar, Defective expression of the interleukin-2/interleukin-15 receptor β subunit leads to a natural killer cell–deficient form of severe combined immunodeficiency, Blood 98 (3) (2001) 877–879.

[112] Z. Zhang, F. Gothe, P. Pennamen, J.R. James, D. McDonald, C.P. Mata, et al., Human interleukin-2 receptor β mutations associated with defects in immunity and peripheral tolerance, J. Exp. Med. 216 (6) (2019) 1311–1327.

[113] A.M. Alazami, M. Al-Helale, S. Alhissi, B. Al-Saud, H. Alajlan, D. Monies, et al., Novel CARMIL2 mutations in patients with variable clinical dermatitis, infections, and combined immunodeficiency, Front. Immunol. 9 (2018) 203.

[114] C. Fournier, Where do T cells stand in rheumatoid arthritis? Joint Bone Spine 72 (6) (2005) 527–532.

[115] S.Y. Kawashiri, A. Kawakami, A. Okada, T. Koga, M. Tamai, S. Yamasaki, et al., CD4+CD25highCD127low/− Treg cell frequency from peripheral blood correlates with disease activity in patients with rheumatoid arthritis, J. Rheumatol. 38 (12) (2011) 2517–2521.

[116] Z. Jiao, W. Wang, R. Jia, J. Li, H. You, L. Chen, et al., Accumulation of FoxP3-expressing CD4+CD25+ T cells with distinct chemokine receptors in synovial fluid of patients with active rheumatoid arthritis, Scand. J. Rheumatol. 36 (6) (2007) 428–433.

[117] D. Cao, V. Malmström, C. Baecher-Allan, D. Hafler, L. Klareskog, C. Trollmo, Isolation and functional characterization of regulatory CD25brightCD4+ T cells from the target organ of patients with rheumatoid arthritis, Eur. J. Immunol. 33 (1) (2003) 215–223.

[118] M.-F. Liu, C.-R. Wang, L.-L. Fung, L.-H. Lin, C.-N. Tsai, The presence of cytokine-suppressive CD4+CD25+ T cells in the peripheral blood and synovial fluid of patients with rheumatoid arthritis, Scand. J. Immunol. 62 (3) (2005) 312–317.

[119] J.M.R. Amelsfort, K.M.G. Jacobs, J.W.J. Bijlsma, F.P.J.G. Lafeber, L.S. Taams, CD4+CD25+ regulatory T cells in rheumatoid arthritis: differences in the presence, phenotype, and function between peripheral blood and synovial fluid, Arthritis Rheum. 50 (9) (2004) 2775–2785.

[120] G.J. Walter, H.G. Evans, B. Menon, N.J. Gullick, B.W. Kirkham, A.P. Cope, et al., Interaction with activated monocytes enhances cytokine expression and suppressive activity of human CD4+CD45ro+CD25+CD127(low) regulatory T cells, Arthritis Rheum. 65 (3) (2013) 627–638.

[121] B. Prakken, E. Wehrens, F. van Wijk, Editorial: quality or quantity? Unraveling the role of Treg cells in rheumatoid arthritis, Arthritis Rheum. 65 (3) (2013) 552–554.

[122] H. Nie, Y. Zheng, R. Li, T.B. Guo, D. He, L. Fang, et al., Phosphorylation of FOXP3 controls regulatory T cell function and is inhibited by TNF-α in rheumatoid arthritis, Nat. Med. 19 (3) (2013) 322–328.

[123] I. Woodman, Rheumatoid arthritis: TNF disables TREG-cell function through FOXP3 modification, Nat. Rev. Rheumatol. 9 (4) (2013) 197.

[124] D.C. Baumgart, S.R. Carding, Inflammatory bowel disease: cause and immunobiology, Lancet 369 (9573) (2007) 1627–1640.

[125] A. Geremia, P. Biancheri, P. Allan, G.R. Corazza, A. Di Sabatino, Innate and adaptive immunity in inflammatory bowel disease, Autoimmunity Rev. 13 (1) (2014) 3–10.

[126] J. Cho, S. Kim, D.H. Yang, J. Lee, K.W. Park, J. Go, et al., Mucosal immunity related to FOXP3+ regulatory T cells, Th17 cells and cytokines in pediatric inflammatory bowel disease, J. Korean Med. Sci. 33 (52) (2018), e336.

[127] E. Godefroy, J. Alameddine, E. Montassier, J. Mathé, J. Desfrançois-Noël, N. Marec, et al., Expression of CCR6 and CXCR6 by gut-derived CD4+/CD8α+ T-regulatory cells, which are decreased in blood samples from patients with inflammatory bowel diseases, Gastroenterology 155 (4) (2018) 1205–1217.

[128] C. Smids, C.S.H.T. Horje, J. Drylewicz, B. Roosenboom, M.J.M. Groenen, E. van Koolwijk, et al., Intestinal T cell profiling in inflammatory bowel disease: linking T cell subsets to disease activity and disease course, J. Crohns Colitis 12 (4) (2018) 465–475.

[129] K. Sznurkowska, A. Żawrocki, J. Sznurkowski, E. Iżycka-Świeszewska, P. Landowski, A. Szlagatys-Sidorkiewicz, et al., Indoleamine 2,3-dioxygenase and regulatory t cells in intestinal mucosa in children with inflammatory bowel disease, J. Biol. Regul. Homeost. Agents 31 (1) (2017) 125–131.

[130] Y.K. Lee, R. Mukasa, R.D. Hatton, C.T. Weaver, Developmental plasticity of Th17 and Treg cells, Curr. Opin. Immunol. 21 (3) (2009) 274–280.

[131] A. Ueno, H. Jijon, R. Chan, K. Ford, C. Hirota, G.G. Kaplan, et al., Increased prevalence of circulating novel IL-17 secreting Foxp3 expressing CD4+ T cells and defective suppressive function of circulating Foxp3+ regulatory cells support plasticity between Th17 and regulatory T cells in inflammatory bowel disease patients, Inflamm. Bowel Dis. 19 (12) (2013) 2522–2534.

[132] Z. Hovhannisyan, J. Treatman, D.R. Littman, L. Mayer, Characterization of interleukin-17-producing regulatory T cells in inflamed intestinal mucosa from patients with inflammatory bowel diseases, Gastroenterology 140 (3) (2011) 957–965.

[133] G. Monteleone, A. Kumberova, N.M. Croft, C. McKenzie, H.W. Steer, T.T. MacDonald, Blocking Smad7 restores TGF-beta1 signaling in chronic inflammatory bowel disease, J. Clin. Invest. 108 (4) (2001) 601–609.

[134] L. Fahlén, S. Read, L. Gorelik, S.D. Hurst, R.L. Coffman, R.A. Flavell, et al., T cells that cannot respond to TGF-beta escape control by CD4(+)CD25(+) regulatory T cells, J. Exp. Med. 201 (5) (2005) 737–746.

[135] M.C. Fantini, A. Rizzo, D. Fina, R. Caruso, M. Sarra, C. Stolfi, et al., Smad7 controls resistance of colitogenic T cells to regulatory T cell-mediated suppression, Gastroenterology 136 (4) (2009) 1308–1316. e1–3.

[136] L. Zhou, C. Chu, F. Teng, N.J. Bessman, J. Goc, E.K. Santosa, et al., Innate lymphoid cells support regulatory T cells in the intestine through interleukin-2, Nature 568 (7752) (2019) 405–409.

[137] K.M. Danikowski, S. Jayaraman, B.S. Prabhakar, Regulatory T cells in multiple sclerosis and myasthenia gravis, J. Neuroinflammation 14 (1) (2017) 117.

[138] A. Ma, Z. Xiong, Y. Hu, S. Qi, L. Song, H. Dun, et al., Dysfunction of IL-10-producing type 1 regulatory T cells and CD4(+)CD25(+) regulatory T cells in a mimic model of human multiple sclerosis in Cynomolgus monkeys, Int. Immunopharmacol. 9 (5) (2009) 599–608.

[139] S.S. Duffy, B.A. Keating, G. Moalem-Taylor, Adoptive transfer of regulatory T cells as a promising immunotherapy for the treatment of multiple sclerosis, Front. Neurosci. 13 (2019) 1107.

[140] F.F. Ni, C.R. Li, Q. Li, Y. Xia, G.B. Wang, J. Yang, Regulatory T cell microRNA expression changes in children with acute Kawasaki disease, Clin. Exp. Immunol. 178 (2) (2014) 384–393.

[141] S. Jia, C. Li, G. Wang, J. Yang, Y. Zu, The T helper type 17/regulatory T cell imbalance in patients with acute Kawasaki disease, Clin. Exp. Immunol. 162 (1) (2010) 131–137.

[142] M.M.H. Guo, W.N. Tseng, C.H. Ko, H.M. Pan, K.S. Hsieh, H.C. Kuo, Th17- and Treg-related cytokine and mRNA expression are associated with acute and resolving Kawasaki disease, Allergy 70 (3) (2015) 310–318.

[143] M. Rasouli, B. Heidari, M. Kalani, Downregulation of Th17 cells and the related cytokines with treatment in Kawasaki disease, Immunol. Lett. 162 (1 Pt. A) (2014) 269–275.

[144] Y. Hirabayashi, Y. Takahashi, Y. Xu, K. Akane, I.B. Villalobos, Y. Okuno, et al., Lack of CD4$^+$CD25$^+$FOXP3$^+$ regulatory T cells is associated with resistance to intravenous immunoglobulin therapy in patients with Kawasaki disease, Eur. J. Pediatr. 172 (6) (2013) 833–837.

[145] J.C. Burns, R. Touma, Y. Song, R.L. Padilla, A.H. Tremoulet, J. Sidney, et al., Fine specificities of natural regulatory T cells after IVIG therapy in patients with Kawasaki disease, Autoimmunity 48 (3) (2015) 181–188.

[146] M. Romano, G. Fanelli, C.J. Albany, G. Giganti, G. Lombardi, Past, present, and future of regulatory T cell therapy in transplantation and autoimmunity, Front. Immunol. 10 (2019) 43.

[147] M. Tenspolde, K. Zimmermann, L.C. Weber, M. Hapke, M. Lieber, J. Dywicki, et al., Regulatory T cells engineered with a novel insulin-specific chimeric antigen receptor as a candidate immunotherapy for type 1 diabetes, J. Autoimmun. 103 (2019) 102289.

[148] A. Hartemann, G. Bensimon, C.A. Payan, S. Jacqueminet, O. Bourron, N. Nicolas, et al., Low-dose interleukin 2 in patients with type 1 diabetes: a phase 1/2 randomised, double-blind, placebo-controlled trial, Lancet Diabetes Endocrinol. 1 (4) (2013) 295–305.

[149] N. Marek-Trzonkowska, M. Myśliwiec, A. Dobyszuk, M. Grabowska, I. Derkowska, J. Juścińska, et al., Therapy of type 1 diabetes with CD4(+)CD25(high)CD127-regulatory T cells prolongs survival of pancreatic islets—results of one year follow-up, Clin. Immunol. 153 (1) (2014) 23–30.

[150] M. Dall'Era, M.L. Pauli, K. Remedios, K. Taravati, P.M. Sandova, A.L. Putnam, et al., Adoptive Treg cell therapy in a patient with systemic lupus erythematosus, Arthritis Rheumatol. 71 (3) (2019) 431–440.

[151] D. Saadoun, M. Rosenzwajg, F. Joly, A. Six, F. Carrat, V. Thibault, et al., Regulatory T-cell responses to low-dose Interleukin-2 in HCV-induced Vasculitis, N. Engl. J. Med. 365 (22) (2011) 2067–2077.

[152] Y. Chen, Z. Xu, R. Liang, J. Wang, A. Xu, N. Na, et al., CD4+CD126low/− Foxp3+ cell population represents a superior subset of regulatory T cells in treating autoimmune diseases, Mol. Ther. (2020), https://doi.org/10.1016/j.ymthe.2020.07.020. S1525-0016(20)30371-3. Epub ahead of print.

[153] A. Sharma, D. Rudra, Regulatory T cells as therapeutic targets and mediators, Int. Rev. Immunol. 38 (5) (2019) 183–203.

CHAPTER

5

Application of IL-6 antagonists in autoimmune disorders

Tiago Borges[a,*], *Arsénio Barbosa*[b] *and Sérgio Silva*[a]

[a]Department of Internal Medicine, Trofa Saúde Private Hospital,
Vila Nova de Gaia, Portugal [b]Department of Internal Medicine, University Hospital
Center of São João, Porto, Portugal
*Corresponding author

Abstract

This chapter explores the role of interleukin (IL)-6 in autoimmune disorders. It starts by providing a historical perspective and exploring the mechanisms responsible for IL-6 signaling. It then describes the pleiotropic effects of IL-6 and several autoimmune and autoimmune-related disorders where IL-6 expression is deregulated, along with laboratory clues of IL-6 overexpression. In the second part of this chapter, the role of IL-6 blockade in autoimmune disorders is explored. For tocilizumab and sarilumab, important studies that have led to their approval in rheumatoid arthritis, juvenile idiopathic arthritis, and giant cell arteritis are briefly presented. For these two anti-IL-6 drugs, data is also presented regarding safety, contraindications, pharmacodynamics, pharmacokinetics, drug interactions, warnings, and immunogenicity. Finally, IL-6 blockade off-label use is discussed, pointing to the most valuable evidence not only in the abovementioned disorders but also in other autoimmune diseases whose management may be achieved by specifically blocking IL-6 signaling.

Keywords

Adaptive immunity, Autoimmune diseases, Immunosuppressive agents, Interleukin-6, Monoclonal antibodies

1 Introduction

Interleukin (IL)-6 is a four-helix protein of 184 amino acids that was originally identified by Kishimoto as a T-cell-derived factor inducing the final maturation of activated B cells into antibody-producing plasma cells [1, 2]. The IL-6 gene is located at 7p15-p21 and cloning of its complementary DNA by Hirano in 1986 revealed that IL-6 had been studied under 36 different names, including B cell stimulatory factor (BSF)-2, interferon (IFN)-β2, hepatocyte-stimulating factor (HSF), hybridoma/plasmacytoma growth factor (HPGF), macrophage granulocyte inducer type 2 (MGI-2A), and thrombopoietin [3–7]. The designation "IL-6" was finally chosen in 1988 to avoid confusion at a conference held in New York [3].

IL-6 is a positive growth regulator [4]. The major source of IL-6 are monocytes but many other cells express IL-6, as seen in Table 1 [8, 9].

IL-6 expression is induced by several factors, including IL-1, tumor necrosis factor (TNF), platelet-derived growth factor (PDGF), and microbial components like lipopolysaccharide (LPS) [5]. IL-6 stimuli can be either physiological or nonphysiological, as shown in Table 2 [10].

The suggestion that IL-6 was involved in autoimmunity was originally derived from the fact that patients with cardiac myxoma often exhibit autoimmune features and myxoma cells produce large amounts of IL-6 [3, 6]. Deregulation of IL-6 production has been observed in several autoimmune disorders (ADs), vasculitides, and other autoimmune-related disorders. However, hematological disorders (e.g., Castleman's disease, graft-versus-host disease), infections (e.g., AIDS), autoinflammatory diseases and other disorders (e.g., cytokine release syndrome, amyloidosis) with autoimmune features have not been considered here.

TABLE 1   Cell types able to express interleukin-6.

Adipocytes	Keratinocytes
Alveolar macrophages	Kupffer cells
Amnion	Macrophages
Astrocytes	Mast cells
B lymphocytes	Mesangial cells
Bone marrow stromal cells	Microglial cells
Bronchial epithelial cells	Monocytes
Chondrocytes	Neutrophils
Endometrial cells	Osteoblast-like cells
Endothelial cells	Osteoclasts
Enterocytes	Pancreatic β cells
Eosinophils	Smooth muscle cells
Epithelial cells	Synoviocytes
Fibroblasts	T lymphocytes
Glial cells	Tumor cells (hematopoietic and non-hematopoietic)
Hepatocytes	

TABLE 2 Physiological and nonphysiological interleukin-6 stimuli.

Physiological	Bacterial lipopolysaccharide
	Viruses
	Cytokines (e.g., IL-1, IL-2, TNF, PDGF, IFN)
	Trauma
	Others (e.g., prostaglandin E1)
Nonphysiological	Ca^{2+} elevating agents (e.g., A23187)
	cAMP agonists (e.g., cholera toxin)
	Protein kinase c activators (e.g., diC8)
	Others (e.g., actinomycin D, anti-C3 antibody)

A23187, calcium ionophore; *diC8*, 1,2-dioctanoylglycerol; *IL*, interleukin; *IFN*, interferons; *PDGF*, platelet-derived growth factor; *TNF*, tumor necrosis factor.

2 Signaling

IL-6 binds to IL-6 receptor (IL-6R), which is a type I transmembrane protein consisting of a 130 kDa signal transducer (gp130) and an 80 kDa receptor (IL-6Rα) that exists in two (transmembrane and soluble) forms [5, 6]. IL-6Rα is expressed by phagocytes, hepatocytes, and a few lymphocytes, while gp130 is expressed ubiquitously in tissues [3]. IL-6 binds first to the α chain but classic (cis) signaling only starts when the IL-6-IL-6R complex binds to gp130 [1, 3, 11]. IL-11, IL-27, ciliary neurotrophic factor (CNTF), leukemia inhibitory factor (LIF), oncostatin M (OM), and cardiotropin 1 (CT-1) belong to the IL-6 family of cytokines that use gp130 as a component of their receptor and own similar biological activities to IL-6 [5, 6, 12, 13]. After dimerization, gp130 activates constitutively bound Janus kinases (JAKs), which then phosphorylate its cytoplasmic portion on tyrosine residues, allowing SHP2 to stimulate the mitogen-activated protein kinase (MAPK) and phosphatidylinositol-4,5-biphosphate 3-kinase (PI3K) pathways. Furthermore, another major pathway related to gp130 takes place when other tyrosine residues are phosphorylated and signal transducer and activator of transcription 3 (STAT3) is recruited, phosphorylated, and dimerized, stimulating the transcription of nuclear genes, as shown in Fig. 1 [1, 4, 12]. The gp130-JAK-STAT pathway upregulates the expression of suppressor of cytokine signaling (SOCS3) protein, which in turn inhibits JAKs and functions as negative feedback, along with protein inhibitors of activated STATs (PIAS) [1, 6].

IL-6 expression is regulated at several stages, including gene polymorphisms, chromatin remodeling, transcription, and posttranscription levels [14]. A nuclear factor for controlling IL-6 expression, NF-IL6, or C/EBPβ is induced by inflammatory signals like IL-6 through gp130, following a Ras/MAP kinase cascade to positively regulate the expression of acute-phase genes [5, 15]. Although C/EBP is constitutively expressed and regulates the albumin gene, NF-IL6 is predominantly expressed in macrophages after stimulation with IL-6, IL-1, TNF, and LPS [5, 16].

The majority of body cells do not express IL-6R but a soluble form of IL-6R (sIL-6R) is responsible for "IL-6 trans-signaling," allowing cells that do not express IL-6Rα to respond to IL-6. IL-6 binds to sIL-6R with the same affinity, forming an IL-6-sIL-6R complex, which is able to stimulate endothelial and smooth muscle cells [1, 3]. Membrane-bound disintegrin and metalloproteinase domain-containing proteins 10 and 17 (ADAM10/17) are proteases that cleave membrane-bound IL-6R to generate sIL-6R (90%), which can also be generated

5. Application of IL-6 antagonists in autoimmune disorders

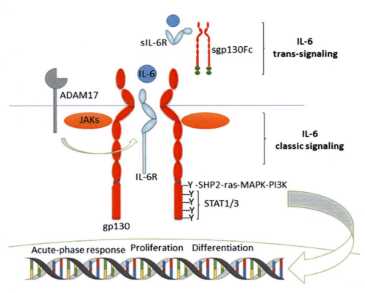

FIG. 1   Interleukin-6 signaling.

by translation of an alternatively spiced mRNA (10%) [1, 4, 17]. Soluble gp130 (sgp130Fc) is generated by alternative splicing, neutralizes the complex formed by IL-6 and sIL-6R, and blocks IL-6 trans-signaling without affecting the classic IL-6 signaling, so sIL-6R and sgp130 constitute a serum buffer for circulating IL-6 [1, 2, 17].

A third signaling pathway, termed IL-6 trans-presentation or cluster signaling, has been described: IL-6 that is intracellularly bound to the IL-6R in dendritic cells is transported to the plasma membrane after antigen presentation so that the membrane-bound IL-6/mIL-6R complex interacts with gp130 on T cells [17, 18]. Sgp130 cannot interfere with cluster signaling and this pathway generates pathogenic Th17 cells by STAT3 induction and IL-23R upregulation in the presence of transforming growth factor-β1 (TGF-β1) [18].

3 Roles of IL-6

In steady-state, IL-6 is not usually produced constitutively by cells [7]. Different designations of IL-6 derive from the fact that it is able to promote the maturation of B cells into antibody-producing cells (BSF-2), induce acute-phase proteins (APPs) in the liver (HSF), stimulate the growth of plasmacytomas (HPGF) and the differentiation of myeloid precursors (MGI-2A), even though IFN activity has not been confirmed (IFN-β2) [6]. IL-6 is a pleiotropic cytokine regulating three main processes: the acute-phase inflammatory reaction, immune response, and hematopoiesis [15]. These pleiotropic effects are summarized in Fig. 2 and are supported by the ubiquitous expression of gp130 and by the IL-6 trans-signaling pathway [19].

IL-6 plays a crucial role in host defense mechanisms including antiviral antibody responses, coordinating the activity of the innate and adaptive immune systems [2, 5, 20]. Neutrophils, monocytes, and macrophages are able to secrete IL-6 after stimulation of Toll-like receptors, and IL-6 stimulation is exerted on endothelial and smooth muscle cells, B cells,

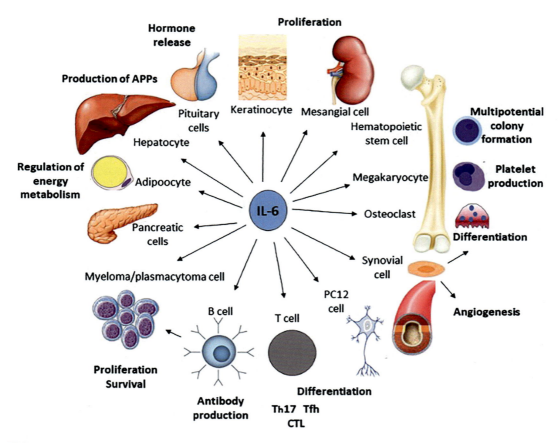

FIG. 2 Pleyotropic effects of interleukin-6.

and hepatocytes [1]. Peripheral neutrophilia induced by IL-6 is caused by demargination of intravascular neutrophils [21]. In the liver, IL-6 induces the expression of C-reactive protein (CRP), serum amyloid A (SAA), fibrinogen, hepcidin, and zinc transporter 14, decreasing the production of albumin, transferrin, and cytochrome p450 [22].

IL-6 acts on hematopoietic stem cells by inducing megakaryocyte maturation and synergizes with macrophage colony-stimulating factor (M-CSF) and granulocyte-macrophage colony-stimulating factor (GM-CSF) to induce megakaryocytic colony-forming cells (CFU-M) [3, 20]. There is also a synergistic effect with IL-3, which induces the proliferation of multipotential hematopoietic progenitors [20]. IL-6 can induce the differentiation of leukemic cells and inhibit the growth of myeloid leukemia cells [3, 20].

IL-6 induces the final maturation of activated B cells into antibody-producing cells, acting synergistically with IL-1 [1, 20]. During systemic autoimmunity, B-cell-derived IL-6 probably drives spontaneous germinal center formation [23]. IL-6 can also induce the growth and differentiation of T cells, increasing IL-2 production and IL-2R expression [6]. Through the expression of orphan nuclear receptors (RORγt and RORα), IL-6 acts synergistically with TGF-β and sIL-6R to induce the differentiation of Th0 naïve T cells into Th17 cells, whose function is directly correlated with autoimmunity and inflammation, particularly defense mechanisms against bacteria and fungi [1, 3, 4]. It also inhibits Treg differentiation in T cells, aggravating the Th17/Treg imbalance, as shown in Fig. 3 [4].

IL-6 is able to induce CD8$^+$ T cells to generate cytotoxic T cells [16, 24]. The role of IL-6 in lymphoid cells is summarized in Table 3.

IL-6 is able to promote the differentiation and activation of macrophages, stimulating osteoclast formation and activity [16, 24]. IL-6 production in bone marrow stromal cells generates the receptor activator of NF-κβ ligand (RANKL), while vascular endothelial growth factor (VEGF) is induced by IL-6 and promotes vascular permeability and angiogenesis [24]. IL-6 is also able to decrease the production of type II collagen and aggrecans by chondrocytes and is responsible for keratinocyte proliferation, increased production of collagen by dermal fibroblasts, hormone release (ACTH, GH, prolactin, LH), and nerve cell differentiation [3, 9, 25]. IL-6 is a physiological regulator of energy metabolism; positive metabolic effects (e.g., protection from insulin resistance, fatty acid oxidation) have been linked to classic signaling, while negative effects (e.g., induction of lipoprotein (a), increased serum triglyceride, and cholesterol levels, increased body weight) may be caused by trans-signaling [2]. Co-agonistic effects of IL-6 have been described with IL-2 (development of cytotoxic cells from immature T cells), IL-3 (proliferation of pluripotent precursors), glucocorticoids (induction of APPs), and IL-6 itself [10].

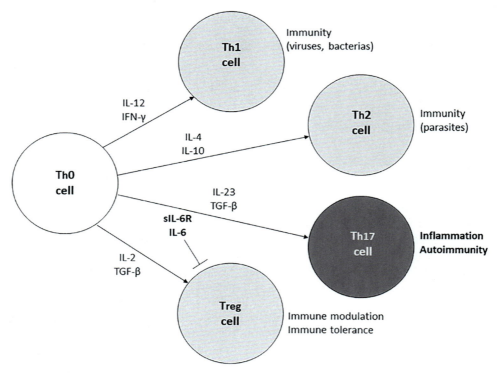

FIG. 3 Role of the interleukin-6 system in T cell differentiation.

TABLE 3 Effects of interleukin-6 on lymphoid cells.

B cells	↑ Antibody production
Plasmablast cells	↑ Survival
Myeloma cells	↑ Proliferation
CD4 T cells	↑ Th17 differentiation ↓ Treg differentiation ↑ T follicular helper cell differentiation
CD8 T cells	↑ Cytotoxic T cells

4 IL-6 in ADs and autoimmune-related disorders

More than other cytokines and chemokines, IL-6, TNF, and probably GM-CSF are crucial to inflammatory pathogenic processes in rheumatoid arthritis (RA) [26]. Both serum and synovial IL-6 levels are increased and induce B cell proliferation and antibody production, activation of T cells and osteoclasts, differentiation to Th17 cells, elevation of APPs, thrombocytosis, and amyloidosis [3, 15, 20]. Serum IL-6 levels are often elevated from 10 to 100 pg/mL and correlate with disease activity, duration of morning stiffness, and radiographic scores [14, 27]. IL-6 is produced by fibroblastic synovial cells and in lesser amounts by lymphocytes and macrophages, activating local endothelial cells that produce chemokines and adhesion molecules for leukocyte recruitment [3]. Local effects of IL-6 also include osteoclast differentiation and fibroblastic cell activation that promote synovial pannus formation and breakdown of the cartilage and bone [3]. IL-6 is also able to induce VEGF in synovial fibroblasts [14]. Systemic effects of IL-6 are explained by its effects not only on hepatocytes through acute-phase response, but also on the hypothalamus-pituitary-adrenal (HPA) axis [3]. Translational effects of IL-6 in RA include pain, fatigue, and mood disorders and are probably related to the ubiquitous expression of gp130 and IL-6 trans-signaling [19].

In systemic lupus erythematosus (SLE), IL-6 has a direct role in B cell hyperactivity and differentiation, controlling autoantibody production, mainly anti-DNA antibodies, while these also upregulate IL-6 expression in endothelial cells [8]. B cells spontaneously express IL-6R and produce large amounts of IL-6, like autoreactive T cells [8]. IL-6 accelerates the progression of proteinuria, playing an important role in the pathogenesis of mesangial proliferative glomerulonephritis and IgA nephropathy [8]. Correlation with disease activity is more consistent with urinary than serum IL-6 levels, especially in nephritis [8, 28, 29].

In systemic sclerosis (SSc), IL-6 gene polymorphisms are important in disease susceptibility [30]. Not only serum IL-6 levels are increased, but also sIL-6R and anti-IL-6 autoantibodies [31]. Spontaneous production of IL-6 and IL-6R by peripheral blood leukocytes is increased, while IL-6 trans-signaling appears to be the dominant pathway for increased collagen synthesis and fibrosis, possibly driving the differentiation of cardiac fibroblasts into pathogenic myofibroblasts [30, 31]. Serum pathogenic IL-17 cells are also increased [30, 32]. Elevated serum levels of IL-6 predict worse outcomes in SSc, including the severity of skin thickening, progression of interstitial lung disease, and cardiac involvement [30, 31].

IL-6 concentrations are elevated in the serum, saliva, and tears of patients with Sjögren's syndrome (SS) [33, 34]. IL-6 has also been found to be highly expressed in serum and peripheral lymphocytes, correlating with extraglandular symptoms and the degree of glandular infiltration [34]. In primary SS, IL-6 not only induces polyclonal activation of B cells but also generates Th17 cells, while IL-6R is mostly expressed in B cells of patients with active disease [35].

IL-6 has been detected in the blood and tissues of all subtypes of juvenile idiopathic arthritis (JIA), but concentrations in synovial fluid are much higher and IL-6 is involved differently according to each subtype [36]. A G/C polymorphism at position 174 in the IL-6 flanking region has been linked to systemic JIA (SJIA) [14]. IL-6 serum levels are elevated in active SJIA, correlating with joint involvement and laboratory parameters of disease activity [37, 38]. Th17 cells are a major pathogenic driver in polyarticular JIA (PJIA), while dysfunction of NK cells is a characteristic of SJIA [36]. Serum IL-6 concentrations are also elevated in both polyarticular and active systemic phenotypes of adult-onset Still's disease (AOSD), but this is probably specific to a subset of patients with arthritis [39, 40]. IL-6 levels are also highly expressed in cutaneous lesions [41].

Phenotypic presentation in giant cell arteritis (GCA) and polymyalgia rheumatica (PMR) may be related to IL-6 polymorphisms and specific genotypes [42–44]. Even though both BAFF and IL-6 show the strongest association with disease activity and hyperproduction of IL-6 characterizes both syndromes, proinflammatory cytokines are more preponderant in PMR, while IFN-γ-producing T cells are prominent in GCA [39, 44, 45]. A marked shift toward Th17 cell response is promoted by IL-6 [39, 42]. IL-6 is expressed in symptomatic muscles of PMR patients, temporal artery walls of GCA patients, and even some patients with PMR without evidence of GCA [39, 42]. In GCA, serum IL-6 levels correlate with clinical symptoms and disease severity [46]. In PMR, serum IL-6 levels are associated with clinical relapse and a need for increased steroid dose, while sIL-6R constitutes a potential prognostic marker for relapse [44]. IL-6 activity is also increased in both serum and synovial fluid of patients with remitting seronegative symmetrical synovitis with pitting edema (RS3PE) syndrome [47]. In Takayasu arteritis (TA), elevated levels of IL-6 have been detected in aortic tissues and peripheral blood, along with IL-17 and Th17 cells [48]. mRNA levels of IL-6 are significantly higher during active phases, so IL-6 may be a biomarker for monitoring disease activity and predicting relapse [49, 50].

Elevated serum IL-6 levels have also been described in Henoch-Schönlein purpura (HSP), IgA vasculitis, acute Kawasaki disease (KD), and polyarteritis nodosa (PAN) [51–54]. Elevated serum IL-6 levels have been associated with an increased risk of developing KD shock syndrome and may predict a bad response to intravenous (IV) immunoglobulin [55, 56]. In ANCA-associated vasculitis (AAV), IL-6 serum levels are significantly increased, being produced at sites of active vasculitis, mainly in granulomatosis with polyangiitis (GPA), correlating with specific clinical manifestations (fever, pulmonary nodules and/or cavities, conductive deafness, and absence of renal involvement) [57]. Increases in serum IL-6 during remission are associated with severe relapse in rituximab-treated patients, but not in those treated with cyclophosphamide or azathioprine [57]. Increased serum levels of IL-6 have also been described in hepatitis C virus (HCV)-related and non-HCV-related mixed cryoglobulinemia [58–60].

In early spondyloarthritis, IL-6 is detected in sacroiliac joints [36]. Elevated serum IL-6 levels have been described in ankylosing spondylitis (AS), correlating with Bath Ankylosing

Spondylitis Disease Activity Score (BASDAI) and Bath Ankylosing Spondylitis Functional Index (BASFI) scores in patients with pure axial involvement, despite not being a reliable predictor of disease progression [61–63]. IL-6 serum levels are elevated in reactive arthritis (ReA), while synovial levels are probably higher than those seen in RA [64, 65]. Innate immune activation through IL-6 is also important in psoriatic patients that develop psoriatic arthritis (PsA) [36]. Increased production of IL-6 occurs in both disorders and serum levels correlate with disease severity in PsA, even though IL-6 does not appear to be involved in the effector phase of PsA [66]. Serum and skin IL-6 levels are also increased in psoriasis and the former correlate with disease activity and treatment response [67, 68]. IL-6 polymorphisms are associated with a predisposition of developing psoriasis [69]. IL-6 is produced mainly by keratinocytes in psoriatic plaques, inhibiting effector T cell suppression and leading to STAT3 activation that induces the IL-23/Th17 signaling cascade [68]. IL-17 and IL-23 are also expressed in the joints of PsA patients [70].

IL-6 levels are elevated in the serum and intestinal tissues of patients with active Crohn's disease (CD), particularly those with colonic involvement, but elevations of serum IL-6 concentrations in inactive CD and both active and inactive ulcerative colitis (UC) are much less pronounced [71–74]. Nevertheless, IL-6 also constitutes the main cytokine expressed in inflamed tissues of UC patients [75]. Specific IL-6R gene polymorphisms (e.g., rs2228145) are associated with increased levels of sIL-6R, reduced IL-6R signaling, and probably a reduced risk of inflammatory bowel disorders (IBD) [76]. IL-6 induces enhanced T cell survival and apoptosis resistance in the lamina propria of inflamed tissues, which are also rich in Th17 cells [74, 75, 77]. Serum IL-6 levels appear to be correlated not only with disease activity in IBD but also with clinical relapse, treatment failure, and response to anti-TNF drugs in UC [74, 78, 79].

In neuromyelitis optica (NMO), IL-6 is increased in both serum and cerebrospinal fluid (CSF) [80]. CSF IL-6 levels are particularly elevated during the initial flares and are superior to those seen in optic neuritis and relapsing-remitting multiple sclerosis (MS), while CSF/serum IL-6 ratio is significantly elevated in NMO comparing to other noninflammatory neurological disorders [80]. In NMO, CSF IL-6 levels probably correlate with Expanded Disability Status Scale (EDSS) scores, recovery from relapse, and duration to next relapse [80]. The effect of IL-6 on autoreactive effector T cells has been demonstrated in MS and IL-6 may interfere with neuroinflammation and be elevated in both MS and autoimmune encephalitis [81, 82]. Anti-AchR antibodies probably affect IL-6 production by muscle cells in myasthenia gravis [83]. IL-6 may also be elevated in the CSF of patients with inflammatory polyneuropathies such as Guillain-Barré syndrome and chronic inflammatory demyelinating polyradiculoneuropathy [84].

Polymorphisms in IL-6 gene are a risk factor for autoimmune thyroid disease [85]. IL-6 serum levels are elevated in Graves' ophthalmopathy (GO) comparing to Graves' patients without ocular involvement [86]. IL-6 is able to stimulate thyrotropin receptor (TSHR) expression in human orbital preadipocyte fibroblasts toward adipogenesis [87, 88]. Serum sIL-6R is also elevated in GO and correlates with disease activity [88].

Autoimmune-related uveitic disorders in which IL-6 plays a role in pathogenesis include Vogt-Koyanagi-Harada syndrome, Behçet's syndrome (BS), sarcoidosis, and idiopathic uveitis and IL-6 concentrations have been described to be increased not only in the vitreous fluid, particularly in cases of active intermediate or posterior uveitis, but also in the serum of active cases [89]. IL-6 probably induces ocular inflammation through Th17 differentiation [90].

5. Application of IL-6 antagonists in autoimmune disorders

TABLE 4   Autoimmune-related disorders with deregulated interleukin-6 expression.

Adult-onset Still disease	Multiple sclerosis
Alopecia areata	Myasthenia gravis
ANCA-associated vasculitis	Noninfectious uveitis
Acquired hemophilia	Neuromyelitis optica
Ankylosing spondylitis	Pemphigus
Antiphospholipid syndrome	Polymyalgia rheumatica
Autoimmune hepatitis (type 2)	Psoriasis
Autoimmune hemolytic anemia	Psoriatic arthritis
Autoimmune encephalitis	Reactive arthritis
Behçet's syndrome	Relapsing polychondritis
Bullous pemphigoid	Remitting seronegative symmetrical synovitis with pitting edema
Celiac disease	
Crohn's disease	Rheumatoid arthritis
Cryoglobulinemia	Rheumatic fever
Graves' ophthalmopathy	Sarcoidosis
Giant cell arteritis	Sjögren's syndrome
Guillain-Barré syndrome	Systemic sclerosis
Henoch-Schönlein purpura	Systemic lupus erythematosus
Inflammatory myopathies	Takayasu arteritis
Juvenile idiopathic arthritis	Type 1 diabetes mellitus
Kawasaki disease	Ulcerative colitis
Mixed connective tissue disease	Vitiligo

IL-6 appears to be increased not only in peripheral blood mononuclear cells but also in plasma of patients with active BS, particularly in those with neurological involvement showing increased IL-6 levels in the CSF [91–93].

Increased expression and/or serum levels of IL-6 have also been described in other ADs and autoimmune-related syndromes as described in Table 4 [94–102].

5 Laboratory clues

Reference values of soluble components of the IL-6 system and APPs are reflected in Table 5 [1]. Serum IL-6 levels may be elevated in patients with several ADs as described above. However, IL-6 is also secreted by muscle cells upon exercise and by adipocytes in

TABLE 5 Reference levels for soluble components of the interleukin-6 system and acute-phase proteins in human blood.

IL-6	1–5 pg/mL
sIL-6R	40–80 ng/mL
sgp130	250–5400 ng/mL
C-reactive protein	<10 mg/L
Fibrinogen	200–400 mg/dL
Haptoglobin	40–200 mg/dL
Serum amyloid A	<10 mg/L

obese patients [1]. In chronic diseases characterized by elevated serum IL-6 concentrations, a negative correlation between hemoglobin and IL-6 levels has been demonstrated, which may be due to upregulation of hepcidin [103]. In RA, IL-6 induces the production of hepcidin by hepatocytes, which decreases serum iron levels and promotes anemia [3]. IL-6 is also able to induce megakaryocyte differentiation and thrombocytosis, correlating with platelet counts [3]. Serum IL-6 concentrations have long been correlated with inflammatory markers and autoantibodies like rheumatoid factor. IL-6R-specific monoclonal antibodies (mAbs) like tocilizumab (TCZ) may further increase serum IL-6 levels and these are suppressed by methotrexate (MTX) in RA and by steroids in PMR [3, 104].

In SLE, elevated serum levels of IL-6 correlate with other laboratory parameters such as anemia [105, 106]. Urinary IL-6 is elevated in patients with active lupus nephritis (World Health Organization Class III and IV), correlating with mesangial proliferation and anti-DNA antibody levels [8, 28]. Increased serum IL-6 levels appear to be correlated with thrombocytosis in SJIA [38]. In AAV, serum IL-6 concentrations correlate with PR3-ANCA titers [57, 107]. In sarcoidosis, elevated serum IL-6 levels correlate with forced vital capacity (FVC) independent of age, gender, and other pulmonary parameters, while IL-6 production by alveolar macrophages appears to be correlated with the CD4/CD8 ratio in bronchoalveolar lavage [95, 108]. Increased IL-6 CSF levels in BS correlate with CSF cell counts and total protein levels [93]. Serum IL-6 concentrations negatively correlate with albumin serum levels in active CD [73]. In NMO, serum IL-6 levels correlate with IL-32, while CSF IL-6 levels appear to correlate with AQP4 antibodies positivity, CSF cells, protein levels, glial fibrillary acidic protein (GFAP), and high-mobility group box-1 (HMGB1) levels [80].

During acute inflammation, IL-6 acts as a hepatocyte-stimulating factor and induces a decrease in several proteins (albumin, transferrin, apolipoprotein A1) and elevations in serum levels of APPs such as CRP, ferritin, fibrinogen, haptoglobin, α1-acid glycoprotein, and SAA [3, 5, 16]. CRP is usually used as a marker of inflammation or infection in clinical practice [1]. IL-6 is considered as the primary inducer of APPs and serum levels are often correlated with erythrocyte sedimentation rate (ESR) and/or CRP, as in GCA and acute KD [6, 16, 42, 53]. However, even when serum levels of IL-6 are significantly increased, CRP levels may not be increased [109].

5. Application of IL-6 antagonists in autoimmune disorders

6 IL-6 blockade

Inhibition of IL-6 trans-signaling in mouse models has been sufficient to block the disease, including RA, IBD, asthma, pancreatitis and related lung injury, peritonitis, and colon cancer, but such effect has not been reproduced in mouse models of *Listeria* infection [1]. Therefore, IL-6 classic signaling has been regarded to be responsible for protective and regenerative functions, while trans-signaling probably corresponds to the proinflammatory activity of IL-6 and is directly related to its translational activity [1, 19]. In fact, global blockade of IL-6 in mouse models of IBD has induced increased disease susceptibility, but since STAT3 activity induced by IL-6 appears to be important for the regeneration of intestinal epithelium, specific blockade of IL-6 trans-signaling is probably more beneficial than global blockade [1]. IL-6 blockade can be achieved at several levels as shown in Table 6. All neutralizing antibodies against IL-6 and IL-6R block both IL-6 classic and trans-signaling [1]. Since the JAK/STAT signaling pathway is common to several cytokines, colony-stimulating factors, prolactin, and GH, targeted synthetic disease-modifying antirheumatic drugs (DMARDs) have not been considered in this chapter.

TABLE 6   Targeting levels of interleukin-6 blockade.

	Specificity	Drugs
JAKs	JAK1, JAK2, JAK3	Baricitinib Filgotinib PF-04965842 Ruxolitinib Tofacitinib Upadacitinib
STAT	STAT3	Stattic CpG-STAT3 decoys or small interfering RNA
IL-6	IL-6 specific monoclonal antibody	Clazakizumab (ALD518, BMS-945429) Elsilimomab (B-E8) EBI-031 FE301 FM101 Gerilimzumab (ARGX 109, GB 224, RYI 008) MEDI5117 (WBP216) Olokizumab (CDP6038) PF-04236921 Siltuximab (CNTO 328) Sirukumab (CNTO-136)
IL-6R	IL-6R-specific monoclonal antibody	Levilimab (BCD 089) NI-1202 Sarilumab (REGN88, SAR153191) Satralizumab (SA237, sapelizumab) Tocilizumab (atlizumab) Vobarilizumab (ALX-0061)
IL-6-IL-6R complex	Soluble gp130 Fc fusion protein	Olamkicept (TJ301, FE999301)

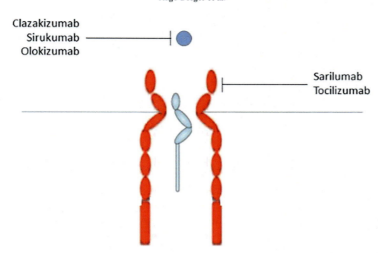

FIG. 4 Targeting interleukin-6 or interleukin-6 receptor.

The initial binding of IL-6 to IL-6R is mediated through site I, triggering homodimerization of gp130 and IL-6 binding to gp130 receptor through site II and to the second gp130 molecule via site III [2]. mAbs targeting IL-6 site I include clazakizumab (CLZ, humanized rabbit mAb), siltuximab (chimeric), and siltuximab (chimeric), while EBI-031 targets site II and olokizumab targets site III (OKZ, humanized mAb and immunomodulator) [2, 110–112]. TCZ, sarilumab (SRL), and satralizumab (STL) are humanized mAbs targeting IL-6R that block IL-6 classic signaling, trans-signaling, and trans-presentation and, unlike anti-IL-6 antibodies, resulting in only mild elevations of serum IL-6 levels due to reduced cellular IL-6R-dependent internalization, as represented in Fig. 4 [2]. Vobarilzumab (VBR) is a bispecific antibody-derived therapeutic protein (Nanobody) with a high affinity to IL-6R [46, 113]. Instead, olamkicept is an sgp130 protein targeting the IL-6/sIL-6R complex that does not interfere with IL-6 classic signaling [2, 114].

6.1 Approved treatments

6.1.1 *Efficacy*

After phase I and II clinical trials reported between 2002 and 2006, the phase II CHARISMA study demonstrated that IL-6 blockade with IV TCZ was highly effective in patients with active RA, achieving ACR20 responses in more than 60% of cases, either as monotherapy or in combination with MTX [115, 116]. While the phase III OPTION trial demonstrated that TCZ-MTX combination was effective and safe in patients with moderate-to-severe RA and lack of response to MTX, the phase III AMBITION trial showed that TCZ monotherapy is better than MTX monotherapy in achieving clinical remission in patients without previous therapeutic failure with MTX or biologics [117, 118]. Radiographic benefits of TCZ monotherapy at 52 weeks on DMARD-refractory patients were also demonstrated in the phase III

SAMURAI trial, while the phase III RADIATE trial demonstrated the efficacy of TCZ (ACR20 response: 50% at week 24) and 4 mg/kg (30.4%) comparing to controls (10.1%) in RA patients refractory to TNF inhibitors, achieving significant dose-related DAS28 remission rates (30.1% vs 7.6% vs 1.6%) [119, 120]. The phase III LITHE trial showed that TCZ 8 mg/kg is associated with less radiographic progression at week 52 compared to placebo in RA patients with the moderate-to-severe disease and inadequate response to MTX, besides achieving significantly higher ACR20, ACR50, and ACR70 response and DAS28 remission rates and improving physical function [121]. Since then, several phase III and IV clinical trials (e.g., TOWARD, SATORI, ROSE, ACT-RAY, ACT-STAR) have demonstrated that both TCZ add-on and switch strategies result in clinical and radiographic responses with favorable safety profiles [116, 122–124]. Almost similar efficacy is to be expected with TCZ monotherapy in patients unable to tolerate conventional synthetic DMARDs (csDMARDs) compared to inadequate responders switching to add-on combination therapy in the management of active RA [125]. The FUNCTION trial has also demonstrated that TCZ is effective for the treatment of early RA either alone or in combination with MTX [126]. The phase IV ADACTA trial demonstrated the superiority of IV TCZ monotherapy in relation to adalimumab therapy for the reduction of RA signs and symptoms in patients for whom MTX was deemed inappropriate, including significantly higher DAS28 improvements with TCZ [127].

The SARIL-RA-MOBILITY Part A phase II randomized controlled trial (RCT) compared five doses of subcutaneous (SC) SRL and placebo in patients with active RA with a duration of at least three months that had been treated with MTX for at least 12 weeks, demonstrating that the primary endpoint ACR20 response was significantly achieved in a higher proportion of patients with SRL 150 mg qw (72%), q2w (67%) and 200 mg q2w (65%) comparing to placebo (46.2%) [128]. SRL 150 and 200 mg q2w were also significantly more effective than placebo in improving DAS28 and HAQ-DI scores, while SRL ≥ 150 mg q2w reduced CRP levels [27, 128]. The SARIL-RA-MOBILITY Part B phase III trial confirmed that SRL 150 and 200 mg q2w plus MTX were significantly more effective than placebo at 24 weeks regarding ACR20 (58% vs 66.4% vs 33.4%, respectively) and ACR50 response rates and DAS28 scores, while the reduction of radiographic progression was only statistically significant with SRL 200 mg q2w [129]. The MOBILITY study has also demonstrated significant improvements in fatigue and mood, as assessed by the FACIT-F and mental component summary (MCS) of the 36-item Short-Form Health Survey (SF-36) [19]. The SARIL-RA-TARGET phase III study demonstrated that SRL 150 and 200 mg q2w are able to achieve significantly higher ACR20 response rates at week 24 comparing to placebo (55.8% vs 60.9% vs 33.7%, respectively) in patients with active moderate-to-severe RA that were inadequate responders or intolerant to anti-TNF drugs [130]. The MONARCH phase III trial demonstrated that 200 mg q2w SRL monotherapy is statistically superior to adalimumab monotherapy, as reflected in higher ACR20 (71.7% vs 58.4%), ACR50 (45.7% vs 29.7%), and ACR70 (23.4% vs 11.9%) response rates and greater HAQ-DI scores in patients with active RA that were unable to take MTX [131]. The EXTEND trial confirmed that better radiographic scores at year two were observed in patients initially randomized to SRL 200 mg q2w [132]. The phase III SARIL-RA-KAKEHASI trial demonstrated sustained clinical efficacy with SRL 150 and 200 mg q2w comparing to placebo in RA patients with inadequate responses to MTX (ACR20 responses at week 24 of 67.9%, 57.5%, and 14.8%, respectively) [133]. The phase III RA-COMPARE trial was terminated due to an internal company decision unrelated to safety issues [11].

The 2019 update of EULAR recommendations for the management of RA synthetic and biological DMARDs have suggested that when poor prognostic factors are present (persistently moderate or high disease activity despite csDMARDs, high APPs, high swollen joint count, high-level rheumatoid factor, and/or anticitrullinated protein antibodies, early erosions or failure of at least two csDMARDs) biological DMARDs or JAK-inhibitor should be used and combined with csDMARDs; when patients are unable to use csDMARDs (TCZ, SRL) and targeted synthetic DMARDs (baricitinib, tofacitinib, and upadacitinib) may have advantages in relation to other biologics [134]. It is assumed that TCZ and SRL as a monotherapy are more efficacious than adalimumab [134]. When a biological DMARD or tsDMARD has failed, treatment with another biological DMARD or a tsDMARD should be considered and SRL may have some efficacy after the failure of TCZ [134, 135]. The efficacy of TCZ is similar to that described with SRL when comparing TCZ 8 mg/kg q4w and SRL 200 mg q2w [27].

A phase II double-blind placebo RCT published in 2016 first demonstrated the efficacy of IV TCZ in inducing and maintaining remission in patients with GCA. This study reported that remission and relapse-free survival was achieved in 85% of 20 patients receiving TCZ compared to 40% and 20%, respectively, of ten patients given placebo [136]. The phase III GiACTA trial was a one-year large-scale RCT that confirmed TCZ (qw or q2w) as the first treatment, besides steroids, to show effectiveness in GCA, leading more patients in remission than prednisone alone (about 50% at 52 weeks vs 14%–18% with prednisone) and helping to reduce the total dose of prednisone [137].

In JIA, TCZ is licensed to treat both systemic-onset and polyarticular subtypes [1]. Japanese phase III trials demonstrated the efficacy of TCZ in children with SJIA and PJIA, leading to its approval in Japan in 2008 [138, 139]. The phase III TENDER placebo-controlled RCT demonstrated the efficacy of TCZ in 112 children aged 2 to 17 years with SJIA refractory to conventional treatment, while the phase III CHERISH placebo-controlled RCT has also demonstrated good efficacy in children with PJIA refractory to MTX [140, 141]. The 2013 update of ACR recommendations for the treatment of SJIA has incorporated anti-IL-6 biologics in its management [1, 37, 142]. Approval of anti-IL-6 drugs in ADs and autoimmune-related disorders is described in Table 7.

6.1.2 *Adverse effects and contraindications*

RA patients taking TCZ are 1.2 more likely to have adverse effects (AEs) and 0.6 less likely to be withdrawn from treatment [116, 143]. The available evidence does not confirm unacceptable AEs with IL-6 blockade and several studies show a good safety profile [144–146].

TABLE 7   Interleukin-6 blockade approved drugs in autoimmune disorders.

Drug	Disorder	Region (year)
Tocilizumab (Actemra)	Rheumatoid arthritis	EU (2009), United States (2010)
	Systemic juvenile idiopathic arthritis	EU (2011), United States (2011)
	Polyarticular juvenile idiopathic arthritis	EU (2013), United States (2013)
	Giant cell arteritis	EU (2017), United States (2017)
Sarilumab (Kevzara)	Rheumatoid arthritis	EU (2017), United States (2017)

TCZ has also been approved for Castleman's disease and chimeric antigen receptor (CAR) T-cell-induced cytokine release syndrome. Siltuximab has been approved for Castleman's disease.

5. Application of IL-6 antagonists in autoimmune disorders

TABLE 8 Adverse event profile of interleukin-6 blockade.

Infections	Very common (>10%): upper respiratory
	Common (1%–10%): cellulitis, pneumonia, oral herpes simplex, herpes zoster
	Uncommon (0.1%–1%): diverticulitis
	Serious: 3.5/100 patient-years
	Opportunistic: 0.23/100 patient-years
Cardiovascular events	Myocardial infarction: 0.25/100 patient-years
	Stroke: 0.19/100 patient-years
Gastrointestinal complications	Common: abdominal pain, mouth ulcers, gastritis, diarrhea
	Uncommon: perforations (0.28/100 patient-years), stomatitis, gastric ulcer
Laboratory parameters	Very common: hypercholesterolemia, elevated transaminases
	Common: leukopenia (grade 4: 0.6%), neutropenia
	Uncommon: thrombocytopenia (grade 3 or 4: <0.1%)
Others	Very common: injection site reactions
	Common: cough, dizziness, dyspnea, headache, hypertension, hypersensitivity reactions, peripheral edema, pruritus, rash, weight gain
	Uncommon: conjunctivitis, exacerbation of autoimmune disorders, hypertriglyceridemia, hypothyroidism, pancreatitis, nephrolithiasis, new-onset sarcoidosis

Most results are obtained from RCTs including patients with RA.

Hypersensitivity constitutes the only absolute contraindication, but relevant comorbidities should be always considered, such as serious infections [147, 148]. The most common (>5%) treatment-related AEs include upper respiratory tract infections, hypercholesterolemia, and injection site reactions with SC formulations, as described in Table 8 [39]. Safety data for SRL have been consistent with IL-6 blockade, as demonstrated by the phase III SARIL-RA-HARUKA trial, and the most frequent AEs are neutropenia increased liver function tests (LFTs), injection site erythema, and upper respiratory tract infections [27, 149, 150]. The ASCERTAIN trial showed no clinically meaningful differences in treatment-emergent AEs between TCZ and SRL in patients with RA and laboratory changes were within comparable ranges [151]. Most withdrawals for AEs are due to neutropenia and increased alanine aminotransferase levels [27, 50].

IL-6 blockade has been associated with an increase in serious infections at rates similar to those seen with TNF inhibitors in RA, including *Mycobacterium tuberculosis* (0.23 per 100 patient-years), but not increasing over time and often occurring when co-administered with immunosuppressants [1, 150]. Infections, mainly of upper respiratory origin, probably constitute more than one-third of reported AEs with TCZ [142]. For skin and/or soft tissue infections, antibiotic therapy and omission of infusion for four weeks are recommended during TCZ therapy [147].

TCZ is associated with elevations in lipoproteins, which are often greater than those seen with other biological agents (e.g., increase of low-density cholesterol of 15% to 20% on average), even though a reversal of insulin resistance after 12 weeks of therapy has been documented [1]. TCZ may also increase antiatherogenic high-density cholesterol more than TNF blockade, decreasing the cardiovascular risk [1]. Increases in total and low-density lipoprotein (LDL) cholesterol also occur with SRL, but serum lipid alterations have been reported only in 1.6% of patients on SRL comparing to 4.3% on adalimumab and the risk also seems to be lower comparing to TCZ [27]. A baseline fasting lipid profile should be obtained and monitoring two to three times during the first six months and then every 12 months is recommended [119].

Gastrointestinal perforations associated with IL-6 blockade tend to mainly affect the large bowel and are probably related to IL-6 classic signaling inhibition, even though confounding factors such as steroids, nonsteroidal inflammatory drugs (NSAIDs) and concomitant diverticulosis should be taken into account [1, 27]. The development of PF-04236921 has been halted due to the association with gastrointestinal perforations in different populations [152, 153].

Neutropenia has been often reported following IL-6 blockade, but it appears to be clinically irrelevant, transient, and not associated with infections rate or severity (even with neutrophil counts <1000 cell/mm^3) [27, 46, 154]. The risk of other cytopenias is much lower, but the risk of neutropenia appears to be higher with SRL than TCZ [27]. Increased LFTs are probably dose-dependent and more prevalent in patients taking MTX [115]. Both LFTs and neutropenia should be monitored for the first six months and no action should be taken if LFTs are less than three the upper limit of normal range (ULN) or neutrophils >1×10^9/L; stopping TCZ is mandatory if LFTs are more than five times the ULN or neutrophils are <0.5×10^9/L [38]. TCZ should not be initiated if LFTs are more than 1.5 the ULN [155].

Even though an increased risk of malignancies has been reported with several biological agents and an incidence rate of 0.5% has been reported with TCZ, no trend in cancer types or consistent higher rates of malignancies have been established (overall 1.1/100 patients-year) [1, 156, 157].

Although it is unlikely that TCZ induces macrophage activation syndrome (MAS), it can mask the symptoms of SJIA-associated MAS and CRP cannot be used as a reliable marker [37, 158]. Increased death rates in relation to placebo lead to the decline of SRK approval in RA by the US Food and Drug Administration (FDA) in 2017 [159, 160].

6.1.3 *Pharmacodynamics and pharmacokinetics*

TCZ is a humanized IgG1κ monoclonal antibody that binds to the α chain of both membrane-bound and soluble forms of the IL-6R [46]. Changes in pharmacodynamics (PD) are to be expected shortly after administration, including decreases in CRP (normalizing as early as two weeks and maintained as long as free TCZ concentrations remain above 1 µg/mL), SAA and ESR levels (normalizing within 6 weeks) and increase in hemoglobin [24, 154, 155, 161]. TCZ may also lower fibrinogen, C3, and C4 serum levels [162, 163]. TCZ paradoxically increases serum levels of IL-6 and sIL-6R without altering IL-6 mRNA expression, since TCZ saturates sIL-6 and prolongs the elimination half-life of sIL-6, besides decreasing the usual route of elimination (IL-6R mediated consumption), therefore the measurements of IL-6 serum levels during TCZ therapy cannot be used for monitoring disease activity [46, 109]. Steady-state concentrations are often achieved around week 12 [155]. Pharmacokinetic (PK) data for approved anti-IL-6 drugs are described in Table 9.

The elimination of TCZ is slow and concentration-dependent [26]. TCZ undergoes biphasic elimination, including parallel linear (predominant at low concentrations via lysosomal destruction) and dose-dependent nonlinear clearances (usually at higher concentrations through the reticuloendothelial system) [154, 155]. Therefore, TCZ has a nonlinear PK profile, since the area under the curve (AUC) increases disproportionately with dose increments

5. Application of IL-6 antagonists in autoimmune disorders

TABLE 9   Pharmacokinetics of anti-interleukin-6 approved drugs.

	Bioavailability	Vd	Half-life	Route	Doses
TCZ	~79.5%	~6.4 L	~1–2 weeks (concentration-dependent)	IV SC	JIA[a]: 12 mg/kg q2w (<30 kg) JIA[a]: 8 mg/kg q2w (>30 kg) RA: 8 mg/kg q4w with a possible reduction to 4 mg/kg q4w (EU) RA: 4 mg/kg q4w with a possible increase to 8 mg/kg q4w (United States) RA: 162 mg qw with a possible decrease to q2w (EU) RA: 162 mg q2w with a possible increase to qw (United States)
SRL	80%	7.3–8.3 L	~3 weeks	SC	RA: 200 mg q2w with a possible reduction to 150 mg q2w in case of neutropenia, thrombocytopenia, or elevated LFTs

EU, European Union; *IV*, intravenous; *JIA*, juvenile idiopathic arthritis; *LFTs*, liver function tests; *RA*, rheumatoid arthritis; *SC*, subcutaneous; *SRL*, sarilumab; *TCZ*, tocilizumab; *Vd*, volume of distribution at steady-state.
[a] *In children above 2 years of age.*

that proportionally increase the maximum concentration of TCZ in the plasma (C_{max}) and its receptor binding becomes saturable at approximately 0.1 μg/mL [107, 154]. PK of TCZ is not affected by ethnicity, gender, age, mild renal impairment, treatment with NSAIDs, steroids, or MTX [83]. However, PD responses are probably less pronounced with q2w SC regimens, mainly in obese patients [164]. Monoclonal antibodies are not eliminated through renal or hepatic pathways and no dosage recommendations are provided in renal or hepatic impairments [27, 96]. Doses greater than 800 mg are not associated with increased efficacy [64]. The SUMMACTA study demonstrated that SC TCZ 162 mg q1w has comparable efficacy to IV TCZ 8 mg/kg q4w and a comparable rate of AEs except for injection site reactions [165].

SRL is a recombinant human IgG1 monoclonal antibody consisting of two human heavy chains linked to one κ light chain through a disulfide covalent bond, binding to soluble and membrane-bound IL-6R (sIL-6Rα and mIL-6Rα) with higher affinity than TCZ [27, 150]. It inhibits both trans- and cis-signaling [11, 27]. SRL is available as a single-dose prefilled syringe and exhibits similar PD effects during the first week to those seen with IV TCZ 4–8 mg/kg, including reduced neutrophil counts and CRP levels and increased IL-6 and sIL-6R concentrations [150]. With recommended doses, it reaches the maximum concentration in two to four days and steady-state concentration in 14–16 weeks, being eliminated through a linear nonsaturable proteolytic pathway at higher doses and a nonlinear saturable target-medication elimination pathway at lower doses [27, 150, 166]. SRL is not eliminated through renal or hepatic pathways and does not need dose adjustments [27, 150]. It is also eliminated by linear (nonsaturable, proteolytic, at higher concentrations) and nonlinear (saturable, target-mediated, at lower concentrations) pathways, resulting in an initial elimination half-life of eight to ten days and a terminal concentration-dependent half-life of two to four days [150]. Age, gender, race, and body weight are irrelevant in terms of PK, but patients with severe renal impairment have not been studied [150].

Certain IL-6R polymorphisms have been associated with lower responses to IL-6 blockade [167]. A strong acute-phase response (baseline ESR >30 mm/h or CRP >10 mg/L) and the presence of extra-articular manifestations have been associated with a rapid response at the observational level, while the combination of IL-6 and sIL-6R may be a more trustful predictive tool to ascertain response than serum IL-6 levels alone [154, 168, 169].

6.1.4 *Drug interactions, warnings, and immunogenicity*

TCZ inhibits the down-regulation of the CYP system caused by IL-6, including CYP1A2, 2C9, 2C19, and 3A4, thus potential interactions include cyclosporine, phenytoin, warfarin, and theophylline [147]. SRL may modulate IL-6 to restore the activity of CYP3A4 and decrease serum concentrations of warfarin, oral contraceptives, theophylline, and statins, reducing exposure to simvastatin by 45% [27, 150, 166].

TCZ is classified as category C in the FDA classification for use in pregnancy and a low rate of congenital malformations (4.5%) and a higher proportion of preterm birth have been described [154].

TCZ should not be administered with other biological DMARDs due to the risk of immunosuppression [155]. A black box warning associated with TCZ points to an increased risk of serious infections, including tuberculosis, invasive fungal infections, sepsis, and MAS [155]. The same boxed warning for SRL only excludes MAS [27].

The incidence of anti-TCZ antibodies appears to be low (1.2%–1.5%) and not related to monotherapy vs combination therapy, loss of efficacy, or injection reactions, but SRL monotherapy may induce an antidrug antibody response in more than 9% of patients (vs 1%–1.6% of patients on SLR plus DMARD) [150, 154].

Inactive vaccines should be administered prior to IL-6 blockade and live vaccines should not be used in patients on anti-IL-6 drugs [27]. A good antibody response is to be expected with pneumococcal and influenza vaccination [154].

6.2 Off-label use

Phase III SIRROUND trials demonstrated the efficacy of sirukumab (SRK) in active RA, not only in patients refractory to csDMARDs (SIRROUND-D), but also in patients who were intolerant or inappropriate to MTX (SIRROUND-H, comparing to adalimumab), MTX or sulfasalazine (SIRROUND-M), and patients who were intolerant or refractory to anti-TNF blockade (SIRROUND-T) [159, 170–172]. Therefore, SRK has shown a largely similar efficacy compared to TCZ in clinical trials and such benefits also appear to be sustained, even though a metaanalysis has suggested that TCZ may have the highest performance based on ACR50 response rate [160, 173, 174]. SRK may also have a good impact on specific RA-related complications, such as depression and cardiovascular disease [159]. In fact, SIRROUND-T has demonstrated significant improvements not only in the MCS component of SF-36, but also fatigue as evaluated by FACIT-F scores [19]. A phase IIb RCT in patients with RA and an inadequate response to MTX induced significant improvements in disease activity and higher rates of remission with CLZ, either alone or in combination with MTX [110]. OKZ has induced significant reductions in activity score in phase II trials, including in patients that had previously failed anti-TNF therapy, and a recent phase III has confirmed that OKZ significantly improves clinical manifestations and physical functioning in RA patients receiving concomitant MTX therapy [175,

176]. VBR has been given to patients with active RA with significant improvements in disease activity in a phase IIb trial that included patients who were intolerant or discontinued MTX, showing similar efficacy and tolerability to TCZ [177]. MEDI5117 is also currently being studied in RA, while levilimab (LVL) was recently evaluated in the phase II AURORA trial not only meeting the primary endpoint (ACR20 response rate at week 12), but also showing sustained (up to week 52) efficacy with LVL-MTX combination in MTX-refractory RA patients [178]. Elsilimomab has been administrated to RA patients with transitory clinical improvements, but trials have been undertaken mainly in patients with lymphoma and myeloma [111, 179]. Only IL-6R antagonists are approved in RA because of safety concerns about direct IL-6 inhibitors, but these may own a higher potency in treating depression and cardiovascular disease [160]. In case of reports, TCZ has also been effective in treating rheumatoid vasculitis, cryoglobulinemic vasculitis, AA amyloidosis, and SS complicating RA [60, 180].

A phase II placebo-controlled trial with PF-04236921 in active SLE patients did not show a significant difference from placebo for the primary efficacy endpoint, even though an effect with the lower dose was observed in a post hoc analysis [181]. A phase II RCT in patients with class III and IV lupus nephritis was unable to confirm both an acceptable safety profile and efficacy of SRK, while VBR failed to meet the primary endpoint in phase II STEADY trial [113, 182].

The phase II faSScinate RCT found that patients with SSc receiving TCZ had a less pronounced decline in forced vital capacity at 48 weeks, despite not being associated with significant differences in skin thickening comparing to placebo [183, 184]. These findings were replicated in phase III focuSSced trial [184, 185]. Considering these studies, FDA has granted breakthrough therapy designation (BTD) status to TCZ in SSc.

A phase III RCT in steroid-refractory AOSD patients demonstrated that IV TCZ 8 mg/kg q2w achieved nonsignificant ACR50 response rates at week 4, but changes in systemic feature score at week 12 and decrease in dose of glucocorticoids constituted secondary endpoints with statistically significant differences between arms [186]. Chronic articular involvement has been associated with significant responses to TCZ in retrospective studies [187].

In PMR, studies have used IV TCZ 8 mg/kg q4w [188]. The TENOR study was the first prospective nonrandomized study to demonstrate that TCZ is effective in recent-onset PMR without previous steroid therapy [189]. A phase IIa study has confirmed that TCZ is effective in newly diagnosed PMR previously treated with steroids for less than one month, allowing a robust steroid-sparing effect [190]. A prospective study has also suggested that TCZ may induce sustained remission (at week 52) in most patients [191]. TCZ monotherapy has been associated with relapses and low disease activity scores in only small percentages of patients and many of the studies that led to the approval of TCZ in GCA also included patients with PMR [39, 188].

A multicenter retrospective study has suggested that TCZ is efficient and may reduce the incidence of relapses in TA [192]. The phase III TAKT trial has favored SC TCZ 162 mg q1w over placebo in TA, although the primary endpoint (time to relapse) was not met [193]. Follow-up of these patients for up to 96 weeks or longer has demonstrated a steroid-sparing effect and improvements in well-being, as previously suggested in relation to cyclophosphamide by retrospective direct comparison [194, 195].

Phase II ANDANTE I and II trials have demonstrated that PF-04236921 induces clinical response and remission in anti-TNF-refractory patients with moderate-to-severe CD, being significantly better than placebo at weeks 8 and 12 [152].

TCZ is probably effective in NMO, but evidence derives mostly from another IL-6R inhibitor [196, 197]. STL induced a significant reduction (55%) in the risk of relapse compared to placebo in the SakuraStar phase III trial, which may be almost 75% in AQP4-positive patients [196, 198]. The SakuraSky phase III RCT demonstrated that STL added to immunosuppressant therapy results in a lower risk of relapse (62% reduction overall and 79% in AQP4-positive patients) [199]. Following these results, FDA has accepted Biologics License Application for STL for NMO in 2019 after granting BTD in 2018. A retrospective cohort study has suggested a beneficial effect of TCZ in rituximab-refractory autoimmune encephalitis [200].

A phase III RCT in moderate-to-severe steroid-resistant GO revealed that IV TCZ 8 mg/kg is associated with significant reductions in the clinical activity score (93.3% vs 58.8% in the placebo group at week 16) and improvement in exophthalmos (− 1.5 vs 0.0 mm) [201].

After several reports of favorable results of IL-6 blockade in noninfectious uveitis (birdshot chorioretinopathy, idiopathic uveitis, BS), a retrospective study suggested that TCZ is effective in cystoid macular edema, while a multicenter study pointed that TCZ may be useful even in patients with JIA-associated uveitis refractory to anti-TNF drugs [202, 203]. The phase II STOP-Uveitis trial demonstrated the efficacy of IV TCZ 4 and 8 mg/kg in improving visual acuity and reducing vitreous haze and central macular thickness in patients with noninfectious intermediate uveitis [204]. The phase II SATURN study also demonstrated that SC SRL 200 mg q2w is able to reduce the vitreous haze at week 16 (64% vs 35% comparing to placebo), particularly in posterior uveitis with macular edema [205]. Evidence for efficacy in other cases of uveitis (e.g., BS) comes from case reports and case series that have suggested that TCZ may be useful in BS patients refractory to anti-TNF drugs and particularly those with skin/mucosal manifestations, neurological involvement, or uveitis [89, 92, 206, 207].

Based on case reports and/or series, IL-6 blockade has been reported to yield favorable outcomes in acquired hemophilia, autoimmune hemolytic anemia, cryoglobulinemia, inflammatory myopathies, KD, limbic encephalitis, MCTD and overlap syndrome, MS, myasthenia gravis, myeloperoxidase (MPO)-ANCA-positive AAV, noninfectious aortitis, PAN, pemphigus, plantar pustular psoriasis, ReA, RP, RS3PE syndrome, sarcoidosis, UC and vitiligo [1, 24, 39, 82, 208–229]. Conflicting results with TCZ have been reported in axial spondyloarthritis, psoriasis and PsA, since most beneficial effects seen in case reports have not been confirmed in clinical trials [1, 36, 64]. Phase II/III BUILDER-1 and 2 trials were terminated precociously due to lack of significant response comparing IV TCZ to placebo in AS patients naïve to TNF inhibitors [230]. The phase II ALIGN trial also failed to show the efficacy of SRL in AS, while a phase IIb trial suggested that IL-6 blockade produces only modest efficacy in the treatment of musculoskeletal manifestations of PsA, without difference in skin outcomes or a dose response [231, 232].

7 Conclusion

IL-6 blockade has been approved in a minority of autoimmune-related disorders that include RA, JIA, and GCA. It is probable that in the future anti-IL-6 drugs will become available in the management of disorders such as SSc, PMR, NMO, GO, posterior autoimmune uveitis or neuro-Behçet and may even constitute the primary biological choice. Furthermore, other anti-IL-6 drugs besides TCZ and SRL will probably become widely available (e.g., SRK, CLZ,

OKZ, VBR). Nevertheless, it is expected that, in specific disorders, anti-IL-6 agents may be approved as secondary biological options. For example, unlike GCA, anti-TNF agents appear to be effective in treating TA and constitute the primary biological choice [233].

Approved anti-IL-6 drugs target IL-6R and block IL-6 classic signaling, trans-signaling, and trans-presentation. Instead, olamkicept targets the IL-6/sIL-6R complex and does not interfere with IL-6 classic signaling. If positive metabolic effects of IL-6 have been linked to classic signaling and negative effects with trans-signaling, it is clinically relevant to know if using olamkicept in the management of ADs instead of TCZ or SRL translates into clinical benefits regarding not only metabolic balance and cardiovascular outcomes, but also by specifically addressing the proinflammatory activity of IL-6 and its translational consequences. Moreover, most of the growing body of evidence regarding IL-6 blockade is directly related to RA patients and more studies are needed, particularly in other ADs and autoimmune-related disorders.

References

[1] L.H. Calabrese, S. Rose-John, IL-6 biology: implications for clinical targeting in rheumatic disease, Nat. Rev. Rheumatol. 10 (12) (2014) 720–727.

[2] C. Garbers, S. Heink, T. Korn, S. Rose-John, Interleukin-6: designing specific therapeutics for a complex cytokine, Nat. Rev. Drug Discov. 17 (6) (2018) 395–412.

[3] E. Assier, M.-C. Boissier, J.-M. Dayer, Interleukin-6: from identification of the cytokine to development of targeted treatments, Joint Bone Spine 77 (6) (2010) 532–536.

[4] C. Zhang, X. Zhang, X.-H. Chen, Inhibition of the interleukin-6 signaling pathway: a strategy to induce immune tolerance, Clin. Rev. Allergy Immunol. 47 (2) (2014) 163–173.

[5] T. Kishimoto, Interleukin-6: from basic science to medicine—40 years in immunology, Annu. Rev. Immunol. 23 (2005) 1–21.

[6] T. Kishimoto, Interleukin-6: discovery of a pleiotropic cytokine, Arthritis Res. Ther. 8 (Suppl. 2) (2006) S2.

[7] J. Van Snick, Interleukin-6: an overview, Annu. Rev. Immunol. 8 (1990) 253–278.

[8] E. Tackey, P.E. Lipsky, G.G. Illei, Rationale for interleukin-6 blockade in systemic lupus erythematosus, Lupus 13 (5) (2004) 339–343.

[9] W.L. Biffl, E.E. Moore, F.A. Moore, V.M. Peterson, Interleukin-6 in the injured patient. Marker of injury or mediator of inflammation? Ann. Surg. 224 (5) (1996) 647–664.

[10] M.C. Wolvekamp, R.L. Marquet, Interleukin-6: historical background, genetics and biological significance, Immunol. Lett. 24 (1) (1990) 1–9.

[11] M.G. Raimondo, M. Biggioggero, C. Crotti, A. Becciolini, E.G. Favalli, Profile of sarilumab and its potential in the treatment of rheumatoid arthritis, Drug Des. Devel. Ther. 11 (2017) 1593–1603.

[12] T. Hirano, Interleukin 6 in autoimmune and inflammatory diseases: a personal memoir, Proc. Jpn. Acad. Ser. B Phys. Biol. Sci. 86 (7) (2010) 717–730.

[13] P.C. Heinrich, I. Behrmann, S. Haan, H.M. Hermanns, G. Müller-Newen, F. Schaper, Principles of interleukin (IL)-6-type cytokine signalling and its regulation, Biochem. J. 374 (Pt 1) (2003) 1–20.

[14] M. Narazaki, T. Tanaka, T. Kishimoto, The role and therapeutic targeting of IL-6 in rheumatoid arthritis, Expert. Rev. Clin. Immunol. 13 (6) (2017) 535–551.

[15] T. Kishimoto, Interleukin-6 and its receptor in autoimmunity, J. Autoimmun. 5 (Suppl. A) (1992) 123–132.

[16] S. Akira, T. Kishimoto, Role of interleukin-6 in macrophage function, Curr. Opin. Hematol. 3 (1) (1996) 87–93.

[17] P. Uciechowski, W.C.M. Dempke, Interleukin-6: a masterplayer in the cytokine network, Oncology 98 (3) (2020) 131–137.

[18] B.E. Jones, M.D. Maerz, J.H. Buckner, IL-6: a cytokine at the crossroads of autoimmunity, Curr. Opin. Immunol. 55 (2018) 9–14.

[19] E.H.S. Choy, L.H. Calabrese, Neuroendocrine and neurophysiological effects of interleukin 6 in rheumatoid arthritis, Rheumatology (Oxford) 57 (11) (2018) 1885–1895.

[20] T. Matsuda, T. Hirano, Interleukin 6 (IL-6), Biotherapy 2 (4) (1990) 363–373.

[21] M. Mihara, M. Hashizume, H. Yoshida, M. Suzuki, M. Shiina, IL-6/IL-6 receptor system and its role in physiological and pathological conditions, Clin. Sci. (Lond.) 122 (4) (2012) 143–159.

[22] T. Tanaka, M. Narazaki, A. Ogata, T. Kishimoto, A new era for the treatment of inflammatory autoimmune diseases by interleukin-6 blockade strategy, Semin. Immunol. 26 (1) (2014) 88–96.

[23] T. Arkatkar, S.W. Du, H.M. Jacobs, E.M. Dam, B. Hou, J.H. Buckner, et al., B cell-derived IL-6 initiates spontaneous germinal center formation during systemic autoimmunity, J. Exp. Med. 214 (11) (2017) 3207–3217.

[24] T. Tanaka, T. Kishimoto, Targeting interleukin-6: all the way to treat autoimmune and inflammatory diseases, Int. J. Biol. Sci. 8 (9) (2012) 1227–1236.

[25] M. Lotz, Interleukin-6, Cancer Investig. 11 (6) (1993) 732–742.

[26] J.S. Smolen, D. Aletaha, I.B. McInnes, Rheumatoid arthritis, Lancet 388 (10055) (2016) 2023–2038.

[27] E.G. Boyce, E.L. Rogan, D. Vyas, N. Prasad, Y. Mai, Sarilumab: review of a second IL-6 receptor antagonist indicated for the treatment of rheumatoid arthritis, Ann. Pharmacother. 52 (8) (2018) 780–791.

[28] A. Dima, C. Jurcut, P. Balanescu, E. Balanescu, C. Badea, S. Caraiola, et al., Clinical significance of serum and urinary interleukin-6 in systemic lupus erythematosus patients, Egypt. Rheumatol. 39 (1) (2016) 1–6.

[29] E. Peterson, A.D. Robertson, W. Emlen, Serum and urinary interleukin-6 in systemic lupus erythematosus, Lupus 5 (6) (1996) 571–575.

[30] S. O'Reilly, R. Cant, M. Ciechomska, J.M. van Laar, Interleukin-6: a new therapeutic target in systemic sclerosis? Clin. Transl. Immunol. 2 (4) (2013) e4.

[31] Y. Kawaguchi, Contribution of interleukin-6 to the pathogenesis of systemic sclerosis, J. Scleroderma Relat. Disord. 2 (Suppl. 2) (2017) S6–S12.

[32] C. Chizzolini, A.M. Dufour, N.C. Brembilla, Is there a role for IL-17 in the pathogenesis of systemic sclerosis? Immunol. Lett. 195 (2018) 61–67.

[33] M.M. Grisius, D.K. Bermudez, P.C. Fox, Salivary and serum interleukin 6 in primary Sjögren's syndrome, J. Rheumatol. 24 (6) (1997) 1089–1091.

[34] N. Roescher, P.P. Tak, G.G. Illei, Cytokines in Sjögren's syndrome, Oral Dis. 15 (8) (2009) 519–526.

[35] P. Youinou, J.-O. Pers, Disturbance of cytokine networks in Sjögren's syndrome, Arthritis Res. Ther. 13 (4) (2011) 227.

[36] S. Akioka, Interleukin-6 in juvenile idiopathic arthritis, Mod. Rheumatol. 29 (2) (2019) 275–286.

[37] S. Grevich, S. Shenoi, Update on the management of systemic juvenile idiopathic arthritis and role of IL-1 and IL-6 inhibition, Adolesc. Health Med. Ther. 8 (2017) 125–135.

[38] S. Yokota, Interleukin 6 as a therapeutic target in systemic-onset juvenile idiopathic arthritis, Curr. Opin. Rheumatol. 15 (5) (2003) 581–586.

[39] S. Castañeda, N. García-Castañeda, D. Prieto-Peña, D. Martínez-Quintanilla, E.F. Vicente, R. Blanco, et al., Treatment of polymyalgia rheumatica, Biochem. Pharmacol. 165 (2019) 221–229.

[40] M.G. Ahmed, Clinical significance of interleukin-18 and interleukin-6 on disease course of adult-onset Still's disease, Ann. Rheum. Dis. 77 (Suppl. 2) (2018) 1162.

[41] E. Zuelgaray, M. Battistella, M.-D. Vignon-Pennamen, J.-D. Bouaziz, L. Michel, Cytokine levels in persistent skin lesions of adult-onset Still disease, J. Am. Acad. Dermatol. 79 (5) (2018) 947–949.

[42] É. Toussirot, A. Régent, V. Devauchelle-Pensec, A. Saraux, X. Puéchal, Interleukin-6: a promising target for the treatment of polymyalgia rheumatica or giant cell arteritis? RMD Open 2 (2) (2016) e000305.

[43] L. Boiardi, B. Casali, E. Farnetti, N. Pipitone, D. Nicoli, F. Cantini, et al., Relationship between interleukin 6 promoter polymorphism at position -174, IL-6 serum levels, and the risk of relapse/recurrence in polymyalgia rheumatica, J. Rheumatol. 33 (4) (2006) 703–708.

[44] S. Mori, Y. Koga, Glucocorticoid-resistant polymyalgia rheumatica: pretreatment characteristics and tocilizumab therapy, Clin. Rheumatol. 35 (5) (2016) 1367–1375.

[45] K.S.M. van der Geest, W.H. Abdulahad, A. Rutgers, G. Horst, J. Bijzet, S. Arends, et al., Serum markers associated with disease activity in giant cell arteritis and polymyalgia rheumatica, Rheumatology (Oxford) 54 (8) (2015) 1397–1402.

[46] V.J. Mariano, W.H. Frishman, Tocilizumab in giant cell arteritis, Cardiol. Rev. 26 (6) (2018) 321–330.

[47] T. Oide, S. Ohara, K. Oguchi, M. Maruyama, M. Yazawa, K. Inoue, et al., Remitting seronegative symmetrical synovitis with pitting edema (RS3PE) syndrome in Nagano, Japan: clinical, radiological, and cytokine studies of 13 patients, Clin. Exp. Rheumatol. 22 (1) (2004) 91–98.

[48] X. Kong, Y. Sun, L. Ma, H. Chen, L. Wei, W. Wu, et al., The critical role of IL-6 in the pathogenesis of Takayasu arteritis, Clin. Exp. Rheumatol. 34 (3 Suppl. 97) (2016) S21–S27.

5. Application of IL-6 antagonists in autoimmune disorders

[49] Q. Gao, N. Lv, A. Dang, Z. Li, J. Ye, D. Zheng, Association of interleukin-6 and interleukin-10 expression, gene polymorphisms, and Takayasu arteritis in a Chinese Han population, Clin. Rheumatol. 38 (1) (2019) 143–148.

[50] Y. Sun, X. Kong, X. Cui, X. Dai, L. Ma, H. Chen, et al., The value of interleukin-6 in predicting disease relapse for Takayasu arteritis during 2-year follow-up, Clin. Rheumatol. 39 (11) (2020) 3417–3425.

[51] C.-Y. Lin, Y.-H. Yang, C.-C. Lee, C.-L. Huang, L.-C. Wang, B.-L. Chiang, Thrombopoietin and interleukin-6 levels in Henoch-Schönlein purpura, J. Microbiol. Immunol. Infect. 39 (6) (2006) 476–482.

[52] T. Kuret, K. Lakota, P. Žigon, M. Ogric, S. Sodin-Semrl, S. Cucnik, et al., Insight into inflammatory cell and cytokine profiles in adult IgA vasculitis, Clin. Rheumatol. 38 (2) (2019) 331–338.

[53] D.S. Kim, Serum interleukin-6 in Kawasaki disease, Yonsei Med. J. 33 (2) (1992) 183–188.

[54] T. Kawakami, S. Takeuchi, Y. Soma, Serum levels of interleukin-6 in patients with cutaneous polyarteritis nodosa, Acta Derm. Venereol. 92 (3) (2012) 322–323.

[55] Y. Li, Q. Zheng, L. Zou, J. Wu, L. Guo, L. Teng, et al., Kawasaki disease shock syndrome: clinical characteristics and possible use of IL-6, IL-10 and IFN-γ as biomarkers for early recognition, Pediatr. Rheumatol. Online J. 17 (1) (2019) 1.

[56] Y. Wu, F.F. Liu, Y. Xu, J.J. Wang, S. Samadli, Y.F. Wu, et al., Interleukin-6 is prone to be a candidate biomarker for predicting incomplete and IVIG nonresponsive Kawasaki disease rather than coronary artery aneurysm, Clin. Exp. Med. 19 (2) (2019) 173–181.

[57] A. Berti, G. Cavalli, C. Campochiaro, B. Guglielmi, E. Baldissera, S. Cappio, et al., Interleukin-6 in ANCA-associated vasculitis: rationale for successful treatment with tocilizumab, Semin. Arthritis Rheum. 45 (1) (2015) 48–54.

[58] A. Antonelli, C. Ferri, S.M. Ferrari, E. Ghiri, F. Goglia, A. Pampana, et al., Serum levels of proinflammatory cytokines interleukin-1beta, interleukin-6, and tumor necrosis factor alpha in mixed cryoglobulinemia, Arthritis Rheum. 60 (12) (2009) 3841–3847.

[59] G.M. Sousa, I.S. Oliveira, L.J.O. Andrade, M.L.B. Sousa-Atta, R. Paraná, A.M. Atta, Serum levels of Th17 associated cytokines in chronic hepatitis C virus infection, Cytokine 60 (1) (2012) 138–142.

[60] L. Kaly, I. Rosner, Tocilizumab—a novel therapy for non-organ-specific autoimmune diseases, Best Pract. Res. Clin. Rheumatol. 26 (1) (2012) 157–165.

[61] W. Liu, Y.-H. Wu, L. Zhang, X.-Y. Liu, B. Xue, Y. Wang, et al., Elevated serum levels of IL-6 and IL-17 may associate with the development of ankylosing spondylitis, Int. J. Clin. Exp. Med. 8 (10) (2015) 17362–17376.

[62] S.K. Sharma, S. Ahmad, S.K. Sharma, Serum IL-6 level as a marker of disease activity in ankylosing spondylitis patients with pure axial involvement, Indian J. Rheumatol. 9 (3) (2014) 115–119.

[63] A. Falkenbach, M. Herold, R. Wigand, Interleukin-6 serum concentration in ankylosing spondylitis: a reliable predictor of disease progression in the subsequent year? Rheumatol. Int. 19 (4) (2000) 149–151.

[64] H. Zeng, B. Luo, Y. Zhang, Z. Xie, Z. Ye, Treatment of reactive arthritis with biological agents: a review, Biosci. Rep. 40 (2) (2020). BSR20191927.

[65] L. Graeve, M. Baumann, P.C. Heinrich, Interleukin-6 in autoimmune diseases. Role of IL-6 in physiology and pathology of the immune defense, Clin. Investig. 71 (1993) 664–671.

[66] A. Ogata, A. Kumanogoh, T. Tanaka, Pathological role of interleukin-6 in psoriatic arthritis, Arthritis 2012 (2012) 713618.

[67] O. Arican, M. Aral, S. Sasmaz, P. Ciragil, Serum levels of TNF-α, IFN-γ, IL-6, IL-8, IL-12, IL-17, and IL-18 in patients with active psoriasis and correlation with disease severity, Mediat. Inflamm. 2005 (5) (2005) 273–279.

[68] A. Saggini, S. Chimenti, A. Chiricozzi, IL-6 as a druggable target in psoriasis: focus on pustular variants, J Immunol Res 2014 (2014) 964069.

[69] A.N. Boca, M. Talamont, M. Galluzzo, E. Botti, S.C. Vesa, S. Chimenti, et al., Genetic variations in IL6 and IL12B decreasing the risk for psoriasis, Immunol. Lett. 156 (1–2) (2013) 127–131.

[70] F. Atzeni, D. Ventura, A. Batticciotto, L. Boccassini, P. Sarzi-Puttini, Interleukin 6 blockade: tocilizumab in psoriatic arthritis, J. Rheumatol. Suppl. 89 (2012) 97–99.

[71] H. Ito, IL-6 and Crohn's disease, Curr. Drug Targets Inflamm. Allergy 2 (2) (2003) 125–130.

[72] S. Nikolaus, G.H. Waetzig, S. Butzin, M. Ziolkiewicz, N. Al-Massad, F. Thieme, et al., Evaluation of interleukin-6 and its soluble receptor components sIL-6R and sgp130 as markers of inflammation in inflammatory bowel diseases, Int. J. Color. Dis. 33 (7) (2018) 927–936.

[73] Y.R. Mahida, L. Kurlac, A. Gallagher, C.J. Hawkey, High circulating concentrations of interleukin-6 in active Crohn's disease but not ulcerative colitis, Gut 32 (12) (1991) 1531–1534.

[74] J. Mudter, M.F. Neurath, Il-6 signaling in inflammatory bowel disease: pathophysiological role and clinical relevance, Inflamm. Bowel Dis. 13 (8) (2007) 1016–1023.

[75] D. Bernardo, S. Vallejo-Díez, E.R. Mann, H.O. Al-Hassi, B. Martínez-Abad, E. Montalvillo, et al., IL-6 promotes immune responses in human ulcerative colitis and induces a skin-homing phenotype in the dendritic cells and Tcells they stimulate, Eur. J. Immunol. 42 (5) (2012) 1337–1353.

[76] C.A. Parisinos, S. Serghiou, M. Katsoulis, M.J. George, R.S. Patel, H. Hemingway, et al., Variation in interleukin 6 receptor gene associates with risk of Crohn's disease and ulcerative colitis, Gastroenterology 155 (2) (2018) 303–306.e302.

[77] P. Desreumaux, Specific targeting of IL-6 signalling pathway: a new way to treat IBD? Gut 47 (4) (2000) 465–466.

[78] Y. Nishida, S. Hosomi, K. Watanabe, K. Watanabe, T. Yukawa, K. Otani, et al., Serum interleukin-6 level is associated with response to infliximab in ulcerative colitis, Scand. J. Gastroenterol. 53 (5) (2018) 579–585.

[79] E. Wine, D.R. Mack, J. Hyams, A.R. Otley, J. Markowitz, W.V. Crandall, et al., Interleukin-6 is associated with steroid resistance and reflects disease activity in severe pediatric ulcerative colitis, J. Crohns Colitis 7 (11) (2013) 916–922.

[80] A. Uzawa, M. Mori, S. Kuwabara, Role of interleukin-6 in the pathogenesis of neuromyelitis optica, Clin. Exp. Neurol. 4 (2) (2013) 167–172.

[81] F. Petkovic, B. Castellano, The role of interleukin-6 in central nervous system demyelination, Neural Regen. Res. 11 (12) (2016) 1922–1923.

[82] R.C. Dale, Interleukin-6 blockade as rescue therapy in autoimmune encephalitis, Neurotherapeutics 13 (4) (2016) 821–823.

[83] M. Maurer, S. Bougoin, T. Feferman, M. Frenkian, J. Bismuth, V. Mouly, et al., IL-6 and Akt are involved in muscular pathogenesis in myasthenia gravis, Acta Neuropathol. Commun. 3 (2015) 1.

[84] D. Maimone, P. Annunziata, I.L. Simone, P. Livrea, G.C. Guazzi, Interleukin-6 levels in the cerebrospinal fluid and serum of patients with Guillain-Barré syndrome and chronic inflammatory demyelinating polyradiculoneuropathy, J. Neuroimmunol. 47 (1) (1993) 55–61.

[85] C. Durães, C.S. Moreira, I. Alvelos, A. Mendes, L.R. Santos, J.C. Machado, et al., Polymorphisms in the TNFA and IL6 genes represent risk factors for autoimmune thyroid disease, PLoS One 9 (8) (2014) e105492.

[86] I. Molnár, C. Balázs, High circulating IL-6 level in Graves' ophthalmopathy, Autoimmunity 25 (2) (1997) 91–96.

[87] S.C. Jyonouchi, R.W. Valyasevi, D.A. Harteneck, C.M. Dutton, R.S. Bahn, Interleukin-6 stimulates thyrotropin receptor expression in human orbital preadipocyte fibroblasts from patients with Graves' ophthalmopathy, Thyroid 11 (10) (2001) 929–934.

[88] D. Łacheta, P. Miśkiewicz, A. Głuszko, G. Nowicka, M. Struga, I. Kantor, et al., Immunological aspects of Graves' ophthalmopathy, Biomed. Res. Int. 2019 (2019) 7453260.

[89] P. Lin, Targeting interleukin-6 for noninfectious uveitis, Clin. Ophthalmol. 9 (2015) 1697–1702.

[90] T. Yoshimura, K.-H. Sonoda, N. Ohguro, Y. Ohsugi, T. Ishibashi, D.J. Cua, et al., Involvement of Th17 cells and the effect of anti-IL-6 therapy in autoimmune uveitis, Rheumatology (Oxford) 48 (4) (2009) 347–354.

[91] Y. Yamakawa, Y. Sugita, T. Nagatani, S. Takahashi, T. Yamakawa, S. Tanaka, et al., Interleukin-6 (IL-6) in patients with Behçet's disease, J. Dermatol. Sci. 11 (3) (1996) 189–195.

[92] F. Caso, L. Costa, D. Rigante, O.M. Lucherini, P. Caso, V. Bascherini, et al., Biological treatments in Behçet's disease: beyond anti-TNF therapy, Mediat. Inflamm. 2014 (2014) 107421.

[93] G. Akman-Demir, E. Tüzün, S. İçöz, N. Yesilot, S.P. Yentür, M. Kürtüncü, et al., Interleukin-6 in neuro-Behçet's disease: association with disease subsets and long-term outcome, Cytokine 44 (3) (2008) 373–376.

[94] K.A. Bain, E. McDonald, F. Moffat, M. Tutino, M. Castelino, A. Barton, et al., Alopecia areata is characterized by dysregulation in systemic type 17 and type 2 cytokines, which may contribute to disease-associated psychological morbidity, Br. J. Dermatol. 182 (1) (2020) 130–137.

[95] O. Denisova, K. Egorova, G. Chernogoryuk, TNF-α, IL-8, IL-6 levels in serum of sarcoidosis patients with different clinical course, Eur. Respir. J. 42 (Suppl. 57) (2013) P3787.

[96] S. Singh, U. Singh, S.S. Pandey, Serum concentration of IL-6, IL-2, TNF-α, and IFNγ in Vitiligo patients, Indian J. Dermatol. 57 (1) (2012) 12–14.

[97] P. Thomas-Dupont, J.M. Remes-Troche, I.Y. Izaguirre-Hernández, L.A. Sánchez-Vargas, M.-J. Maldonado-Rentería, K.G. Hernández-Flores, et al., Elevated circulating levels of IL-21 and IL-22 define a cytokine signature profile in type 2 autoimmune hepatitis patients, Ann. Hepatol. 15 (4) (2016) 550–558.

5. Application of IL-6 antagonists in autoimmune disorders

[98] Y. Yang, Y. Liu, L. Huang, L. Wang, K. Liu, M. Liu, et al., Clinical features and cytokine profile in myositis patients with anti-EJ autoantibodies detected by a novel immunoprecipation assay, Biomed. Res. Int. 2019 (2019) 1856180.

[99] E. Schmidt, B. Bastian, R. Dummer, H.P. Tony, E.B. Bröcker, D. Zillikens, Detection of elevated levels of IL-4, IL-6, and IL-10 in blister fluid of bullous pemphigoid, Arch. Dermatol. Res. 288 (7) (1996) 353–357.

[100] J.S. Manavalan, L. Hernandez, J.G. Shah, J. Konikkara, A.J. Naiyer, A.R. Lee, et al., Serum cytokine elevations in celiac disease: association with disease presentation, Hum. Immunol. 71 (1) (2010) 50–57.

[101] P. Soltesz, H. Der, K. Veres, R. Laczik, S. Sipka, G. Szegedi, et al., Immunological features of primary anti-phospholipid syndrome in connection with endothelial dysfunction, Rheumatology (Oxford) 47 (11) (2008) 1628–1634.

[102] O. Yeğin, M. Coşkun, H. Ertuğ, Cytokines in acute rheumatic fever, Eur. J. Pediatr. 156 (1) (1997) 25–29.

[103] P.E. Lipsky, Interleukin-6 and rheumatic diseases, Arthritis Res. Ther. 8 (Suppl 2) (2006) S4.

[104] D. Camellino, S. Soldano, M. Cutolo, M.A. Cimmino, Dissecting the inflammatory response in polymyalgia rheumatica: the relative role of IL-6 and its inhibition, Rheumatol. Int. 38 (9) (2018) 1699–1704.

[105] B.J.M. Ripley, B. Goncalves, D.A. Isenberg, D.S. Latchman, A. Rahman, Raised levels of interleukin 6 in systemic lupus erythematosus correlate with anaemia, Ann. Rheum. Dis. 64 (6) (2005) 849–853.

[106] S.M.A. Galil, N. Ezzeldin, M.E. El-Boshy, The role of serum IL-17 and IL-6 as biomarkers of disease activity and predictors of remission in patients with lupus nephritis, Cytokine 76 (2) (2015) 280–287.

[107] K. Takenaka, T. Ohba, K. Suhara, Y. Sato, K. Nagasaka, Successful treatment of refractory aortitis in antineutrophil cytoplasmic antibody-associated vasculitis using tocilizumab, Clin. Rheumatol. 33 (2014) 287–289.

[108] K. Sahashi, Y. Ina, K. Takada, T. Sato, M. Yamamoto, M. Morishita, Significance of interleukin 6 in patients with sarcoidosis, Chest 106 (1) (1994) 156–160.

[109] N. Nishimoto, K. Terao, T. Mima, H. Nakahara, N. Takagi, T. Kakehi, Mechanisms and pathologic significances in increase in serum interleukin-6 (IL-6) and soluble IL-6 receptor after administration of an anti-IL-6 receptor antibody, tocilizumab, in patients with rheumatoid arthritis and Castleman disease, Blood 112 (10) (2008) 3959–3964.

[110] M.E. Weinblatt, P. Mease, E. Mysler, T. Takeuchi, E. Drescher, A. Berman, et al., The efficacy and safety of subcutaneous clazakizumab in patients with moderate-to-severe rheumatoid arthritis and an inadequate response to methotrexate: results from a multinational, phase IIb, randomized, double-blind, placebo/active-controlled, dose-ranging study, Arthritis Rheum. 67 (10) (2015) 2591–2600.

[111] D. Wendling, E. Racadot, J. Wijdenes, Treatment of severe rheumatoid arthritis by anti-interleukin 6 monoclonal antibody, J. Rheumatol. 20 (2) (1993) 259–262.

[112] S. Shaw, T. Bourne, C. Meier, B. Carrington, R. Gelinas, A. Henry, et al., Discovery and characterization of olokizumab: a humanized antibody targeting interleukin-6 and neutralizing gp130-signaling, MAbs 6 (3) (2014) 774–782.

[113] M. Van Roy, C. Ververken, E. Beirnaert, S. Hoefman, J. Kolkman, M. Vierboom, et al., The preclinical pharmacology of the high affinity anti-IL-6R Nanobody® ALX-0061 supports its clinical development in rheumatoid arthritis, Arthritis Res. Ther. 17 (1) (2015) 135.

[114] T.-H. Heo, J. Wahler, N. Suh, Potential therapeutic implications of IL-6/IL-6R/gp130-targeting agents in breast cancer, Oncotarget 7 (13) (2016) 15460–15473.

[115] R.N. Maini, P.C. Taylor, J. Szechinski, K. Pavelka, J. Bröll, G. Balint, et al., Double-blind randomized controlled clinical trial of the interleukin-6 receptor antagonist, tocilizumab, in European patients with rheumatoid arthritis who had an incomplete response to methotrexate, Arthritis Rheum. 54 (9) (2006) 2817–2829.

[116] A. Ogata, T. Hirano, Y. Hishitani, T. Tanaka, Safety and efficacy of tocilizumab for the treatment of rheumatoid arthritis, Clin. Med. Insights Arthritis Musculoskelet. Disord. 5 (2012) 27–42.

[117] J.S. Smolen, A. Beaulieu, A. Rubbert-Roth, C. Ramos-Remus, J. Rovensky, E. Alecock, et al., Effect of interleukin-6 receptor inhibition with tocilizumab in patients with rheumatoid arthritis (OPTION study): a double-blind, placebo-controlled, randomised trial, Lancet 371 (9617) (2008) 987–997.

[118] G. Jones, A. Sebba, J. Gu, M.B. Lowenstein, A. Calvo, J.J. Gomez-Reino, et al., Comparison of tocilizumab monotherapy versus methotrexate monotherapy in patients with moderate to severe rheumatoid arthritis: the AMBITION study, Ann. Rheum. Dis. 69 (1) (2010) 88–96.

[119] N. Nishimoto, J. Hashimoto, N. Miyasaka, K. Yamamoto, S. Kawai, T. Takeuchi, et al., Study of active controlled monotherapy used for rheumatoid arthritis, an IL-6 inhibitor (SAMURAI): evidence of clinical and

radiographic benefit from an X ray reader-blinded randomised controlled trial of tocilizumab, Ann. Rheum. Dis. 66 (9) (2007) 1162–1167.

[120] P. Emery, E. Keystone, H.P. Tony, A. Cantagrel, R. van Vollenhoven, A. Sanchez, et al., IL-6 receptor inhibition with tocilizumab improves treatment outcomes in patients with rheumatoid arthritis refractory to anti-tumour necrosis factor biologicals: results from a 24-week multicentre randomised placebo-controlled trial, Ann. Rheum. Dis. 67 (11) (2008) 1516–1523.

[121] J.M. Kremer, R. Blanco, M. Brzosko, R. Burgos-Vargas, A.-M. Halland, E. Vernon, et al., Tocilizumab inhibits structural joint damage in rheumatoid arthritis patients with inadequate responses to methotrexate: results from the double-blind treatment phase of a randomized placebo-controlled trial of tocilizumab safety and prevention of structural joint damage at one year, Arthritis Rheum. 63 (3) (2011) 609–621.

[122] M. Dougados, K. Kissel, T. Sheeran, P.P. Tak, P.G. Conaghan, E.M. Mola, et al., Adding tocilizumab or switching to tocilizumab monotherapy in methotrexate inadequate responders: 24-week symptomatic and structural results of a 2-year randomised controlled strategy trial in rheumatoid arthritis (ACT-RAY), Ann. Rheum. Dis. 72 (1) (2013) 43–50.

[123] Y. Yazici, J.R. Curtis, A. Ince, H. Baraf, R.L. Malamet, L.L. Teng, et al., Efficacy of tocilizumab in patients with moderate to severe active rheumatoid arthritis and a previous inadequate response to disease-modifying antirheumatic drugs: the ROSE study, Ann. Rheum. Dis. 71 (2) (2012) 198–205.

[124] T. Tanaka, A. Ogata, M. Narazaki, Tocilizumab for the treatment of rheumatoid arthritis, Expert. Rev. Clin. Immunol. 6 (6) (2010) 843–854.

[125] X.M. Teitsma, A.K.A. Marijnissen, J.W.J. Bijlsma, F.P.J. Lafeber, J.W.G. Jacobs, Tocilizumab as monotherapy or combination therapy for treating active rheumatoid arthritis: a meta-analysis of efficacy and safety reported in randomized controlled trials, Arthritis Res. Ther. 18 (1) (2016) 211.

[126] G.R. Burmester, W.F. Rigby, R.F. van Vollenhoven, J. Kay, A. Rubbert-Roth, A. Kelman, et al., Tocilizumab in early progressive rheumatoid arthritis: FUNCTION, a randomised controlled trial, Ann. Rheum. Dis. 75 (6) (2016) 1081–1091.

[127] C. Gabay, P. Emery, R. van Vollenhoven, A. Dikranian, R. Alten, K. Pavelka, et al., Tocilizumab monotherapy versus adalimumab monotherapy for treatment of rheumatoid arthritis (ADACTA): a randomised, double-blind, controlled phase 4 trial, Lancet 381 (9877) (2013) 1541–1550.

[128] T.W.J. Huizinga, R.M. Fleischmann, M. Jasson, A.R. Radin, J. van Adelsberg, S. Fiore, et al., Sarilumab, a fully human monoclonal antibody against IL-6Rα in patients with rheumatoid arthritis and an inadequate response to methotrexate: efficacy and safety results from the randomised SARIL-RA-MOBILITY Part A trial, Ann. Rheum. Dis. 73 (9) (2014) 1626–1634.

[129] M.C. Genovese, R. Fleischmann, A.J. Kivitz, M. Rell-Bakalarska, R. Martincova, et al., Sarilumab plus methotrexate in patients with active rheumatoid arthritis and inadequate response to methotrexate: results of a phase III study, Arthritis Rheum. 67 (6) (2015) 1424–1437.

[130] R. Fleischmann, J. van Adelsberg, Y. Lin, G.R. Castelar-Pinheiro, J. Brzezicki, P. Hrycaj, et al., Sarilumab and nonbiologic disease-modifying antirheumatic drugs in patients with active rheumatoid arthritis and inadequate response or intolerance to tumor necrosis factor inhibitors, Arthritis Rheum. 69 (2) (2017) 277–290.

[131] G.R. Burmester, Y. Lin, R. Patel, J. van Adelsberg, E.K. Mangan, N.M.H. Graham, et al., Efficacy and safety of sarilumab monotherapy versus adalimumab monotherapy for the treatment of patients with active rheumatoid arthritis (MONARCH): a randomised, double-blind, parallel-group phase III trial, Ann. Rheum. Dis. 76 (5) (2017) 840–847.

[132] M.C. Genovese, J. van Adelsberg, C. Fan, N.M.H. Graham, H. van Hoogstraten, J. Parrino, et al., Two years of sarilumab in patients with rheumatoid arthritis and an inadequate response to MTX: safety, efficacy and radiographic outcomes, Rheumatology (Oxford) 57 (8) (2018) 1423–1431.

[133] Y. Tanaka, K. Wada, Y. Takahashi, O. Hagino, H. van Hoogstraten, N.M.H. Graham, et al., Sarilumab plus methotrexate in patients with active rheumatoid arthritis and inadequate response to methotrexate: results of a randomized, placebo-controlled phase III trial in Japan, Arthritis Res. Ther. 21 (1) (2019) 79.

[134] J.S. Smolen, R.B.M. Landewé, J.W.J. Bijlsma, G.R. Burmester, M. Dougados, A. Kerschbaumer, et al., EULAR recommendations for the management of rheumatoid arthritis with synthetic and biological disease-modifying antirheumatic drugs: 2019 update, Ann. Rheum. Dis. 79 (6) (2020) 685–699.

[135] P. Verschueren, P. Emery, H. van Hoogstraten, Q. Dong, E.K. Mangan, A. den Broeder, Efficacy of sarilumab in patients with rheumatoid arthritis with and without previous response to tocilizumab, Ann. Rheum. Dis. 77 (Suppl. 2) (2018) 327–328.

[136] P.M. Villiger, S. Adler, S. Kuchen, F. Wermelinger, D. Dan, V. Fiege, et al., Tocilizumab for induction and maintenance of remission in giant cell arteritis: a phase 2, randomised, double-blind, placebo-controlled trial, Lancet 387 (10031) (2016) 1921–1927.

[137] J.H. Stone, K. Tuckwell, S. Dimonaco, M. Klearman, M. Aringer, D. Blockmans, et al., Trial of tocilizumab in giant-cell arteritis, N. Engl. J. Med. 377 (4) (2017) 317–328.

[138] S. Yokota, T. Imagawa, M. Mori, T. Miyamae, Y. Aihara, S. Takei, et al., Efficacy and safety of tocilizumab in patients with systemic-onset juvenile idiopathic arthritis: a randomised, double-blind, placebo-controlled, withdrawal phase III trial, Lancet 371 (9617) (2008) 998–1006.

[139] T. Imagawa, S. Yokota, M. Mori, T. Miyamae, S. Takei, H. Imanaka, et al., Safety and efficacy of tocilizumab, an anti-IL-6-receptor monoclonal antibody, in patients with polyarticular-course juvenile idiopathic arthritis, Mod. Rheumatol. 22 (1) (2012) 109–115.

[140] F. De Benedetti, H.I. Brunner, N. Ruperto, A. Kenwright, S. Wright, I. Calvo, et al., Randomized trial of tocilizumab in systemic juvenile idiopathic arthritis, N. Engl. J. Med. 367 (25) (2012) 2385–2395.

[141] H.I. Brunner, N. Ruperto, Z. Zuber, C. Keane, O. Harari, A. Kenwright, et al., Efficacy and safety of tocilizumab in patients with polyarticular-course juvenile idiopathic arthritis: results from a phase 3, randomised, double-blind withdrawal trial, Ann. Rheum. Dis. 74 (6) (2015) 1110–1117.

[142] J.E. Frampton, Tocilizumab: a review of its use in the treatment of juvenile idiopathic arthritis, Paediatr. Drugs 15 (6) (2013) 515–531.

[143] J.A. Singh, S. Beg, M.A. Lopez-Olivo, Tocilizumab for rheumatoid arthritis: a Cochrane systematic review, J. Rheumatol. 38 (1) (2011) 10–20.

[144] N. Nishimoto, N. Miyasaka, K. Yamamoto, S. Kawai, T. Takeuchi, J. Azuma, Long-term safety and efficacy of tocilizumab, an anti-IL-6 receptor monoclonal antibody, in monotherapy, in patients with rheumatoid arthritis (the STREAM study): evidence of safety and efficacy in a 5-year extension study, Ann. Rheum. Dis. 68 (10) (2009) 1580–1584.

[145] G.G. Illei, Y. Shirota, C.H. Yarboro, J. Daruwalla, E. Tackey, K. Takada, et al., Tocilizumab in systemic lupus erythematosus: data on safety, preliminary efficacy, and impact on circulating plasma cells from an open-label phase I dosage-escalation study, Arthritis Rheum. 62 (2) (2010) 542–552.

[146] M. Aringer, J.S. Smolen, Safety of off-label biologicals in systemic lupus erythematosus, Expert Opin. Drug Saf. 14 (2) (2015) 243–251.

[147] M. Sheppard, F. Laskou, P.P. Stapleton, S. Hadavi, B. Dasgupta, Tocilizumab (Actemra), Hum. Vaccin. Immunother. 13 (9) (2017) 1972–1988.

[148] J.S. Smolen, M.M. Schoels, N. Nishimoto, F.C. Breedveld, G.R. Burmester, M. Dougados, et al., Consensus statement on blocking the effects of interleukin-6 and in particular by interleukin-6 receptor inhibition in rheumatoid arthritis and other inflammatory conditions, Ann. Rheum. Dis. 72 (4) (2013) 482–492.

[149] H. Kameda, K. Wada, Y. Takahashi, O. Hagino, H. van Hoogstraten, N. Graham, et al., Sarilumab monotherapy or in combination with non-methotrexate disease-modifying antirheumatic drugs in active rheumatoid arthritis: a Japan phase 3 trial (HARUKA), Mod. Rheumatol. 30 (2) (2020) 239–248.

[150] L.J. Scott, Sarilumab: first global approval, Drugs 77 (6) (2017) 705–712.

[151] P. Emery, J. Rondon, J. Parrino, Y. Lin, C. Pena-Rossi, H. van Hoogstraten, et al., Safety and tolerability of subcutaneous sarilumab and intravenous tocilizumab in patients with rheumatoid arthritis, Rheumatology (Oxford) 58 (5) (2019) 849–858.

[152] S. Danese, S. Vermeire, P. Hellstern, R. Panaccione, G. Rogler, G. Fraser, et al., Randomised trial and open-label extension study of an anti-interleukin-6 antibody in Crohn's disease (ANDANTE I and II), Gut 68 (1) (2019) 40–48.

[153] J. Sabino, B. Verstockt, S. Vermeire, M. Ferrante, New biologics and small molecules in inflammatory bowel disease: an update, Ther. Adv. Gastroenterol. 12 (2019). 1756284819853208.

[154] R. Sanmartí, V. Ruiz-Esquide, C. Bastida, D. Soy, Tocilizumab in the treatment of adult rheumatoid arthritis, Immunotherapy 10 (6) (2018) 447–464.

[155] K. Decelle, E.R. Horton, Tocilizumab for the treatment of juvenile idiopathic arthritis, Ann. Pharmacother. 46 (6) (2012) 822–829.

[156] T. Koike, M. Harigai, S. Inokuma, N. Ishiguro, J. Ryu, T. Takeuchi, et al., Postmarketing surveillance of tocilizumab for rheumatoid arthritis in Japan: interim analysis of 3881 patients, Ann. Rheum. Dis. 70 (12) (2011) 2148–2151.

[157] L. Campbell, C. Chen, S.S. Bhagat, R.A. Parker, A.J.K. Östör, Risk of adverse events including serious infections in rheumatoid arthritis patients treated with tocilizumab: a systematic literature review and meta-analysis of randomized controlled trials, Rheumatology (Oxford) 50 (3) (2011) 552–562.

[158] M. Shimizu, Y. Nakagishi, K. Kasai, Y. Yamasaki, M. Miyoshi, S. Takei, et al., Tocilizumab masks the clinical symptoms of systemic juvenile idiopathic arthritis-associated macrophage activation syndrome: the diagnostic significance of interleukin-18 and interleukin-6, Cytokine 58 (2) (2012) 287–294.

[159] F. Bartoli, S. Bae, L. Cometi, M.M. Cerinic, D.E. Furst, Sirukumab for the treatment of rheumatoid arthritis: update on sirukumab, 2018, Expert. Rev. Clin. Immunol. 14 (7) (2018) 539–547.

[160] A.B. Avci, E. Feist, G.R. Burmester, Targeting IL-6 or IL-6 receptor in rheumatoid arthritis: what's the difference? BioDrugs 32 (6) (2018) 531–546.

[161] L.J. Scott, Tocilizumab: a review in rheumatoid arthritis, Drugs 77 (17) (2017) 1865–1879.

[162] C. Romano, A.D. Mastro, A. Sellitto, E. Solaro, S. Esposito, G. Cuomo, Tocilizumab reduces complement C3 and C4 serum levels in rheumatoid arthritis patients, Clin. Rheumatol. 37 (6) (2018) 1695–1700.

[163] N. Martis, D. Chirio, V. Queyrel-Moranne, M.-C. Zenut, F. Rocher, J.-G. Fuzibet, Tocilizumab-induced hypofibrinogenemia: a report of 7 cases, Joint Bone Spine 84 (3) (2017) 369–370.

[164] H. Abdallah, J.C. Hsu, P. Lu, S. Fettner, X. Zhang, W. Douglass, et al., Pharmacokinetic and pharmacodynamic analysis of subcutaneous tocilizumab in patients with rheumatoid arthritis from 2 randomized, controlled trials: SUMMACTA and BREVACTA, J. Clin. Pharmacol. 57 (4) (2017) 459–468.

[165] G.R. Burmester, A. Rubbert-Roth, A. Cantagrel, S. Hall, P. Leszczynski, D. Feldman, et al., A randomised, double-blind, parallel-group study of the safety and efficacy of subcutaneous tocilizumab versus intravenous tocilizumab in combination with traditional disease-modifying antirheumatic drugs in patients with moderate to severe rheumatoid arthritis (SUMMACTA study), Ann. Rheum. Dis. 73 (1) (2014) 69–74.

[166] Y.N. Lamb, E.D. Deeks, Sarilumab: a review in moderate to severe rheumatoid arthritis, Drugs 78 (9) (2018) 929–940.

[167] C. Enevold, B. Baslund, L. Linde, N.L. Josephsen, U. Tarp, H. Lindegaard, et al., Interleukin-6-receptor polymorphisms rs12083537, rs2228145, and rs4329505 as predictors of response to tocilizumab in rheumatoid arthritis, Pharmacogenet. Genomics 24 (8) (2014) 401–405.

[168] J. Narváez, B. Magallares, C.D. Torné, M.V. Hernández, D. Reina, H. Corominas, et al., Predictive factors for induction of remission in patients with active rheumatoid arthritis treated with tocilizumab in clinical practice, Semin. Arthritis Rheum. 45 (4) (2016) 386–390.

[169] C. Diaz-Torne, M.D.A. Ortiz, P. Moya, M.V. Hernandez, D. Reina, et al., The combination of IL-6 and its soluble receptor is associated with the response of rheumatoid arthritis patients to tocilizumab, Semin. Arthritis Rheum. 47 (6) (2018) 757–764.

[170] T. Takeuchi, C. Thorne, G. Karpouzas, S. Sheng, W. Xu, R. Rao, et al., Sirukumab for rheumatoid arthritis: the phase III SIRROUND-D study, Ann. Rheum. Dis. 76 (12) (2017) 2001–2008.

[171] D. Aletaha, C.O. Bingham 3rd, Y. Tanaka, P. Agarwal, R. Kurrasch, P.P. Tak, et al., Efficacy and safety of sirukumab in patients with active rheumatoid arthritis refractory to anti-TNF therapy (SIRROUND-T): a randomised, double-blind, placebo-controlled, parallel-group, multinational, phase 3 study, Lancet 389 (10075) (2017) 1206–1217.

[172] P.C. Taylor, M.H. Schiff, Q. Wang, Y. Jiang, Y. Zhuang, R. Kurrasch, et al., Efficacy and safety of monotherapy with sirukumab compared with adalimumab monotherapy in biologic-naïve patients with active rheumatoid arthritis (SIRROUND-H): a randomised, double-blind, parallel-group, multinational, 52-week, phase 3 study, Ann. Rheum. Dis. 77 (5) (2018) 658–666.

[173] C. Thorne, T. Takeuchi, G.A. Karpouzas, S. Sheng, R. Kurrasch, K. Fei, et al., Investigating sirukumab for rheumatoid arthritis: 2-year results from the phase III SIRROUND-D study, RMD Open 4 (2) (2018) e000731.

[174] S.-C. Bae, Y.H. Lee, Comparison of the efficacy and tolerability of tocilizumab, sarilumab, and sirukumab in patients with active rheumatoid arthritis: a Bayesian network meta-analysis of randomized controlled trials, Clin. Rheumatol. 37 (6) (2018) 1471–1479.

[175] M.C. Genovese, R. Fleischmann, D. Furst, N. Janssen, J. Carter, B. Dasgupta, et al., Efficacy and safety of olokizumab in patients with rheumatoid arthritis with an inadequate response to TNF inhibitor therapy: outcomes of a randomised Phase IIb study, Ann. Rheum. Dis. 73 (9) (2014) 1607–1615.

[176] T. Takeuchi, Y. Tanaka, H. Yamanaka, K. Amano, R. Nagamine, W. Park, et al., Efficacy and safety of olokizumab in Asian patients with moderate-to-severe rheumatoid arthritis, previously exposed to anti-TNF therapy: results from a randomized phase II trial, Mod. Rheumatol. 26 (1) (2016) 15–23.

5. Application of IL-6 antagonists in autoimmune disorders

[177] T. Dörner, M. Weinblatt, K. Van Beneden, E.J. Dombrecht, K. De Beuf, P. Schoen, et al., Results of a phase 2b study of vobarilizumab, an anti-interleukin-6 receptor nanobody, as monotherapy in patients with moderate to severe rheumatoid arthritis, Ann. Rheum. Dis. 76 (Suppl. 2) (2017) 575.

[178] V. Mazurov, E. Zotkin, E. Ilivanova, T. Kropotina, T. Plaksina, O. Nesmeyanova, et al., Efficacy of levilimab, novel monoclonal anti-IL-6 receptor antibody, in combination with methotrexate in patients with rheumatoid arthritis: 1-year results of phase 2 AURORA study, Ann. Rheum. Dis. 79 (Suppl. 1) (2020) 637–638.

[179] R. Burger, A. Günther, K. Klausz, M. Staudinger, M. Peipp, E.M.M. Penas, et al., Due to interleukin-6 type cytokine redundancy only glycoprotein 130 receptor blockade efficiently inhibits myeloma growth, Haematologica 102 (2) (2017) 381–390.

[180] H. Nakahara, K. Kawamoto, H. Mori, S. Nozato, M. Hirai, H. Matuoka, et al., Tocilizumab is effective for the patient with Sjögren's syndrome complicated with rheumatoid arthritis, Ann. Rheum. Dis. 73 (Suppl. 2) (2014) 967–968.

[181] D.J. Wallace, V. Strand, J.T. MerrillT, S. Popa, A.J. Spindler, A. Eimon, et al., Efficacy and safety of an interleukin 6 monoclonal antibody for the treatment of systemic lupus erythematosus: a phase II dose-ranging randomised controlled trial, Ann. Rheum. Dis. 76 (3) (2017) 534–542.

[182] B.H. Rovin, R.F. van Vollenhoven, C. Aranow, C. Wagner, R. Gordon, Y. Zhuang, et al., A multicenter, randomized, double-blind, placebo-controlled study to evaluate the efficacy and safety of treatment with sirukumab (CNTO 136) in patients with active lupus nephritis, Arthritis Rheum. 68 (9) (2016) 2174–2183.

[183] D. Khanna, C.P. Denton, A. Jahreis, J.M. van Laar, T.M. Frech, M.E. Anderson, et al., Safety and efficacy of subcutaneous tocilizumab in adults with systemic sclerosis (faSScinate): a phase 2, randomised, controlled trial, Lancet 387 (10038) (2016) 2630–2640.

[184] D. Khanna, C.P. Denton, C.J.F. Lin, J.M. van Laar, T.M. Frech, M.E. Anderson, et al., Safety and efficacy of subcutaneous tocilizumab in systemic sclerosis: results from the open-label period of a phase II randomised controlled trial (faSScinate), Ann. Rheum. Dis. 77 (2) (2018) 212–220.

[185] C.J.F. Lin, M. Kuwana, Y. Allanore, A. Batalov, I. Butrimiene, P. Carreira, et al., Efficacy and safety of tocilizumab for the treatment of systemic sclerosis: results from a phase 3 randomized controlled trial, in: ACR/ARHP Annual Meeting, 2018. Abstract Number 898.

[186] Y. Kaneko, H. Kameda, K. Ikeda, T. Ishii, K. Murakami, H. Takamatsu, et al., Tocilizumab in patients with adult-onset Still's disease refractory to glucocorticoid treatment: a randomised, double-blind, placebo-controlled phase III trial, Ann. Rheum. Dis. 77 (12) (2018) 1720–1729.

[187] F. Vercruysse, T. Barnetche, E. Lazaro, E. Shipley, F. Lifermann, A. Balageas, et al., Adult-onset Still's disease biological treatment strategy may depend on the phenotypic dichotomy, Arthritis Res. Ther. 21 (1) (2019) 53.

[188] M. Akiyama, Y. Kaneko, T. Takeuchi, Tocilizumab in isolated polymyalgia rheumatica: a systematic literature review, Semin. Arthritis Rheum. 50 (3) (2020) 521–525.

[189] V. Devauchelle-Pensec, M. Berthelot, D. Cornec, Y. Renaudineau, T. Marhadour, S. Jousse-Joulin, et al., Efficacy of first-line tocilizumab therapy in early polymyalgia rheumatica: a prospective longitudinal study, Ann. Rheum. Dis. 75 (8) (2016) 1506–1510.

[190] L. Lally, L. Forbess, C. Hatzis, R. Spiera, Brief report: a prospective open-label phase IIa trial of tocilizumab in the treatment of polymyalgia rheumatica, Arthritis Rheum. 68 (10) (2016) 2550–2554.

[191] K. Chino, T. Kondo, R. Sakai, S. Saito, Y. Okada, A. Shibata, et al., Tocilizumab monotherapy for polymyalgia rheumatica: a prospective, single-center, open-label study, Int. J. Rheum. Dis. 22 (12) (2019) 2151–2157.

[192] A. Mekinian, M. Resche-Rigon, C. Comarmond, A. Soriano, J. Constans, L. Alric, et al., Efficacy of tocilizumab in Takayasu arteritis: multicenter retrospective study of 46 patients, J. Autoimmun. 91 (2018) 55–60.

[193] Y. Nakaoka, M. Isobe, S. Takei, Y. Tanaka, T. Ishii, S. Yokota, et al., Efficacy and safety of tocilizumab in patients with refractory Takayasu arteritis: results from a randomised, double-blind, placebo-controlled, phase 3 trial in Japan (the TAKT study), Ann. Rheum. Dis. 77 (3) (2018) 348–354.

[194] Y. Nakaoka, M. Isobe, Y. Tanaka, T. Ishii, S. Ooka, H. Niiro, et al., Long-term efficacy and safety of tocilizumab in refractory Takayasu arteritis: final results of the randomized controlled phase 3 TAKT study, Rheumatology (Oxford) 59 (9) (2020) 2427–2434.

[195] H. Liao, L.L. Pan, J. Du, N. Gao, T. Wang, Efficacy and safety of tocilizumab in patients with Takayasu arteritis, Abstract, Zhonghua Nei Ke Za Zhi 58 (6) (2019) 444–448.

[196] M. Araki, Blockade of IL-6 signaling in neuromyelitis optica, Neurochem. Int. 130 (2019) 104315.

[197] E.C. Guarnizo, R.H. Clares, T.C. Triviño, V.M. Lallana, V.A. Casañ, F.I. Martínez, et al., Experience with tocilizumab in patients with neuromyelitis optica spectrum disorders, Neurologia S0213-4853 (19) (2019) 30033–30037.

[198] A. Traboulsee, B. Greenberg, J.L. Bennett, L. Szczechowski, E. Fox, S. Shkrobot, et al., Safety and efficacy of satralizumab in neuromyelitis optica spectrum disorder: a randomised, double-blind, multicentre, placebo-controlled phase 3 trial, Lancet Neurol. 19 (5) (2020) 402–412.

[199] T. Yamamura, I. Kleiter, K. Fujihara, J. Palace, B. Greenberg, B. Zakrzewska-Pniewska, et al., Trial of satralizumab in neuromyelitis optica spectrum disorder, N. Engl. J. Med. 381 (22) (2019) 2114–2124.

[200] W.-J. Lee, S.-T. Lee, J. Moon, J.-S. Sunwoo, J.-I. Byun, J.-A. Lim, et al., Tocilizumab in autoimmune encephalitis refractory to rituximab: an institutional cohort study, Neurotherapeutics 13 (4) (2016) 824–832.

[201] J.V. Perez-Moreiras, J.J. Gomez-Reino, J.R. Maneiro, E. Perez-Pampin, A.R. Lopez, F.M.R. Alvarez, et al., Efficacy of tocilizumab in patients with moderate to severe corticosteroid resistant Graves´ orbitopathy: a randomized clinical trial, Am J. Ophthalmol. 195 (2018) 181–190.

[202] M. Mesquida, A. Leszczynska, V. Llorenç, A. Adán, Interleukin-6 blockade in ocular inflammatory diseases, Clin. Exp. Immunol. 176 (3) (2014) 301–309.

[203] V. Calvo-Río, M. Santos-Gómez, I. Calvo, M.I. González-Fernández, B. López-Montesinos, M. Mesquida, et al., Anti-interleukin-6 receptor tocilizumab for severe juvenile idiopathic arthritis-associated uveitis refractory to anti-tumor necrosis factor therapy: a multicenter study of twenty-five patients, Arthritis Rheum. 69 (3) (2017) 668–675.

[204] Y.J. Sepah, M.A. Sadiq, D.S. Chu, M. Dacey, R. Gallemore, P. Dayani, et al., Primary (month-6) outcomes of the STOP-uveitis study: evaluating the safety, tolerability, and efficacy of tocilizumab in patients with noninfectious uveitis, Am J. Ophthalmol. 183 (2017) 71–80.

[205] J. Heissigerová, D. Callanan, M.D. de Smet, S.K. Srivastava, M. Karkanová, O. Garcia-Garcia, et al., Efficacy and safety of sarilumab for the treatment of posterior segment noninfectious uveitis (SARIL-NIU): the phase 2 SATURN study, Ophthalmology 126 (3) (2019) 428–437.

[206] A. Deroux, C. Chiquet, L. Bouillet, Tocilizumab in severe and refractory Behcet's disease: four cases and literature review, Semin. Arthritis Rheum. 45 (6) (2016) 733–737.

[207] B. Atienza-Mateo, V. Calvo-Río, E. Beltrán, L. Martínez-Costa, E. Valls-Pascual, M. Hernández-Garfella, et al., Anti-interleukin 6 receptor tocilizumab in refractory uveitis associated with Behçet's disease: multicentre retrospective study, Rheumatology (Oxford) 57 (5) (2018) 856–864.

[208] T. Tanaka, T. Kishimoto, Immunotherapeutic implication of IL-6 blockade, Immunotherapy 4 (1) (2012) 87–105.

[209] S. Nishida, T. Kawasaki, H. Kashiwagi, A. Morishima, Y. Hishitani, M. Kawai, et al., Successful treatment of acquired hemophilia A, complicated by chronic GVHD, with tocilizumab, Mod. Rheumatol. 21 (4) (2011) 420–422.

[210] F.J. García-Hernández, R. González-León, M.J. Castillo-Palma, C. Ocaña-Medina, J. Sánchez-Román, Tocilizumab for treating refractory haemolytic anaemia in a patient with systemic lupus erythematosus, Rheumatology 51 (10) (2012) 1918–1919.

[211] C. Cohen, A. Mekinian, N. Saidenberg-Kermanac'h, J. Stirnemann, P. Fenaux, R. Gherardi, et al., Efficacy of tocilizumab in rituximab-refractory cryoglobulinemia vasculitis, Ann. Rheum. Dis. 71 (4) (2012) 628–629.

[212] A. Beaumel, O. Muis-Pistor, J.-G. Tebib, F. Coury, Antisynthetase syndrome treated with tocilizumab, Joint Bone Spine 83 (3) (2016) 361–362.

[213] S.M. Murphy, J.B. Lilleker, P. Helliwell, H. Chinoy, The successful use of tocilizumab as third-line biologic therapy in a case of refractory anti-synthetase syndrome, Rheumatology (Oxford) 55 (12) (2016) 2277–2278.

[214] T. Nozawa, T. Imagawa, S. Ito, Coronary-artery aneurysm in tocilizumab-treated children with Kawasaki's disease, N. Engl. J. Med. 377 (19) (2017) 1894–1896.

[215] M. Benucci, L. Tramacere, M. Infantino, M. Manfredi, V. Grossi, A. Damiani, et al., Efficacy of tocilizumab in limbic encephalitis with anti-CASPR2 antibodies, Case Rep. Neurol. Med. 2020 (2020) 5697670.

[216] N. Cabrera, A. Duquesne, M. Desjonquères, J.-P. Larbre, J.-C. Lega, N. Fabien, et al., Tocilizumab in the treatment of mixed connective tissue disease and overlap syndrome in children, RMD Open 2 (2) (2016) e000271.

[217] H. Hoshino, Y. Shirai, H. Konishi, T. Yamamura, N. Shimizu, Efficacy of tocilizumab for fulminant multiple sclerosis with a tumefactive cervical lesion: a 12-year-old boy, Mult. Scler. Relat. Disord. 37 (2020) 101460.

[218] D.I. Jonsson, R. Pirskanen, F. Piehl, Beneficial effect of tocilizumab in myasthenia gravis refractory to rituximab, Neuromuscul. Disord. 27 (6) (2017) 565–568.

[219] R. Sakai, T. Kondo, T. Kurasawa, E. Nishi, A. Okuyama, K. Chino, et al., Current clinical evidence of tocilizumab for the treatment of ANCA-associated vasculitis: a prospective case series for microscopic polyangiitis in a combination with corticosteroids and literature review, Clin. Rheumatol. 36 (10) (2017) 2383–2392.

5. Application of IL-6 antagonists in autoimmune disorders

[220] J. Loricera, R. Blanco, S. Castañeda, A. Humbría, N. Ortego-Centeno, J. Narváez, et al., Tocilizumab in refractory aortitis: study on 16 patients and literature review, Clin. Exp. Immunol. 32 (3 Suppl. 82) (2014) S79–S89.

[221] L. Bodoki, E. Végh, Z. Szekanecz, G. Szűcs, Tocilizumab treatment in polyarteritis nodosa, Isr. Med. Assoc. J. 21 (8) (2019) 560–562.

[222] F. Caso, L. Iaccarino, S. Bettio, F. Ometto, L. Costa, L. Punzi, et al., Refractory pemphigus foliaceus and Behçet's disease successfully treated with tocilizumab, Immunol. Res. 56 (2–3) (2013) 390–397.

[223] P. Jayasekera, R. Parslew, A. Al-Sharqi, A case of tumour necrosis factor-α inhibitor- and rituximab-induced plantar pustular psoriasis that completely resolved with tocilizumab, Br. J. Dermatol. 171 (6) (2014) 1546–1549.

[224] T. Tanaka, Y. Kuwahara, Y. Shima, T. Hirano, M. Kawai, M. Ogawa, et al., Successful treatment of reactive arthritis with a humanized anti-interleukin-6 receptor antibody, tocilizumab, Arthritis Rheum. 61 (12) (2009) 1762–1764.

[225] M. Kawai, K. Hagihara, T. Hirano, Y. Shima, Y. Kuwahara, J. Arimitsu, et al., Sustained response to tocilizumab, anti-interleukin-6 receptor antibody, in two patients with refractory relapsing polychondritis, Rheumatology (Oxford) 48 (3) (2009) 318–319.

[226] T. Tanaka, K. Hagihara, Y. Shima, M. Narazaki, A. Ogata, I. Kawase, et al., Treatment of a patient with remitting seronegative, symmetrical synovitis with pitting oedema with a humanized anti-interleukin-6 receptor antibody, tocilizumab, Rheumatology (Oxford) 49 (4) (2010) 824–826.

[227] M. Sharp, S.C. Donnelly, D.R. Moller, Tocilizumab in sarcoidosis patients failing steroid sparing therapies and anti-TNF agents, Respir. Med. X 1 (2019) 100004.

[228] M.C.H. Szeto, M.D. Yalçın, A. Khan, A. Piotrowicz, Successful use of tocilizumab in a patient with coexisting rheumatoid arthritis and ulcerative colitis, Case Reports Immunol. 2016 (2016) 7562123.

[229] C.B. Bunker, J. Manson, Vitiligo remitting with tocilizumab, J. Eur. Acad. Dermatol. Venereol. 33 (1) (2019), e20.

[230] J. Sieper, J. Braun, J. Kay, S. Badalamenti, A.R. Radin, L. Jiao, et al., Sarilumab for the treatment of ankylosing spondylitis: results of a phase II, randomised, double-blind, placebo-controlled study (ALIGN), Ann. Rheum. Dis. 74 (6) (2015) 1051–1057.

[231] J. Sieper, B. Porter-Brown, L. Thompson, O. Harari, M. Dougados, Assessment of short-term symptomatic efficacy of tocilizumab in ankylosing spondylitis: results of randomised, placebo-controlled trials, Ann. Rheum. Dis. 93 (1) (2014) 95–100.

[232] A. Kerschbaumer, J.S. Smolen, M. Dougados, M. de Wit, J. Primdahl, I. McInnes, et al., Pharmacological treatment of psoriatic arthritis: a systematic literature research for the 2019 update of the EULAR recommendations for the management of psoriatic arthritis, Ann. Rheum. Dis. 79 (6) (2020) 778–786.

[233] M. Samson, G. Espígol-Frigolé, N. Terrades-García, S. Prieto-González, M. Corbera-Bellalta, R. Alba-Rovira, et al., Biological treatments in giant cell arteritis & Takayasu arteritis, Eur. J. Intern. Med. 50 (2018) 12–19.

CHAPTER 6

The search for monomer-interaction-based alternative TNF-α therapies

Mark Farrugia and Byron Baron*

Centre for Molecular Medicine and Biobanking, University of Malta, Msida, Malta
***Corresponding author**

Abstract

Inflammation is regulated by tumor necrosis factor alpha (TNF-α), which as such plays a major role in various autoimmune disorders. High levels of TNF-α induce a wide range of inflammatory phenotypes according to the autoimmune disease in question. Regulating the amount of TNF-α in the body is one of the main treatments administered in order to help alleviate the inflammation that ensues in such conditions. The two autoimmune diseases which will be considered here are psoriasis and rheumatoid arthritis in the contexts of pregnancy and old age. These are particularly sensitive situations as the flare up or development of new inflammatory conditions in these contexts could be associated with serious complications since there are limited treatment options available on the market. Inflammation is elicited by a cascade resulting from the binding of active TNF-α, which is a trimer, to the TNF-α receptor. Most available TNF-α therapies address receptor-binding rather than the TNF-α molecule production or multimerization. The formation of the TNF-α trimer also includes posttranslational modifications but very few have been identified so far, and hence their link to human disease is not characterized. Understanding the trigger, production, assembly, and binding of TNF-α would allow the development of allosteric TNF-α inhibitors to be used in complicated contexts including during pregnancy and old age.

Keywords

TNF-α, Inflammation, Autoimmune disorders, Inhibitors, Posttranslational modifications

1 Introduction

Inflammation is a reactive response of the body, which occurs in the vascularized connective tissue, with the aim of protecting the vital organ tissues. The immune response is triggered by a stimulus usually associated with the presence of a foreign or damaging entity [1]. Through inflammation, the immune system tries to get rid of this entity (such as microbes or toxins) and the consequences of the invasion of that stimulus to the body and the following immune response (such as necrotic cells and tissues). Inflammation thus blocks, reduces, or eliminates the injurious agent, and at the same time starts a series of events aimed at healing and regenerating the damaged tissue [1].

A critical function of inflammation is the delivery of leukocytes to the site of injury. This is achieved by increased local blood flow, structural changes in the microvasculature to allow leukocyte emigration and accumulation at the site of the inflammatory response. Leukocytes ingest offending agents, kill or deactivate microbes, and degrade necrotic tissue and foreign antigens, while at the same help in the prolongation and maintenance of the inflammation through the release of various cytokines, enzymes, and toxic oxygen radicals [2]. Although inflammation is a protective response, uncontrolled inflammation may be potentially harmful and may underlie the pathogenesis of many acute and chronic diseases. Moreover, inflammation may be caused by nondamaging entities or even through a reaction to self-antigens causing autoimmune responses [3].

Inflammation can be either acute or chronic. Acute inflammation is of relatively short duration, lasting from minutes up to a few days, mainly characterized by the slow release of fluids and plasma proteins in the area (exudation), which could lead to swelling (edema) and the introduction of leukocytes in the area, predominantly neutrophils. Chronic inflammation takes place over a longer period and is associated with the presence of lymphocytes and macrophages in the inflamed regions coupled with angiogenesis, which stimulate a further increase in fibrosis and tissue necrosis, caused by the presence of these same leukocytes. In chronic inflammation, active inflammation, tissue destruction, and attempts at regeneration all proceed simultaneously [4]. Chronic inflammation may follow acute inflammation, but it often begins as a nondetectable asymptomatic response, which in most cases the etiology is still unknown. Some known causes include persistent infection by certain microorganisms (such as tubercle bacilli and *Treponema pallidum* causing syphilis), prolonged exposure to potentially toxic agents (either exogenous such as silica or endogenous such as plasma lipid components resulting in atherosclerosis), and autoimmune responses as in psoriasis or rheumatoid arthritis [2].

Mononuclear phagocytes, especially monocytes and macrophages, were thought to be the most important executers of chronic inflammation. In fact, monocytes transform into phagocytic macrophages that secrete a wide variety of biological compounds resulting in tissue injury and fibrosis characteristic of chronic inflammation. However, more insight has been recently gained into the role played by other actors of inflammation, including leukocyte subtypes such as T regulatory (Treg) cells that are critical in controlling the inflammation homeostasis [5]. Moreover, the pivotal role of cytokines in both the maintenance and shift in the balance of the immune microenvironment, with particular interest in tumor necrosis factor alpha (TNF-α) has been investigated through different studies [6–10].

1.1 Role of TNF-α in inflammation

TNF-α is a proinflammatory cytokine that plays a vital role in various facets of inflammation as described in this section.

During vasodilation, TNF-α acts by stimulating nitric oxide (NO) synthesis via inducible nitric oxide synthase (iNOS) expression in macrophages and other leukocytes [11]. TNF-α has the opposite effect on endothelial nitric oxide synthase (eNOS) by suppressing its expression. The NO produced by eNOS is critical for physiological functions of the endothelium [12]. TNF-α also increases the production of prostanoids such as prostaglandin E_2 (PGE2), prostaglandin F2α (PGF2α), and prostacyclin (also known as prostaglandin PGI2) via stimulation of cyclooxygenase 2 (COX-2).

TNF-α also induces edema. Edema develops as a consequence of higher vessel permeability, temporarily increased pressure in the capillaries, and decreased oncotic blood plasma pressure; with the balance created between these three factors, the transfer of transvascular liquid and protein and thus the access of antibodies and acute phase proteins to the site of the inflammation are facilitated [13]. TNF-α contributes to the creation of edema by disrupting the structure of the vessels' endothelium, which is achieved by degrading the glycocalyx layer that keeps healthy endothelium strengthened, thus increasing permeability of the vessels [14]. TNF-α also disturbs the integrity of the endothelial cell cytoskeleton by increasing the tyrosine phosphorylation of the adhesive molecule, cadherin, at endothelial cell junctions, opening the paracellular passage for solutes and macromolecules and thus forming intercellular gaps [15]. Up to 60% of the disintegration of the endothelial barrier is caused by these mechanisms [16].

Furthermore, TNF-α affects selectins, which are cell adhesion molecules (CAMs) with pivotal roles in the interaction between leukocytes and endothelial cells. TNF-α increases the expression of E-selectin and P-selectin, which are involved in the adhesion of neutrophils, monocytes, and memory T cells to the stimulated platelets and endothelial cells [17]. TNF-α also stimulates the expression of intercellular adhesion molecule 1 (ICAM-1) and vascular cell adhesion molecule 1 (VCAM-1), which contribute to leukocyte-leukocyte, leukocyte-endothelium, and leukocyte-epithelium interactions and transendothelial migration as well as mediating the binding of lymphocytes, monocytes, basophiles, and eosinophils to the endothelium.

A study performed on isolated human coronary endothelial cells concluded that TNF-α increases the expression of the nicotinamide adenine dinucleotide phosphate (NADPH) oxidase (NOX) family (NOX4A, p47phox, p67phox, and p22phox), which results in up to three times more NOX activity [18]. NOX produce reactive oxygen species (ROS) and these play an important role in inflammatory signal transduction by triggering some redox-dependent cell signal pathways which catalyze electron transfer from reduced NADPH to molecular oxygen, aiding in creating superoxide radicals and hydrogen peroxide [19].

TNF-α serves a key role in the pathogenesis of a variety of immunological diseases, such as rheumatoid arthritis (RA) [5] and psoriasis [20]. The high levels of TNF-α play a role in the inflammatory phenotypes that come with such diseases. Regulating the amount of TNF-α in the body would help to alleviate the inflammation that comes with these conditions.

1.2 Inflammation and TNF-α in psoriasis

Psoriasis is a common chronic autoimmune skin disease characterized by skin redness (erythema), epidermal hyperplasia, abnormal differentiation of keratinocytes, and scaling. The histological analysis of the affected areas presents accumulation of inflammatory molecules and angiogenesis [21]. Such changes are mediated by abnormal T cell cytokine production [22]. Psoriasis is a relatively common condition affecting up to 2% of Europeans [23].

T helper 1 (Th1) and T helper 17 (Th17) cells are the main cells responsible for the inflammatory immune response in psoriasis by inducing a cascade of inflammatory cytokines, notably TNF-α [24, 25]). However, various cells involved in the pathophysiology of psoriasis, such as keratinocytes, dendritic cells (DCs), and natural killer T (NKT) cells, Th1, Th17, and Th22 cells produce TNF-α. In keratinocytes, apart from immune and inflammatory responses, TNF-α induces tissue remodeling, cell motility, cell cycling, and apoptosis [26]. Additionally, activated keratinocytes also produce many chemokines responsible for the recruitment of neutrophils, macrophages, and skin-specific memory T cells [26]. TNF-α induces a number of cytokines including interleukin (IL)-19, IL-20, IL-22, and IL-24, which contribute to the initiation and progress of the disease; for instance, IL-24 appears to be required for the initiation phase of psoriasis [27–30].

A meta-analysis study indicated that certain single nucleotide polymorphisms (SNPs) of TNF-α can increase (238G/A) or decrease (308G/A) the risk of psoriasis by affecting the transcription and regulation of *TNF* and other susceptibility genes, such as *STAT4*, *IL10*, and vitamin receptor D (*VDR*) [31]. Similarly, polymorphisms in TNF-α-related genes such as *TNFAIP3* may affect the response to anti-TNF-α treatment by limiting nuclear factor kappa-light-chain-enhancer of activated B-cells (NF-κB) mediated inflammation [32].

Despite all the above-mentioned data, the underlying mechanism of psoriasis is still unclear. However, it appears to be more complex than initially believed, with TNF-α being implicated in both the initial and chronic phase of psoriasis, affecting various processes resulting in the pathogenesis. Moreover, a large proportion of psoriasis patients also present other chronic inflammatory disease such as inflammatory bowel disease (IBD) and RA as well as obesity, hypertension, diabetes mellitus, and depression, all of which have been associated with adverse pregnancy and birth outcomes [33], which will be discussed in Section 2.1.

Psoriasis has been shown to develop as a side effect to anti-TNF-α therapies in some patients with IBD or RA. While the actual cause remains unclear, it is thought to be a class effect (based on the similarity between the drugs) and may be relate to the alteration in immunity induced by the inhibition of TNF-α activity in predisposed individuals [34, 35]. The incidence rate of psoriasis in such patients has been found to be 0.53% per patient-year of anti-TNF-α treatment, with a cumulative incidence of psoriasis of 1.0% at 1 year, 2.5% at 5 years, and 4.5% at 10 years. Women and smokers (or former smokers) were found to have an increased risk of psoriasis induced by anti-TNF-α drugs [36].

1.3 Inflammation and TNF-α in rheumatoid arthritis

RA is an autoimmune disorder brought about by the chronic inflammation of the lining of the joints, with significant morbidity and mortality rates if left untreated [37]. RA is characterized by synovial inflammation and hyperplasia (swelling), autoantibody production (rheumatoid factor (RF) and anticitrullinated protein antibodies (ACPAs)), cartilage and bone destruction, besides the systemic features including cardiovascular, pulmonary, psychological, and skeletal complications [38].

Several of the risk alleles linked to RA are functionally linked to immune regulation, including the NF-κB-dependent signaling and T-cell stimulation, activation, and functional differentiation. This suggests that these immunologic pathways are among the main modulators of the development of the autoimmune inflammation observed in RA [5]. The interactions among DCs, T cells, and B cells are thought to occur primarily in the lymph nodes, generating an autoimmune response to citrulline containing self-proteins [38]. The inflammation of the synovial membrane (synovitis) is then caused by the infiltration and buildup of leukocytes in the synovial cavity. This hyperplastic synovium is the major contributor to the cartilage damage in RA.

The inflammation is brought about by the activation and costimulation of various leukocyte types present. Innate effector cells, such as macrophages, mast cells, and NK cells, are found in the synovial membrane, while neutrophils are found mainly in the synovial fluid. The main role of macrophages in this scenario is that of releasing cytokines (e.g., TNF-α and interleukins), reactive oxygen intermediates, nitrogen intermediates, production of prostanoids (including prostaglandins) and matrix-degrading enzymes. The classic macrophage-associated roles of phagocytosis and antigen presentation also play a role in inducing synovitis [39]. These findings provided evidence that activation of the innate immune pathways, driven by cytokines such as TNF-α, contributes to synovitis and the physiopathology of RA [40].

TNF-α thus plays a fundamental role in RA through the activation of cytokine and chemokine expression, expression of endothelial cell adhesion molecules, protection of synovial fibroblasts, promotion of angiogenesis, suppression of Treg cells, and induction of pain [41, 42].

2 TNF-α in relation to stages in life

So far we have focused on two main autoimmune diseases and how inflammatory cytokines, mainly TNF-α, play important roles in their pathology. However, it is important to consider the role of TNF-α in a systematic manner at different stages of life.

2.1 TNF-α in pregnancy

Normal pregnancy can be considered as a controlled state of mild systemic inflammation in mother, with circulating proinflammatory cytokines including TNF-α, which is detectable at higher levels compared to the nonpregnant state [43].

In the first and early second trimester of pregnancy, TNF-α is mainly found in the cytotrophoblastic cell columns as invasion occurs [44]. In the placenta, both the extra-embryonic membranes and maternal tissues express TNF-α throughout pregnancy, depending on the gestational age [45]. The importance of TNF-α in placental function is demonstrated through the expression of tumor necrosis factor receptor 1 (TNFR1) in all of the placenta's cell types; meanwhile, the expression levels increase as pregnancy progresses [46].

In the circulation, the levels of TNF-α and other proinflammatory cytokines decrease as pregnancy progresses, while antiinflammatory cytokines (such as IL-10 and IL-6) increase [47], although another study found that plasma levels of TNF-α increase till the second trimester, and then decrease [48]. Inversely, TNF-α and other proinflammatory cytokine levels in the amniotic fluid increase toward term [49] and are high during the labor [50]. The increase in TNF-α level and Matrix metallopeptidase (MMP)-9 activity in the amniochorionic membranes [51] is important for parturition.

An increase in TNF-α levels produced by peripheral blood mononuclear cells is associated with adverse pregnancy outcomes, including miscarriage, premature rupture of fetal membranes, intrauterine fetal growth retardation (IUGR), and preeclampsia [52]. Similarly, an increase in TNF-α and proinflammatory cytokines in amniotic fluid is associated with preterm labor, and preterm premature rupture of membranes [50, 53–56]. High levels of TNF-α and proinflammatory cytokines in women with late miscarriages or premature labor, initiate the production of stimulatory molecules required for triggering the onset of labor and delivery such as prostaglandins, MMP-2, MMP-9, vascular endothelial growth factor (VEGF), the progesterone receptor C isoform, and cortisol [57]. Thus, women presenting recurrent spontaneous miscarriages have been treated with TNF-α inhibitors to increase the rate of live births [58] by controlling the increased levels of TNF-α and proinflammatory cytokines [59].

Preeclampsia is considered as a state of exaggerated systemic inflammation, in excess of the baseline inflammatory state of normal pregnancy due to endothelial dysfunction [60]. TNF-α mediates the systemic effects of preeclampsia that is resulted from endothelial dysfunction [61]. Therefore, the balance is very fine between the initial importance of TNF-α in effective placentation and excess levels that is linked to endothelial dysfunction.

In cases of the combination of an autoimmune disease such as psoriasis with pregnancy, the process is not the same. Psoriasis represent in different manifestations in pregnancy since 55% of women with psoriasis reported an improvement in skin symptoms, while 23% reported worsening of their disease, and 21% reported no change [62]. Those that showed flare up or developing new onset psoriasis may require treatment and TNF inhibitors are the only current noncontraindicated systemic treatment option during pregnancy.

Psoriasis is associated with adverse pregnancy outcomes. For instance, women with psoriasis have been shown to have an increased risk of gestational diabetes, gestational hypertension, preeclampsia, and elective or emergency cesarean section. The risks were even higher in women with severe psoriasis (receiving systemic therapy with at least one dispensed prescription), who also had an increased risk of preterm birth and low birth weight [63].

Since pregnant and breastfeeding women are excluded from trials of anti-TNF-α therapies to protect the fetus from potential risks, concrete recommendations during pregnancy are limited to the results of small cohorts study or case reports of women who inadvertently became pregnant while on anti-TNF-α therapies. Despite the conflicting literature, there seems to be some degree of consensus that the chances of undesired outcomes of pregnancy and birth for pregnant women with autoimmune disorders including psoriasis on anti-TNF-α therapies during pregnancy appear to be similar to those for women who stopped their anti-TNF-α treatment, although more data is still required [64–70]. It is important for studies to stratify their cohorts for drug use in order to reach a better understanding of the effects of the various therapies on pregnancy outcomes [70, 71].

2.2 Inflammation (TNF-α) in aging

Aging is a complex process with the contribution of environmental, genetic, and epigenetic factors. Chronic inflammation is a persistent feature of aging and represents a significant risk factor for morbidity and mortality in the elderly. Several possible causes have been recently proposed to explain the chronic inflammation observed during aging and age-related diseases [72]. Cell senescence and dysregulation of innate immunity is one such mechanism by which persistent prolonged inflammation occurs even after the initial stimulus has been removed. Many tissues in the elderly are chronically inflamed and inflammatory cytokines such as IL-6, IL-1β, and TNF-α are known to weaken the anabolic signaling cascade, including insulin and erythropoietin signaling [73].

Changes due to aging are evident all over the body. The barrier of the oral and gut mucosa against bacterial infection gets weaker by aging and the gut microbiota of the elderly is less diverse [74]. This is reflected in a reduction in antiinflammatory microbes, such as members of *Clostridium* cluster XIVa, *Bifidobacterium* spp., and *Faecalibacterium prausnitzii*. Data supports the trend that the level of *Bifidobacterium* is inversely correlated with serum levels of inflammatory cytokines, such as TNF-α and IL-1β [75]. Conversely, inflammatory and pathogenic microbes such as *Streptococcus* spp., *Staphylococcus* spp., *Enterococcus* spp., and *Enterobacter* spp. are more common with older ages. Their presence would further trigger the induction of inflammatory cytokines and the onset of chronic inflammation.

Studies on mice provide further evidence on the important nature of inflammatory cytokines, such as TNF-α, in aging. It was shown that TNF-α plays an important role in the development of platelet hyperreactivity during aging. Platelet hyperreactivity is one of the most important factors in the initiation of thrombotic accidents leading to heart attack and ischemic stroke and is a life-threatening complication of diabetes [76].

Another study demonstrates that in aged mice, spontaneously elevated TNF-α represents a priming signal that functions to control nucleotide-binding and oligomerization domain (NOD)-like receptors (NLRs) family pyrin domain containing 3 (NLRP3) inflammasome activation. The NLRP3 inflammasome pathway has been identified as an important driver of sterile inflammatory processes through NLRP3 mediated caspase-1 cleavage and inflammasome activation. Elevated systemic TNF-α level was responsible for increased NLRP3 expression and caspase-1 activity in adipose tissues and the liver, which resulted in impaired glucose tolerance that could be attributed to peripheral insulin resistance [77].

A novel TNF-α–extracellular signal-regulated kinases (ERK)–*ETS1*–*IL27Ra* pathway, which potentially contributes to aging phenotypes of hematopoietic stem cells (HSCs) was recently described by Hu et al. [78]. It was shown that TNF-α, ERK, and ETS1 are each necessary (and TNF-α is sufficient) for the induction of IL27Ra in HSCs. Old IL27Ra knockout mice avoided most of the known aging-associated changes in their HSCs [79].

3 Structure of TNF-α

As discussed earlier, TNF-α plays a key role in the pathogenesis of several autoimmune diseases and the onset of conditions which themselves promote immune-related illnesses. The study of the structure of TNF-α and the mechanisms by which this immune mediator interacts with its receptors was thus vital in the field of drug discovery and development.

3.1 TNF-α complex structure and receptor-binding

TNF-α is the main member of the TNF superfamily in human [80, 81]. TNF-α is produced as a 26 kDa type II transmembrane (i.e., intracellular N-terminus and extracellular C-terminus) protein (tmTNF-α). The extracellular domain of tmTNF-α can then be proteolytically cleaved by the matrix metalloproteinase TNF-α converting enzyme (TACE; ADAM17) into soluble TNF-α (sTNF-α), which is a 17 kDa protein [82–84]. Both forms bind to the receptors TNFR1 and TNFR2, however, TNFR2 can only be activated fully by tmTNF [85]. Besides their different function, sTNF-α and tmTNF-α show different biological activities as tmTNF-α is more active than the sTNF-α [86].

TNF-α has a critical structural motif in its C-terminus called the TNF homology domain (THD), which consists of a 150 amino acid sequence made up of highly conserved aromatic and hydrophobic residues that are responsible for receptor-binding [80]. The crystal structures generated for TNF-α show that the TNF-α monomer has a core consisting of 4 b-strands arranged as an antiparallel sheet, creating a sandwiched structure which has been described as a "jelly-roll" structure [80, 86, 87]. Three such monomers interact in the quaternary structure making TNF-α a homotrimer. The three monomers interact together through the inner sheet of each subunit, which consists of mostly hydrophobic residues, while the outer sheet of each subunit is involved in solvent interaction [88]. The threefold axis of symmetry within the trimer does not have equivalent packing environments, with two b-strands making up the majority of the trimer interface. The top of the trimer forms polar interactions, with Glu104 of one subunit and Arg103 of another subunit possibly forming a salt bridge. The center consists of hydrophobic interactions involving Tyr119, Leu57, and Leu157, as well as between Tyr59, Tyr119, and Tyr153 of one subunit and Phe124 of another subunit. The bottom of the trimer contains a salt bridge between Lys11 of one subunit and the terminal carboxylate group of Leu156 of another subunit [86].

The TNF receptors, TNFR1 (55 kDa) and TNFR2 (75 kDa), are composed of preassembled trimers with their extracellular region containing cysteine-rich domains (CRDs) [80, 89]. TNFR1 and TNFR2 have four CRDs each containing six cysteines and three disulfide bonds. The TNF-binding domains are CRD2 and CRD4 [90], while CRD1 is required for the formation of TNF receptor self-complex on the surface of cells [87]. TNFR1 and TNFR2 also have a conserved domain in the extracellular region called the preligand-binding assembly domain (PLAD), which is necessary for ligand-independent assembly of the receptor trimer [89]. The soluble forms of these receptors (sTNFR1 and sTNFR2) are created from the membrane receptor counterparts by the TACE enzyme (the same enzyme responsible for generating sTNF-α). These soluble receptors can reduce the effect of TNF-α by competition, besides stabilizing TNF-α to protect it from degradation [91, 92].

TNFR1 is expressed on the surface of most human cell types and can be activated by both tmTNF-α and sTNF-α. However, TNFR2 is located mainly on immune and endothelial cells, can only be fully activated by tmTNF-α, and has a lower binding affinity for TNF-α [93]. The signaling pathways of TNFR1 and TNFR2 are distinct but also overlapping [94]. Although TNFR1 is the major mediator of TNF-α action for most cells, TNFR2 plays an equivalent role in leukocytes and also acts as an accessory receptor for TNFR1, which can enhance or synergize the effect of TNFR1 [95].

The formation of the TNF-α-TNF receptor complex involves the formation of a TNF-α homotrimer surrounded by three TNF receptor molecules, with two TNF-α monomers interacting with one TNFR monomer [87, 90]. Through mutational analysis, it was determined that TNF-α residue, Tyr87, is essential for the interaction with both TNF receptors, while conservation of the sequence near residue 140 is important for TNFR1-binding and conservation of the sequence near residue 30 is important for TNFR2-binding. These findings suggest a difference between the binding interfaces of TNFR1 and TNFR2 [96,97].

The differences in the binding of TNF to the two receptors are significant enough to be therapeutically exploited [97]. Similarly, inhibitory molecules that distinguish between tmTNF-α and sTNF-α may have less side effects [98, 99].

3.2 Posttranslational modifications of TNF-α

So far, the only information available about posttranslational modifications (PTMs) on the TNF-α monomers in humans are phosphorylation at Ser162 and Ser171, identified by high-throughput mass spectrometry [100]. There are probably many more phosphorylation sites still unidentified. Phosphorylation of serine, threonine, and tyrosine can mediate the formation of complexes and regulate the function. For this reason, phosphorylation sites are generally found at the binding interfaces of the monomers within a complex. As a result, phosphorylation may modulate the strength of monomeric interactions at such interfaces and in some cases greatly affect the binding energy [101]. Phosphorylation is known to be essential for cytokine production through its role in interferon (IFN) production, where it affects interferon regulatory factor 3 (IRF3) recruitment (for phosphorylation by TANK-binding kinase 1, TBK1) to the innate immune adaptor proteins including mitochondrial antiviral signaling protein (MAVS), stimulator of interferon genes (STING), or Toll-like receptor adaptor molecule (TRIF), which are also activated by phosphorylation. Once phosphorylated IRF3 dissociates from the adaptor protein, it dimerizes using the same phospho-binding domain and translocates into the nucleus, where it induces IFN [102].

Other PTMs on the soluble form of TNF-α, such as acetylation, methylation, and ubiquitination, have not yet been identified, and their functions remain uncharacterized. Acetylation of lysine, not so common in ligand-receptor interactions, however is a good example of the role of acetylation that can be seen in the interaction between the mineralocorticoid receptor (MR) of aldosterone and heat-shock protein 90 (HSP90). Acetylation of HSP90 at Lys295 in the cytosolic heterocomplex formed with MR maintains the receptor in a competent conformation for ligand-binding and regulates ligand-induced shuttling from the cytoplasm to the nucleus and consequently gene transactivation, similar to how HSP90 regulates its interaction with the androgen and glucocorticoid receptors [103]. Another protein that binds acetylated ligands is the lysine acetyltransferase p300, which interacts with acetylated proteins such as histones (e.g., histone H4 acetylated at Lys20), myoblast determination protein 1 (MyoD; acetylated at Lys99 and Lys102), signal transducer and activator of transcription 3 (STAT3; acetylated at Lys49 and Lys87), tumor protein 53 (p53; acetylated at Lys382), and HIV Tat (acetylated at Lys50) through the bromodomain in the N-terminal side [104].

Protein methylation, which occurs mainly on lysine and arginine, is known to affect the molecule's function via domain activity, interaction strength, localization, and protein stability [105]. While in general, a specific PTM can cause only one or a few of the above effects, protein methylation can produce a range of outcomes depending on the protein target, residue position, and the cellular context [106]. Despite the functional significance, very little is yet known for most nonhistone proteins due to technical limitations [105]. Considering the context of ligand-binding, methylation of p53 on Lys382 by the methyltransferase Set8 modulates its tumor-suppressing function by affecting the expression of target genes [107]. Similarly, methylation of the Numb protein on Lys158 and Lys163 within the phosphotyrosine-binding

(PTB) domain by Set8 impairs binding to p53 [108]. A different functional outcome can be observed in the transcriptional factor E2F1, where methylation on Lys185 by Set9 brings about increased ubiquitination and degradation [109]. A methylation related to downstream signaling can be seen in β-catenin, which is methylated at Lys133 by SET and MYND domain-containing protein 2 (SMYD2) and affects its nuclear translocation [110].

Of even greater relevance is the fact that the potential role of such PTMs on TNF-α in human disease is unknown. For instance, it is possible that the TNF-α protein overproduction in autoimmune and inflammatory conditions is posttranslationally modified in a different way from normal production of TNF-α, and as a result might affect its binding affinity. Of particular interest for therapeutic applications are those PTMs involved in stabilizing the trimer and making the TNF-α molecule functionally active. These PTMs would provide valuable information on how to design effective inhibitors to mimic such biological processes.

4 TNF-α therapies

4.1 Current TNF-α inhibitors

Current TNF-α inhibitors (TNFi) function by antagonizing and thereby neutralizing the activity of transmembrane and soluble TNF-α, thus preventing its binding to the two different TNF-receptors, TNFR1 and TNFR2. TNF-α inhibitors often work in a dose-dependent manner, blocking the proinflammatory activities of TNF-α [111, 112]. Five biologic agents potentially target TNF-α: infliximab (Remicade), adalimumab (Humira), golimumab (Simponi), certolizumab (Cimzia), and etanercept (Enbrel). The first to be licensed was etanercept, a fusion protein consisting of two soluble p75-TNF-receptor domains and the constant fragment of the IgG1 antibody. Next was the chimeric mouse human antibody infliximab (the first TNF-α inhibitor to be trialed in humans), which inhibits binding of TNF-α to its receptors. Later the fully human antibody, adalimumab, was developed that inhibits binding of TNF-α to both of its receptors and lyses cells that bear TNF-α on their surfaces. Due to lack of enough efficacy, two new TNF-α inhibitors were developed; namely certolizumab pegol and golimumab. Golimumab binds to both soluble and transmembrane forms of TNF-α, while certolizumab pegol binds and neutralizes both soluble and transmembrane TNF-α and inhibits signaling through both TNF-α receptors in vitro [113]. Application of these agents dramatically improved the outcome of inflammatory diseases. However, they give rise to an unwanted immune response, which is described as a result of their immunogenicity. Some studies have indicated that formation of antibodies against these therapeutic agents decreased their efficacy and increased their toxicity. Antidrug antibodies (ADABs) developed in 13% of patients. All five TNF-α inhibitors were associated with ADABs, but to different degrees depending on the specificity of the TNF-α inhibitor and the disease. ADABs are associated with reduced clinical response and an increased incidence of infusion reactions and injection site reactions. Combination treatments including immunosuppressive drugs with TNF-α inhibitors can reduce ADAB formation [114].

TNF-α inhibitors possess different pharmacokinetic properties and potentially different mechanisms of action. For example, the ability of etanercept to inhibit the action of lymphotoxin has been implicated as to the reason of the efficacy of etanercept in patients resistant to infliximab [115]. Moreover, intolerance to TNFi therapy, which would warrant cessation of treatment may be idiosyncratic (rather than a TNFi class effect), thus permitting the use of an alternative TNFi.

Certolizumab pegol is distinct from other TNF-α inhibitors in terms of its structure. It is composed of the antibody-binding fragment (Fab) of a humanized monoclonal antibody against TNF-α conjugated to polyethylene glycol. Thus, unlike other TNF-α inhibitors, it does not contain the constant fragment of immunoglobulin. Attachment of polyethylene glycol to the Fab increases its plasma half-life in comparison to that of whole antibody TNF-α inhibitors such as adalimumab, to approximately 14 days, allowing fortnightly subcutaneous administration [113]. Certolizumab pegol binds both soluble and membrane-bound TNF-α, inhibiting the proinflammatory actions of this cytokine. Unlike other TNF-α inhibitors, owing to its lack of the Fc component, it is incapable of fixing complement or binding to Fc receptors. Unlike monoclonal antibodies, it does not cause antibody-dependent or complement-dependent cytotoxicity in vitro, suggesting this mechanism of action may not be necessary for clinical efficacy of TNF-α inhibitor therapies [116].

When it comes to using these current therapies during pregnancy, the general concern stems from the fact that complete immunoglobulin G (IgG) antibodies (irrespective of whether it is maternal or therapeutic) cross the placenta via active transport, which is facilitated by the neonatal fragment crystallizable (Fc) receptor on the placenta. This transfer increases rapidly between week 22 and 26 of gestation and keeps increasing until term [117]. This is more relevant to adalimumab, golimumab, and infliximab since these are complete IgG1 antibodies, and less relevant to etanercept since it only contains the IgG1 Fc portion. Certolizumab pegol presents least concern since it lacks the Fc moiety and thereby prevents its binding to placental Fc receptor [118,119], and crossing the placenta at a detectable level, unlike infliximab, which has been shown to cross the placenta with high levels detectable in newborns [120]. This may be explained by the fact that, in the second trimester of pregnancy, IgG crosses the placenta via a process mediated through its Fc component. In addition, serum levels of Certolizumab pegol in infants born to mothers receiving certolizumab pegol for IBD suggest certolizumab pegol is not actively transferred across the placenta in the third trimester of pregnancy [121]. Accordingly, the use of infliximab or adalimumab during the third trimester leads to a higher cord blood's drug level compared to the drug level in the peripheral blood of mothers [122, 123]. Furthermore, infliximab administered throughout the third trimester of pregnancy was still detected in the serum of infants 6–12 months after the in utero exposure [124, 125]. Hypersensitivity and reduced response of the infant to intracellular infections are reported as the long-term effect [126].

4.2 Development and application of new TNF-α inhibitors

A new generation of TNF-α inhibitors are being developed which consist of small molecules that can interfere with the symmetrical trimeric structure of TNF-α, reducing its ability to bind to the receptor and weakening its ability to elicit a signaling cascade. While biological therapies exhibit inevitable disadvantages such as increased risk of infection, high costs, and the requirement for intravenous injections, small molecule inhibitors are relatively cheaper and could be taken orally. Therefore, the identification of small molecules that can inhibit the TNF-α regulated pathway presents a promising alternative to currently available

TNF-α inhibitors. This has been attempted with a number of small molecules [127–130] and macrocyclic peptides [131], that destabilize the TNF-α trimer, such that it can no longer bind to the receptor.

Suramin inhibits the TNF-α interaction with its receptor as shown by gel filtration chromatography, where suramin, preincubated with TNF-α, resulted in isolation of trimeric and monomeric TNF-α, while TNF-α alone resulted in isolation of only the trimer [132]. A computational docking study using three structural features of suramin, namely the sulfonic acid groups, molecular length, and symmetry has identified Trypan blue and Evans blue as having an effect on TNF-α [133]. Three residues identified in the crystal structure as playing a role in trimer association [90], namely Arg103, Tyr119, and Lys98, made surface contacts with sulfonic groups and played a role in orientation, in all three active compounds [133]. Later, the compound SPD305, containing dimethylamine-linked trifluoromethyl indole and dimethyl chromone moieties was synthesized [127]. X-ray crystallography for SPD305 revealed that the compound displaced a subunit from the trimer, forms 16 contacts with TNF-α, with all contacts being hydrophobic in nature, including Tyr59 and Tyr119, two of the tyrosines previously identified in the trimeric crystal structure as important factors for trimer association [90, 127]. Two saponins (of the terpenoid class), isolated from the methanolic extract of *Parthenium hysterophorus* (congress grass) were found to have an effect on TNF-α, while in silico docking studies showed that the contact residues of these compounds were very similar to those of SPD305 [134]. A library of 240,000 compounds was screened in silico using the mechanism of binding of SPD305, together with the TNF-α dimer crystal structure and a modified scoring function that included a solvation model for the ability to bind the TNF-α dimer and to the three top isolated compounds that all had a pyrimidine-2,4,6-trione moiety in common [135]. A virtual high-throughput ligand-docking screen based on dimer-SPD305 structure of 20,000 natural product or similar compounds identified quinuclidine and indoloquinolizidine as large, hydrophobic natural products that could mimic the binding of SPD305, using Tyr59, Tyr119, and Tyr159 in hydrophobic interactions [136].

Natural products such as Japonicone A and physcion-8-*O*-β-D-monoglucoside (PMG), which inhibits the preferential binding of TNF-α to TNFR1, have also been investigated [78, 137]. The two mechanisms of action for such molecules are through competition with the receptor-binding site (orthosteric) or noncompetitively by binding at a site that is not involved in receptor-binding (allosteric) [130]. In either cases, the change in spatial arrangement of the TNF-α monomers brought about by small molecule inhibitors, results in distortion of the receptor-binding sites, thus preventing the threefold symmetry required for receptor-binding and initiation of the downstream signaling [130].

Various methods have been established to determine and study possible eligible small molecules to act as TNF-α inhibitors. These include surface plasmon resonance biosensor and ultraperformance liquid chromatography-mass spectrometry (UPLC-MS) [137] and in silico screening [135, 136, 138]. These technologies not only serve as efficient tools to identify novel therapeutic molecules, but could also serve as scientific models to understand the exact action mechanism of already approved therapies. We thus hypothesize that if the TNF-α protein over-produced by autoimmune and inflammatory conditions is posttranslationally modified in order to be functional, then eliminating one or a few of the crucial PTMs would reduce the stability of the TNF-α trimer and its activity, without completely inhibiting its function. The targeted PTMs could be removed by modulating the activity of the enzymes inducing these

PTMs, or competitively by introducing TNF-α monomers that are already decorated with other PTMs at key sites. The overall expected outcome would be a reduction in inflammation, without inducing negative impacts on other biological processes requiring TNF-α for normal function, as in pregnancy.

5 Conclusion

A large proportion of the population is affected by chronic inflammation due to autoimmune diseases, and the available therapeutics do not suffice to effectively treat these conditions in all life contexts. The current knowledge of TNF-α structure and its therapeutic inhibition provides a basis for further research. Mass-spectrometric analysis of TNF-α PTMs could open up a new avenue for research, with significant therapeutic application.

References

[1] T. Lawrence, D.A. Willoughby, D.W. Gilroy, Anti-inflammatory lipid mediators and insights into the resolution of inflammation, Nat. Rev. Immunol. 2 (10) (2002) 787–795.

[2] D. Sarkar, P.B. Fisher, Molecular mechanisms of aging-associated inflammation, Cancer Lett. 236 (1) (2006) 13–23.

[3] C.A. Janeway Jr., P. Travers, M. Walport, M.J. Shlomchik, Autoimmune responses are directed against self antigens, in: Immunobiology: The Immune System in Health and Disease, fifth ed., Garland Science, 2001.

[4] G.L. Larsen, P.M. Henson, Mediators of inflammation, Annu. Rev. Immunol. 1 (1) (1983) 335–359.

[5] M. Farrugia, B. Baron, The role of TNF-α in rheumatoid arthritis: a focus on regulatory T cells, J. Clin. Transl. Res. 2 (3) (2016) 84.

[6] F. Hildebrand, H.C. Pape, C. Krettek, The importance of cytokines in the posttraumatic inflammatory reaction, Unfallchirurg 108 (10) (2005) 793–794.

[7] J.M. Zhang, J. An, Cytokines, inflammation and pain, Int. Anesthesiol. Clin. 45 (2) (2007) 27.

[8] M. Dougan, G. Dranoff, S.K. Dougan, GM-CSF, IL-3, and IL-5 family of cytokines: regulators of inflammation, Immunity 50 (4) (2019) 796–811.

[9] A. Annibaldi, P. Meier, Checkpoints in TNF-induced cell death: implications in inflammation and cancer, Trends Mol. Med. 24 (1) (2018) 49–65.

[10] H. Blaser, C. Dostert, T.W. Mak, D. Brenner, TNF and ROS crosstalk in inflammation, Trends Cell Biol. 26 (4) (2016) 249–261.

[11] D.B. Sanders, D.F. Larson, K. Hunter, M. Gorman, B. Yang, Comparison of tumor necrosis factor-α effect on the expression of iNOS in macrophage and cardiac myocytes, Perfusion 16 (1) (2001) 67–74.

[12] P. Neumann, N. Gertzberg, A. Johnson, TNF-α induces a decrease in eNOS promoter activity, Am. J. Phys. Lung Cell. Mol. Phys. 286 (2) (2004) L452–L459.

[13] E.R. Sherwood, T. Toliver-Kinsky, Mechanisms of the inflammatory response, Best Pract. Res. Clin. Anaesthesiol. 18 (3) (2004) 385–405.

[14] D. Chappell, K. Hofmann-Kiefer, M. Jacob, M. Rehm, J. Briegel, U. Welsch, P. Conzen, B.F. Becker, TNF-α induced shedding of the endothelial glycocalyx is prevented by hydrocortisone and antithrombin, Basic Res. Cardiol. 104 (1) (2009) 78.

[15] S.E. Goldblum, W.L. Sun, Tumor necrosis factor-alpha augments pulmonary arterial transendothelial albumin flux in vitro, Am. J. Phys. Lung Cell. Mol. Phys. 258 (2) (1990) L57–L67.

[16] D.J. Angelini, S.W. Hyun, D.N. Grigoryev, P. Garg, P. Gong, I.S. Singh, A. Passaniti, J.D. Hasday, S.E. Goldblum, TNF-α increases tyrosine phosphorylation of vascular endothelial cadherin and opens the paracellular pathway through fyn activation in human lung endothelia, Am. J. Physiol. Lung Cell. Mol. Physiol. 291 (6) (2006) L1232–L1245.

[17] U.M. Chandrasekharan, M. Siemionow, M. Unsal, L. Yang, E. Poptic, J. Bohn, K. Ozer, Z. Zhou, P.H. Howe, M. Penn, P.E. DiCorleto, Tumor necrosis factor α (TNF-α) receptor-II is required for TNF-α–induced leukocyte-endothelial interaction in vivo, Blood 109 (5) (2007) 1938–1944.

[18] L.S. Yoshida, S. Tsunawaki, Expression of NADPH oxidases and enhanced H_2O_2-generating activity in human coronary artery endothelial cells upon induction with tumor necrosis factor-α, Int. Immunopharmacol. 8 (10) (2008) 1377–1385.

[19] M.J. Morgan, Z.G. Liu, Crosstalk of reactive oxygen species and NF-κB signaling, Cell Res. 21 (1) (2011) 103–115.

[20] F.C. Eberle, J. Brück, J. Holstein, K. Hirahara, K. Ghoreschi, Recent advances in understanding psoriasis, F1000Research 5 (2016). F1000 Faculty Rev-770.

[21] L. Grine, L. Dejager, C. Libert, R.E. Vandenbroucke, An inflammatory triangle in psoriasis: TNF, type I IFNs and IL-17, Cytokine Growth Factor Rev. 26 (1) (2015) 25–33.

[22] G.C. de Gannes, M. Ghoreishi, J. Pope, A. Russell, D. Bell, S. Adams, K. Shojania, M. Martinka, J.P. Dutz, Psoriasis and pustular dermatitis triggered by TNF-α inhibitors in patients with rheumatologic conditions, Arch. Dermatol. 143 (2) (2007) 223–231.

[23] W.H. Boehncke, M.P. Schön, Psoriasis, Lancet 386 (9997) (2015) 983–994.

[24] J.M. Ovigne, B.S. Baker, D.W. Brown, A.V. Powles, L. Fry, Epidermal CD8+ T cells in chronic plaque psoriasis are Tc1 cells producing heterogeneous levels of interferon-gamma, Exp. Dermatol. 10 (3) (2001) 168–174.

[25] J.L. Harden, J.G. Krueger, A.M. Bowcock, The immunogenetics of psoriasis: a comprehensive review, J. Autoimmun. 64 (2015) 66–73.

[26] T. Banno, A. Gazel, M. Blumenberg, Effects of tumor necrosis factor-α (TNFα) in epidermal keratinocytes revealed using global transcriptional profiling, J. Biol. Chem. 279 (31) (2004) 32633–32642.

[27] S.M. Sa, P.A. Valdez, J. Wu, K. Jung, F. Zhong, L. Hall, I. Kasman, J. Winer, Z. Modrusan, D.M. Danilenko, W. Ouyang, The effects of IL-20 subfamily cytokines on reconstituted human epidermis suggest potential roles in cutaneous innate defense and pathogenic adaptive immunity in psoriasis, J. Immunol. 178 (4) (2007) 2229–2240.

[28] M. Tohyama, Y. Hanakawa, Y. Shirakata, X. Dai, L. Yang, S. Hirakawa, S. Tokumaru, H. Okazaki, K. Sayama, K. Hashimoto, IL-17 and IL-22 mediate IL-20 subfamily cytokine production in cultured keratinocytes via increased IL-22 receptor expression, Eur. J. Immunol. 39 (10) (2009) 2779–2788.

[29] S. Kunz, K. Wolk, E. Witte, K. Witte, W.D. Doecke, H.D. Volk, W. Sterry, K. Asadullah, R. Sabat, Interleukin (IL)-19, IL-20 and IL-24 are produced by and act on keratinocytes and are distinct from classical ILs, Exp. Dermatol. 15 (12) (2006) 991–1004.

[30] S. Kumari, M.C. Bonnet, M.H. Ulvmar, K. Wolk, N. Karagianni, E. Witte, C. Uthoff-Hachenberg, J.C. Renauld, G. Kollias, R. Toftgard, R. Sabat, Tumor necrosis factor receptor signaling in keratinocytes triggers interleukin-24-dependent psoriasis-like skin inflammation in mice, Immunity 39 (5) (2013) 899–911.

[31] L. Zhuang, W. Ma, D. Cai, H. Zhong, Q. Sun, Associations between tumor necrosis factor-α polymorphisms and risk of psoriasis: a meta-analysis, PLoS One 8 (12) (2013) e68827.

[32] T. Tejasvi, P.E. Stuart, V. Chandran, J.J. Voorhees, D.D. Gladman, P. Rahman, J.T. Elder, R.P. Nair, TNFAIP3 gene polymorphisms are associated with response to TNF blockade in psoriasis, J. Investig. Dermatol. 132 (3) (2012) 593–600.

[33] C.B. Johansen, E. Jimenez-Solem, A. Haerskjold, F.L. Sand, S.F. Thomsen, The use and safety of TNF inhibitors during pregnancy in women with psoriasis: a review, Int. J. Mol. Sci. 19 (5) (2018) 1349.

[34] P.P. Sfikakis, A. Iliopoulos, A. Elezoglou, C. Kittas, A. Stratigos, Psoriasis induced by anti–tumor necrosis factor therapy: a paradoxical adverse reaction, Arthritis Rheum. 52 (8) (2005) 2513–2518.

[35] I. Guerra, J.P. Gisbert, Onset of psoriasis in patients with inflammatory bowel disease treated with anti-TNF agents, Expert Rev. Gastroenterol. Hepatol. 7 (1) (2013) 41–48.

[36] I. Guerra, T. Pérez-Jeldres, M. Iborra, A. Algaba, D. Monfort, X. Calvet, M. Chaparro, M. Mañosa, E. Hinojosa, M. Minguez, J. Ortiz de Zarate, Incidence, clinical characteristics, and management of psoriasis induced by anti-TNF therapy in patients with inflammatory bowel disease: a nationwide cohort study, Inflamm. Bowel Dis. 22 (4) (2016) 894–901.

[37] D. Aletaha, T. Neogi, A.J. Silman, J. Funovits, D.T. Felson, C.O. Bingham III, N.S. Birnbaum, G.R. Burmester, V.P. Bykerk, M.D. Cohen, B. Combe, 2010 rheumatoid arthritis classification criteria: an American College of Rheumatology/European League Against Rheumatism collaborative initiative, Arthritis Rheum. 62 (9) (2010) 2569–2581.

[38] I.B. McInnes, G. Schett, The pathogenesis of rheumatoid arthritis, N. Engl. J. Med. 365 (23) (2011) 2205–2219.

[39] F.Y. Liew, I.B. McInnes, The role of innate mediators in inflammatory response, Mol. Immunol. 38 (12–13) (2002) 887–890.

[40] Z. Szekanecz, A. Pakozdi, A. Szentpetery, T. Besenyei, A.E. Koch, Chemokines and angiogenesis in rheumatoid arthritis, Front. Biosci. (Elite Ed.) 1 (2009) 44.

[41] M. Feldmann, F.M. Brennan, R.N. Maini, Role of cytokines in rheumatoid arthritis, Annu. Rev. Immunol. 14 (1) (1996) 397–440.

[42] A. Hess, R. Axmann, J. Rech, S. Finzel, C. Heindl, S. Kreitz, M. Sergeeva, M. Saake, M. Garcia, G. Kollias, R.H. Straub, Blockade of TNF-α rapidly inhibits pain responses in the central nervous system, Proc. Natl. Acad. Sci. 108 (9) (2011) 3731–3736.

[43] A. Sharma, A. Satyam, J.B. Sharma, Leptin, IL-10 and inflammatory markers (TNF-α, IL-6 and IL-8) in pre-eclamptic, normotensive pregnant and healthy non-pregnant women, Am. J. Reprod. Immunol. 58 (1) (2007) 21–30.

[44] R. Pijnenborg, P.J. McLaughlin, L. Vercruysse, M. Hanssens, P.M. Johnson, J.C. Keith Jr., F.A. Van Assche, Immunolocalization of tumour necrosis factor-α (TNF-α) in the placental bed of normotensive and hypertensive human pregnancies, Placenta 19 (4) (1998) 231–239.

[45] H.L. Chen, Y.P. Yang, X.L. Hu, K.K. Yelavarthi, J.L. Fishback, J.S. Hunt, Tumor necrosis factor alpha mRNA and protein are present in human placental and uterine cells at early and late stages of gestation, Am. J. Pathol. 139 (2) (1991) 327.

[46] S.L. Opsjøn, D. Novick, N.C. Wathen, A.P. Cope, D. Wallach, D. Aderka, Soluble tumor necrosis factor receptors and soluble interleukin-6 receptor in fetal and maternal sera, coelomic and amniotic fluids in normal and pre-eclamptic pregnancies, J. Reprod. Immunol. 29 (2) (1995) 119–134.

[47] J.M. Denney, E.L. Nelson, P.D. Wadhwa, T.P. Waters, L. Mathew, E.K. Chung, R.L. Goldenberg, J.F. Culhane, Longitudinal modulation of immune system cytokine profile during pregnancy, Cytokine 53 (2) (2011) 170–177.

[48] I. Beckmann, W. Visser, P.C. Struijk, M. van Dooren, J. Glavimans, H.C. Wallenburg, Circulating bioactive tumor necrosis factor-α, tumor necrosis factor-α receptors, fibronectin, and tumor necrosis factor-α inducible cell adhesion molecule VCAM-1 in uncomplicated pregnancy, Am. J. Obstet. Gynecol. 177 (5) (1997) 1247–1252.

[49] J. Halgunset, H. Johnsen, A.M. Kjøllesdal, E. Qvigstad, T. Espevik, R. Austgulen, Cytokine levels in amniotic fluid and inflammatory changes in the placenta from normal deliveries at term, Eur. J. Obstet. Gynecol. Reproduct. Biol. 56 (3) (1994) 153–160.

[50] R. Romero, M. Mazor, W. Sepulveda, C. Avila, D. Copeland, J. Williams, Tumor necrosis factor in preterm and term labor, Am. J. Obstet. Gynecol. 166 (5) (1992) 1576–1587.

[51] S.J. Fortunato, R. Menon, S.J. Lombardi, Role of tumor necrosis factor-α in the premature rupture of membranes and preterm labor pathways, Am. J. Obstet. Gynecol. 187 (5) (2002) 1159–1162.

[52] F.Y. Azizieh, R.G. Raghupathy, Tumor necrosis factor-α and pregnancy complications: a prospective study, Med. Princ. Pract. 24 (2) (2015) 165–170.

[53] A. Shobokshi, M. Shaarawy, Maternal serum and amniotic fluid cytokines in patients with preterm premature rupture of membranes with and without intrauterine infection, Int. J. Gynecol. Obstet. 79 (3) (2002) 209–215.

[54] S.L. Hillier, S.S. Witkin, M.A. Krohn, D.H. Watts, N.B. Kiviat, D.A. Eschenbach, The relationship of amniotic fluid cytokines and preterm delivery, amniotic fluid infection, histologic chorioamnionitis, and chorioamnion infection, Obstet. Gynecol. 81 (6) (1993) 941–948.

[55] M.L. Houben, P.G. Nikkels, G.M. Van Bleek, G.H. Visser, M.M. Rovers, H. Kessel, W.J. de Waal, L. Schuijff, A. Evers, J.L. Kimpen, L. Bont, The association between intrauterine inflammation and spontaneous vaginal delivery at term: a cross-sectional study, PLoS One 4 (8) (2009) e6572.

[56] E. Maymon, F. Ghezzi, S.S. Edwin, M. Mazor, B.H. Yoon, R. Gomez, R. Romero, The tumor necrosis factor α and its soluble receptor profile in term and preterm parturition, Am. J. Obstet. Gynecol. 181 (5) (1999) 1142–1148.

[57] I. Christiaens, D.B. Zaragoza, L. Guilbert, S.A. Robertson, B.F. Mitchell, D.M. Olson, Inflammatory processes in preterm and term parturition, J. Reprod. Immunol. 79 (1) (2008) 50–57.

[58] E.E. Winger, J.L. Reed, Treatment with tumor necrosis factor inhibitors and intravenous immunoglobulin improves live birth rates in women with recurrent spontaneous abortion, Am. J. Reprod. Immunol. 60 (1) (2008) 8–16.

[59] M. Shaarawy, A.R. Nagui, Enhanced expression of cytokines may play a fundamental role in the mechanisms of immunologically mediated recurrent spontaneous abortion, Acta Obstet. Gynecol. Scand. 76 (3) (1997) 205–211.

[60] M. Portelli, B. Baron, Clinical presentation of preeclampsia and the diagnostic value of proteins and their methylation products as biomarkers in pregnant women with preeclampsia and their newborns, J. Pregnancy 2018 (2018) 1–23.

[61] D.F. Lewis, B.J. Canzoneri, Y. Wang, Maternal circulating TNF-α levels are highly correlated with IL-10 levels, but not IL-6 and IL-8 levels, in women with pre-eclampsia, Am. J. Reprod. Immunol. 62 (5) (2009) 269–274.

[62] J.E. Murase, K.K. Chan, T.J. Garite, D.M. Cooper, G.D. Weinstein, Hormonal effect on psoriasis in pregnancy and post partum, Arch. Dermatol. 141 (5) (2005) 601–606.

[63] G. Bröms, A. Haerskjold, F. Granath, H. Kieler, L. Pedersen, I.A. Berglind, Effect of maternal psoriasis on pregnancy and birth outcomes: a population-based cohort study from Denmark and Sweden, Acta Derm. Venereol. 98 (7–8) (2018) 728–734.

[64] L. Puig, D. Barco, A. Alomar, Treatment of psoriasis with anti-TNF drugs during pregnancy: case report and review of the literature, Dermatology 220 (1) (2010) 71–76.

[65] E. Vinet, C. Pineau, C. Gordon, A.E. Clarke, S. Bernatsky, Anti-TNF therapy and pregnancy outcomes in women with inflammatory arthritis, Expert. Rev. Clin. Immunol. 5 (1) (2009) 27–34.

[66] S.M. Verstappen, Y. King, K.D. Watson, D.P. Symmons, K.L. Hyrich, BSRBR Control Centre Consortium and BSR Biologics Register, Anti-TNF therapies and pregnancy: outcome of 130 pregnancies in the British Society for Rheumatology Biologics Register, Ann. Rheum. Dis. 70 (5) (2011) 823–826.

[67] N. Khan, H. Asim, G.R. Lichtenstein, Safety of anti-TNF therapy in inflammatory bowel disease during pregnancy, Expert Opin. Drug Saf. 13 (12) (2014) 1699–1708.

[68] M. Seirafi, B. De Vroey, A. Amiot, P. Seksik, X. Roblin, M. Allez, L. Peyrin-Biroulet, P. Marteau, G. Cadiot, D. Laharie, A. Boureille, Factors associated with pregnancy outcome in anti-TNF treated women with inflammatory bowel disease, Aliment. Pharmacol. Ther. 40 (4) (2014) 363–373.

[69] J.P. Gisbert, M. Chaparro, Safety of anti-TNF agents during pregnancy and breastfeeding in women with inflammatory bowel disease, Am. J. Gastroenterol. 108 (9) (2013) 1426–1438.

[70] R. Bobotsis, W.P. Gulliver, K. Monaghan, C. Lynde, P. Fleming, Psoriasis and adverse pregnancy outcomes: a systematic review of observational studies, Br. J. Dermatol. 175 (3) (2016) 464–472.

[71] E. Pottinger, R.T. Woolf, L.S. Exton, A.D. Burden, C. Nelson-Piercy, C.H. Smith, Exposure to biological therapies during conception and pregnancy: a systematic review, Br. J. Dermatol. 178 (1) (2018) 95–102.

[72] F. Sanada, Y. Taniyama, J. Muratsu, R. Otsu, H. Shimizu, H. Rakugi, R. Morishita, Source of chronic inflammation in aging, Front. Cardiovasc. Med. 5 (2018) 12.

[73] I. Beyer, T. Mets, I. Bautmans, Chronic low-grade inflammation and age-related sarcopenia, Curr. Opin. Clin. Nutr. Metab. Care 15 (1) (2012) 12–22.

[74] J. Kinross, J.K. Nicholson, Gut microbiota: dietary and social modulation of gut microbiota in the elderly, Nature Rev. Gastroenterol. Hepatol. 9 (10) (2012) 563.

[75] R. Toward, S. Montandon, G. Walton, G.R. Gibson, Effect of prebiotics on the human gut microbiota of elderly persons, Gut Microbes 3 (1) (2012) 57–60.

[76] P. Davizon-Castillo, B. McMahon, S. Aguila, D. Bark, K. Ashworth, A. Allawzi, R.A. Campbell, E. Montenont, T. Nemkov, A. D'Alessandro, N. Clendenen, TNF-α–driven inflammation and mitochondrial dysfunction define the platelet hyperreactivity of aging, Blood 134 (9) (2019) 727–740.

[77] F. Bauernfeind, S. Niepmann, P.A. Knolle, V. Hornung, Aging-associated TNF production primes inflammasome activation and NLRP3-related metabolic disturbances, J. Immunol. 197 (7) (2016) 2900–2908.

[78] Z. Hu, J. Qin, H. Zhang, D. Wang, Y. Hua, J. Ding, L. Shan, H. Jin, J. Zhang, W. Zhang, Japonicone A antagonizes the activity of TNF-α by directly targeting this cytokine and selectively disrupting its interaction with TNF receptor-1, Biochem. Pharmacol. 84 (11) (2012) 1482–1491.

[79] J. DeGregori, Aging, inflammation, and HSC, Blood 136 (2) (2020) 153–154.

[80] J.L. Bodmer, P. Schneider, J. Tschopp, The molecular architecture of the TNF superfamily, Trends Biochem. Sci. 27 (1) (2002) 19–26.

[81] R.M. Locksley, N. Killeen, M.J. Lenardo, The TNF and TNF receptor superfamilies: integrating mammalian biology, Cell 104 (4) (2001) 487–501.

[82] M. Kriegler, C. Perez, K. DeFay, I. Albert, S.D. Lu, A novel form of TNF/cachectin is a cell surface cytotoxic transmembrane protein: ramifications for the complex physiology of TNF, Cell 53 (1) (1988) 45–53.

[83] B. Luettig, T. Decker, M.L. Lohmann-Matthes, Evidence for the existence of two forms of membrane tumor necrosis factor: an integral protein and a molecule attached to its receptor, J. Immunol. 143 (12) (1989) 4034–4038.

[84] R.A. Black, C.T. Rauch, C.J. Kozlosky, J.J. Peschon, J.L. Slack, M.F. Wolfson, B.J. Castner, K.L. Stocking, P. Reddy, S. Srinivasan, N. Nelson, A metalloproteinase disintegrin that releases tumour-necrosis factor-α from cells, Nature 385 (6618) (1997) 729–733.

[85] M. Grell, E. Douni, H. Wajant, M. Löhden, M. Clauss, B. Maxeiner, S. Georgopoulos, W. Lesslauer, G. Kollias, K. Pfizenmaier, P. Scheurich, The transmembrane form of tumor necrosis factor is the prime activating ligand of the 80 kDa tumor necrosis factor receptor, Cell 83 (5) (1995) 793–802.

[86] M.J. Eck, S.R. Sprang, The structure of tumor necrosis factor-alpha at 2.6 A resolution. Implications for receptor binding, J. Biol. Chem. 264 (29) (1989) 17595–17605.

[87] D.W. Banner, A. D'Arcy, W. Janes, R. Gentz, H.J. Schoenfeld, C. Broger, H. Loetscher, W. Lesslauer, Crystal structure of the soluble human 55 kd TNF receptor-human TNFα complex: implications for TNF receptor activation, Cell 73 (3) (1993) 431–445.

[88] J.M. Davis, J. Colangelo, Small-molecule inhibitors of the interaction between TNF and TNFR, Future Med. Chem. 5 (1) (2013) 69–79.

[89] F.K.M. Chan, H.J. Chun, L. Zheng, R.M. Siegel, K.L. Bui, M.J. Lenardo, A domain in TNF receptors that mediates ligand-independent receptor assembly and signaling, Science 288 (5475) (2000) 2351–2354.

[90] Y. Mukai, T. Nakamura, M. Yoshikawa, Y. Yoshioka, S.I. Tsunoda, S. Nakagawa, Y. Yamagata, Y. Tsutsumi, Solution of the structure of the TNF-TNFR2 complex, Sci. Signal. 3 (148) (2010) ra83.

[91] D. Aderka, H. Engelmann, Y. Maor, C. Brakebusch, D. Wallach, Stabilization of the bioactivity of tumor necrosis factor by its soluble receptors, J. Exp. Med. 175 (2) (1992) 323–329.

[92] A.H. Hajeer, I.V. Hutchinson, TNF-α gene polymorphism: clinical and biological implications, Microsc. Res. Tech. 50 (3) (2000) 216–228.

[93] D. Tracey, L. Klareskog, E.H. Sasso, J.G. Salfeld, P.P. Tak, Tumor necrosis factor antagonist mechanisms of action: a comprehensive review, Pharmacol. Ther. 117 (2) (2008) 244–279.

[94] M.A. Palladino, F.R. Bahjat, E.A. Theodorakis, L.L. Moldawer, Anti-TNF-α therapies: the next generation, Nat. Rev. Drug Discov. 2 (9) (2003) 736–746.

[95] M. Grell, H. Wajant, G. Zimmermann, P. Scheurich, The type 1 receptor (CD120a) is the high-affinity receptor for soluble tumor necrosis factor, Proc. Natl. Acad. Sci. 95 (2) (1998) 570–575.

[96] H. Loetscher, D. Stueber, D. Banner, F. Mackay, W. Lesslauer, Human tumor necrosis factor alpha (TNF alpha) mutants with exclusive specificity for the 55-kDa or 75-kDa TNF receptors, J. Biol. Chem. 268 (35) (1993) 26350–26357.

[97] Y. Mukai, H. Shibata, T. Nakamura, Y. Yoshioka, Y. Abe, T. Nomura, M. Taniai, T. Ohta, S. Ikemizu, S. Nakagawa, S.I. Tsunoda, Structure–function relationship of tumor necrosis factor (TNF) and its receptor interaction based on 3D structural analysis of a fully active TNFR1-selective TNF mutant, J. Mol. Biol. 385 (4) (2009) 1221–1229.

[98] M.G. Tansey, D.E. Szymkowski, The TNF superfamily in 2009: new pathways, new indications, and new drugs, Drug Discov. Today 14 (23–24) (2009) 1082–1088.

[99] R.E. Kontermann, P. Scheurich, K. Pfizenmaier, Antagonists of TNF action: clinical experience and new developments, Expert Opin. Drug Discovery 4 (3) (2009) 279–292.

[100] P.V. Hornbeck, B. Zhang, B. Murray, J.M. Kornhauser, V. Latham, E. Skrzypek, PhosphoSitePlus, 2014: mutations, PTMs and recalibrations, Nucleic Acids Res. 43 (2015) D512–D520.

[101] H. Nishi, K. Hashimoto, A.R. Panchenko, Phosphorylation in protein-protein binding: effect on stability and function, Structure 19 (12) (2011) 1807–1815.

[102] S. Liu, X. Cai, J. Wu, Q. Cong, X. Chen, T. Li, F. Du, J. Ren, Y.T. Wu, N.V. Grishin, Z.J. Chen, Phosphorylation of innate immune adaptor proteins MAVS, STING, and TRIF induces IRF3 activation, Science 347 (6227) (2015) 2630-1–2630-14.

[103] D. Alvarez de la Rosa, R. Jimenez-Canino, F. Lorenzo-Diaz, T. Giraldez, Hsp90 acetylation regulates mineralocorticoid receptor subcellular dynamics and aldosterone-induced promoter transactivation (1097.15), FASEB J. 28 (2014) 1097-15.

[104] B.M. Dancy, P.A. Cole, Protein lysine acetylation by p300/CBP, Chem. Rev. 115 (6) (2015) 2419–2452.

[105] B. Baron, Lysine methylation of non-histone proteins, Biochem. Mod. Appl. 1 (2015) 1–2.

[106] B. Baron, The lysine multi-switch: the impact of lysine methylation on transcription factor properties, Biohelikon: Cell Biol. 2 (2014) a13.

[107] X. Shi, I. Kachirskaia, H. Yamaguchi, L.E. West, H. Wen, E.W. Wang, S. Dutta, E. Appella, O. Gozani, Modulation of p53 function by SET8-mediated methylation at lysine 382, Mol. Cell 27 (4) (2007) 636–646.

6. Monomer-interaction-based alternative TNF-α therapies

[108] G.K. Dhami, H. Liu, M. Galka, C. Voss, R. Wei, K. Muranko, T. Kaneko, S.P. Cregan, L. Li, S.S.C. Li, Dynamic methylation of Numb by Set8 regulates its binding to p53 and apoptosis, Mol. Cell 50 (4) (2013) 565–576.

[109] H. Kontaki, I. Talianidis, Lysine methylation regulates E2F1-induced cell death, Mol. Cell 39 (1) (2010) 152–160.

[110] X. Deng, R. Hamamoto, T. Vougiouklakis, R. Wang, Y. Yoshioka, T. Suzuki, N. Dohmae, Y. Matsuo, J.H. Park, Y. Nakamura, Critical roles of SMYD2-mediated β-catenin methylation for nuclear translocation and activation of Wnt signaling, Oncotarget 8 (34) (2017) 55837.

[111] T. Vergou, A.E. Moustou, P.P. Sfikakis, C. Antoniou, A.J. Stratigos, Pharmacodynamics of TNF-α inhibitors in psoriasis, Expert. Rev. Clin. Pharmacol. 4 (4) (2011) 515–523.

[112] P.P. Sfikakis, The first decade of biologic TNF antagonists in clinical practice: lessons learned, unresolved issues and future directions, in: TNF Pathophysiology, vol. 11, Karger Publishers, 2010, pp. 180–210.

[113] S.C. Horton, S. Das, P. Emery, Certolizumab pegol in rheumatoid arthritis: a review of phase III clinical trials and its role in real-life clinical practice, Int. J. Clin. Rheumatol. 6 (5) (2011) 517.

[114] S.S. Thomas, N. Borazan, N. Barroso, L. Duan, S. Taroumian, B. Kretzmann, R. Bardales, D. Elashoff, S. Vangala, D.E. Furst, Comparative immunogenicity of TNF inhibitors: impact on clinical efficacy and tolerability in the management of autoimmune diseases. A systematic review and meta-analysis, BioDrugs 29 (4) (2015) 241–258.

[115] M.H. Buch, P.G. Conaghan, M.A. Quinn, S.J. Bingham, D. Veale, P. Emery, True infliximab resistance in rheumatoid arthritis: a role for lymphotoxin α? Ann. Rheum. Dis. 63 (10) (2004) 1344–1346.

[116] A. Nesbitt, G. Fossati, M. Bergin, P. Stephens, S. Stephens, R. Foulkes, D. Brown, M. Robinson, T. Bourne, Mechanism of action of certolizumab pegol (CDP870): in vitro comparison with other anti-tumor necrosis factor α agents, Inflamm. Bowel Dis. 13 (11) (2007) 1323–1332.

[117] N.E. Simister, Placental transport of immunoglobulin G, Vaccine 21 (24) (2003) 3365–3369.

[118] C. Porter, S. Armstrong-Fisher, T. Kopotsha, B. Smith, T. Baker, L. Kevorkian, A. Nesbitt, Certolizumab pegol does not bind the neonatal Fc receptor (FcRn): consequences for FcRn-mediated in vitro transcytosis and ex vivo human placental transfer, J. Reprod. Immunol. 116 (2016) 7–12.

[119] F. Förger, P.M. Villiger, Treatment of rheumatoid arthritis during pregnancy: present and future, Expert. Rev. Clin. Immunol. 12 (9) (2016) 937–944.

[120] C. Porter, T. Kopotsha, B.J. Smith, A.M. Nesbitt, S.J. Urbaniak, S.S. Armstrong-Fisher, W1208 No significant transfer of certolizumab pegol compared with IgG in the perfused human placenta in vitro, Gastroenterology 138 (5) (2010) S-674.

[121] D. Wolf, U. Mahadevan, Certolizumab pegol use in pregnancy: low levels detected in cord blood, Arthritis Rheum. 62 (Suppl. 10) (2010) 718.

[122] Z. Zelinkova, C. de Haar, L. de Ridder, M.J. Pierik, E.J. Kuipers, M.P. Peppelenbosch, C.J. Van Der Woude, High intra-uterine exposure to infliximab following maternal anti-TNF treatment during pregnancy, Aliment. Pharmacol. Ther. 33 (9) (2011) 1053–1058.

[123] Z. Zelinkova, C. van der Ent, K.F. Bruin, O. van Baalen, H.G. Vermeulen, H.J. Smalbraak, R.J. Ouwendijk, A.C. Hoek, S.D. van der Werf, E.J. Kuipers, C.J. van der Woude, Effects of discontinuing anti-tumor necrosis factor therapy during pregnancy on the course of inflammatory bowel disease and neonatal exposure, Clin. Gastroenterol. Hepatol. 11 (3) (2013) 318–321.

[124] E.A. Vasiliauskas, J.A. Church, N. Silverman, M. Barry, S.R. Targan, M.C. Dubinsky, Case report: evidence for transplacental transfer of maternally administered infliximab to the newborn, Clin. Gastroenterol. Hepatol. 4 (10) (2006) 1255–1258.

[125] M. Julsgaard, L.A. Christensen, P.R. Gibson, R.B. Gearry, J. Fallingborg, C.L. Hvas, B.M. Bibby, N. Uldbjerg, W.R. Connell, O. Rosella, A. Grosen, Concentrations of adalimumab and infliximab in mothers and newborns, and effects on infection, Gastroenterology 151 (1) (2016) 110–119.

[126] A. Esteve-Solé, À. Deyà-Martínez, I. Teixidó, E. Ricart, M. Gompertz, M. Torradeflot, N. de Moner, E.A. Gonzalez, A.M. Plaza-Martin, J. Yagüe, M. Juan, Immunological changes in blood of newborns exposed to anti-TNF-α during pregnancy, Front. Immunol. 8 (2017) 1123.

[127] M.M. He, A.S. Smith, J.D. Oslob, W.M. Flanagan, A.C. Braisted, A. Whitty, M.T. Cancilla, J. Wang, A.A. Lugovskoy, J.C. Yoburn, A.D. Fung, Small-molecule inhibition of TNF-α, Science 310 (5750) (2005) 1022–1025.

[128] P. Alexiou, A. Papakyriakou, E. Ntougkos, C.P. Papaneophytou, F. Liepouri, A. Mettou, I. Katsoulis, A. Maranti, K. Tsiliouka, S. Strongilos, S. Chaitidou, Rationally designed less toxic SPD-304 analogs and preliminary evaluation of their TNF inhibitory effects, Arch. Pharm. 347 (11) (2014) 798–805.

132

[129] C. Papaneophytou, P. Alexiou, A. Papakyriakou, E. Ntougkos, K. Tsiliouka, A. Maranti, F. Liepouri, A. Strongilos, A. Mettou, E. Couladouros, E. Eliopoulos, Synthesis and biological evaluation of potential small molecule inhibitors of tumor necrosis factor, MedChemComm 6 (6) (2015) 1196–1209.

[130] J. O'Connell, J. Porter, B. Kroeplien, T. Norman, S. Rapecki, R. Davis, D. McMillan, T. Arakaki, A. Burgin, D. Fox Iii, T. Ceska, Small molecules that inhibit TNF signalling by stabilising an asymmetric form of the trimer, Nat. Commun. 10 (1) (2019) 1–12.

[131] S. Luzi, Y. Kondo, E. Bernard, L.K. Stadler, M. Vaysburd, G. Winter, P. Holliger, Subunit disassembly and inhibition of TNFα by a semi-synthetic bicyclic peptide, Protein Eng. Des. Sel. 28 (2) (2015) 45–52.

[132] R. Alzani, A. Corti, L. Grazioli, E. Cozzi, P. Ghezzi, F. Marcucci, Suramin induces deoligomerization of human tumor necrosis factor alpha, J. Biol. Chem. 268 (17) (1993) 12526–12529.

[133] F. Mancini, C.M. Toro, M. Mabilia, M. Giannangeli, M. Pinza, C. Milanese, Inhibition of tumor necrosis factor-α (TNF-α)/TNF-α receptor binding by structural analogues of suramin, Biochem. Pharmacol. 58 (5) (1999) 851–859.

[134] B.A. Shah, R. Chib, P. Gupta, V.K. Sethi, S. Koul, S.S. Andotra, A. Nargotra, S. Sharma, A. Pandey, S. Bani, B. Purnima, Saponins as novel TNF-α inhibitors: isolation of saponins and a nor-pseudoguaianolide from Parthenium hysterophorus, Org. Biomol. Chem. 7 (16) (2009) 3230–3235.

[135] H. Choi, Y. Lee, H. Park, D.S. Oh, Discovery of the inhibitors of tumor necrosis factor alpha with structure-based virtual screening, Bioorg. Med. Chem. Lett. 20 (21) (2010) 6195–6198.

[136] D.S.H. Chan, H.M. Lee, F. Yang, C.M. Che, C.C. Wong, R. Abagyan, C.H. Leung, D.L. Ma, Structure-based discovery of natural-product-like TNF-α inhibitors, Angew. Chem. Int. Ed. 49 (16) (2010) 2860–2864.

[137] Y. Cao, Y.H. Li, D.Y. Lv, X.F. Chen, L.D. Chen, Z.Y. Zhu, Y.F. Chai, J.P. Zhang, Identification of a ligand for tumor necrosis factor receptor from Chinese herbs by combination of surface plasmon resonance biosensor and UPLC-MS, Anal. Bioanal. Chem. 408 (19) (2016) 5359–5367.

[138] Q. Shen, J. Chen, Q. Wang, X. Deng, Y. Liu, L. Lai, Discovery of highly potent TNFα inhibitors using virtual screen, Eur. J. Med. Chem. 85 (2014) 119–126.

Further reading

J.M. Blevitt, M.D. Hack, K.L. Herman, P.F. Jackson, P.J. Krawczuk, A.D. Lebsack, A.X. Liu, T. Mirzadegan, M.I. Nelen, A.N. Patrick, S. Steinbacher, Structural basis of small-molecule aggregate induced inhibition of a protein–protein interaction, J. Med. Chem. 60 (8) (2017) 3511–3517.

G. Bröms, F. Granath, A. Ekbom, K. Hellgren, L. Pedersen, H.T. Sørensen, O. Stephansson, H. Kieler, Low risk of birth defects for infants whose mothers are treated with anti-tumor necrosis factor agents during pregnancy, Clin. Gastroenterol. Hepatol. 14 (2) (2016) 234–241.

D.S.H. Chan, H.M. Lee, F. Yang, C.M. Che, C.C. Wong, R. Abagyan, C.H. Leung, D.L. Ma, Structure-based discovery of natural-product-like TNF-α inhibitors, Angew. Chem. Int. Ed. 49 (16) (2010) 2860–2864.

C. Chen, T.J. Nott, J. Jin, T. Pawson, Deciphering arginine methylation: Tudor tells the tale, Nat. Rev. Mol. Cell Biol. 12 (10) (2011) 629–642.

H. He, P. Xu, X. Zhang, M. Liao, Q. Dong, T. Cong, B. Tang, X. Yang, M. Ye, Y.J. Chang, W. Liu, Aging-induced IL27Ra signaling impairs hematopoietic stem cells, Blood 136 (2) (2020) 183–198.

A. Malek, R. Sager, H. Schneider, Maternal—fetal transport of immunoglobulin G and its subclasses during the third trimester of human pregnancy, Am. J. Reprod. Immunol. 32 (1) (1994) 8–14.

A.J. Schottelius, L.L. Moldawer, C.A. Dinarello, K. Asadullah, W. Sterry, C.K. Edwards III, Biology of tumor necrosis factor-α–implications for psoriasis, Exp. Dermatol. 13 (4) (2004) 193–222.

T.P. Shanley, R.L. Warner, P.A. Ward, The role of cytokines and adhesion molecules in the development of inflammatory injury, Mol. Med. Today 1 (1) (1995) 40.

C.M. Story, J.E. Mikulska, N.E. Simister, A major histocompatibility complex class I-like Fc receptor cloned from human placenta: possible role in transfer of immunoglobulin G from mother to fetus, J. Exp. Med. 180 (6) (1994) 2377–2381.

H. Wajant, K. Pfizenmaier, P. Scheurich, Tumor necrosis factor signaling, Cell Death Differ. 10 (1) (2003) 45–65.

CHAPTER
7

Generation of thymic cells from pluripotent stem cells for basic research and cell therapy

Stephan Ramos* and Holger A. Russ*

Barbara Davis Center for Diabetes, Department of Pediatrics, School of Medicine, University of Colorado Anschutz Medical Campus, Aurora, CO, United States
*Corresponding author

Abstract

The thymus is the central organ facilitating the development of the adaptive immune system to effectively recognize foreign antigens while being tolerant to self-peptides. This critical function is achieved by educating developing T cells via interaction with thymic stromal cells. The thymus is most active during the first years of life and involutes at the time of adolescence, severely reducing naïve T cell output. This age-related decrease in thymic function is further accelerated by certain clinical interventions including chemotherapy. Thus, there is a great interest in developing an abundant source of functional, human thymic cells, both for future cell therapy and to investigate human thymus biology. Pluripotent stem cells (PSCs) have the ability to differentiate into every cell found in the human body, given appropriate stimuli are provided. Based on knowledge largely gained from studies in animal model systems, direct differentiation of human PSCs (hPSCs) for the generation of distinct differentiated cell types have been developed. Here we review recent progress in generating functional thymic cells from hPSCs by direct differentiation approaches and discuss remaining challenges and opportunities in the field.

Keywords

Human thymus development and function, T cell education, Positive and negative selection, Thymic epithelial cells (TECs) and thymic epithelial progenitor cells (TEPs), Pluripotent stem cells, Direct differentiation

7. Generation of thymic cells from pluripotent stem cells

1 Introduction

The thymus gland is the essential organ for the education of developing T cell which constitutes the adaptive arm of the immune system. The thymus is most active during early childhood and involutes during adolescence resulting in a rapid decline of naïve T cell output, reducing the ability to fight off new infections and transformed cells. Reduced thymic function can be further exacerbated by clinical treatments, e.g., chemotherapy or congenital thymus defects. Cell therapy employing a functional thymus equivalent to patients could provide an effective treatment or cure. Thus, recent research efforts have focused on the generation of a thymus from pluripotent stem cells. Here, we provide a concise review of thymus function, how this organ develops and common thymic diseases. We discuss how comprehensive knowledge of thymus biology has informed approaches to direct the differentiation of human pluripotent stem cells into thymic cell types and highlight emerging concepts in this regenerative research field.

2 Thymus organogenesis

The thymus is a bi-lobed endoderm-derived organ located in the central chest cavity, and develops from the third pharyngeal pouch endoderm [1]. The functional thymus is organized into central medullary structures surrounded by cortical regions, both with distinct functions in educating developing T cells. Studies carried out in mouse models have demonstrated critical molecular pathways necessary for the development of a functional thymus. Transcription factors and signaling molecules such as; Hoxa3, Pax1, Eya1, Six1/4, Tbx1, Foxn1, Bmp4, Fgf8, Shh, and Wnt5b have been identified as regulators of pharyngeal pouch, and subsequently, thymus development [1, 2]. During development, the third pharyngeal pouch serves as the primordium for both the thymus, and a pair of parathyroid glands [3]. A well-balanced interplay between a number of signaling molecules; such as sonic hedgehog (Shh) from the pharynx and bone morphogenic protein 4 (Bmp4) and patched from surrounding neural crest cells; as well as cell intrinsic regulation by transcription factors such as Gcm2, Tbx1, and Foxn1, act to segregate the third pharyngeal pouch into two distinct dorsal and ventral primordia, which will become the parathyroid and thymus, respectively. After patterning and specification of the parathyroid and thymic primordia, the paired primordia detach from the pharynx, and eventually from each other, by apoptosis and begin to migrate to their final locations in the central chest cavity [2]. While the exact cellular and molecular mechanisms that drive the migration of the thymic lobes to their proper final location are not fully known, evidence demonstrates that thymic epithelial cells (TECs) of the thymus maintain expression of E-cadherin and do not undergo epithelial-mesenchymal transition [4]. Additionally, studies support a role for ephrin B2 expressing neural crest cells in acting to "pull" the developing thymic lobes to their proper final locations [5]. Both before and after migrating to the central chest cavity, the thymus primordium secretes chemokines, such as CCL21/25, which attract hematopoietic stem cells (HSCs)/lymphoid progenitor cells (LPCs) to the thymus [6, 7]. While the presence of LPCs is not strictly required for complete differentiation and organogenesis of the thymus, further TEC differentiation from TEPs, and the formation of a functional thymic medulla require TEC/LPC crosstalk [8, 9]. Mouse models have provided a wealth of information and insight into the cellular and molecular mechanisms of thymus development.

While these aspects of thymic development seem to be well conserved in human thymus development [10], aspects of T cell development are known to differ between mouse and human [11, 12]. Thus, the development of human-based model systems for studying human thymic and T cell development would be an invaluable resource in efforts to identify the cellular and molecular mechanisms that drive pathogenic thymic and T cell disorders, such as immunodeficiencies and autoimmune diseases, in the human context.

3 Thymus function

T cells comprise a specific and critical arm of the adaptive immune system and function in the immunological response toward pathogens, allergens, and tumors [13]. T cell development occurs in the thymus; a glandular organ, for which T cells are named after, that serves as the primary location for the development of functional T cells [14]. The thymus is organized in a cortical/medullary structure, comprised of cortical and medullary thymic epithelial cells (cTECs and mTECs), respectively, as well as other stromal cell types [15, 16]. While c/mTECs comprise the most-characterized stromal population in the thymus, recent advances in single-cell omics have uncovered a plethora of additional cell types that are starting to be characterized and appreciated, including distinct cTEC and mTEC subpopulations, thymic nurse cells, tuft cells, and Hassell's corpuscles [17–19]. Hematopoietic stem cells (HSCs) develop in the bone marrow and migrate to the thymus, directed by chemotactic signals provided by cTECs and mTECs [13]. In the cortex, cTECs express delta-like ligand 4 (DLL4) and signal through NOTCH receptors on HSCs to commit multipotent HSCs to the T cell lineage [15]. In conjunction to participating in the process of T cell commitment, cTECs also express peptide/ major histocompatibility complexes (MHC) on their surface. This allows for positive selection of developing T cells to ensure the proper recombination of the developing T cell's T cell receptor (TCR) and appropriate expression of costimulatory molecules, CD3, 4, and 8 [15, 16]. Developing T cells that do not bind strongly enough to peptide/ MHC complexes presented on cTECs, fail to induce the appropriate survival signals, and die by neglect [16]. T cells that properly recombine their TCR and successfully pass through positive selection migrate to the thymic medulla. In the medulla, mTECs and resident dendritic cells negatively select autoreactive T cells [16]. Negative selection is primarily driven by two key transcription factors expressed by mTECs, autoimmune regulator (Aire) and Fezf2 [20, 21]. These factors promote the ectopic expression of self-antigens, which are processed and presented on the MHC of mTECs and thymic dendritic cells [20, 21]. T cells that react moderately to self-antigens differentiate to regulatory T cells that migrate to the periphery and provide peripheral tolerance [22], while T cells that react too strongly to self-antigens, thus being overtly autoreactive, are deleted via apoptosis [16]. This process of negative selection ensures a peripheral T cell repertoire that is able to respond to foreign antigens, while being tolerant to self.

4 Common thymic disorders

As the thymus plays an integral role in the formation, function, and homeostasis of the adaptive immune system, thymic defects can have devastating effects on the health of affected individuals. Thymic deficiencies can arise as a congenital status or as the result of an acute or chronic insult, such as chemotherapy or radiation therapy in the treatment of cancers. Congenital deficiencies primarily arise from mutations in *TBX1*, a transcription factor that is integral for the formation of the third pharyngeal pouch, or in the key thymic transcription factor FOXN1. Individuals deficient in TBX1, a result of the deletion of chromosome 22q11.2, present with DiGeorge syndrome, which is a condition that results in congenital thymic hypoplasia [23–25]. Likewise, mutations in *FOXN1* also result in severe thymic hypoplasia (known as the *nude* phenotype) in mouse and human [26–28]. Both of these conditions result in a severe decrease, or complete absence, of peripheral T cells and the development of primary immunodeficiency. In addition to mutations that cause severe thymic hypoplasia, mutations in *AIRE* result in the development of autoimmune polyendocrine syndrome-1 (APS-1), also known as autoimmune polyendocrinopathy-candidiasis-ectodermal dystrophy (APECED), a condition characterized by systemic autoimmune attack, primarily affecting endocrine organs [29].

For reasons yet unknown, the thymus undergoes age-related atrophy beginning at the time of puberty [30]. Thus, as we age, we gradually lose the ability to generate new naïve T cells, and thus, our ability to effectively respond to new infections and transformed cells [31–33]. This issue can be exacerbated in individuals who have undergone lymphoablative treatments such as chemotherapy or radiation therapy [34]. Taken together, the critical importance of the thymus and T cell function for human health, and the devastating outcomes when these processes are disrupted, have triggered an increased interest in investigating human thymus homeostasis and pathology.

5 Human pluripotent stem cells to TECs: A new frontier

Human pluripotent stem cells (hPSC) come in two flavors; human embryonic stem cells (hESC) and human-induced pluripotent stem cells (hiPSC); based on how each pluripotent cell type is derived. hESCs are derived from pluripotent cells, cells with the ability to generate any cell type in the human body, of the inner cell mass of early human embryos at the blastocyst stage [35]. Meanwhile, hiPSCs are generated by forcing the expression of pluripotency reprogramming factors in somatic human cells [36], thus, allowing for the generation of patient-specific hPSCs. Both hESCs and hiPSCs are able to undergo directed differentiation to a variety of cell types, if provided with the proper developmental cues and signaling molecules. However, it is critical to first understand the molecular and signaling pathways directing the development of the tissue of interest in vivo, to allow for effective translation of this knowledge to directed differentiation approaches of hPSCs in vitro. Extensive studies conducted in various vertebrate models reviewed here [3] have provided a framework of the developmental pathways and requirements as a foundation for the formulation of directed differentiation protocols for human stem cells into different endodermal lineages. Directed differentiation protocols typically follow in vivo development in a step-wise manner, mimicking key developmental stages in vitro by providing recombinant growth factors, signaling molecules and to a lesser degree, extracellular matrix components.

6 Mimicking development in vitro to generate hPSC-derived anterior foregut endoderm

As the thymus is an endodermal-derived organ, it is imperative to be able to generate definitive endoderm cells from hPSCs at high efficiency. High levels of nodal signaling, a member of the TGF-β superfamily, have been shown to be necessary for the development of endoderm in mice [37, 38]. Accordingly, it has been demonstrated that high levels of the TGF-β superfamily member, ActivinA, in conjugation with severe reduction of fetal bovine serum or serum replacement knock out added to media, can be utilized to generate quasipure definitive endoderm cells (DEs) from hPSCs. DEs express all of the known canonical markers of definitive endoderm after just 3–5 days of direct differentiation [39]. After differentiation to definitive endoderm in vivo, DEs acquire an anteroposterior axis identity, and form the gut tube [3]. The gut tube can be segregated into fore, mid, and hindgut, found anterior to posterior, respectively [3]. The foregut itself can be further divided along the anterior-posterior axis based on distinct tissues that arise from a specific location, starting anterior with the middle ear, trachea, lung, esophagus, and thymus, while the posterior foregut endoderm gives rise to the stomach, duodenum, pancreas, and liver [3, 40]. The anterior foregut endoderm further undergoes dorsoventral patterning to generate the lung buds, trachea, and pharyngeal pouches. A multitude of transcription factors and signaling pathways regulate this anteroposterior axis of the foregut endoderm, and knowledge of pertinent pathways can be leveraged in vitro to differentiate DEs toward a specific subsequent cell fate [41, 42]. Inhibition of both BMP4 and ActivinA/nodal signaling has been demonstrated to trigger the differentiation of hPSC-derived DEs into anterior foregut endoderm cells (AFEs) [41]. Of note, the differentiation of hPSCs to both DEs and AFE is quite efficient, with over 90% of all cells expressing respective lineage markers after differentiation [41]. As during in vivo development, the timing of when specific signaling molecules are added to differentiating hPSC cultures in vitro, has critical effects on the cell type generated. For example, when AFEs are treated with a combination of WNT3a, FGF10, KGF, BMP4, and EGF during days 7–13, cells effectively specify their further development into a ventral identity, while AFE cells treated with the same factors from days 9 to 13 did not [41]. Interestingly, while the differentiation efficiency of AFEs was very high (over 90%), the subsequent generation of ventral anterior foregut endoderm (vAFE) dropped to about 37% [41], suggesting that normal vAFE development is only partially recapitulated using described differentiation conditions. Thus, a deeper understanding of the signaling molecules driving each lineage decision during direct differentiation into thymic cells is needed to achieve highly efficient generation of target cells. As each subsequent developmental stage mimicked in vitro bears the possibility of off target differentiation, this is especially the case for the later differentiation stages. Indeed, current differentiation protocols to generate vAFE derivatives utilize combinations of many different factors which make further optimization challenging and time-consuming [41].

7 Generating thymic epithelial progenitor cells in vitro

In mouse and human, the pharyngeal pouches develop from the ventral anterior foregut endoderm, with the thymus being a derivative of the third pharyngeal pouch [2, 3, 10].

Utilizing developmental knowledge primarily derived from vertebrate model systems, as well as some degree of trial and error, two groups demonstrated the ability to generate third pharyngeal pouch endoderm, and subsequent thymic epithelial progenitors (TEPs) from hESCs through directed differentiation in vitro [43, 44]. Both studies employed somewhat similar strategies to achieve this feat, by testing specific combination of key signaling molecules involved in anterior-posterior and ventral-dorsal patterning of AFEs. Bmp4, Fgf8, Wnt, and Shh molecules act to control pharyngeal pouch and thymus development in the mouse [2, 45]. Bmp4 functions to control thymic morphogenesis [2, 45], Fgf8 acts on early pouch formation [2], Wnt protein function thought to promote Foxn1 expression [2, 45], and Shh plays a role in driving parathyroid fate [2, 45]. Interestingly, while Parent et al. uses BMP4, retinoic acid, Wnt3a, FGF8, and SHH inhibition to generate ventral pharyngeal pouch cells marked by HOXA3 and subsequently TEPs marked by FOXN1 expression, Sun et al. merely uses retinoic acid signaling in combination with WNT inhibition to first generate pharyngeal pouch-like cells from DE, followed by the addition of BMP4 and Wnt3a to specify TEPs. Collectively both studies point toward a critical role for precise manipulation of both BMP and WNT signaling during the later stages of direct differentiation to generate human thymic cells in vitro. In both studies, retinoic acid appears to have an important role in the generation of thymic cells, but the exact mechanisms and timing is not clear. Retinoic acid has previously been demonstrated to play a key role in lung development, in both mouse and human, and addition of all-trans retinoic acid to NOGGIN/SB-431542-induced AFE cultures, results in a decrease in pharyngeal pouch marker while increasing lung markers [41, 46]. However, retinoic acid has also been implicated in acting to control pharyngeal pouch patterning, and has been shown to be necessary for the proper development of the pharyngeal pouches [47]. Indeed, retinoic acid is necessary for efficient directed differentiation of TEPs from hPSCs, with differentiation conditions lacking retinoic acid during pharyngeal pouch formation resulting in lower expression of pharyngeal pouch markers [43, 44]. Based on HOXA3 protein staining, a marker for third pharyngeal poach cells, approximately 45%–65% of all cells adopted the desired developmental phenotype at day 9 of differentiation, indicating an opportunity to further improve these published protocols. However, utilizing FOXN1 mRNA levels as a readout for TEP differentiation in the absence of a reliable FOXN1 antibody, both protocols show reproducible induction of this critical key thymic transcription factor at the end of the differentiation [43, 44]. Of note, both thymic protocols result in cell populations with moderate levels of parathyroid markers *TBX1* or *GCM2* [43, 44], indicating either a low degree of off-target differentiation toward a parathyroid fate or inefficient generation of pharyngeal poach cells competent to give rise to subsequent tissue types. Interestingly, Soh et al. demonstrated that hESCs could be differentiated into TEP-like cells after prolonged treatment of embryoid bodies (clusters of undifferentiated hPSCs cultured in suspension) with just ActivinA and BMP4. Notably, WNT and retinoic acid signaling was not modulated in these experiments. However, the efficiency of TEP generation using this approach was low during the initial differentiation period, indicating considerable off-target differentiation, but TEP numbers increased notably by extending the differentiation duration. To overcome the challenges of detecting FOXN1 protein, these researchers created and utilized a $FOXN1^{GFP/W}$ reporter hPSC line, where GFP is inserted into the endogenous *FOXN1* locus, allowing for flow-based quantification of TEP generation. To determine whether FOXN1-GFP$^+$ cells were capable of supporting T cell development in vitro, purified FOXN1-GFP$^+$ cells were cocultured with umbilical cord blood-derived CD34/CD7$^+$ T cell progenitors. However, co-culture experiments did not result in the development of T cells, but rather, CD14$^+$ myeloid cells; indicating that the TEP-like cells may have been too immature to properly support in vitro T cell development [48]. Using fluorescence-activated cell sorting, followed by global transcriptomic analysis of FOXN$^-$GFP$^+$ cells resulted in the identification of specific TEP surface markers, HLA-DR and ITGB4, that could be used in conjugation with unmodified hPSCs, thus carrying considerable therapeutic potential. However, the usefulness of both markers to either further optimize direct differentiation approaches or isolate live TEP cells for downstream culture and analysis needs to be demonstrated in the future.

8 hPSC-derived thymic epithelial cells

As TEPs require interactions with developing hematopoietic stem cells/thymic seeding progenitors (HSC/TSPs) in order to undergo complete maturation [8, 9], two groups transplanted hESC-derived TEPs under the kidney capsule of nude (athymic) mice and allowed grafts to mature in vivo for 12–28 weeks [43, 44]. Indeed, explanted grafts displayed further thymic differentiation with areas of developing TECs, double positive for the cTEC and mTEC markers, keratin 8 and 5, respectively, and single positive cells, indicating the generation of mature c- and mTECs within transplants. Explanted grafts showed increased expression of critical TEC markers including HLA-DR and DLL4, as well as chemokines to attract TSP at the RNA and protein level. Additionally, developing T cells were present in grafts and single positive T cells, including Tregs, were found in the periphery of transplanted nude mice. Peripheral mouse T cells developed in the hESC-derived TEP grafts exhibit a diverse TCR repertoire and can respond to allogenic stimuli [43, 44]. Taken together, these results indicate that hES-derived TEPs have the capacity to further differentiate into functional TECs in a xenogeneic model system and thus, provide a framework for future studies aimed at developing patient-specific thymic cells for basic research and therapeutic approaches.

Indeed, the use of hESCs does not allow for the investigation of thymic development and function in a patient-specific context. Thus, recent work by two independent groups has demonstrated the ability to generate functional TEPs/TECs from hiPSCs using slightly modified directed differentiation protocols based on the previous work by Parent et al. [49, 50]. Chhatta et al. optimized the TEP directed differentiation protocol using a commercially available kit for DE formation from hiPSCs, and adding EC23 (a retinoic acid receptor agonist) starting at day 5, instead of day 4 as described in Parent et al. [43]. More importantly, differentiating cultures were transduced with a lentiviral FOXN1 overexpression construct at day 9, in an attempt to increase TEP differentiation efficiency. However, the efficiency of TEP generation remained low, indicating that cells at this stage might not be competent to differentiate into TEPs or that FOXN1 alone is not sufficient to drive further thymus differentiation at this stage. *FOXN1* levels detected in these experiments were much lower than what is present in primary neonatal thymus potentially indicating an additional caveat [43, 44, 49]. Furthermore, whether these results are the consequence of many cells expressing low levels of *FOXN1*, or few cells expressing high *FOXN1* levels, remains to be determined. Regardless of the challenges in achieving high differentiation efficiency and *FOXN1* expression levels, iPSC-derived TEPs from this study are also able to support mouse T cell development in vivo,

7. Generation of thymic cells from pluripotent stem cells

providing a proof of principle for the generation of patient-specific TECs [49]. While these studies represent significant advances toward the goal of generating a human patient-specific thymus in vitro, the models and approaches employed still contain caveats that need to be overcome. First, transplantation of TEPs into mice to generate functional TECs relies on the interactions of human TEPs/TECs with developing mouse T cells that can potentially inhibit or confound results due to mismatches in interacting proteins. Indeed, *AIRE* expression is not detected using the nude mouse model, likely due to differences in human and mouse RANK and ligand interactions [43]. The maturation of TEPs to TECs by engraftment in mice requires considerable time (months) and exhibits substantial variability in TEC maturation and consequently in the kinetics of peripheral T cell emergence. Furthermore, using xenogeneic model systems impairs the utility of hPSC-derived thymic cells for therapeutic approaches. Thus, recent work has largely focused on the development of in vitro human thymus models (Fig. 1).

9 In vitro coculture systems to model thymic function

An in vitro system to mature TEPs to TECs and generate T cells in the dish is an attractive goal that would have many implications in both, basic mechanistic studies of human thymus development and in the therapeutic cell therapy context. Reaggregated thymic organotypic cultures (RTOCs) represent an elegant, early approach to investigate human thymic development and function in vitro. Thymic mesenchyme plays a critical role in the development and function of the thymus; thus, RTOCs are generated by mixing TECs and thymic mesenchyme cell populations expanded from primary neonatal thymus samples with allogenic HSCs. To specifically isolate TECs and mesenchyme from primary thymus samples, neonatal thymi, removed during cardiac surgeries, are mechanically dissociated into fragments smaller than $1\,mm^3$ and plated in growth medium supplemented with either low or high percentages of fetal bovine serum to promote TEC or mesenchymal cell expansion, respectively. TECs and thymic mesenchyme can be expanded for up to 3 weeks, after which, cell populations are aggregated and cocultured with allogenic umbilical cord blood-derived HSCs (CB-HSCs) on a cell culture membrane, at the air-liquid interface [51]. Using this system, researchers were able to obtain human T cell development after 4 weeks of coculture in vitro.

Another major, early development toward the ability to generate human T cells from HSCs in vitro was the development of the OP9-DLL1 system. As NOTCH signaling is required to specify HSCs to the T-cell lineage, this system utilizes OP9 mouse bone marrow stromal cells transduced with a retroviral construct to constitutively express DLL1 to facilitate the development of human T cells from HSCs in vitro [52]. Building on this system, researchers at the University of California, Los Angeles, developed artificial thymic organoids (ATOs), that use MS5 mouse bone marrow stromal cells genetically engineered to express human DLL4 at high levels. When MS5-DLL4 are cocultured with either umbilical cord blood-derived HSCs, or hPSC-derived human embryonic mesoderm progenitors (hEMPs) at the air-liquid interface, efficient T cell development is observed within a few weeks [53, 54]. Most notably, this approach can be used to generate functional, patient-specific naïve T cells with a desired TCR sequence via retroviral transduction. While these powerful model systems allow the de novo generation of human T cells from umbilical cord blood and hPSC-derived sources, they do not provide a human thymic compartment and thus have critical shortcomings. For example,

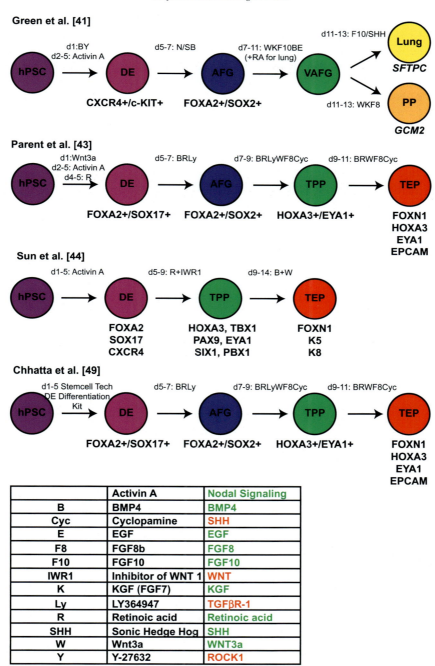

FIG. 1 Overview of direct differentiation protocols to generate thymic cells in vitro. Schematic outlining the stepwise differentiation approach published by different groups. Different molecules and their incubation times to generate subsequent, differentiated cell types identified by key marker expression are provided. *hPSC*, human pluripotent stem cells; *DE*, definitive endoderm; *AFG*, anterior foregut; *VAFG*, ventral anterior foregut; *PP*, pharyngeal pouch; *TPP*, third pharyngeal pouch; *TEP*, thymic epithelial cells.

these approaches do not allow the investigation of thymus-mediated mechanisms of T cell development, such as negative selection and as such, preclude the utilization for potential future treatment of thymic or autoimmune disorders. Additionally, in xenogeneic systems, human T cells are educated on mouse MHC class I expressed on the OP9 or MS5 murine cell lines, resulting in the skewing of T cell development toward CD8 expressing T cells [54, 55].

Taking the recent developments into account, the coculture of hPSC-derived TEPs with CB-HSCs would be an attractive first step in the generation of a patient-specific thymus model in vitro. Much progress has been achieved in our ability to generate HSCs from hPSC sources [56–59]. However, it must be noted that different blood cell types are derived from different HSCs, with erythroid and myeloid cells being derived from the primitive HSC program, and B and T cells being derived from the definitive HSC program [60]. Despite much effort, many groups have struggled to efficiently differentiate multipotent HSCs capable of developing into functional T cells, with some protocols only supporting primitive HSC development, and some supporting definitive HSC development, but with low efficiency [56–58]. Recently, Motazedian et al. demonstrated the ability to efficiently generate functional T cells from hPSC-derived hematopoietic organoids [59]. The ability to generate hPSC-derived HSCs allows the possibility of generating isogenic hPSC-derived TEP/HSC cocultures, potentially allowing the generation of a patient specific functional thymus in vitro. Such stem cell derived thymic organoid cultures would provide unprecedented possibilities for their use in basic research studies, as well as a potential attractive tissue source for cell therapy of patients with thymic and autoimmune disorders. Furthermore, STOCs could be utilized to generate novel preclinical animal models that harbor a patient-specific human adaptive immune system. We predict that such efforts will soon allow for further investigation into the mechanisms of human T cell selection, autoimmune disorders, thymic disorders, and immune system/tumor interactions.

10 Conclusion

Rigorously mediated processes of positive and negative selection in the thymus ensure the generation of a peripheral T cell population that expresses TCRs that are able to recognize foreign antigens, while being tolerant to self-antigens mounted on MHCs. Negative T cell selection is primarily mediated by mTECs, as well as by resident dendritic cells in the thymic medulla [16]. Various studies in mouse models have demonstrated that presentation of self-antigens by mTECs is mediated by two known transcription factors, AIRE and Fezf2 [20, 21]. During development, T cells that react at moderate to strong levels to self-antigens are induced to develop into regulatory T cells or deleted by apoptosis [16]. While these processes have been studied and characterized in various mouse models, we currently lack an adequate model to study human thymic negative selection in a physiological context. Recent progress in the generation of TEPs and T cells from human hPSC sources has made the potential of an in vitro patient-specific thymus model a feasible goal. Multiple groups have demonstrated the ability to generate TEPs from hPSCs that are able to mature to functional TECs capable of supporting T cell development in vivo [43, 44, 49]. Additionally, multiple groups have demonstrated the ability to generate hematopoietic stem cells and T cells from hPSC [56–59]. Such advances present an attractive platform for the investigation of the mechanisms of negative T cell selection and autoimmunity in the human context.

Acknowledgments

Work in the laboratory of HAR is supported by the Children's Diabetes Foundation, NIH/NIDDK grant R01DK120444 and NIH/NIAID grant R21AI140044, a new investigator award from the NIH/NIDDK supported Human Islet Research Network (HIRN, RRID:SCR_014393; UC24 DK104162), the Culshaw Junior Investigator Award in Diabetes, a CU Grubstake award and the JDRF (2-SRA-2019-781-S-B).

References

[1] N.R. Manley, B.G. Condie, Transcriptional regulation of thymus organogenesis and thymic epithelial cell differentiation, Prog. Mol. Biol. Transl. Sci. 92 (2010) 103–120.

[2] J. Gordon, N.R. Manley, Mechanisms of thymus organogenesis and morphogenesis, Development 138 (2011) 3865–3878.

[3] A.M. Zorn, J.M. Wells, Vertebrate endoderm development and organ formation, Annu. Rev. Cell Dev. Biol. 25 (2009) 221–251.

[4] J. Gordon, S.R. Patel, Y. Mishina, N.R. Manley, Evidence for an early role for BMP4 signaling in thymus and parathyroid morphogenesis, Dev. Biol. 339 (1) (2010) 141–154.

[5] K.E. Foster, et al., EphB-ephrin-B2 interactions are required for thymus migration during organogenesis, Proc. Natl. Acad. Sci. U. S. A. 107 (30) (2010) 13414–13419.

[6] C. Liu, et al., The role of CCL21 in recruitment of T-precursor cells to fetal thymi, Blood 105 (1) (2005) 31–39.

[7] C. Liu, et al., Coordination between CCR7- and CCR9-mediated chemokine signals in prevascular fetal thymus colonization, Blood 108 (8) (2006) 2531–2539.

[8] T. Nitta, I. Ohigashi, Y. Nakagawa, Y. Takahama, Cytokine crosstalk for thymic medulla formation, Curr. Opin. Immunol. 23 (2) (2011) 190–197.

[9] M.A. Ritter, R.L. Boyd, Development in the thymus: it takes two to tango, Immunol. Today 14 (9) (1993) 462–469.

[10] A.M. Farley, et al., Dynamics of thymus organogenesis and colonization in early human development, Development 140 (9) (2013) 2015–2026.

[11] F. Famili, A.S. Wiekmeijer, F.J. Staal, The development of T cells from stem cells in mice and humans, Future Sci. OA 3 (3) (2017).

[12] J. Halkias, et al., Conserved and divergent aspects of human T-cell development and migration in humanized mice, Immunol. Cell Biol. 93 (8) (2015) 716–726.

[13] B.V. Kumar, T.J. Connors, D.L. Farber, Human T cell development, localization, and function throughout life, Immunity 48 (2018) 202–213.

[14] H.J. Vaidya, A. Briones Leon, C.C. Blackburn, FOXN1 in thymus organogenesis and development, Eur. J. Immunol. 46 (8) (2016) 1826–1837.

[15] H.-R. Rodewald, Thymus organogenesis, Annu. Rev. Immunol. 26 (2008) 355–388.

[16] L. Klein, B. Kyewski, P.M. Allen, K.A. Hogquist, Positive and negative selection of the T cell repertoire: what thymocytes see and don't see, Nat. Rev. Immunol. 14 (6) (2014) 377–391.

[17] N. Kadouri, S. Nevo, Y. Goldfarb, J. Abramson, Thymic epithelial cell heterogeneity: TEC by TEC, Nat. Rev. Immunol. 20 (2020) 239–253.

[18] C. Bornstein, et al., Single-cell mapping of the thymic stroma identifies IL-25-producing tuft epithelial cells, Nature 559 (2018) 622–626.

[19] C.N. Miller, et al., Thymic tuft cells promote an IL-4-enriched medulla and shape thymocyte development, 559, Nature, 2018, pp. 627–631.

[20] H. Takaba, H. Takayanagi, The mechanisms of T cell selection in the thymus, Trends Immunol. 38 (11) (2017) 805–816.

[21] G.A. Passos, C.A. Speck-Hernandez, A.F. Assis, D.A. Mendes-Da-Cruz, Update on Aire and thymic negative selection, Immunology 153 (2017) 10–20.

[22] Í. Caramalho, H. Nunes-Cabaço, R.B. Foxall, A.E. Sousa, Regulatory T-cell development in the human thymus, Front. Immunol. 6 (2015) 395.

[23] S. Merscher, et al., TBX1 is responsible for cardiovascular defects in velo-cardio-facial/DiGeorge syndrome, Cell 104 (2001) 619–629.

[24] E.A. Lindsay, et al., Tbx1 haploinsufficiency in the DiGeorge syndrome region causes aortic arch defects in mice, Nature 410 (2001) 97–101.

[25] L.A. Jerome, V.E. Papaioannou, DiGeorge syndrome phenotype in mice mutant for the T-box gene, Tbx1, Nat. Genet. 27 (2001) 286–291.

[26] M. Nehls, D. Pfeifer, M. Schorpp, H. Hedrich, T. Boehm, New member of the winged-helix protein family disrupted in mouse and rat nude mutations, Nature 372 (1994) 103–107.

[27] M. Nehls, et al., Two genetically separable steps in the differentiation of thymic epithelium, Science (80-.) 272 (1996) 886–889.

[28] M. Adriani, et al., Ancestral founder mutation of the Nude (FOXN1) gene in congenital severe combined immunodeficiency associated with alopecia in Southern Italy population, Ann. Hum. Genet. 68 (2004) 265–268.

[29] L. De Martino, et al., Novel findings into AIRE genetics and functioning: clinical implications, Front. Pediatr. 4 (2016) 86.

[30] D.H.D. Gray, et al., Developmental kinetics, turnover, and stimulatory capacity of thymic epithelial cells, Blood 108 (2006) 3777–3785.

[31] I.K. Chinn, C.C. Blackburn, N.R. Manley, G.D. Sempowski, Changes in primary lymphoid organs with aging, Semin. Immunol. 24 (5) (2012) 309–320.

[32] L. Haynes, A.C. Maue, Effects of aging on T cell function, Curr. Opin. Immunol. 21 (2009) 414–417.

[33] J. Nikolich-Žugich, G. Li, J.L. Uhrlaub, K.R. Renkema, M.J. Smithey, Age-related changes in CD8 T cell homeostasis and immunity to infection, Semin. Immunol. 24 (2012) 356–364.

[34] K.M. Williams, F.T. Hakim, R.E. Gress, T cell immune reconstitution following lymphodepletion, Semin. Immunol. 19 (2007) 318–330.

[35] J.A. Thomson, et al., Embryonic stem cell lines derived from human blastocysts, Science (80-.) 282 (5391) (1998) 1145–1147.

[36] K. Takahashi, et al., Induction of pluripotent stem cells from adult human fibroblasts by defined factors, Cell 131 (5) (2007) 861–872.

[37] L.A. Lowe, S. Yamada, M.R. Kuehn, Genetic dissection of nodal function in patterning the mouse embryo, Development 128 (10) (2001) 1831–1843.

[38] S.D. Vincent, N.R. Dunn, S. Hayashi, D.P. Norris, E.J. Robertson, Cell fate decisions within the mouse organizer are governed by graded Nodal signals, Genes Dev. 17 (13) (2003) 1646–1662.

[39] K.A. D'Amour, A.D. Agulnick, S. Eliazer, O.G. Kelly, E. Kroon, E.E. Baetge, Efficient differentiation of human embryonic stem cells to definitive endoderm, Nat. Biotechnol. 23 (12) (2005) 1534–1541.

[40] L. Han, et al., Single cell transcriptomics identifies a signaling network coordinating endoderm and mesoderm diversification during foregut organogenesis, Nat. Commun. 11 (2020) 4158.

[41] M.D. Green, et al., Generation of anterior foregut endoderm from human embryonic and induced pluripotent stem cells, Nat. Biotechnol. 29 (3) (2011) 267–272.

[42] K.M. Loh, et al., Efficient endoderm induction from human pluripotent stem cells by logically directing signals controlling lineage bifurcations, Cell Stem Cell 14 (2) (2014) 237–252.

[43] A.V. Parent, et al., Generation of functional thymic epithelium from human embryonic stem cells that supports host T cell development, Cell Stem Cell 13 (2) (2013) 219–229.

[44] X. Sun, et al., Directed differentiation of human embryonic stem cells into thymic epithelial progenitor-like cells reconstitutes the thymic microenvironment in vivo, Cell Stem Cell 13 (2) (2013) 230–236.

[45] L. Palamaro, R. Romano, A. Fusco, G. Giardino, V. Gallo, C. Pignata, FOXN1 in organ development and human diseases, Int. Rev. Immunol. 33 (2014) 83–93.

[46] F. Chen, Y. Cao, J. Qian, F. Shao, K. Niederreither, W.V. Cardoso, A retinoic acid-dependent network in the foregut controls formation of the mouse lung primordium, J. Clin. Invest. 120 (6) (2010) 2040–2048.

[47] A. Graham, M. Okabe, R. Quinlan, The role of the endoderm in the development and evolution of the pharyngeal arches, J. Anat. 207 (5) (2005) 479–487.

[48] C.-L. Soh, et al., FOXN1 GFP/w reporter hESCs enable identification of integrin-b4, HLA-DR, and EpCAM as markers of human PSC-derived FOXN1 + thymic epithelial progenitors, Stem Cell Rep. 2 (2014) 925–937.

[49] A.R. Chhatta, et al., De novo generation of a functional human thymus from induced pluripotent stem cells, J. Allergy Clin. Immunol. 144 (5) (2019) 1416–1419. e7.

[50] Y. Yamazaki, et al., PAX1 is essential for development and function of the human thymus, Sci. Immunol. 5 (2020).

[51] B. Chung, et al., Engineering the human thymic microenvironment to support thymopoiesis in vivo, Stem Cells 32 (9) (2014) 2386–2396.

[52] R.N. La Motte-Mohs, E. Herer, J.C. Zuniga-Pflucker, Induction of T-cell development from human cord blood hematopoietic stem cells by Delta-like 1 in vitro, Blood 105 (2005) 1431–1439.

[53] C.S. Seet, et al., Generation of mature T cells from human hematopoietic stem and progenitor cells in artificial thymic organoids, Nat. Methods 14 (2017) 521.

[54] A. Montel-Hagen, et al., Organoid-induced differentiation of conventional T cells from human pluripotent stem cells, Cell Stem Cell 24 (3) (2019) 376–389. e8.

[55] C.S. Seet, et al., Generation of mature T cells from human hematopoietic stem and progenitor cells in artificial thymic organoids, Nat. Methods 14 (5) (2017) 5–8.

[56] A. Ditadi, C.M. Sturgeon, Directed differentiation of definitive hemogenic endothelium and hematopoietic progenitors from human pluripotent stem cells, Methods 101 (2016) 65–72.

[57] R. Sugimura, et al., Haematopoietic stem and progenitor cells from human pluripotent stem cells, Nature 545 (7655) (2017) 432–438.

[58] S. Doulatov, et al., Induction of multipotential hematopoietic progenitors from human pluripotent stem cells via respecification of lineage-restricted precursors human pluripotent stem cells (hPSCs) represent a promising source of patient-specific cells for disease modeling, Cell Stem Cell 13 (2013) 459–470.

[59] A. Motazedian, et al., Multipotent RAG1+ progenitors emerge directly from haemogenic endothelium in human pluripotent stem cell-derived haematopoietic organoids, Nat. Cell Biol. 22 (2020) 60–73.

[60] A. Medvinsky, S. Rybtsov, S. Taoudi, Embryonic origin of the adult hematopoietic system: advances and questions, Development 138 (2011) 1017–1031.

CHAPTER 8

The NLRP3 inflammasome pathway in autoimmune diseases: a chronotherapeutic perspective?

Cécilia Bellengier[a,b,c,d], Hélène Duez[a,b,c,d], and Benoit Pourcet[a,b,c,d,]*

[a]Univ. Lille, U1011 – EGID, Lille, France [b]Inserm, U1011, Lille, France
[c]CHU Lille, Lille, France [d]Institut Pasteur de Lille, Lille, France
*Corresponding author

Abstract

Innate and adaptive immune cells cooperate to protect the host from exogenous invaders and to maintain body integrity. However, in autoimmune diseases, the immune system turns against the host himself leading to dramatic tissue damage and loss-of-function. The NLRP3 inflammasome is a master regulator of the innate immune system, especially in macrophages, and a key sensor involved in maintaining cellular health in response to cytolytic pathogens or stress signals. Deficiency or overactivation of such important sensor leads to critical diseases including rheumatoid arthritis, spondylarthritis, systemic lupus erythematosus, inflammatory bowel diseases, systemic sclerosis, and type 1 diabetes. Targeting the NLRP3 inflammasome and the production of IL-1β has proven to be a promising approach for autoimmune disease management in humans and animal models. Our immune system is controlled by a circadian clock, which anticipates cyclic environmental changes and allows the adaptation of immune cell behavior to these daily cycles. Recently, the biological clock was demonstrated to control NLRP3 expression and activation. Accordingly, circadian oscillations of NLRP3 signaling are lost in models of clock disruption, thereby contributing to the development of autoimmune diseases. This report will discuss the role of the NLRP3 inflammasome in the pathogenesis of autoimmune diseases, the putative beneficial effect of new modulators of inflammasomes in the treatment of autoimmune diseases, and the opportunity to use a chrono-pharmacological approach in such strategies.

Keywords

NLRP3 inflammasome, Circadian rhythm, Clock, Circadian immunity, Chronotherapy, Autoimmune disease, Atherosclerosis, Systemic lupus erythematosus, Rheumatoid arthritis, Type 1 diabetes

1 Introduction

Autoimmune diseases encompass numerous chronic and systemic inflammatory pathological conditions among which rheumatoid arthritis, spondylarthritis, systemic lupus erythematosus, inflammatory bowel diseases, systemic sclerosis, and type 1 diabetes are the most common ones. Although these autoimmune disorders are mainly characterized by an inappropriate autoreactive immune response and the production of autoantibodies leading to organ damage, the precise pathogenic mechanisms still need to be elucidated. Autoimmune diseases were primarily characterized by aberrant cellular and humoral immune responses to self-antigens. The adaptive immune system was then first incriminated in the onset of these diseases and was thus the main immune disease-related research focus to elucidate the molecular and cellular mechanisms involved. However, since the adaptive immune system collaborate intricately with the innate immune system to maintain body integrity, it was hypothesized a decade ago that autoimmune diseases might also originate from innate immune system failure. Accordingly, rheumatoid arthritis, multiple sclerosis, systemic lupus erythematosus, as well as autoinflammatory diseases, can be treated with agents blocking innate cells-derived cytokines [1].

The innate immune system is the first line of defense involved in the clearing of exogenous invaders including viruses, bacteria, parasites, and in the removal of abnormally accumulated self-components released by damaged or dying cells following tissue injury. At the molecular level, infectious agents-derived molecules, namely pathogen-associated molecular patterns (PAMPs) and noninfectious endogenous danger molecules or damage-associated molecular patterns (DAMPs) are specifically recognized by innate immune cells expressing pattern recognition receptors (PRRs). Five main classes of PRRs may be distinguished depending on their subcellular localization such as membrane-inserted Toll-like receptors (TLRs) and C-type lectin receptors (CLRs), cytoplasmic nucleotide-binding and oligomerization domain (NOD)-like Receptors (NLR), retinoid acid-inducible gene I (RIG-1)-like receptors (RLRs), and multiple intracellular DNA sensors (CDSs) including cyclic GMP-AMP synthase (cGAS) and absent in melanoma 2 (AIM2) [2]. DAMPs or PAMPs-mediated activation of PRRs results, among others, in the release of proinflammatory cytokines including interleukins (IL)-1β, IL-6, IL-17, interferons (IFNs) and tumor-necrosis factor alpha (TNF-α). Interestingly, TLRs may be activated not only by bacterial wall components such as Lipopolysaccharide (LPS) or proteoglycans, but also by DAMPs including intracellular proteins and extracellular matrix components released after tissue damage that induces a TLR2 or a TLR4-dependent signaling cascade [2]. Additionally, cytoplasmic NLRs can detect both bacterial compounds such as flagellin, and endogenous crystals, ATP, amyloid fibers, or mitochondrial DNA. Extracellular signals are usually recognized as resolvable low-threat while intracellular signals represent high-threats that may induce pyroptosis, a process known as an IL-1β and IL-18-triggered cell death program induced by cytosolic PRRs only and mainly inflammasomes [3]. Importantly, the chronic and aberrant activation of such related inflammatory pathways triggers tissue pathology and clinical manifestations. For instance, altered regulation of proinflammatory cytokines such as IL-1β may be involved in susceptibility or resistance to autoimmunity as shown for arthritis [4]. IL-1β belongs to the IL-1 cytokine family. As such, it is produced as an inactive pro-IL-1β cytokine that requires maturation by enzymatic cleavage to generate a biologically active form. The Caspase 1 is the predominant IL-1 processing protease, whose activity is controlled by cytosolic PRR-constituted inflammasome complexes. Among inflammasomes, the nucleotide-binding domain (NOD)-, Leucine-rich repeat (LRR)- and pyrin domain-containing protein 3 (NLRP3) inflammasome is unique as it is not only activated by microbial and environmental molecules but also by several metabolic products including ATP, cholesterol crystals, and β amyloid fibers. Therefore, NLRP3 is able to sense a wide range of threats, while its erratic activation leads to numerous NLRP3-driven diseases including autoimmune diseases.

2 The NLRP3 inflammasome

The NLRP3 inflammasome was first identified in the cryopyrin-associated periodic syndrome (CAPS) and was later recognized to be involved in many other inflammatory/metabolic diseases [5,6] and autoimmune diseases [7,8]. The NLRP3 inflammasome is not only expressed by leukocytes (macrophages, dendritic cells, and neutrophils) but also by hepatocytes, neurons, endothelial cells, cardiomyocytes, and pancreatic beta cells [6].

2.1 Structure and function

The NLRP3 inflammasome is a large complex consisting of a sensor (NLRP3), an adaptor (apoptosis-associated speck-like protein containing a Caspase recruitment domain (ASC) encoded by *PYCARD*) and an effector (Caspase 1) [9] (Fig. 1). Upon stimulation, NLRP3 oligomerizes through homotypic interactions between NACHT domains of two NLRP3 proteins and promotes the recruitment of ASC proteins, which produce helical ASC filaments that form ASC specks [10–12]. Assembled ASC then recruits pro-caspase-1 enabling the self-cleavage of pro-caspase 1 to produce p20-p10 active caspase 1 complex [13]. In addition, the NIMA-related kinase 7 (NEK7) specifically oligomerizes with NLRP3, but not with other inflammasomes, by bridging the gaps between adjacent NLRP3 subunits to mediate NLRP3 oligomerization (Fig. 1). This association is essential for ASC speck formation and caspase 1 activation [14–16]. Activated-Caspase 1 is then able to process pro-IL-1β and pro-IL-18 into mature and functional IL-1β and IL-18.

In addition to the regulation of proinflammatory cytokine maturation, the NLRP3 inflammasome is also involved in the control of pyroptosis, an inflammatory programmed cell death. Pyroptosis results from the caspase 1, 4, 5, 11-mediated cleavage of the pro-Gasdermin D (GSDMD) where the C_{ter} autoinhibition domain is removed from the N_{ter} cell death domain. GSDMD^{Nterm} then binds to the inner leaflet of the cell membrane and forms a pore with other protomers that kills the cell [17] (Fig. 1).

2.2 Priming of the NLRP3 inflammasome

The activation of the NLRP3 inflammasome is a two-step activation process consisting of a priming step and an activation step. The priming step encompasses both transcriptional induction of the inflammasome complex components and the induction of NLRP3 posttranslational modifications. The transcription of NLRP3 components is not only induced by the binding of PAMPs or DAMPs to PRRs including TLRs, but also by cytokine receptors such as TNFR (Fig. 1). The activation of such receptors then triggers the activation of the nuclear

8. The NLRP3 inflammasome pathway in autoimmune diseases

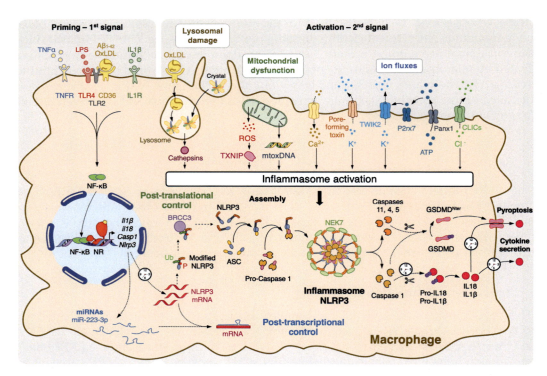

FIG. 1   The NLRP3 inflammasome priming and activations steps. The **priming** (first step) of the NLRP3 inflammasome requires the binding and activation of PRRs (TLRs, …) by PAMPs such as LPS, cytokines or ox-LDL, resulting in the transcription of the NLRP3 inflammasome components. Its **activation** (second step) is the result of recognition of PAMPs (such as the bacterial pore-forming toxin nigericin) or DAMPs which are released by damaged or dying cells (such as ATP) following injury or metabolic imbalance (such as mtROS), or accumulate in tissues (such as crystals). These lead to lysosomal damage, mitochondrial damages (exposition of cardiolipin, mtDNA) which ultimately modify ion (K^+, Ca^{2+}) fluxes. Upon this two-step process, the NLRP3 inflammasome assembles, caspase-1 is activated, Gasdermin-D and pro-IL-1β and pro-IL-18 are cleaved, leading to mature cytokines secretion and cell death by pyroptosis. The activity of nuclear receptors on each step is indicated when appropriate. *ASC*, apoptosis-associated speck-like protein containing a CARD domain; *ATP*, adenosine triphosphate; *BRCC3*, Lys-63-specific deubiquitinase BRCC36; *casp*, caspase; *CLIC*, chloride intracellular channels; *DAMPs*, damage-associated molecular patterns; *GSDMD*, gasdermin-D; *IL*, interleukin; *IL1R*, interleukin-1 receptor; *LPS*, lipopolysaccharide; *mtoxDNA*, mitochondrial oxidized DNA; *NF-κB*, nuclear factor-kappa B; *NLRP3*, nucleotide-binding, LRR and PYD domains-containing protein 3; *OxLDL*, oxidized low-density lipoproteins; *P*, Phosphate; *PAMPs*, pathogen-associated molecular patterns; *Panx1*, Pannexin-1; *PRRs*, Pattern Recognition Receptors; *ROS*, reactive oxygen species; *P2rx7*, purinergic receptor P2X 7; *TLR*, Toll-like receptor; *TNF*, tumor necrosis factor; *TNFR*, tumor necrosis factor receptor; *TWIK2*, two-pore domain weak inwardly rectifying K+ channel; *TXNIP*, Thioredoxin-interacting protein; *Ub*, ubiquitin.

factor κB (NF-κB) transcriptional factor and the subsequent induction of *Nlrp3* and *Il1β* gene transcription. Interestingly, in addition to classical TLRs ligands, metabolic alterations have also been shown to prime the NLRP3 inflammasome. For instance, oxidized LDL, islet amyloid polypeptide and, beta-amyloid peptides (Aβ$_{1-42}$) induce *Nlrp3* and *Il1β* gene expression in a CD36-TLR2-TLR4-dependent manner in primary macrophages [18,19] (Fig. 1).

Interestingly, neutrophil-release of Neutrophils Extracellular Traps (NETs) also prime NLRP3 in macrophages through the activation of several TLRs [20]. These NETs, abundantly found in lupus patients, then leads to organ damage [21]. Finally, members of the nuclear receptor superfamily including Rev-erbα, RORγ, and LXRs have also been shown to control the expression of *Nlrp3* and *Il1β* gene expression [22] (Fig. 1). As these nuclear receptors sense environmental modifications including lipid accumulation, these regulatory pathways thus provide additional mechanisms by which NLRP3 indirectly detects the alteration of body homeostasis [22].

In addition to transcriptional regulatory mechanisms, inflammasome component mRNA may also undergo posttranscriptional control by noncoding RNA [23]. Indeed, several small RNA such as miR-223-3p, are able to target the 3′-untranslated region (UTR) of the *Nlrp3* mRNA and promote its degradation [24]. Accordingly, altered expression of several miRNAs is associated with the development of numerous NLRP3-driven diseases such as rheumatoid arthritis [25], multiple sclerosis [26], and systemic lupus erythematosus [27,28] (Fig. 1).

Finally, additional posttranslational mechanisms maintain the NLRP3 protein in an inactive but poised state allowing a rapid response upon the sensing of an activation signal. This transcription-independent mechanism triggers an instant formation of the NLRP3 inflammasome complex. These posttranslational modifications are mainly ubiquitination, SUMOylation, and phosphorylation [29]. As expected, ubiquitination of NLRP3 promotes its proteasomal degradation while its BRCC3-mediated deubiquitination triggers ASC oligomerization and inflammasome activation [30,31] (Fig. 1).

2.3 Activation of the NLRP3 inflammasome

The activation of the NLRP3 inflammasome consists of the complex assembly. A wide range of stimuli with various chemical properties is able to trigger the NLRP3 inflammasome complex heterodimerization. These include not only exogenous molecules such as environmental particulates or pathogens, but also many endogenous molecules that abnormally accumulate in tissues. Among them, we may distinguish particles leading to lysosomal damage such as crystals, danger molecules originating from cell death, or damaged tissues including ATP or processes promoting mitochondrial dysfunction and Reactive Oxygen Species (ROS) production [32] (Fig. 1). Although lysosomal damage is one of the main processes for NLRP3 activation, downstream mechanisms between lysosome alteration and NLRP3 activation are poorly understood. It is thought however that phagocytosis of crystals (cholesterol, urea, hydroxyapatite crystals) or fibrillar protein aggregates (β-amyloid, IAPP) leads to lysosome disruption and the subsequent release of proteases such as cathepsins, which activate the NLRP3 inflammasome [33]. Interestingly, whereas cathepsin B was once believed to be the only cathepsin responsible for NLRP3 activation, the use of broad spectrum cathepsin inhibitors and individual knock-out models has later confirmed the implication of several cathepsins [34,35] (Fig. 1).

In addition to cathepsins, it is noteworthy that Leu-Leu-OMe-induced lysosomal damage enhances K^+ and Ca^{2+} efflux and may also account for lysosomal damage-controlled NLRP3 activation [36]. This is particularly interesting because ion fluxes are important regulators of NLRP3 inflammasome activation as well. As such that it was even believed that every pathway involved in NLRP3 activation is mediated by ion fluxes. Indeed, changes in ion homeostasis such as increased intracellular Ca^{2+} levels as well as decreased intracellular K^+ and Cl^- levels also appear to play a pivotal role in NLRP3 activation. For instance, nigericin, a K^+ ionophore, as well as the ATP-mediated activation of P2X purinoceptor 7 (P2rx7), a ligand-gated ion channel, promote K^+ efflux-dependent IL-1β maturation [37–39] (Fig. 1). Interestingly, P2rx7 has long been believed to be a receptor involved in K^+ efflux. Actually, P2rx7 promotes Ca^{2+} and Na^{2+} influx after ATP stimulation, which activates the K^+ channel two-pore domain weak inwardly rectifying K^+ channel (TWIK2) to promote K^+ efflux [40]. Finally, Chloride Intracellular Channels (CLICs), especially CLIC1 and CLIC4, mediate NLRP3 activation by promoting Cl^- efflux downstream of nigericin-induced K^+ efflux and mitochondrial ROS production [41,42] (Fig. 1). Interestingly, K^+ seems to drive NLRP3 oligomerization, probably in a NEK7-dependent manner [43,44], while Cl^- efflux is prone to induce ASC polymerization [44]. However, the link between ion fluxes and the inflammasome activation remains to be identified (Table 1).

Finally, K^+ efflux must be associated with Ca^{2+} influx to promote mitochondrial-mediated ROS production [78] and NLRP3 activation [79,80]. Although the source of ROS is still controversial, ROS are considered as critical NLRP3 inducers [81]. At the molecular level, mitochondrial (mt)ROS altogether with Ca^{2+} promote the release of mitochondrial (mt)DNA into the cytosol where it is eventually oxidized [82,83]. Oxidized mtDNA then interacts with NLRP3 and promotes its activation. In addition to mtDNA, mtROS also induces thioredoxin-interacting protein (TXNIP)-NLRP3 interaction and NLRP3 expression [84]. Finally, mtROS promotes K^+ efflux and triggers the fast relocation of NLRP3 from the endoplasmic reticulum (ER) membrane to the mitochondrial membrane where the complex NLRP3-ASC is formed [81].

A caspase 8-dependent alternative inflammasome activation pathway has been demonstrated to induce NLRP3 activation independently of K^+ efflux [85]. Interestingly, this pathway does not induce pyroptosis and cellular death, thus suggesting that the alternative inflammasome pathway is likely involved in cytokine production but preserves cellular integrity.

Bacteria-derived LPS may also be sensed by human caspases 4 and 5, and mouse caspase 11, to induce the noncanonical NLRP3 inflammasome independently of TLR4 signaling [86,87]. In this pathway, caspase-4/5/11 promote pyroptosis by processing pro-GSDMD and pannexin-1, a protein channel that releases ATP from the cell. This extracellular ATP then activates P2xr7 to promote K^+ efflux and NLRP3 activation [88,89] (Fig. 1).

3 NLRP3 and autoimmune diseases

The NLRP3/IL-1β axis is at the crossroad of the innate and adaptive immune systems, and therefore displays a key regulatory function of both systems. IL-1β is a highly potent proinflammatory cytokine, mainly expressed in myeloid cells (monocytes, macrophages, and dendritic cells (DCs)) and prolongs the lifespan of neutrophils and macrophages, thus lasting their functions. IL-1β was originally defined as a costimulatory factor for T cells and is known to induce T cell differentiation and polarization, especially toward Th17 cells [90]. Actually, IL-1β is involved in the overall inflammatory processes by inducing the production of cyclooxygenase type 2, prostaglandin E2 and by promoting fever acute phase response, vasodilation, angiogenesis, and leukocyte activation [90]. In endothelial cells, secretion of IL-1β enhances the production of adhesion molecules and chemokines involved in the recruitment of leukocytes [90]. IL-1β also triggers dendritic cell-mediated IL-12 secretion, which, in turn, enhances T cell-dependent interferon-γ production [90]. IL-1β has finally been shown to stimulate B cells proliferation and antibody production [90]. In the same manner, IL-18 induces IL-12-mediated IFN-γ production in Th1 cells and natural killer cells and promotes Th17 differentiation [7].

NLRP3 inflammasome deregulation was primarily associated with the development of autoinflammatory syndromes collectively defined as cryopyrin-Associated Periodic Syndromes (CAPS), which are inherited autoinflammatory disorders characterized by systemic inflammation with fever, skin rashes, and central nervous system inflammation. More recently, NLRP3 inflammasome-related gene polymorphisms were also associated with the susceptibility and the disease severity of autoimmune diseases including RA and SLE [7]. Autoimmune diseases are a family of chronic and systemic inflammatory disorders (e.g., rheumatoid arthritis (RA), systemic lupus erythematosus (SLE), ankylosing spondylitis (AS), Sjögren's syndrome (SS), and systemic sclerosis (SSc)) and are characterized by the dysfunction of the immune system itself, which ultimately results in the loss of immunological self-tolerance [91]. On the contrary, autoinflammatory diseases are characterized by episodes of sterile inflammation due to dysregulation of the innate immune system without participation of the adaptive immune system, i.e., without autoreactive T cells and autoantibodies. Autoinflammatory diseases thus range from hereditary monogenic diseases (e.g., familial Mediterranean fever) to multifactorial conditions [92]. In numerous studies, aberrant activation of NLRP3 and altered IL-1β or IL-18 production has been associated with excessive inflammation and tissue damage, in both autoimmune and autoinflammatory diseases (Table 1).

TABLE 1   NLRP3 inflammasome activity in autoimmune diseases.

Disease	NLRP3 inflammasome activity	Mechanisms involving NLRP3 inflammasome	Organism	
SLE	Activation	Hyperactivation of NLRP3 in PBMCs	SLE patients	Yang et al. [45]
	Activation	Upregulation of *Nlrp3* in renal cells (tubular cells and podocytes) leading to kidney failure and proteinuria	SLE patients	Fu et al. [46], Huang et al. [47]
	Activation	dsDNA-autoantibodies complex formation, ROS production, K^+ efflux	SLE patients	Shin et al. [48]
	Activation	Activation of NLRP3 in monocytes induced by U1-small nuclear ribonucleoprotein-Antibodies complex formation through the upregulation of ROS production and ion fluxes	SLE patients	Shin et al. [49]
	Activation	NETosis and IL-18 feedback loop	SLE patients	Kahlenberg et al.[21], Mende et al. [50]
	Inhibition	Protective effect of NEK7/NLRP3 axis activation	SLE patients	Ma et al. [99]

Continued

8. The NLRP3 inflammasome pathway in autoimmune diseases

TABLE 1 NLRP3 inflammasome activity in autoimmune diseases—cont'd

Disease	NLRP3 inflammasome activity	Mechanisms involving NLRP3 inflammasome	Organism	
RA	Activation	Dysregulation of NLRP3 pathways in immune (monocytes, macrophages, and dendritic cells) and synovial cells	RA patients	Guo et al. [51], Choulaki et al. [52], Ruscitti et al. [53], Kolly et al. [54]
	Activation	ACPA activates Akt/NF-kB signaling inducing an increase of NLRP3 and IL1-β through CD147/Integrin-β1 interaction	RA patients	Dong et al. [55], Ilchovska et al. [56]
	Activation	A20/Tnfaip3 mediated NLRP3 inflammasome activation and pyroptosis	A20 Myeloid KO	Walle et al. [57]
	Inhibition	Curculigoside A downregulates the NF-kB pathways-mediated NLRP3 pathway	CFA-induced RA in Rat model	Ding et al. [58]
	Activation	HIF-1α activation by synovial accumulation of succinate	CFA-induced RA in Rat model	Li et al. [59]
	Inhibition	miR-20a decreases NLRP3 inflammasome expression through TXNIP inhibition in fibroblast-like synoviocyte	CFA-induced RA in Rat model	Li et al. [60]
	Inhibition	Protective effect of miR-223-3p on NLRP3 inflammasome pathway	Rat model, RA patients	Tian et al. [61], Wu et al. [62]
AS	Activation	Low expression of *A20/Tnfaip* in monocytes is correlated with activation of NLRP3 inflammasome	AS patients	Zhai et al. [63]
	Inhibition	TNFAIP3 promotes autophagy decreasing NLRP3 activation and IL1-β dependent secretion through its interaction with DEPTOR	AS patients	
SSc	Activation	Hyperactivation of NLRP3 inflammasome in skin biopsies correlated with an increase of skin thickness	SSc patients	Martínez-Godínez et al. [64]
	Activation	Hyperactivation of NLRP3 inflammasome-dependent pathways in fibroblasts	SSc patients	Artlett et al. [65]
	Activation	Parvovirus B19 activates NLRP3 inflammasome pathway and increases caspase 1 cleavage and IL-1β maturation in monocytes	SSc patients, human cell line	Zakrzewska et al. [66]

TABLE 1 NLRP3 inflammasome activity in autoimmune diseases—cont'd

Disease	NLRP3 inflammasome activity	Mechanisms involving NLRP3 inflammasome	Organism	
SSc	Activation	Upregulation of mRNA and protein levels of IL-1β, IL18, NLRP3 in tears and conjunctival expression cytology samples	SS patients	Niu et al. [67]
	Inhibition	P2rx7 inhibition promotes saliva secretion and inhibits salivary gland inflammation	Mouse model	Khalafalla MG et al. [68]
	Activation	High levels of cell-free DNA are correlated with an impaired DNAse type1 activity leading to an increase of gene expression of the NLRP3 inflammasome pathway	SS patients	Vakrakou AG et al. [69]
	Activation	Increase in the caspase 1-GSDMD axis-dependent pyroptosis in salivary gland epithelial cells	SS patients	Hong S-M et al. [70]
IBD	Activation	Upregulation of NLRP3, ASC, and IL-1β in the colon mucosa	IBD patients	Liu L et al. [71]
	Inhibition	Protective role of NLRP3 deficiency in dextran sodium sulfate-induced colitis through the inhibition of proinflammatory cytokines expression	DSS-induced Colitis mouse model	Bauer C et al. [72]
	Inhibition	Caspase 1 inhibition	DSS-induced Colitis mouse model	Loher F et al. [73]
	Activation	ROS production and NF-kB pathway controls NLRP3 activation	DSS-induced Colitis mouse model	Shen et al. [8]
	Inhibition	Protective effect of miR-223-3p on NLRP3 inflammasome pathway	Mouse model	Neudecker V et al. [74]
T1D	Activation	mtDNA-dependent NLRP3 activation in a streptozotocin murine model	STZ mouse model	Carlos D et al. [75]
	Activation	Endothelial and vascular dysfunction	T1D patients	Pereira CA et al. [76]
	Activation	Hyperactivated NLRP3 inflammasome pathway in macrophages	STZ mouse model	Davanso MR et al. [77]
	Activation	NO production and increase of the inflammatory cytokines expression	STZ mouse model	

AS, ankylosing spondylitis; *ASC*, apoptosis-associated speck-like protein containing a CARD; *DEPTOR*, DEP domain-containing mTOR-interacting protein; *DSS-induced colitis*, dextran sodium sulfate-induced colitis; *GSDMD*, Gasdermin D; *HIF-1α*, hypoxia-induced factor-1α; *IBD*, inflammatory bowel disease; *iNOS*, inducible nitric oxyde synthase; *IRF-1*: interferon regulatory factor 1; *mtDNA*: Mitochondrial DNA; *NLRP3*, NOD like receptor family pyrin domain-containing 3; *NEK7*, NIMA-related kinases; *NET*, neutrophil extracellular traps; *P2xr7*, P2X purinoceptor 7; *PBMC*, peripheral blood mononuclear cell; *RA*, rheumatoid arthritis; *ROS*, reactive oxygen species; *IL-1β*: interleukine-1β; *SLE*, systemic lupus erythematosus; *SpA*, spondyloarthritis; *SSc*, systemic sclerosis; *SS*, Sjögren's syndrome; *T1D*, type 1 diabete; *Tnfaip*, tumor necrosis factor, alpha-induced protein 3; *TXNIP*, thioredoxin interacting protein.

3.1 NLRP3 in the systemic lupus erythematosus

SLE is a systemic autoimmune disease with multiorgan inflammation, formation of autoantibodies, complement activation, and immune complex depositions [93]. Although the cause of SLE is currently unknown, it results from altered innate and adaptive immune system responses that promote life-threatening symptoms including skin, joints, kidneys, heart, and brain disturbances [93]. NLRP3 is hyperactivated in peripheral blood mononuclear cells (PBMCs) isolated from patients with SLE [45] and in myeloid cells from the experimental lupus mice model [94] (Table 1). Additionally, its expression is upregulated in renal cells, including tubular cells and podocytes, thus provoking kidney failure and proteinuria in SLE patients [46,47].

At the molecular and cellular levels, SLE is characterized by the production of autoantibodies that can actually induce the NLRP3 inflammasome. Autoantibodies form an immune complex with dsDNA, which upregulates NLRP3 and Caspase 1, altogether with NF-κB, ROS production, and K^+ efflux in monocytes from SLE patients, thus worsening IL-1β production [48] (Table 1). Other immune complexes with the U1-small nuclear ribonucleoprotein also activate the NLRP3 inflammasome in SLE patients' monocytes by inducing ROS production and ion fluxes [49]. Neutrophils extracellular traps (NETs) are large extracellular fibrillar networks composed of antimicrobial peptides and enzymes that are assembled on a scaffold of decondensed chromatin [95]. NETs are mainly released by neutrophils undergoing a cell death process named NETosis. This pathway usually serves in the antimicrobial responses by trapping bacteria, fungi, viruses, and parasites [95]. However, if dysregulated, NETs can contribute to the pathogenesis of immune diseases probably by further activating the NLRP3 inflammasome in lupus macrophages [21]. While serum levels of IL-18, but not IL-1β, were found to be abnormally elevated in SLE patients [50], IL-18 promotes NETosis, thus amplifying the NETs' effect in SLE [21] (Table 1).

Type I interferons (IFN-I), especially IFN-α are also important mediators of SLEs [96]. Strikingly, prolonged exposure of monocytes from SLE patients to IFN-α induces the NLRP3 inflammasome activation and the secretion of IL-1β in an IRF-1-dependent manner [97]. In contrast, elevated expression of IFN-I was correlated to decreased NLRP3 levels in SLE patients, [98].

Intriguingly, NEK7, NLRP3, and ASC were decreased while the expression of caspase 1, IL-18, and IL-1β were increased in PBMCs from SLE patients, thus suggesting a protective effect of the NEK7/NLRP3 axis against SLE pathogenesis [99] (Table 1).

3.2 NLRP3 in the rheumatoid arthritis

The rheumatoid arthritis (RA) is a chronic autoinflammatory disease characterized by a synovial inflammation and irreversible multi-joint destruction involving cartilages and bones. RA then results in joint deformity, dysfunction, and even premature death [100]. Accumulated evidences suggest now that the NLRP3 inflammasome displays a critical role in the pathogenesis of RA [101]. Indeed, *NLPR3* gene expression, as well as NLRP3 inflammasome-related proteins, are induced in myeloid cells isolated from RA patients [51–53] (Table 1). Nevertheless, fibroblast-like synoviocytes from RA patients express *NLRP3* mRNA but do not display NLRP3 protein increase or extracellular Caspase 1. This defect in NLRP3 protein upregulation results in the absence of IL-1β processing and secretion in these cells [54] (Table 1). One could hypothesize that RA pathogenesis may rather occur through the deregulation of the NLRP3 pathway in immune cells instead of synovial cells. Expression of *NLRP3* and *ASC* are, however, reduced in neutrophils from RA patients [102]. Then, RA may be due to elevated NLRP3 pathway in monocyte-derived cells including monocyte, macrophages, and dendritic cells but not neutrophils. In an animal study, *Nlrp3* expression is induced in synovial tissue from the collagen-induced arthritis mouse model, although whether this occurs in myeloid cells or others must be determined.

As shown in SLE, autoantibodies also exhibit NLRP3 activating properties in RA. For instance, the anticitrullinated peptide antibody (ACPA) activates the Akt/NF-κB signaling by promoting the interaction between CD147 (extracellular matrix metalloprotease inducer) and integrin β1. This interaction induces the expression of NLRP3 and IL-1β [55]. As expected, the NF-κB signaling pathway participates in RA pathogenesis from proinflammatory cytokine production to joint destruction and synovial proliferation [56]. The deletion of *A20/Tnfaip3*, the negative regulator of NF-κB signaling in macrophages, triggers a spontaneous arthritis in mice that resembles human RA [57]. Interestingly, this phenomenon mainly relies on the NLRP3 inflammasome and the IL-1 receptor signaling [57]. At the cellular level, A20-deficient macrophages exhibit enhanced NLRP3-mediated Caspase 1 activation, pyroptosis, and IL-1β secretion [57]. Accordingly, the curculigoside A (CA) significantly reduces the hind paw swelling, decreases the levels of IL-1β, and downregulates the expression of NF-κB-mediated NLRP3 pathway in Complete Freund's Adjuvant (CFA)-induced arthritis rats [58] (Table 1). In addition to the NF-κB signaling pathway, the hypoxia-inducible factor-1α (HIF-1α) also exhibits RA promoting properties. Indeed, the synovial accumulation of succinate in CFA-induced arthritis rat model induces HIF-1α expression, which in turn activates NLRP3 [59] (Table 1). Finally, the deregulation of microRNA (miRNAs) expression also contributes to RA pathogenesis. For instance, the miRNA-223-3p is downregulated in RA. Because miR-223-3p targets NLRP3 mRNA, its downregulation increases pyroptosis in fibroblast-like synoviocytes and reverses the effect of monosodium urate on RA [61] (Table 1). Consistently, the compound Icariin alleviates RA by inducing miR-223-3p and then reducing NLRP3 [62] (Table 1). Moreover, the miR-20a decreases NLRP3 inflammasome expression by inhibiting TXNIP in fibroblast-like synoviocytes from CFA-induced arthritis rat model [60] (Table 1).

3.3 NLRP3 and the spondyloarthritis/ankylosing spondylitis

In addition to RA, spondyloarthritis (SpA) is a group of chronic inflammatory arthritis such as psoriatic arthritis (PsA), juvenile inflammatory arthritis (JIA), and ankylosing spondylitis (AS). Genetic studies demonstrate that *NLRP3* polymorphisms are associated with psoriatic JIA [103] and AS [104]. Moreover, *NLRP3*, *ASC*, *Caspase 1*, *IL-1β*, *IL-17A*, and *IL-23* mRNA levels are increased in PBMCs from AS patients [105].

As shown in RA, the activation of the NLRP3 inflammasome may be due to decreased expression of *A20/TNFAIP3* [63] (Table 1). TNFAIP3 actually enhances autophagy thus preventing NLRP3 activation and IL-1β secretion [63] (Table 1). At the molecular level, TNFAIP3 physically interacts with DEP domain containing mTOR interacting protein (DEPTOR) to enhance autophagy and inhibits inflammasome-dependent IL-1β secretion [63]. Interestingly, the NOD2 pathway was also involved in the pathogenesis of SA. Indeed, the NOD2 ligand muramyl dipeptide (MDP) further enhances the expression of *NLRP3, IL23A, IL-1β,* and *IL-17A* genes in AS-derived PBMC [106].

3.4 NLRP3 and the systemic sclerosis (SSc)

Systemic Sclerosis (SSc) is a rare chronic profibrotic disease where patients exhibit dramatic collagen accumulation leading to skin fibrosis, vasculopathy, and gastrointestinal alterations [8]. Strikingly, overactivation of the NLRP3 inflammasome in skin biopsies from SSc patients is positively correlated with an increase in skin thickness [64] (Table 1). At the gene expression level, NLRP3 inflammasome pathway-related genes including *NLRP3, IL-1β,* and *IL-18* are upregulated in fibroblasts isolated from SSc patients [65]. Furthermore, *NLRP3* and *ASC* deficiencies promote resistance to bleomycin-induced skin fibrosis, which then suggests a direct role of the NLRP3 inflammasome pathway in SSc [65] (Table 1).

Parvovirus B19 (B19V) is a single-stranded DNA virus involved in arthritis and chronic bone marrow failure [66]. After infection, its presence persists in many tissues including the liver, synovia, and skin. The impact of such persistence was however unknown. A pathogenic role of B19V has, however, been suggested in some autoimmune diseases such as SSC [66]. Recently, B19V has been shown to activate the NLRP3 inflammasome pathway, Caspase 1 cleavage, and IL-1β maturation in THP-1 human macrophage cells line and monocytes from SSc patients [66] (Table 1).

Finally, the inflammasome pathway promotes the expression of miR-155 in SSc, which is associated with fibrosis [107]. Accordingly, miR-155 inhibitor inhibits dermal fibrosis in the scleroderma mouse model, thus highlighting a novel therapeutic perspective [108].

3.5 NLRP3 and the Sjögren's syndrome (SS)

The Sjögren's syndrome (SS) is a systemic autoimmune disease characterized by T and B cells infiltration in the exocrine glands such as lacrimal and salivary glands, which impairs their secretory function and promotes epithelial cell apoptosis. As shown in other autoimmune diseases, mRNAs of inflammasome pathway-related genes, including *IL-1β, ASC, Caspase 1,* and *NLRP3,* were induced in PBMCs isolated from SS patients [109]. Similarly, mRNA and protein levels of IL-1β, IL-18, and NLRP3 were significantly increased in tears and conjunctival cytology samples from SS patients harboring dry eyes [67] (Table 1). Furthermore, elevated levels of *P2xr7, NLRP3, ASC,* and *Caspase 1* gene expression were associated with increased mature IL-18 amount in the salivary gland of SS patients that exhibit high levels of SS-specific autoantibodies [110]. Accordingly, similar expression patterns were observed in SS patients developing a mucosa-associated lymphoid tissue non-Hodgkin's lymphoma [111].

The dependency of P2xr7 in this NLRP3-mediated process was confirmed using the *P2xr7*-deficient mouse model [68]. P2xr7-mediated release of IL-1β from submandibular gland epithelial cells is dependent on ion fluxes, ROS production and Hsp90, involved in activation and stabilization of NLRP3 [68]. Consequently, the inhibition of P2xr7 improves saliva secretion and inhibits salivary gland inflammation in the autoimmune salivary gland exocrinopathy mouse model, thus acknowledging the identification of a putative therapeutic strategy [68] (Table 1). Moreover, elevated cell-free DNA was associated with impaired type I DNase activity in the serum and PBMCs of SS patients [69]. Increased amounts of cytoplasmic DNA deposition led to the activation of inflammasome-related genes, highlighting the DAMP effect of undegraded DNA on the NLRP3 inflammasome activation in the context of SS [69] (Table 1). Finally, as shown in SLE, type I IFN signature genes were correlated with an increase of caspase 1 and GSDMD protein levels in salivary gland epithelial cells from SS patients [70] (Table 1). As expected, the caspase-dependent pyroptosis was then hastened upon inflammasome activation leading to targeted tissue damage, uncovering a new pathogenic role of type I IFN in these patients [70].

3.6 NLRP3 in inflammatory bowel diseases (IBD)

Inflammatory bowel diseases (IBD) are relapsing chronic inflammatory diseases of the small intestine and the colon, which mainly consist of ulcerative colitis and Crohn's disease [112]. Clinical studies evidenced that increase of IL-1β secreted levels from colon tissue macrophages of IBD patients is correlated to the severity of the disease [113]. Accordingly, the expression of NLRP3, ASC, and IL-1β are increased in the colon mucosa of IBD patients [71] (Table 1).

Intriguingly, the deletion of NLRP3, ASC, and Caspase 1 triggered an accentuated deleterious phenotype in experimental colitis mice by aggravating diarrhea, bodyweight loss, rectal bleeding, and mortality [114]. These results obtained in this mouse model then argue for a protective action of NLRP3 in the colon tissue, which may be assigned to IL-18 release, a key regulator of mucosal repair. On the other hand, the deficiency of NLRP3 in dextran sodium sulfate (DSS)-induced colitis model has also been proposed to protect animals from colitis [72]. Indeed, NLRP3-deficient mice exhibit reduced expression of proinflammatory cytokines and lower severe colitis in the DSS-induced model [72] (Table 1). Furthermore, the administration of a caspase 1 inhibitor, the pralnacasan, lowers colon tissue damage [73]. It has been proposed that the discrepancy between protective versus detrimental role of NLRP3 between these studies comes from different experimental conditions [115]. For instance, NLRP3 would play a beneficial effect on the pathogenesis of colitis when DSS is administered for a short time while it would play deleterious effect when colitis is induced for a longer time [115].

At the molecular level, both NF-κB and ROS production control NLRP3 activation in the context of IBD [8]. Finally, the miR-223-3p also regulates intestinal inflammation via the repression of the NLRP3 inflammasome in the DSS-induced colitis mouse model [74] (Table 1).

3.7 NLRP3 in the type 1 diabetes (T1D)

Type 1 diabetes (T1D) is a metabolic disease where autoreactive T cells infiltrate pancreatic islets and induce insulitis that causes β cell death. T1D is then characterized by insulin production deficiency and hyperglycemia. [116]. Two Single Nucleotides Polymorphisms (SNPs) in NLRP3 identified in the northeastern Brazilian population were associated with an increased risk of T1D [117]. Accordingly, IL-1β levels are increased in patients with a newly diagnosed T1D as well as in patients with a settled T1D [118–120]. In addition, at the molecular and cellular levels, IL-1β induces the migration of proinflammatory cells into pancreatic islets, promotes β cell apoptosis, and exerts a cytotoxic effect on these cells [121,122]. Accordingly, NLRP3 deficiency affects the activation, maturation, and migration of T cells to pancreatic islets [122]. Interestingly, the defect of NLRP3 also inhibits the expression of chemokines such as CCL5 and CXCL10 in pancreatic islet cells in an IRF-1 dependent manner [122]. Conversely, activation of NLRP3 with mtDNA contributes to T1D setting in a streptozotocin (STZ) model, thus demonstrating the diabetogenic contribution of NLRP3 [75] (Table 1). Additionally, mtDNA-mediated NLRP3 activation promotes endothelial and vascular dysfunction in mouse and T1D patients, emphasizing the interplay between the NLRP3 inflammasome and diabetic complications [76] (Table 1).

Interestingly, resident macrophages from STZ-induced T1D diabetic mice exhibit an activated NLRP3 inflammasome pathway [77]. This is likely due to advanced glycation end products, thus suggesting that the hyperglycemic state poised macrophages to a proinflammatory state [77]. Indeed, resident peritoneal macrophages from diabetic mice were kept in a proinflammatory state characterized by increased NLRP3/iNOS pathway-mediated NO production and upregulated proinflammatory cytokine expression [77]. As an interesting therapeutic point of view, treatment with docosahexaenoic acid (DHA) improves diabetes in mice and ameliorates the macrophage inflammatory state, but surprisingly in an NLRP3-independent manner [77] (Table 1).

3.8 NLRP3 and autoimmune diseases-induced atherosclerosis

Atherosclerosis is the main cause of cardiovascular diseases and usually affects large vessels, mainly arteries. Atherosclerosis is a lipid-driven inflammatory disease of the vascular wall during which infiltrating LDLs are eventually oxidized, triggering their uptake by macrophages. The plaque progresses toward advanced lesions with necrotic core, degradation of the extracellular matrix, migration of smooth muscle cells, and in some cases calcification and intraplaque neovascularization [123]. Strikingly, ablation of the NLRP3 inflammasome pathway decreases atherosclerosis progression, thus emphasizing the critical role of NLRP3 in atherosclerosis [124,125]. At the molecular level, oxidized LDLs promote both priming and cholesterol crystals-mediated activation of NLRP3 in a CD36-dependent manner in macrophages [18,19].

Patients with autoimmune diseases are at high cardiovascular risk [126]. Indeed, patients with RA exhibit an increased incidence of vulnerable plaque in the left anterior descending coronary artery compared to control [126]. In addition, SLE patients have an almost fourfold increased risk of ischemic heart disease [126]. Accordingly, patients with SLE or RA developed twice more plaques in carotid and femoral arteries. As a result, acute myocardial infarction is the cause of death in 3 to 25% of SLE patients [126].

Finally, atherosclerosis is now considered as a chronic inflammatory disease involving innate and adaptive immune cells such as monocytes, macrophages, neutrophils, mast cells, B cells, and NK cells [127–129]. Interestingly, dendritic cells, CD4, and CD8 cells were found in atherosclerotic plaques [130]. T cells response is usually triggered by dendritic cell-mediated antigen presentation. It is hypothesized that DCs initially phagocytize atherogenic antigens in the arterial intima and transport them to lymph nodes [131]. In addition, it is also believed that local antigen presentation involving macrophages and smooth muscle cells also occurs in lesions and enhances the local T-cell response. Numerous studies have identified candidate antigens such as oxidized-LDL and β2-glycoprotein I (Apolipoprotein H) in mouse and human [131]. Interestingly, autoantibodies against the latter were not only found in patients with atherosclerosis but also in those with SLE [132]. Circulating specific IgG were additionally found in both human and murine models, thus further stressing the role of B cells in atherogenesis [130]. Altogether, atherosclerosis could be characterized by the sustained abnormal activation of the innate and the adaptive immune system associated with the production of autoantibodies, then resuming the definition of autoimmune diseases as recently suggested [133].

4 The clock and autoimmune diseases

Most biological activities oscillate along the day in order to be poised at the most appropriate time window [134]. Among these physiological pathways, immune functions vary according to the time of day [6, 135], a process described as circadian immunity, in which innate immune cells such as macrophages harbor an intrinsic clockwork that drives circadian transcription of genes involved in the response to bacterial challenge [135–137]. Then, the immune features such as trafficking and abundance of blood leukocytes, their recruitment to tissue, their ability to respond to pathogens and to secrete immune molecules vary in a circadian manner [138,139]. Importantly, both innate and adaptive immune cells exhibit circadian variation of their activity and/or tissue abundance [140].

4.1 Structure of the clock

Circadian rhythms are generated by a clock machinery the in most cell types including immune cells [141,142]. The central pacemaker is located in the suprachiasmatic nucleus of the hypothalamus where it received light information and synchronizes clocks throughout the body according to this time cue. Peripheral clocks are also synchronized by other time cues such as food intake and exercise. At the molecular level, the mammalian clock consists of a complex network of transcription factors and interconnected transcriptional feedback loops that orchestrate cellular biological mechanisms on a period of almost 24 h [143]. The positive limb is driven by the heterodimer BMAL1 (Brain and Muscle ARNT-like 1) and CLOCK (circadian locomotor output cycles kaput) which binds to E-boxes in the promoter of its target genes, including *Per* and *Cry* clock genes, to induce their transcription. Period (PER) 1/2/3 and cryptochrome (CRY) 1/2 form the negative limb (Fig. 2). Once they reach a sufficient threshold, PER and CRY heterodimerize and translocate to the nucleus where they quench BMAL1-CLOCK heterodimer to inhibit its transcriptional activity (Fig. 2). In addition, the ligand-activated nuclear receptors Rev-erbs and RORs finely tune the first circuitry [144]. While Rev-erbs act as transcriptional repressors, RORs compete with Rev-erbs for the same response element to induce the transcription of their common target genes (Fig. 2). These transcription factors not only control each other's transcription but also modulate the expression of numerous genes, thereby generating rhythmic transcriptional oscillation in transcriptional programs and specific tissue functions.

4.2 Clock alteration in autoimmune diseases

Our modern lifestyle, including social demands, food habits, and shift work, have dramatically and durably impeded our circadian rhythms. It is now recognized by national health organizations that disruption of the intrinsic cellular clock alters immune response and has severe consequences on health [145]. Disruption of circadian rhythms in humans is indeed

8. The NLRP3 inflammasome pathway in autoimmune diseases

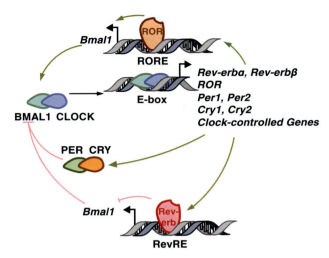

FIG. 2 The molecular clock machinery. The molecular clockwork is formed by transcription–translation feedback loops. The transcription factors BMAL1/CLOCK induce the expression of E-box-containing genes including the negative regulators period (PER) and cryptochrome (CRY). In turn, the PER/CRY heterodimer inhibits the transcriptional activity of BMAL1/CLOCK. Once PER and CRY levels are sufficiently low, a new cycle may start. CLOCK/BMAL1 induce the expression of the nuclear receptors Rev-erbα/β) and retinoid-related orphan receptor α, β, and γ (RORα/β/γ). Rev-erbs and RORs interact with co-repressors (NCoR) and co-activators (NCoA) and compete for the binding of RevRE/RORE elements in common target genes to repress or activate, respectively, their transcription. Rev-erb and ROR are also able to repress E4BP4/Nfil3 which rhythmically inhibits D-box-dependent transcription. Additional layers of regulation of circadian gene expression include rhythmic histone modifications, circadian chromosomal 3D conformation and posttranslational modifications such as acetylation, phosphorylation, SUMOylation, O-GlcNacylation. The clock is involved in the control of so-called circadian immunity.

considered as a new risk factor for neurological, metabolic, and chronic inflammatory disorders [145–147] such as asthma, atherosclerosis, type 2 diabetes, or Alzheimer's Disease [141,147].

Accordingly, clock disruption has been associated with an increased risk to develop autoimmune diseases [148]. For instance, a study performed in a population of 15 to 19-year-old Danish teenagers demonstrated that an alteration of the circadian rhythm provoked by a shift work increases the risk to develop multiple sclerosis (MS) in adulthood [149]. MS is a T cell-mediated brain affection featuring demyelination of neurons in the brain and spinal cord. MS and T cell-induced autoimmune diseases may be mimicked using experimental autoimmune encephalomyelitis, a model of brain inflammation-induced after injection of myelin peptides. In this model, the severity of EAE depends on the time of induction, thus confirming the impact of the circadian clock on the development of this pathology. At the pathophysiological level, demyelination is further increased when EAE is induced in mice at 4 pm compared to mice injected at 4 am. Strikingly, this circadian feature was lost in T cell-specific $Bmal1^{-/-}$, thereby demonstrating the dependency on a functional clock machinery to control the peptide sensitivity in EAE pathogenesis [150]. Interestingly, the expression of $Bmal1$ in myeloid cells also appears to modulate EAE severity. Accordingly, the deletion of $Bmal1$ in myeloid cells prevents diurnal variation of EAE severity with an increased overall severity along the whole day. Accordingly, *Bmal1* and *Rev-erbα* gene expression was downregulated in the spinal cord of mice undergoing EAE, thus suggesting a putative role of the circadian machinery in the development of the disease [151]. At the cellular level, *Bmal1* disruption sets a proinflammatory environment in the central nervous system that facilitates the infiltration of monocytes and increases the presence of pathogenic IL-17$^+$IFNγ$^+$ T cells in the CNS [151]. In addition to Bmal1, global disruption of other core clock components such as Rev-erbα increases CD4$^+$ T cells infiltration into the CNS and EAE severity [152]. Nonetheless, the double RORα/γ knockout protects mice from EAE by preventing Th17 cell development [153]. Interestingly, activation of Rev-erbα with a pharmacological compound protects mice from EAE progression, emphasizing the therapeutic potential of Rev-erbα [152].

Interestingly, patients with RA often feel heightened joint pain and stiffness in the morning, suggesting diurnal variation in their symptoms [154]. This is actually associated with circadian changes in circulating metabolites such as ceramides in RA patients [155]. Accordingly, such a pattern was also found in the collagen-induced arthritis mouse model where joint inflammation is actively repressed during the active phase [156]. Alteration of the circadian clock in *Cry1$^{-/-}$Cry2$^{-/-}$* mice results in an increase in activated T cells and an exacerbation of joint swelling in a collagen-antibody-driven model of arthritis [157], thus supporting the idea that a functional clock protects from RA.

Finally, SNPs in the core clock gene *PER2* were correlated with the susceptibility and clinical manifestation of SLE in genetic studies, thus emphasizing the relationship between the circadian machinery and the onset of SLE [158].

Altogether, these studies highlight the critical role of the clock in autoimmune diseases progression. Although, we may hypothesize that clock components directly control immune cells, whose activity is altered in autoimmune diseases, the actual underlying mechanisms are still unknown. Remarkably, the NLRP3 inflammasome is controlled by the circadian machinery [6] and could therefore be the missing link between autoimmune diseases and clock disruption.

4.3 The NLRP3 inflammasome is a clock-controlled pathway

The control of the NLRP3 inflammasome pathway by the clock was first reported *in vivo* and *in vitro* in both mouse and human primary macrophages [22]. In this context, NLRP3, IL-1β, and IL-18 mRNA exhibit circadian oscillations in mouse peritoneal macrophages and in synchronized primary mouse and human macrophages with a functional consequence on the secretion of these cytokines which display a rhythmic pattern as well [22]. At the molecular level, the oscillation of the NLRP3 inflammasome-related genes depends on the direct binding of both Rev-erbα [22] and RORγ [159] in macrophages. Interestingly, these two nuclear receptors are both recruited to the same site in the promoter of *Nlrp3*, thereby demonstrating that Rev-erbα and RORγ directly control the priming of NLRP3. In addition, Rev-erbα has been suggested to indirectly regulate the inflammasome priming by interacting with the NF-κB signaling pathway [160,161]. Furthermore, Rev-erbα would also prevent the NLRP3 activation step. Indeed, nigericin- and ATP-induced ASC speck formation was increased in *Rev-erbα*- deficient mouse primary macrophages compared to control [22]. However, as this effect may only reflect the increase of *Nlrp3* gene expression, additional experiments are needed to uncover the underlying mechanisms. However, because Rev-erbα regulates mitochondrial function and autophagy processes [162], it may be speculated that Rev-erbα-regulated NLRP3 assembly is mediated by a decrease in ROS production and an enhancement of mitochondrial function. Finally, Rev-erbα is also involved in the control of the circadian expression of the long noncoding RNA *Platr4*, which serves as a circadian repressor of the NLRP3 inflammasome as well [163]. However, because *Platr4* and *Nlrp3* circadian patterns are in phase, further studies are needed to investigate the kinetics of *Platr4*-mediated *Nlrp3* mRNA stability. It is noteworthy that Rev-erbs activation with natural or synthetic ligands reduces the secretion of IL-1β and IL-18 by inhibiting the expression of NLRP3 inflammasome component-related genes [22].

Clock disruption alters NLRP3 circadian oscillations in a mouse model of jetlag or in genetic and pharmacological models of clock alteration, thereby worsening the progression of inflammatory diseases [6] including colitis [160], myocardial infarction/ischemia–reperfusion injury [164], lung injury [161], nonalcoholic steatohepatitis [163] and fulminant hepatitis [22,159]. For instance, as discussed above, NLRP3 is involved in the control of DSS-induced colitis and the severity of DSS-induced colitis is increased when the clock is altered either in environmental or in the genetic model of clock disruption [160]. Confirming previous results obtained in acute hepatic inflammatory diseases [22], the deletion of *Rev-erbα* increases NLRP3 activation, thus worsening DSS-colitis pathogenesis, while the pharmacological activation of Rev-erbα prevents the onset of colitis [160]. These studies then demonstrate a pathogenic repercussion of NLRP3 expression when the clock is altered. However, whether such regulation is involved in the development of other autoimmune diseases still needs to be determined.

5 NLRP3 as a chronotherapeutic target for autoimmune diseases treatment

The NLRP3 inflammasome appears then to be a critical actor of autoimmune disease onset. Then, the NLRP3 inflammasome pathway could be identified as a promising therapeutic target. Until now, few strategies have already been identified, either by directly inhibiting NLRP3, by targeting the NLRP3 inflammasome products IL-1β and IL-18, or by decreasing the Caspase-1 activity. Accordingly, treatment lowering NLRP3 activity brought significant encouraging results for several autoimmune diseases.

5.1 NLRP3 inhibitors

MCC950 is a specific NLRP3 inhibitor, which prevents ASC oligomerization thus abolishing IL-1β and IL-18 secretion in human and mouse macrophages [165]. MCC950 weakens disease severity in animal models of arthritis, lupus nephritis, and EAE [46,51,165]. However, although it can target wild-type NLRP3, MCC950 is unable to bind CAPS-related NLRP3 mutants, disqualifying this strategy in the treatment of CAPS patients [57]. In addition, MCC950 displays hepato-toxicity in a phase II clinical trial for RA, which may then limit its use in human [166]. From then, a plethora of NLRP3 inhibitors has been developed including

IZD334, Inzomelid, Bay11–7082, parthenolide, tranilast, OLT1177, CY-09, 3,4-methylenedioxy-β-nitrostyrene (MNS), and the oridonin [167]. These compounds are currently in clinical development and their use in the treatment of autoimmune diseases has not been reported yet. Finally, two compounds, NU9056 and SP600125, were shown to indirectly inhibit NLRP3 by modulating its posttranslational modifications [167].

5.2 Caspase 1 inhibitors

Caspase 1 is the common IL-1 cytokine processor downstream the activation of all canonical inflammasome pathways. Therefore, targeting Caspase 1 opens an interesting perspective to treat inflammasome-driven diseases. Main strategies explored so far were the development of tetrapeptides that target the conserved Cys285 in the active site of Caspase 1. However, these compounds display low stability, solubility, and selectivity, while their byproducts demonstrate toxicity. Pralnacasan (VX-740) and belnacasan (VX-765) are two Caspase 1 inhibitor prodrugs that are converted in the cytosol. This is supposed to bypass toxicity and bioavailability issues. Pralnacasan reduces joint damage in mouse osteoarthritis models and lowers colon damage in DSS-induced colitis [73,168]. However, it exhibits hepatotoxicity in long-term follow-up animal studies, imposing the end of phase 2 clinical trial in RA patients [169]. On contrary to pralnacasan, belnacasan seems to have a favorable safety profile [167] and improves RA and skin inflammation in mouse models by suppressing the production of proinflammatory factors [170,171].

5.3 IL-1 blockade

IL-1β and IL-18 are the main products of the NLRP3 inflammasome activation and are likely responsible for the main deleterious effects observed when its activation is uncontrolled. Therefore, IL-1 blockade strategies have been developed to treat NLRP3-driven diseases. Anakinra is a recombinant IL-1 receptor antagonist, which is effective in RA, SLE, and JIA [7]. Nevertheless, due to its short plasma half-life, daily subcutaneous administrations of anakinra are required and is then no longer used for these diseases [172]. Instead, canakinumab, a human IL-1β-neutralizing antibody, is preferred as it exhibits a 26 days half-life [173] with antiinflammatory effects in RA [174] and JIA [175]. Rilonercept is a decoy receptor to IL-1β and IL-1α. Several clinical trials demonstrate its efficiency in gout, but not in autoimmune diseases. Finally, the tadekinig alfa, a recombinant version of human IL-18 binding protein is used as IL-18 decoy receptor. Interestingly, it has demonstrated favorable safety profile, but its effect in the pathogenesis of autoimmune diseases has not been reported yet. On the other hand, GSK1070806, an IL-18-neutralizing antibody, is currently evaluated in a phase 2 clinical study for the treatment of Crohn's disease patients [167].

IL-1 blockade strategies may be considered as efficient treatments against autoinflammatory and autoimmune diseases. However, its application remains limited due to the frequency of injection, and mostly, due to the high risk of infections. The identification of novel targets or strategies may be then needed to improve treatments efficacy and safety.

5.4 NLRP3 and chronotherapies

Chronotherapy is defined as the optimal timing of administration of a therapeutic agent such as drug, radiation, or surgery to reduce adverse effects and improve both patient prognosis and treatment efficacy [176]. Because NLRP3 is controlled by the clock machinery, the time of exposure to drugs and their half-lives may have a dramatic impact on the disease outcome and its resolution. As such, a chrono-pharmacological approach targeting NLRP3 may have greater benefits for the treatment of NLRP3-driven diseases and autoimmune diseases.

Berberine is an isoquinoline alkaloid extracted from several herbs used in traditional Chinese medicine. This compound directly targets the NEK7 protein to block its interaction with NLRP3, thus inhibiting the activation of the complex [177]. In addition, berberine has been identified as a Rev-erbα agonist [178]. Interestingly, Rev-erbα-mediated effect of berberine shows better results on DSS-induced colitis when administered during the late resting phase compared early resting phase, thus acknowledging the rationale to target core clock components in NLRP3-driven diseases [178]. Such circadian effect of drug efficiency might be explained by the lower severity of colitis at the late resting phase, which coincides with the maximum expression of Rev-erbα and the minimum expression of NLRP3. Consistently, the time of cardiac ischemia/reperfusion and subsequent SR9009-mediated Rev-erbα activation affects the heart functional recovery, the best response being obtained when Rev-erbα expression is at its highest, i.e., when NLRP3 expression is at its lowest [164].

Intuitively, it then appears that the optimal timing of drug administration coincides with the maximum peak of the target expression. It should be mentioned, however, that pathological tissues may exhibit shifted circadian rhythm compared to healthy regions. For instance, myeloid cells are recruited to atherosclerotic lesions in a circadian manner, with a peak during the active-to-rest transition, through the rhythmic deposit of CCL2 on the arterial endothelium by circulating cells. On the other hand, the circadian oscillation of this cellular recruitment was shifted by 12h in healthy microvascular beds to reach a peak at the early active phase [179]. A chrono-pharmacological approach targeting monocyte recruitment via timed inhibition of the CCR2/CCL2 axis during the active phase dampened atherosclerotic lesions development. This study then acknowledges the rationale of chronotherapy, even in the context of chronic diseases. Since pathological tissues could have distinct circadian oscillation patterns compared to healthy tissues, NLRP3 may then specifically be targeted in pathological areas without affecting the homeostasis of healthy tissues, thereby reducing adverse effects. In addition to NLRP3, several targets should also be considered, i.e., the NLRP3 pathway itself or NLRP3-regulating clock components such as Rev-erbα. Finally, considering that alteration of NLRP3 oscillation observed in elderlies or in shift workers could drive autoimmune diseases, targeting clock components to re-entrain the molecular clock and sustain circadian amplitude of NLRP3 expression may also be considered as an alternative or an additional approach in these patients.

6 Conclusion

Innate and adaptive immune cells collaborate to ensure an efficient defense against microbes and to maintain body homeostasis. When imbalanced, alteration of both innate and adaptive immune systems drives the pathogenesis of autoimmune diseases. However, the uncovering of mechanisms responsible for such deleterious processes is only recent. As a central sensor of DAMPs, the NLRP3 inflammasome is a critical regulator of the innate immune system homeostasis. Alteration of this pathway was associated with the pathogenesis of numerous diseases including autoimmune diseases. Considerable efforts were then made to identify new therapeutic strategies by developing new compounds directly targeting NLRP3 or its products. As other physiological processes, the immune system is controlled by our intrinsic clock machinery. Accordingly, many studies in mouse and human evidence that circadian rhythm alteration drives the onset of autoimmune and autoinflammatory diseases. Remarkably, the NLRP3 inflammasome is regulated by the clock machinery and then exerts key features in the control of the circadian immunity. Consistently, clock alteration drives NLRP3-driven autoimmune diseases. Therefore, targeting NLRP3 at the right time imposes itself as an interesting option to optimally treat patients. With the emergence of new compounds, knowledge, and tools, our further understanding of these processes should provide us with additional clinical benefits and innovative chronotherapy strategies improving the effectiveness of interventions.

Fundings

Some of our work included in this review manuscript was supported by the Fondation pour la Recherche Médicale (FRM, EQU202003010310), INSERM, the Région Hauts-de-France/FEDER (Chronoregeneration), Association Francaise contre les Myopathies (AFM), Fondation de France and the Société Francophone du Diabète (SFD)-SERVIER. This project is cofounded by the European Union under the European Region Development Fund (ERDF) and by the Hauts de France Region Council (contract_20000007), the MEL (contract-2020-ESR-02) and the French State (contract n°2019-R3-CTRL_IPL_Phase3). This project is cofounded by the European Union under the European Region Development Fund (ERDF) and by the Hauts de France Region Council (contract_20002842), the MEL (contract-2020-ESR-06) and the French State (contract n°2020-R3-CTRL_IPL_Phase4). This project is co-funded by the Agence Nationale pour la Recherche (ANR) (ANR-19-CE15-0033-01, ANR-20-CE14-0035). This work was supported by the Agence Nationale de la Recherche (ANR) grants « European Genomic Institute for Diabetes » E.G.I.D, ANR-10-LABX-0046, a French State fund managed by ANR under the frame program Investissements d'Avenir I-SITE ULNE/ANR-16-IDEX-0004 ULNE. The funders were not involved in the study design, collection, analysis, interpretation of data, the writing of this article or the decision to submit it for publication.

References

[1] D. Langan, K.D. Moudgil, N.R. Rose, Common innate pathways to autoimmune disease, Clin. Immunol. 212 (2020) 108361, https://doi.org/10.1016/j.clim.2020.108361.

[2] T. Gong, L. Liu, W. Jiang, R. Zhou, DAMP-sensing receptors in sterile inflammation and inflammatory diseases, Nat. Rev. Immunol. 20 (2020) 95–112, https://doi.org/10.1038/s41577-019-0215-7.

[3] C.L. Evavold, J.C. Kagan, Inflammasomes: threat-assessment organelles of the innate immune system, Immunity 51 (2019) 609–624, https://doi.org/10.1016/j.immuni.2019.08.005.

[4] S. Venkatesha, S. Dudics, E. Weingartner, E. So, J. Pedra, K. Moudgil, Altered Th17/Treg balance and dysregulated IL-1β response influence susceptibility/resistance to experimental autoimmune arthritis, Int. J. Immunopathol. Pharmacol. 28 (2015) 318–328, https://doi.org/10.1177/0394632015595757.

[5] L. Broderick, D.D. Nardo, B.S. Franklin, H.M. Hoffman, E. Latz, The inflammasomes and autoinflammatory syndromes, Annu. Rev. Pathol. 10 (2015) 395–424.

[6] B. Pourcet, H. Duez, Circadian control of inflammasome pathways: implications for circadian medicine, Front. Immunol. 11 (2020) 1630, https://doi.org/10.3389/fimmu.2020.01630.

[7] Z. Li, J. Guo, L. Bi, Role of the NLRP3 inflammasome in autoimmune diseases, Biomed. Pharmacother. 130 (2020) 110542, https://doi.org/10.1016/j.biopha.2020.110542.

[8] H.-H. Shen, Y.-X. Yang, X. Meng, X.-Y. Luo, X.-M. Li, Z.-W. Shuai, et al., NLRP3: A promising therapeutic target for autoimmune diseases, Autoimmun. Rev. 17 (2018) 694–702, https://doi.org/10.1016/j.autrev.2018.01.020.

[9] K.V. Swanson, M. Deng, J.P.-Y. Ting, The NLRP3 inflammasome: molecular activation and regulation to therapeutics, Nat. Rev. Immunol. 19 (2019) 477–489, https://doi.org/10.1038/s41577-019-0165-0.

[10] F.I. Schmidt, A. Lu, J.W. Chen, J. Ruan, C. Tang, H. Wu, et al., A single domain antibody fragment that recognizes the adaptor ASC defines the role of ASC domains in inflammasome assemblyA VHH defines mechanism of inflammasome assembly, J. Exp. Med. 213 (2016) 771–790, https://doi.org/10.1084/jem.20151790.

[11] A. Lu, V.G. Magupalli, J. Ruan, Q. Yin, M.K. Atianand, M.R. Vos, et al., Unified polymerization mechanism for the assembly of ASC-dependent inflammasomes, Cell 156 (2014) 1193–1206, https://doi.org/10.1016/j.cell.2014.02.008.

[12] X. Cai, J. Chen, H. Xu, S. Liu, Q.-X. Jiang, R. Halfmann, et al., Prion-like polymerization Underlies Signal Transduction In Antiviral Immune Defense And Inflammasome Activation, Cell 156 (2014) 1207–1222, https://doi.org/10.1016/j.cell.2014.01.063.

[13] D. Boucher, M. Monteleone, R.C. Coll, K.W. Chen, C.M. Ross, J.L. Teo, et al., Caspase-1 self-cleavage is an intrinsic mechanism to terminate inflammasome activityCaspase-1 protease activity is self-limiting, J. Exp. Med. 215 (2018) 827–840, https://doi.org/10.1084/jem.20172222.

[14] H. Shi, Y. Wang, X. Li, X. Zhan, M. Tang, M. Fina, et al., NLRP3 activation and mitosis are mutually exclusive events coordinated by NEK7, a new inflammasome component, Nat. Immunol. 17 (2016) 250–258, https://doi.org/10.1038/ni.3333.

[15] H. Sharif, L. Wang, W.L. Wang, V.G. Magupalli, L. Andreeva, Q. Qiao, et al., Structural mechanism for NEK7-licensed activation of NLRP3 inflammasome, Nature 570 (2019) 338–343, https://doi.org/10.1038/s41586-019-1295-z.

[16] J.L. Schmid-Burgk, D. Chauhan, T. Schmidt, T.S. Ebert, J. Reinhardt, E. Endl, et al., A genome-wide CRISPR (clustered regularly interspaced short palindromic repeats) screen identifies NEK7 as an essential component of NLRP3 inflammasome activation, J. Biol. Chem. 291 (2016) 103–109, https://doi.org/10.1074/jbc.c115.700492.

[17] J. Ding, K. Wang, W. Liu, Y. She, Q. Sun, J. Shi, et al., Pore-forming activity and structural autoinhibition of the gasdermin family, Nature 535 (2016) 111–116, https://doi.org/10.1038/nature18590.

[18] F.J. Sheedy, A. Grebe, K.J. Rayner, P. Kalantari, B. Ramkhelawon, S.B. Carpenter, et al., CD36 coordinates NLRP3 inflammasome activation by facilitating intracellular nucleation of soluble ligands into particulate ligands in sterile inflammation, Nat. Immunol. 14 (2013) 812–820.

[19] C.R. Stewart, L.M. Stuart, K. Wilkinson, J.M. van Gils, J. Deng, A. Halle, et al., CD36 ligands promote sterile inflammation through assembly of a Toll-like receptor 4 and 6 heterodimer, Nat. Immunol. 11 (2010) 155–161, https://doi.org/10.1038/ni.1836.

[20] A. Warnatsch, M. Ioannou, Q. Wang, V. Papayannopoulos, Inflammation. Neutrophil extracellular traps license macrophages for cytokine production in atherosclerosis, Science 349 (2015) 316–320, https://doi.org/10.1126/science.aaa8064.

[21] J.M. Kahlenberg, C. Carmona-Rivera, C.K. Smith, M.J. Kaplan, Neutrophil extracellular trap–associated protein activation of the NLRP3 inflammasome is enhanced in lupus macrophages, J. Immunol. 190 (2013) 1217–1226, https://doi.org/10.4049/jimmunol.1202388.

[22] B. Pourcet, M. Zecchin, L. Ferri, J. Beauchamp, S. Sitaula, C. Billon, et al., Nuclear receptor subfamily 1 group D member 1 regulates circadian activity of NLRP3 inflammasome to reduce the severity of fulminant hepatitis in mice, Gastroenterology 154 (2018) 1449–1464.e20, https://doi.org/10.1053/j.gastro.2017.12.019.

[23] N. Boxberger, M. Hecker, U.K. Zettl, Dysregulation of inflammasome priming and activation by MicroRNAs in human immune-mediated diseases, J. Immunol. 202 (2019) 2177–2187, https://doi.org/10.4049/jimmunol.1801416.

[24] F. Bauernfeind, A. Rieger, F.A. Schildberg, P.A. Knolle, J.L. Schmid-Burgk, V. Hornung, NLRP3 inflammasome activity is negatively controlled by miR-223, J. Immunol. 189 (2012) 4175–4181, https://doi.org/10.4049/jimmunol.1201516.

[25] H. Shibuya, T. Nakasa, N. Adachi, Y. Nagata, M. Ishikawa, M. Deie, et al., Overexpression of microRNA-223 in rheumatoid arthritis synovium controls osteoclast differentiation, Mod. Rheumatol. 23 (2013) 674–685, https://doi.org/10.1007/s10165-012-0710-1.

[26] M. Meira, C. Sievers, F. Hoffmann, M. Rasenack, J. Kuhle, T. Derfuss, et al., Unraveling natalizumab effects on deregulated miR-17 expression in CD4+ T cells of patients with relapsing-remitting multiple sclerosis, J Immunol Res 2014 (2014) 1–11, https://doi.org/10.1155/2014/897249.

[27] H. Kaga, A. Komatsuda, A. Omokawa, M. Ito, K. Teshima, H. Tagawa, et al., Downregulated expression of miR-155, miR-17, and miR-181b, and upregulated expression of activation-induced cytidine deaminase and interferon-α in PBMCs from patients with SLE, Mod. Rheumatol. 25 (2015) 865–870, https://doi.org/10.3109/14397595.2015.1030102.

[28] R.A. Sarhan, H.R.A. Aboelenein, S.K.N. Sourour, I.O. Fawzy, S. Salah, A.I. Abdelaziz, Targeting E2F1 and c-Myc expression by microRNA-17-5p represses interferon-stimulated gene MxA in peripheral blood mononuclear cells of pediatric systemic lupus erythematosus patients, Discov. Med. 19 (2015) 419–425.

[29] N. Kelley, D. Jeltema, Y. Duan, Y. He, The NLRP3 inflammasome: an overview of mechanisms of activation and regulation, Int. J. Mol. Sci. 20 (2019) 3328, https://doi.org/10.3390/ijms20133328.

[30] B.F. Py, M.S. Kim, H. Vakifahmetoglu-Norberg, J. Yuan, Deubiquitination of NLRP3 by BRCC3 critically regulates inflammasome activity, Mol. Cell 49 (2013) 331–338, https://doi.org/10.1016/j.molcel.2012.11.009.

[31] G. Lopez-Castejon, N.M. Luheshi, V. Compan, S. High, R.C. Whitehead, S. Flitsch, et al., Deubiquitinases regulate the activity of caspase-1 and interleukin-1β secretion via assembly of the inflammasome, J. Biol. Chem. 288 (2013) 2721–2733, https://doi.org/10.1074/jbc.m112.422238.

[32] H. Duez, B. Pourcet, Nuclear receptors in the control of the NLRP3 inflammasome pathway, Front. Endocrinol. 12 (2021) 630536, https://doi.org/10.3389/fendo.2021.630536.

[33] V. Hornung, F. Bauernfeind, A. Halle, E.O. Samstad, H. Kono, K.L. Rock, et al., Silica crystals and aluminum salts activate the NALP3 inflammasome through phagosomal destabilization, Nat. Immunol. 9 (2008) 847–856, https://doi.org/10.1038/ni.1631.

[34] G.M. Orlowski, S. Sharma, J.D. Colbert, M. Bogyo, S.A. Robertson, H. Kataoka, et al., Frontline science: multiple cathepsins promote inflammasome-independent, particle-induced cell death during NLRP3-dependent IL-1β activation, J. Leukoc. Biol. 102 (2017) 7–17, https://doi.org/10.1189/jlb.3hi0316-152r.

[35] G.M. Orlowski, J.D. Colbert, S. Sharma, M. Bogyo, S.A. Robertson, K.L. Rock, Multiple cathepsins promote Pro–IL-1β synthesis and NLRP3-mediated IL-1β activation, J. Immunol. 195 (2015) 1685–1697, https://doi.org/10.4049/jimmunol.1500509.

[36] M.A. Katsnelson, K.M. Lozada-Soto, H.M. Russo, B.A. Miller, G.R. Dubyak, NLRP3 inflammasome signaling is activated by low-level lysosome disruption but inhibited by extensive lysosome disruption: roles for K+ efflux and Ca2+ influx, Am. J. Phys. Cell Phys. 311 (2016) C83–100, https://doi.org/10.1152/ajpcell.00298.2015.

[37] A. Surprenant, F. Rassendren, E. Kawashima, R.A. North, G. Buell, The cytolytic P2Z receptor for extracellular ATP identified as a P2X receptor (P2X7), Science 272 (1996) 735–738, https://doi.org/10.1126/science.272.5262.735.

[38] I. Walev, K. Reske, M. Palmer, A. Valeva, S. Bhakdi, Potassium-inhibited processing of IL-1 beta in human monocytes, EMBO J. 14 (1995) 1607–1614.

[39] D. Perregaux, C.A. Gabel, Interleukin-1 beta maturation and release in response to ATP and nigericin. Evidence that potassium depletion mediated by these agents is a necessary and common feature of their activity, J. Biol. Chem. 269 (1994) 15195–15203.

[40] A. Di, S. Xiong, Z. Ye, R.K.S. Malireddi, S. Kometani, M. Zhong, et al., The TWIK2 potassium efflux channel in macrophages mediates NLRP3 inflammasome-induced inflammation, Immunity 49 (2018) 56–65.e4, https://doi.org/10.1016/j.immuni.2018.04.032.

[41] R. Domingo-Fernández, R.C. Coll, J. Kearney, S. Breit, L.A.J. O'Neill, The intracellular chloride channel proteins CLIC1 and CLIC4 induce IL-1β transcription and activate the NLRP3 inflammasome, J. Biol. Chem. 292 (2017) 12077–12087, https://doi.org/10.1074/jbc.m117.797126.

[42] T. Tang, X. Lang, C. Xu, X. Wang, T. Gong, Y. Yang, et al., CLICs-dependent chloride efflux is an essential and proximal upstream event for NLRP3 inflammasome activation, Nat. Commun. 8 (2017) 202, https://doi.org/10.1038/s41467-017-00227-x.

[43] Y. He, M.Y. Zeng, D. Yang, B. Motro, G. Núñez, NEK7 is an essential mediator of NLRP3 activation downstream of potassium efflux, Nature 530 (2016) 354–357, https://doi.org/10.1038/nature16959.

[44] J.P. Green, S. Yu, F. Martín-Sánchez, P. Pelegrin, G. Lopez-Castejon, C.B. Lawrence, et al., Chloride regulates dynamic NLRP3-dependent ASC oligomerization and inflammasome priming, Proc. Natl. Acad. Sci. U. S. A. 115 (2018) 201812744, https://doi.org/10.1073/pnas.1812744115.

[45] C.-A. Yang, S.-T. Huang, B.-L. Chiang, Sex-dependent differential activation of NLRP3 and AIM2 inflammasomes in SLE macrophages, Rheumatology 54 (2015) 324–331, https://doi.org/10.1093/rheumatology/keu318.

[46] R. Fu, C. Guo, S. Wang, Y. Huang, O. Jin, H. Hu, et al., Podocyte activation of NLRP3 inflammasomes contributes to the development of proteinuria in lupus nephritis, Arthritis Rheum. 69 (2017) 1636–1646, https://doi.org/10.1002/art.40155.

[47] T. Huang, H. Yin, W. Ning, X. Wang, C. Chen, W. Lin, et al., Expression of inflammasomes NLRP1, NLRP3 and AIM2 in different pathologic classification of lupus nephritis, Clin. Exp. Rheumatol. 38 (2020) 680–690.

[48] M.S. Shin, Y. Kang, N. Lee, E.R. Wahl, S.H. Kim, K.S. Kang, et al., Self double-stranded (ds)DNA induces IL-1β production from human monocytes by activating NLRP3 inflammasome in the presence of anti–dsDNA antibodies, J. Immunol. 190 (2013) 1407–1415, https://doi.org/10.4049/jimmunol.1201195.

[49] M.S. Shin, Y. Kang, N. Lee, S.H. Kim, K.S. Kang, R. Lazova, et al., U1-small nuclear ribonucleoprotein activates the NLRP3 inflammasome in human monocytes, J. Immunol. 188 (2012) 4769–4775, https://doi.org/10.4049/jimmunol.1103355.

[50] R. Mende, F.B. Vincent, R. Kandane-Rathnayake, R. Koelmeyer, E. Lin, J. Chang, et al., Analysis of serum interleukin (IL)-1β and IL-18 in systemic lupus erythematosus, Front. Immunol. 9 (2018) 1250, https://doi.org/10.3389/fimmu.2018.01250.

[51] C. Guo, R. Fu, S. Wang, Y. Huang, X. Li, M. Zhou, et al., NLRP3 inflammasome activation contributes to the pathogenesis of rheumatoid arthritis, Clin. Exp. Immunol. 194 (2018) 231–243, https://doi.org/10.1111/cei.13167.

[52] C. Choulaki, G. Papadaki, A. Repa, E. Kampouraki, K. Kambas, K. Ritis, et al., Enhanced activity of NLRP3 inflammasome in peripheral blood cells of patients with active rheumatoid arthritis, Arthritis Res. Ther. 17 (2015) 257, https://doi.org/10.1186/s13075-015-0775-2.

[53] P. Ruscitti, P. Cipriani, P.D. Benedetto, V. Liakouli, O. Berardicurti, F. Carubbi, et al., Monocytes from patients with rheumatoid arthritis and type 2 diabetes mellitus display an increased production of interleukin (IL)-1β via the nucleotide-binding domain and leucine-rich repeat containing family pyrin 3(NLRP3)-inflammasome activation: a possible implication for therapeutic decision in these patients, Clin. Exp. Immunol. 182 (2015) 35–44, https://doi.org/10.1111/cei.12667.

[54] L. Kolly, N. Busso, G. Palmer, D. Talabot-Ayer, V. Chobaz, A. So, Expression and function of the NALP3 inflammasome in rheumatoid synovium, Immunology 129 (2010) 178–185, https://doi.org/10.1111/j.1365-2567.2009.03174.x.

[55] X. Dong, Z. Zheng, P. Lin, X. Fu, F. Li, J. Jiang, et al., ACPAs promote IL-1β production in rheumatoid arthritis by activating the NLRP3 inflammasome, Cell. Mol. Immunol. 17 (2020) 261–271, https://doi.org/10.1038/s41423-019-0201-9.

[56] D. Ilchovska, M. Barrow, An overview of the NF-kB mechanism of pathophysiology in rheumatoid arthritis, investigation of the NF-kB ligand RANKL and related nutritional interventions, Autoimmun. Rev. 20 (2020) 102741, https://doi.org/10.1016/j.autrev.2020.102741.

[57] L.V. Walle, N.V. Opdenbosch, P. Jacques, A. Fossoul, E. Verheugen, P. Vogel, et al., Negative regulation of the NLRP3 inflammasome by A20 protects against arthritis, Nature 512 (2014) 69–73.

[58] H. Ding, G. Gao, L. Zhang, G. Shen, W. Sun, Z. Gu, et al., The protective effects of curculigoside A on adjuvant-induced arthritis by inhibiting NF-κB/NLRP3 activation in rats, Int. Immunopharmacol. 30 (2016) 43–49, https://doi.org/10.1016/j.intimp.2015.11.026.

[59] Y. Li, J.-Y. Zheng, J.-Q. Liu, J. Yang, Y. Liu, C. Wang, et al., Succinate/NLRP3 inflammasome induces synovial fibroblast activation: therapeutical effects of clematichinenoside AR on arthritis, Front. Immunol. 7 (2016) 532, https://doi.org/10.3389/fimmu.2016.00532.

[60] X.-F. Li, W.-W. Shen, Y.-Y. Sun, W.-X. Li, Z.-H. Sun, Y.-H. Liu, et al., MicroRNA-20a negatively regulates expression of NLRP3-inflammasome by targeting TXNIP in adjuvant-induced arthritis fibroblast-like synoviocytes, Joint Bone Spine 83 (2016) 695–700, https://doi.org/10.1016/j.jbspin.2015.10.007.

[61] J. Tian, D. Zhou, L. Xiang, X. Liu, H. Zhang, B. Wang, et al., MiR-223-3p inhibits inflammation and pyroptosis in monosodium urate-induced rats and fibroblast-like synoviocytes by targeting NLRP3, Clin. Exp. Immunol. (2021), https://doi.org/10.1111/cei.13587.

[62] Z.-M. Wu, J. Luo, X.-D. Shi, S.-X. Zhang, X.-B. Zhu, J. Guo, Icariin alleviates rheumatoid arthritis via regulating miR-223-3p/NLRP3 signalling axis, Autoimmunity (2020) 1–9, https://doi.org/10.1080/08916934.2020.1836488.

[63] Y. Zhai, P. Lin, Z. Feng, H. Lu, Q. Han, J. Chen, et al., TNFAIP3-DEPTOR complex regulates inflammasome secretion through autophagy in ankylosing spondylitis monocytes, Autophagy 14 (2018) 1629–1643, https://doi.org/10.1080/15548627.2018.1458804.

[64] M.A. Martínez-Godínez, M.P. Cruz-Domínguez, L.J. Jara, A. Domínguez-López, R.A. Jarillo-Luna, O. Vera-Lastra, et al., Expression of NLRP3 inflammasome, cytokines and vascular mediators in the skin of systemic sclerosis patients, Isr. Med. Assoc. J. 17 (2015) 5–10.

[65] C.M. Artlett, S. Sassi-Gaha, J.L. Rieger, A.C. Boesteanu, C.A. Feghali-Bostwick, P.D. Katsikis, The inflammasome activating caspase 1 mediates fibrosis and myofibroblast differentiation in systemic sclerosis, Arthritis Rheum. 63 (2011) 3563–3574, https://doi.org/10.1002/art.30568.

[66] K. Zakrzewska, R. Arvia, M.G. Torcia, A.M. Clemente, M. Tanturli, G. Castronovo, et al., Effects of parvovirus B19 in vitro infection on monocytes from patients with systemic sclerosis: enhanced inflammatory pathways by caspase-1 activation and cytokine production, J. Invest. Dermatol. 139 (2019) 2125–2133.e1, https://doi.org/10.1016/j.jid.2019.03.1144.

[67] L. Niu, S. Zhang, J. Wu, L. Chen, Y. Wang, Upregulation of NLRP3 inflammasome in the tears and ocular surface of dry eye patients, PLoS One 10 (2015), https://doi.org/10.1371/journal.pone.0126277, e0126277.

[68] M.G. Khalafalla, L.T. Woods, J.M. Camden, A.A. Khan, K.H. Limesand, M.J. Petris, et al., P2X7 receptor antagonism prevents IL-1β release from salivary epithelial cells and reduces inflammation in a mouse model of autoimmune exocrinopathy, J. Biol. Chem. 292 (2017) 16626–16637, https://doi.org/10.1074/jbc.m117.790741.

[69] A.G. Vakrakou, S. Boiu, P.D. Ziakas, E. Xingi, H. Boleti, M.N. Manoussakis, Systemic activation of NLRP3 inflammasome in patients with severe primary Sjögren's syndrome fueled by inflammagenic DNA accumulations, J. Autoimmun. 91 (2018) 23–33, https://doi.org/10.1016/j.jaut.2018.02.010.

[70] S.-M. Hong, J. Lee, S.G. Jang, J. Lee, M.-L. Cho, S.-K. Kwok, et al., Type I interferon increases inflammasomes associated pyroptosis in the salivary glands of patients with primary Sjögren's syndrome, Immune Netw. 20 (2020), https://doi.org/10.4110/in.2020.20.e39, e39.

[71] L. Liu, Y. Dong, M. Ye, S. Jin, J. Yang, M.E. Joosse, et al., The pathogenic role of NLRP3 inflammasome activation in inflammatory bowel diseases of both mice and humans, J. Crohn's Colitis 11 (2017) 737–750, https://doi.org/10.1093/ecco-jcc/jjw219.

[72] C. Bauer, P. Duewell, C. Mayer, H.A. Lehr, K.A. Fitzgerald, M. Dauer, et al., Colitis induced in mice with dextran sulfate sodium (DSS) is mediated by the NLRP3 inflammasome, Gut 59 (2010) 1192–1199, https://doi.org/10.1136/gut.2009.197822.

[73] F. Loher, C. Bauer, N. Landauer, K. Schmall, B. Siegmund, H.A. Lehr, et al., The interleukin-1β-converting enzyme inhibitor pralnacasan reduces dextran sulfate sodium-induced murine colitis and T helper 1 T-cell activation, J. Pharmacol. Exp. Ther. 308 (2004) 583–590, https://doi.org/10.1124/jpet.103.057059.

[74] V. Neudecker, M. Haneklaus, O. Jensen, L. Khailova, J.C. Masterson, H. Tye, et al., Myeloid-derived miR-223 regulates intestinal inflammation via repression of the NLRP3 inflammasomemiR-223 control of NLRP3 activation during colitis, J. Exp. Med. 214 (2017) 1737–1752, https://doi.org/10.1084/jem.20160462.

[75] D. Carlos, F.R.C. Costa, C.A. Pereira, F.A. Rocha, J.N.U. Yaochite, G.G. Oliveira, et al., Mitochondrial DNA activates the NLRP3 inflammasome and predisposes to type 1 diabetes in murine model, Front. Immunol. 8 (2017) 164, https://doi.org/10.3389/fimmu.2017.00164.

[76] C.A. Pereira, D. Carlos, N.S. Ferreira, J.F. Silva, C.Z. Zanotto, D.S. Zamboni, et al., Mitochondrial DNA promotes NLRP3 inflammasome activation and contributes to endothelial dysfunction and inflammation in type 1 diabetes, Front. Physiol. 10 (2020) 1557, https://doi.org/10.3389/fphys.2019.01557.

[77] M.R. Davanso, A.R. Crisma, T.T. Braga, L.N. Masi, C.L. do Amaral, V.N.C. Leal, et al., Macrophage inflammatory state in Type 1 diabetes: triggered by NLRP3/iNOS pathway and attenuated by docosahexaenoic acid, Clin. Sci. 135 (2021) 19–34, https://doi.org/10.1042/cs20201348.

[78] J.R. Yaron, S. Gangaraju, M.Y. Rao, X. Kong, L. Zhang, F. Su, et al., K+ regulates Ca2+ to drive inflammasome signaling: dynamic visualization of ion flux in live cells, Cell Death Dis. 6 (2015) e1954, https://doi.org/10.1038/cddis.2015.277.

[79] T. Murakami, J. Ockinger, J. Yu, V. Byles, A. McColl, A.M. Hofer, et al., Critical role for calcium mobilization in activation of the NLRP3 inflammasome, Proc. Natl. Acad. Sci. U. S. A. 109 (2012) 11282–11287, https://doi.org/10.1073/pnas.1117765109.

[80] G.-S. Lee, N. Subramanian, A.I. Kim, I. Aksentijevich, R. Goldbach-Mansky, D.B. Sacks, et al., The calcium-sensing receptor regulates the NLRP3 inflammasome through Ca2+ and cAMP, Nature 492 (2012) 123–127, https://doi.org/10.1038/nature11588.

[81] R. Zhou, A.S. Yazdi, P. Menu, J. Tschopp, A role for mitochondria in NLRP3 inflammasome activation, Nature 469 (2011) 221–225, https://doi.org/10.1038/nature09663.

[82] K. Nakahira, J.A. Haspel, V.A. Rathinam, S.J. Lee, T. Dolinay, H.C. Lam, et al., Autophagy proteins regulate innate immune responses by inhibiting the release of mitochondrial DNA mediated by the NALP3 inflammasome, Nat. Immunol. 12 (2011) 222–230, https://doi.org/10.1038/ni.1980.

[83] K. Shimada, T.R. Crother, J. Karlin, J. Dagvadorj, N. Chiba, S. Chen, et al., Oxidized mitochondrial DNA activates the NLRP3 inflammasome during apoptosis, Immunity 36 (2012) 401–414, https://doi.org/10.1016/j.immuni.2012.01.009.

[84] R. Zhou, A. Tardivel, B. Thorens, I. Choi, J. Tschopp, Thioredoxin-interacting protein links oxidative stress to inflammasome activation, Nat. Immunol. 11 (2010) 136–140, https://doi.org/10.1038/ni.1831.

[85] M.M. Gaidt, T.S. Ebert, D. Chauhan, T. Schmidt, J.L. Schmid-Burgk, F. Rapino, et al., Human monocytes engage an alternative inflammasome pathway, Immunity 44 (2016) 833–846, https://doi.org/10.1016/j.immuni.2016.01.012.

[86] N. Kayagaki, S. Warming, M. Lamkanfi, L.V. Walle, S. Louie, J. Dong, et al., Non-canonical inflammasome activation targets caspase-11, Nature 479 (2011) 117–121, https://doi.org/10.1038/nature10558.

[87] P.J. Baker, D. Boucher, D. Bierschenk, C. Tebartz, P.G. Whitney, D.B. D'Silva, et al., NLRP3 inflammasome activation downstream of cytoplasmic LPS recognition by both caspase-4 and caspase-5, Eur. J. Immunol. 45 (2015) 2918–2926, https://doi.org/10.1002/eji.201545655.

[88] P. Pelegrin, A. Surprenant, Pannexin-1 mediates large pore formation and interleukin-1β release by the ATP-gated P2X7 receptor, EMBO J. 25 (2006) 5071–5082, https://doi.org/10.1038/sj.emboj.7601378.

[89] D. Yang, Y. He, R. Muñoz-Planillo, Q. Liu, G. Núñez, Caspase-11 requires the pannexin-1 channel and the purinergic P2X7 pore to mediate pyroptosis and endotoxic shock, Immunity 43 (2015) 923–932, https://doi.org/10.1016/j.immuni.2015.10.009.

[90] C.A. Dinarello, Immunological and inflammatory functions of the interleukin-1 family, Annu. Rev. Immunol. 27 (2009) 519–550, https://doi.org/10.1146/annurev.immunol.021908.132612.

[91] A.N. Theofilopoulos, D.H. Kono, R. Baccala, The multiple pathways to autoimmunity, Nat. Immunol. 18 (2017) 716–724, https://doi.org/10.1038/ni.3731.

[92] G. Cavalli, C.A. Dinarello, Anakinra therapy for non-cancer inflammatory diseases, Front. Pharmacol. 9 (2018) 1157, https://doi.org/10.3389/fphar.2018.01157.

[93] G.C. Tsokos, Autoimmunity and organ damage in systemic lupus erythematosus, Nat. Immunol. 21 (2020) 605–614, https://doi.org/10.1038/s41590-020-0677-6.

[94] A. Lu, H. Li, J. Niu, S. Wu, G. Xue, X. Yao, et al., Hyperactivation of the NLRP3 inflammasome in myeloid cells leads to severe organ damage in experimental lupus, J. Immunol. 198 (2017) 1119–1129, https://doi.org/10.4049/jimmunol.1600659.

[95] V. Papayannopoulos, Neutrophil extracellular traps in immunity and disease, Nat. Rev. Immunol. 18 (2018) 134–147, https://doi.org/10.1038/nri.2017.105.

[96] M.-L. Eloranta, L. Rönnblom, Cause and consequences of the activated type I interferon system in SLE, J. Mol. Med. 94 (2016) 1103–1110, https://doi.org/10.1007/s00109-016-1421-4.

[97] J. Liu, C.C. Berthier, J.M. Kahlenberg, Enhanced inflammasome activity in systemic lupus erythematosus is mediated via type I interferon–induced up-regulation of interferon regulatory factor 1, Arthritis Rheum. 69 (2017) 1840–1849, https://doi.org/10.1002/art.40166.

[98] Q. Yang, C. Yu, Z. Yang, Q. Wei, K. Mu, Y. Zhang, et al., Deregulated NLRP3 and NLRP1 inflammasomes and their correlations with disease activity in systemic lupus erythematosus, J. Rheumatol. 41 (2013) 444–452, https://doi.org/10.3899/jrheum.130310.

[99] Z.-Z. Ma, H.-S. Sun, J.-C. Lv, L. Guo, Q.-R. Yang, Expression and clinical significance of the NEK7-NLRP3 inflammasome signaling pathway in patients with systemic lupus erythematosus, J. Inflamm. 15 (2018) 16, https://doi.org/10.1186/s12950-018-0192-9.

[100] J.S. Smolen, D. Aletaha, I.B. McInnes, Rheumatoid arthritis, Lancet 388 (2016) 2023–2038, https://doi.org/10.1016/s0140-6736(16)30173-8.

[101] H.W. Kim, Y.-J. Kwon, B.W. Park, J.J. Song, Y.-B. Park, M.C. Park, Differential expressions of NOD-like receptors and their associations with inflammatory responses in rheumatoid arthritis, Clin. Exp. Rheumatol. 35 (2017) 630–637.

[102] M. Bakele, M. Joos, S. Burdi, N. Allgaier, S. Pöschel, B. Fehrenbacher, et al., Localization and Functionality of the Inflammasome in Neutrophils*, J. Biol. Chem. 289 (2014) 5320–5329, https://doi.org/10.1074/jbc.m113.505636.

[103] T.G. Day, A.V. Ramanan, A. Hinks, R. Lamb, J. Packham, C. Wise, et al., Autoinflammatory genes and susceptibility to psoriatic juvenile idiopathic arthritis, Arthritis Rheum. 58 (2008) 2142–2146, https://doi.org/10.1002/art.23604.

[104] S. Zhao, H. Chen, G. Wu, C. Zhao, The association of NLRP3 and TNFRSF1A polymorphisms with risk of ankylosing spondylitis and treatment efficacy of etanercept, J. Clin. Lab. Anal. 31 (2017), https://doi.org/10.1002/jcla.22138, e22138.

[105] S.-K. Kim, Y.J. Cho, J.-Y. Choe, NLRP3 inflammasomes and NLRP3 inflammasome-derived proinflammatory cytokines in peripheral blood mononuclear cells of patients with ankylosing spondylitis, Clin. Chim. Acta 486 (2018) 269–274, https://doi.org/10.1016/j.cca.2018.08.022.

[106] N. Vanaki, T. Golmohammadi, A. Jamshidi, M. Akhtari, M. Vojdanian, S. Mostafaei, et al., Increased inflammatory responsiveness of peripheral blood mononuclear cells (PBMCs) to in vitro NOD2 ligand stimulation in patients with ankylosing spondylitis, Immunopharmacol. Immunotoxicol. 40 (2018) 1–8, https://doi.org/10.1080/08923973.2018.1510963.

[107] C.M. Artlett, S. Sassi-Gaha, J.L. Hope, C.A. Feghali-Bostwick, P.D. Katsikis, Mir-155 is overexpressed in systemic sclerosis fibroblasts and is required for NLRP3 inflammasome-mediated collagen synthesis during fibrosis, Arthritis Res. Ther. 19 (2017) 144, https://doi.org/10.1186/s13075-017-1331-z.

[108] Q. Yan, J. Chen, W. Li, C. Bao, Q. Fu, Targeting miR-155 to treat experimental scleroderma, Sci. Rep. 6 (2016) 20314, https://doi.org/10.1038/srep20314.

[109] S.-K. Kim, J.-Y. Choe, G.H. Lee, Enhanced expression of NLRP3 inflammasome-related inflammation in peripheral blood mononuclear cells in Sjögren's syndrome, Clin. Chim. Acta 474 (2017) 147–154, https://doi.org/10.1016/j.cca.2017.09.019.

[110] C. Baldini, C. Rossi, F. Ferro, E. Santini, V. Seccia, V. Donati, et al., The P2X7 receptor–inflammasome complex has a role in modulating the inflammatory response in primary Sjögren's syndrome, J. Intern. Med. 274 (2013) 480–489, https://doi.org/10.1111/joim.12115.

[111] C. Baldini, E. Santini, C. Rossi, V. Donati, A. Solini, The P2X7 receptor–NLRP3 inflammasome complex predicts the development of non-Hodgkin's lymphoma in Sjögren's syndrome: a prospective, observational, single-centre study, J. Intern. Med. 282 (2017) 175–186, https://doi.org/10.1111/joim.12631.

[112] M.F. Neurath, Cytokines in inflammatory bowel disease, Nat. Rev. Immunol. 14 (2014) 329–342, https://doi.org/10.1038/nri3661.

[113] M. Coccia, O.J. Harrison, C. Schiering, M.J. Asquith, B. Becher, F. Powrie, et al., IL-1β mediates chronic intestinal inflammation by promoting the accumulation of IL-17A secreting innate lymphoid cells and CD4+ Th17 cells, J. Exp. Med. 209 (2012) 1595–1609, https://doi.org/10.1084/jem.20111453.

[114] S.A. Hirota, J. Ng, A. Lueng, M. Khajah, K. Parhar, Y. Li, et al., NLRP3 inflammasome plays a key role in the regulation of intestinal homeostasis, Inflamm. Bowel Dis. 17 (2010) 1359–1372, https://doi.org/10.1002/ibd.21478.

[115] R. Fusco, R. Siracusa, T. Genovese, S. Cuzzocrea, R.D. Paola, Focus on the role of NLRP3 inflammasome in diseases, Int. J. Mol. Sci. 21 (2020) 4223, https://doi.org/10.3390/ijms21124223.

[116] X. Sun, H. Pang, J. Li, S. Luo, G. Huang, X. Li, et al., The NLRP3 inflammasome and its role in T1DM, Front. Immunol. 11 (2020) 1595, https://doi.org/10.3389/fimmu.2020.01595.

[117] A. Pontillo, L. Brandao, R. Guimaraes, L. Segat, J. Araujo, S. Crovella, Two SNPs in NLRP3 gene are involved in the predisposition to type-1 diabetes and celiac disease in a pediatric population from northeast Brazil, Autoimmunity 43 (2010) 583–589, https://doi.org/10.3109/08916930903540432.

[118] E.M. Bradshaw, K. Raddassi, W. Elyaman, T. Orban, P.A. Gottlieb, S.C. Kent, et al., Monocytes from patients with type 1 diabetes spontaneously secrete proinflammatory cytokines inducing Th17 cells, J. Immunol. 183 (2009) 4432–4439, https://doi.org/10.4049/jimmunol.0900576.

[119] Y. Dogan, S. Akarsu, B. Ustundag, E. Yilmaz, M.K. Gurgoze, Serum IL-1β, IL-2, and IL-6 in insulin-dependent diabetic children, Mediat. Inflamm. 2006 (2006) 59206, https://doi.org/10.1155/mi/2006/59206.

[120] E.C. Kaizer, C.L. Glaser, D. Chaussabel, J. Banchereau, V. Pascual, P.C. White, Gene expression in peripheral blood mononuclear cells from children with diabetes, J. Clin. Endocrinol. Metab. 92 (2007) 3705–3711, https://doi.org/10.1210/jc.2007-0979.

[121] E.K. Grishman, P.C. White, R.C. Savani, Toll-like receptors, the NLRP3 inflammasome, and interleukin-1β in the development and progression of type 1 diabetes, Pediatr. Res. 71 (2012) 626–632, https://doi.org/10.1038/pr.2012.24.

[122] C. Hu, H. Ding, Y. Li, J.A. Pearson, X. Zhang, R.A. Flavell, et al., NLRP3 deficiency protects from type 1 diabetes through the regulation of chemotaxis into the pancreatic islets, Proc. Natl. Acad. Sci. U. S. A. 112 (2015) 11318–11323, https://doi.org/10.1073/pnas.1513509112.

[123] A.J. Lusis, Atherosclerosis, Nature 407 (2000) 233–241, https://doi.org/10.1038/35025203.

[124] P. Duewell, H. Kono, K.J. Rayner, C.M. Sirois, G. Vladimer, F.G. Bauernfeind, et al., NLRP3 inflammasomes are required for atherogenesis and activated by cholesterol crystals, Nature 464 (2010) 1357–1361, https://doi.org/10.1038/nature08938.

[125] T. van der Heijden, E. Kritikou, W. Venema, J. van Duijn, P.J. van Santbrink, B. Slütter, et al., NLRP3 inflammasome inhibition by MCC950 reduces atherosclerotic lesion development in apolipoprotein E-deficient mice-brief report, Arterioscler. Thromb. Vasc. Biol. 37 (2017) 1457–1461, https://doi.org/10.1161/atvbaha.117.309575.

[126] R.O. Escárcega, M.J. Lipinski, M. García-Carrasco, C. Mendoza-Pinto, J.L. Galvez-Romero, R. Cervera, Inflammation and atherosclerosis: cardiovascular evaluation in patients with autoimmune diseases, Autoimmun. Rev. 17 (2018) 703–708, https://doi.org/10.1016/j.autrev.2018.01.021.

[127] M. Bäck, A. Yurdagul, I. Tabas, K. Öörni, P.T. Kovanen, Inflammation and its resolution in atherosclerosis: mediators and therapeutic opportunities, Nat. Rev. Cardiol. 16 (2019) 389–406, https://doi.org/10.1038/s41569-019-0169-2.

[128] P. Libby, Inflammation in atherosclerosis, Nature 420 (2002) 868–874.

[129] E. Galkina, K. Ley, Immune and inflammatory mechanisms of atherosclerosis*, Annu. Rev. Immunol. 27 (2009) 165–197, https://doi.org/10.1146/annurev.immunol.021908.132620.

[130] H. Ait-Oufella, A.P. Sage, Z. Mallat, A. Tedgui, Adaptive (T and B Cells) immunity and control by dendritic cells in atherosclerosis, Circ. Res. 114 (2014) 1640–1660, https://doi.org/10.1161/circresaha.114.302761.

[131] M. Subramanian, I. Tabas, Dendritic cells in atherosclerosis, Semin. Immunopathol. 36 (2014) 93–102, https://doi.org/10.1007/s00281-013-0400-x.

[132] J. Rauch, D. Salem, R. Subang, M. Kuwana, J.S. Levine, β2-glycoprotein I-reactive T cells in autoimmune disease, Front. Immunol. 9 (2018) 2836, https://doi.org/10.3389/fimmu.2018.02836.

[133] P. Sima, L. Vannucci, V. Vetvicka, Atherosclerosis as autoimmune disease, Ann. Transl. Med. 6 (2018) 116, https://doi.org/10.21037/atm.2018.02.02.

[134] J. Bass, Circadian topology of metabolism, Nature 491 (2012) 348–356.

[135] M.M. Bellet, E. Deriu, J.Z. Liu, B. Grimaldi, C. Blaschitz, M. Zeller, et al., Circadian clock regulates the host response to Salmonella, Proc. Natl. Acad. Sci. U. S. A. 110 (2013) 9897–9902.

[136] J.E. Gibbs, J. Blaikley, S. Beesley, L. Matthews, K.D. Simpson, S.H. Boyce, et al., The nuclear receptor REV-ERBα mediates circadian regulation of innate immunity through selective regulation of inflammatory cytokines, Proc. Natl. Acad. Sci. U. S. A. 109 (2012) 582–587, https://doi.org/10.1073/pnas.1106750109.

[137] M. Keller, J. Mazuch, U. Abraham, G.D. Eom, E.D. Herzog, H.D. Volk, et al., A circadian clock in macrophages controls inflammatory immune responses, Proc. Natl. Acad. Sci. U. S. A. 106 (2009) 21407–21412.

[138] J.O. Early, A.M. Curtis, Immunometabolism: is it under the eye of the clock? Semin. Immunol. (2016), https://doi.org/10.1016/j.smim.2016.10.006.

[139] K. Man, A. Loudon, A. Chawla, Immunity around the clock, Science 354 (2016) 999–1003, https://doi.org/10.1126/science.aah4966.

[140] W. He, S. Holtkamp, S.M. Hergenhan, K. Kraus, A. de Juan, J. Weber, et al., Circadian expression of migratory factors establishes lineage-specific signatures that guide the homing of leukocyte subsets to tissues, Immunity 49 (2018) 1175–1190.e7, https://doi.org/10.1016/j.immuni.2018.10.007.

[141] A.M. Curtis, M.M. Bellet, P. Sassone-Corsi, L.A. O'Neill, Circadian clock proteins and immunity, Immunity 40 (2014) 178–186.

[142] N. Labrecque, N. Cermakian, Circadian clocks in the immune system, J. Biol. Rhythm. 30 (2015) 277–290, https://doi.org/10.1177/0748730415577723.

[143] F. Rijo-Ferreira, J.S. Takahashi, Genomics of circadian rhythms in health and disease, Genome Med. 11 (2019) 82, https://doi.org/10.1186/s13073-019-0704-0.

[144] J. Bass, M.A. Lazar, Circadian time signatures of fitness and disease, Science 354 (2016) 994–999, https://doi.org/10.1126/science.aah4965.

[145] M. Cuesta, P. Boudreau, G. Dubeau-Laramee, N. Cermakian, D.B. Boivin, Simulated night shift disrupts circadian rhythms of immune functions in humans, J. Immunol. 196 (2016) 2466–2475, https://doi.org/10.4049/jimmunol.1502422.

[146] C.J. Morris, T.E. Purvis, K. Hu, F.A. Scheer, Circadian misalignment increases cardiovascular disease risk factors in humans, Proc. Natl. Acad. Sci. U. S. A. 113 (2016) E1402–E1411, https://doi.org/10.1073/pnas.1516953113.

[147] A. Videnovic, A.S. Lazar, R.A. Barker, S. Overeem, 'The clocks that time us'—circadian rhythms in neurodegenerative disorders, Nat. Rev. Neurol. 10 (2014) 683–693, https://doi.org/10.1038/nrneurol.2014.206.

[148] C.C. Nobis, N. Labrecque, N. Cermakian, From immune homeostasis to inflammation, a question of rhythms, Curr. Opin. Physiol. 5 (2018) 90–98, https://doi.org/10.1016/j.cophys.2018.09.001.

[149] S. Gustavsen, H.B. Søndergaard, D.B. Oturai, B. Laursen, J.H. Laursen, M. Magyari, et al., Shift work at young age is associated with increased risk of multiple sclerosis in a Danish population, Mult. Scler. Relat. Disord. 9 (2016) 104–109, https://doi.org/10.1016/j.msard.2016.06.010.

[150] D. Druzd, O. Matveeva, L. Ince, U. Harrison, W. He, C. Schmal, et al., Lymphocyte circadian clocks control lymph node trafficking and adaptive immune responses, Immunity 46 (2017) 120–132, https://doi.org/10.1016/j.immuni.2016.12.011.

[151] C.E. Sutton, C.M. Finlay, M. Raverdeau, J.O. Early, J. DeCourcey, Z. Zaslona, et al., Loss of the molecular clock in myeloid cells exacerbates T cell-mediated CNS autoimmune disease, Nat. Commun. 8 (2017) 1923, https://doi.org/10.1038/s41467-017-02111-0.

[152] M. Amir, S. Chaudhari, R. Wang, S. Campbell, S.A. Mosure, L.B. Chopp, et al., REV-ERBα regulates TH17 cell development and autoimmunity, Cell Rep. 25 (2018) 3733–3749.e8, https://doi.org/10.1016/j.celrep.2018.11.101.

[153] X.O. Yang, B.P. Pappu, R. Nurieva, A. Akimzhanov, H.S. Kang, Y. Chung, et al., T Helper 17 lineage differentiation is programmed by orphan nuclear receptors RORα and RORγ, Immunity 28 (2008) 29–39, https://doi.org/10.1016/j.immuni.2007.11.016.

[154] J.A. Harkness, M.B. Richter, G.S. Panayi, K.V. de Pette, A. Unger, R. Pownall, et al., Circadian variation in disease activity in rheumatoid arthritis, Br. Med. J. (Clin. Res. Ed.) 284 (1982) 551, https://doi.org/10.1136/bmj.284.6315.551.

[155] T.M. Poolman, J. Gibbs, A.L. Walker, S. Dickson, L. Farrell, J. Hensman, et al., Rheumatoid arthritis reprograms circadian output pathways, Arthritis Res. Ther. 21 (2019) 47, https://doi.org/10.1186/s13075-019-1825-y.

[156] L.E. Hand, T.W. Hopwood, S.H. Dickson, A.L. Walker, A.S.I. Loudon, D.W. Ray, et al., The circadian clock regulates inflammatory arthritis, FASEB J. 30 (2016) 3759–3770, https://doi.org/10.1096/fj.201600353r.

[157] A. Hashiramoto, T. Yamane, K. Tsumiyama, K. Yoshida, K. Komai, H. Yamada, et al., Mammalian clock gene cryptochrome regulates arthritis via proinflammatory cytokine TNF-α, J. Immunol. 184 (2010) 1560–1565, https://doi.org/10.4049/jimmunol.0903284.

[158] Y.-L. Dan, C.-N. Zhao, Y.-M. Mao, Q. Wu, Y.-S. He, Y.-Q. Hu, et al., Association of PER2 gene single nucleotide polymorphisms with genetic susceptibility to systemic lupus erythematosus, Lupus (2021), https://doi.org/10.1177/0961203321989794, 096120332198979.

[159] C. Billon, M.H. Murray, A. Avdagic, T.P. Burris, RORγ regulates the NLRP3 inflammasome, J. Biol. Chem. 294 (2019) 10–19, https://doi.org/10.1074/jbc.ac118.002127.

[160] S. Wang, Y. Lin, X. Yuan, F. Li, L. Guo, B. Wu, REV-ERBα integrates colon clock with experimental colitis through regulation of NF-κB/NLRP3 axis, Nat. Commun. 9 (2018) 4246, https://doi.org/10.1038/s41467-018-06568-5.

[161] D. Yu, X. Fang, Y. Xu, H. Xiao, T. Huang, Y. Zhang, et al., Rev-erbα can regulate the NF-κB/NALP3 pathway to modulate lipopolysaccharide-induced acute lung injury and inflammation, Int. Immunopharmacol. 73 (2019) 312–320, https://doi.org/10.1016/j.intimp.2019.04.035.

[162] E. Woldt, Y. Sebti, L.A. Solt, C. Duhem, S. Lancel, J. Eeckhoute, et al., Rev-erb-alpha modulates skeletal muscle oxidative capacity by regulating mitochondrial biogenesis and autophagy, Nat. Med. 19 (2013) 1039–1046.

[163] Y. Lin, S. Wang, L. Gao, Z. Zhou, Z. Yang, J. Lin, et al., Oscillating lncRNA Platr4 regulates NLRP3 inflammasome to ameliorate nonalcoholic steatohepatitis in mice, Theranostics 11 (2021) 426–444, https://doi.org/10.7150/thno.50281.

[164] C.J. Reitz, F.J. Alibhai, T.N. Khatua, M. Rasouli, B.W. Bridle, T.P. Burris, et al., SR9009 administered for one day after myocardial ischemia-reperfusion prevents heart failure in mice by targeting the cardiac inflammasome, Commun. Biol. 2 (2019) 353, https://doi.org/10.1038/s42003-019-0595-z.

[165] R.C. Coll, A.A. Robertson, J.J. Chae, S.C. Higgins, R. Munoz-Planillo, M.C. Inserra, et al., A small-molecule inhibitor of the NLRP3 inflammasome for the treatment of inflammatory diseases, Nat. Med. 21 (2015) 248–255.

[166] M.S.J. Mangan, E.J. Olhava, W.R. Roush, H.M. Seidel, G.D. Glick, E. Latz, Targeting the NLRP3 inflammasome in inflammatory diseases, Nat. Rev. Drug Discov. 17 (2018) 688, https://doi.org/10.1038/nrd.2018.149.

[167] D. Chauhan, L.V. Walle, M. Lamkanfi, Therapeutic modulation of inflammasome pathways, Immunol. Rev. 297 (2020) 123–138, https://doi.org/10.1111/imr.12908.

[168] K. Rudolphi, N. Gerwin, N. Verzijl, P. van der Kraan, W. van den Berg, Pralnacasan, an inhibitor of interleukin-1β converting enzyme, reduces joint damage in two murine models of osteoarthritis, Osteoarthr. Cartil. 11 (2003) 738–746, https://doi.org/10.1016/s1063-4584(03)00153-5.

[169] S.H. MacKenzie, J.L. Schipper, A.C. Clark, The potential for caspases in drug discovery, Curr. Opin. Drug Discov. Devel. 13 (2010) 568–576.

[170] Y. Zhang, Y. Zheng, Effects and mechanisms of potent caspase-1 inhibitor VX765 treatment on collagen-induced arthritis in mice, Clin. Exp. Rheumatol. 34 (2016) 111–118.

[171] W. Wannamaker, R. Davies, M. Namchuk, J. Pollard, P. Ford, G. Ku, et al., (S)-1-((S)-2-{[1-(4-Amino-3-chloro-phenyl)-methanoyl]-amino}-3,3-dimethyl-butanoyl)-pyrrolidine-2-carboxylic acid ((2R,3S)-2-ethoxy-5-oxo-tetrahydro-furan-3-yl)-amide (VX-765), an orally available selective interleukin (IL)-converting enzyme/caspase-1 inhibitor, exhibits potent anti-inflammatory activities by inhibiting the release of IL-1β and IL-18, J. Pharmacol. Exp. Ther. 321 (2007) 509–516, https://doi.org/10.1124/jpet.106.111344.

[172] E.V. Granowitz, R. Porat, J.W. Mier, J.P. Pribble, D.M. Stiles, D.C. Bloedow, et al., Pharmacokinetics, safety and immunomodulatory effects of human recombinant interleukin-1 receptor antagonist in healthy humans, Cytokine 4 (1992) 353–360, https://doi.org/10.1016/1043-4666(92)90078-6.

[173] A. Chakraborty, S. Tannenbaum, C. Rordorf, P.J. Lowe, D. Floch, H. Gram, et al., Pharmacokinetic and pharmacodynamic properties of canakinumab, a human anti-interleukin-1β monoclonal antibody, Clin. Pharmacokinet. 51 (2012) e1–18, https://doi.org/10.2165/11599820-000000000-00000.

[174] R. Alten, J. Gomez-Reino, P. Durez, A. Beaulieu, A. Sebba, G. Krammer, et al., Efficacy and safety of the human anti-IL-1beta monoclonal antibody canakinumab in rheumatoid arthritis: results of a 12-week, phase II, dose-finding study, BMC Musculoskelet. Disord. 12 (2011) 153, https://doi.org/10.1186/1471-2474-12-153.

[175] J.E. Orrock, N.T. Ilowite, Canakinumab for the treatment of active systemic juvenile idiopathic arthritis, Expert. Rev. Clin. Pharmacol. 9 (2016) 1–10, https://doi.org/10.1080/17512433.2016.1204910.

[176] G. Sulli, E.N.C. Manoogian, P.R. Taub, S. Panda, Training the circadian clock, clocking the drugs, and drugging the clock to prevent, manage, and treat chronic diseases, Trends Pharmacol. Sci. 39 (2018) 812–827, https://doi.org/10.1016/j.tips.2018.07.003.

[177] Q. Zeng, H. Deng, Y. Li, T. Fan, Y. Liu, S. Tang, et al., Berberine directly targets the NEK7 protein to block the NEK7–NLRP3 interaction and exert anti-inflammatory activity, J. Med. Chem. 64 (2020) 768–781, https://doi.org/10.1021/acs.jmedchem.0c01743.

[178] Z. Zhou, Y. Lin, L. Gao, Z. Yang, S. Wang, B. Wu, Circadian pharmacological effects of berberine on chronic colitis in mice: Role of the clock component Rev-erbα, Biochem. Pharmacol. 172 (2020) 113773, https://doi.org/10.1016/j.bcp.2019.113773.

[179] C. Winter, C. Silvestre-Roig, A. Ortega-Gomez, P. Lemnitzer, H. Poelman, A. Schumski, et al., Chrono-pharmacological targeting of the CCL2-CCR2 axis ameliorates atherosclerosis, Cell Metab. 28 (2018) 175–182. e5, https://doi.org/10.1016/j.cmet.2018.05.002.

CHAPTER

9

Plasmocyte depletion in autoimmune diseases

Nathalie Sturm[a,b] and Bertrand Huard[b,*]

[a]Department of Pathology, University Hospital, Grenoble, France
[b]TIMC-IMAG Laboratory, CNRS UMR5525, University Grenoble-Alpes, La Tronche, France
*Corresponding author

Abstract

B-cells have recently been successfully targeted in autoimmune diseases. Indeed, depletion of the mature B-cell pool with cytotoxic antibodies directed against CD20/CD19 and antagonism of the B-cell activating factor from the TNF family led to drug approval in several diseases. Notably, this success was achieved with reagents not impacting directly the autoantibody-secreting effector plasmocytes. Here, we are listing the candidate targets that may be used to deplete plasmocytes. We are also discussing the benefits provided to autoimmunity by such putative treatments.

Keywords

B-cell therapies, CD19, CD20, BAFF, Plasmocytes, Autoimmunity

1 Introduction

Our immune system is sometimes dysfunctioning by reacting against our own body, conducting to a so-called autoimmune disease. Outcome of these diseases may be fatal to patients when associated with the failure of the targeted organ. The adaptive arm of the immune system plays the main pathogenic role in an autoimmune reaction. CD8[+] and to a lesser extent CD4[+] T cells will immediately display cytotoxic functions when recognizing self-antigens presented at the surface of host cells. The humoral immunity with the high and constitutive secretion of antibodies by plasmocytes also mediates cytotoxic functions. The latter is done indirectly when the antibody is bound at the host cell surface and triggers natural killer cells/macrophages and the complement system to mediate antibody-dependent cellular and complement dependent, respectively, cytotoxicities. One may also notice that antibodies may induce organ dysfunction by modulating the physiological function of a key receptor at the surface of a host cell without inducing any death.

Drugs classified under the generic term immunosuppressive are used to control most of the autoimmune diseases. Two main categories exist, corticoids and anti-mitotic reagents. Corticoids act via a specific cytoplasmic receptor, which shuts down the transcription of many inflammatory genes when stimulated by a membrane permeable reagent. In effector T cells, it will diminish the production of many cytokines including IL-2, their main growth factor. The cytotoxic perforin/granzyme pathway is also impaired by glucocorticoids [1]. In addition, corticoids decrease the overall inflammation of the tissue leading to decrease in access to blood leukocytes. Anti-mitotic reagents as their name indicate inhibit cell proliferation. They may act in different manners, by suppressing nucleotide synthesis (methotrexate, mycophenolate mofetil, hydroxyurea, 5-fluorouracil), by being nucleotide substitutes (azathioprine) and by alkylating the DNA (cyclophosphamide). These reagents will dampen the massive T-and B-cell proliferation induced during an autoimmune immune response so that the pool of autoreactive cells generated will be extensively contracted. Based on their action mode, it is obvious to conclude that all these reagents are not specific to immune cells, and adverse effects are frequently seen in patients. In addition, none of these drugs directly impact plasmocytes. Indeed, corticoids have never been shown to act on immunoglobulin synthesis. Furthermore, anti-mitotic reagents are also not efficient on plasmocytes, which are, by definition for terminally differentiated cells, quiescent. The lack of plasmocyte susceptibility to these reagents has been well documented in animal models [2,3]. Taken together, these highlight the fact that autoimmune diseases are treated by regimen sparing one harmful autoimmune effector cell, the plasmocyte. Leaving alive autoimmune effector cells able by themselves to trigger the disease may conduct to a lifelong treatment and/or relapses at treatment withdrawal. These two situations are frequently seen in autoimmune patients. The aim of this chapter is to translate the knowledge acquired on plasmocyte biology into druggable targets, review the drugs available or currently in clinical trials to achieve this effect and ideally suggest new targets. Finally, a list of autoimmune diseases that may benefit of plasmocyte targeting will be presented.

2 The plasmocyte

Plasmocytes are the effector cells of the humoral immunity own to their ability to constitutively secrete a high amount of antibodies. They represent the terminal differentiation stage of this humoral response. Plasmocytes are derived from mature B-lymphocytes activated once their receptor, the B-cell receptor (BCR), encounters its cognate antigen. This activation occurs in secondary lymphoid organs and the activated B cells differentiate into several stages before becoming an antibody-producing cells. At first, activated B cells enter a neostructure build in secondary lymphoid organs draining an inflamed tissue, the germinal center (GC). In GCs, the fittest B-lymphocytes, selected according to the affinity of its BCR for the antigen, are able to leave the structure, and start producing antibodies. At that stage, the cells called plasmablasts are proliferative. Plasmablasts in secondary lymphoid organs are short-lived due to the lack of survival factors provided by the environment. Hence, plasmablasts must leave the secondary lymphoid organ to find a supportive environment enabling them to survive. The selection of the fittest B cells is T-cell dependent since it relies on a CD4$^+$ T-cell subset, the follicular helper subset, specific for the BCR-cognate antigen presented by the B cells onto their major histocompatibility complex of class II. Before all this sophisticated response, there is a first wave of plasmablasts produced in draining secondary lymphoid organs that does not pass through GCs, and are produced independently of T cells. They are the source of an early production of low-affinity antibodies. Note that in some nonlymphoid tissues usually highly inflamed, structures called ectopic GCs fulfill the same function to deliver antibody-producing cells directly in the tissue. Finally, B cells may also respond in a T-cell independent way for some peculiar antigens. These antigens must highly crosslink the BCR or give a costimulatory signal to B cells by triggering their Toll-like receptors.

Plasmablasts rapidly leave secondary lymphoid organs by reaching the blood circulation and will respond to the chemotactic signal provided by tissues. Most of the cells will be unable to achieve this and will dye in the secondary lymphoid tissue. The inflamed tissue will produce chemokines able to recruit plasmablasts. These chemokines are from the CXCL class, CXCL-9, −10, and −11 [4]. While it has been demonstrated that these three chemokines are interferon inducible, their cellular source in tissue remains poorly described. The receptor responding to these chemokines expressed by plasmablasts is CXCR3 [5]. This homing pathway dependent on inflammation is insuring a local function for antibodies. The inflamed tissue is not the only homing site for effector antibody-producing cells, and this is a specificity of the humoral response. Indeed, a fraction of the blood circulating plasmablasts ends up in the bone marrow under the chemoattraction of another CXCL chemokine, CXCL-12 [4]. On the contrary to the other chemokines, CXCL-12 is produced constitutively by the bone marrow in the steady state, because it has to fulfill several hematopoietic functions. Bone marrow stromal cells produce CXCL-12. The responding receptor expressed by plasmablasts is CXCR-4. Once homed in the bone marrow, plasmablasts become quiescent and persist at a terminally differentiated stage, the plasmocyte, in structures called niches, which provide them constitutively with survival factors. It is thought that bone marrow plasmocytes persist for decades in a single niche, for this reason, they are called memory plasmocytes. In a niche, they lose their ability to respond to a chemotactic signal. Own to a highly sophisticated intravital imaging experimentation, it has been possible to record nonmotile plasmocytes in bone marrow niches for up to 30 min in mouse [6].

As said previously, plasmocytes rely on survival factors provided by the environment to persist. Numerous factors able to transmit a survival signal to plasmocytes have been identified. The best-known survival factor is a proliferation inducing ligand (APRIL), member 13 of the tumor necrosis factor superfamily (TNFSF13) [7]. It is probably the most specific for plasmocytes since expression of its cognate receptor the transmembrane activator and calcium modulator and cyclophilin ligand interactor (TACI) and the B-cell maturation antigen (BCMA) are quite restricted to late differentiation stages of B-lymphocytes. TACI and BCMA are part of the TNF-receptor superfamily, TNFRSF13b and TNFRSF17, respectively. Many cell types from the bone marrow have been identified as producing APRIL. This includes megakaryocytes, resident eosinophils, and myeloid precursor cells [8–10]. Other factors classified as growth factors display a similar function. If one considers the growth factors identified with the use of multiple myeloma cells, the most common form of plasmocyte neoplasms, this concerns at least five molecules, the vascular endothelial growth factor, the heparin-binding epidermal growth factor, the hepatocyte growth factor, the fibroblast growth factor, and the insulin-like growth factor-binding protein. The source of these factors in the bone marrow has not been extensively studied. Notably, all these growth factors require the binding to heparan sulfate proteoglycan (HSPG) to efficiently signal into target cells [11]. This requirement is also shared by APRIL [12]. As a consequence, plasmocytes express a cognate receptor for all these factors as one unique HSPG, syndecan-1 also called CD138 [13]. CD138 is expressed on all differentiated plasmocytes and is a common marker used to identify these cells in the hematopoietic lineage [14]. In total, the chemokine responsible for the homing of plasmocytes in the bone marrow is unique, but many survival factors contribute to the long-term maintenance of these cells. The number of survival niches is thought to be limited [15]. This is well in agreement with the restricted number (range of 0.1–0.5% of the total cellularity) of plasmocytes that may be detected in the steady state from the bone marrow. However, this is in disagreement with observations regarding the abundant presence of key factors defining the niches. As two relevant examples, APRIL production peaks in myeloid precursor cells, which represent the most abundant hematopoietic cells in the bone marrow, and CXCL-12 should be massively produced to perform one of its hematopoietic functions, the retention of myeloid precursor cells during their maturation process. Detailed analysis of the plasmocyte population in the bone marrow revealed that it is not solely constituted by long-lived established plasmocytes. Indeed, it contains also newly formed plasmocytes from ongoing immune responses [16]. If one considers that the number of niches in bone marrow is limiting, this suggest that newly generated plasmocytes may replace old ones. Indeed, the replacement of established cells by newly generated plasmocytes was probed in an animal model [17]. Taken together, this is unlikely that the restricted pool of plasmocytes existing at a given time in a bone marrow will solely be responsible for the high concentration of antibodies that could be measured in the human population long after exposure to an infection or a vaccination. One explanation for that could be a recirculation pathway of established plasmocytes after a "rest" time from the bone marrow to the blood. Of note, cells close and/or constituting the blood vessels, perisinusoidal mesenchymal stem cells and endothelial cells, are the main source of CXCL-12 in the bone marrow. Hence, plasmocytes may transiently transit via the bone marrow by exiting the blood circulation to gain access to survival signals. Such a pathway has been well described for leukemic cells. In the gut, an organ also known to host plasmocytes, long-lived plasmocytes also exist [18]. Regarding inflamed nonlymphoid tissues, much less is known. It is even not yet sure whether antibody-secreting cells frequently infiltrating autoimmune tissues are plasmablasts or fully differentiated plasmocytes. One study performed in multiple sclerosis showed that they are more on the plasmocyte side due to their lack of the proliferative marker Ki67 [19]. On the other hand, another study performed in neuromyelitis optica showed that antibody-secreting cells in the cerebrospinal fluid are related to the plasmablast stage own to their expression of major histocompatibility complex of class II [20]. This is definitely the main black box, and efforts have to be made to characterize in more details antibody-secreting cells infiltrating autoimmune tissues.

Plasmocytes are best-known as effector cells producing antibodies. However, one should be aware that this is not their unique effector function. Indeed, plasmocytes have been described to produce toxic factors such as nitric oxide [21]. This has been demonstrated in the gut and may contribute to their pathogenic role in autoimmunity, although not yet demonstrated.

At variance, plasmocytes may exert regulatory functions by secreting the immunosuppressive cytokines IL-10 and IL-35 [22].

3 New drugs targeting the humoral immunity

As stated in the introduction, drugs applied to patients may be classified as nonspecific immunosuppressive agents, since they do act on nonimmune cells. These drugs are timely replaced by more specific reagents that are only targeting the immune system. They are either antibodies or solubilized receptors targeting immune molecules. This applies to the humoral immunity with the approval of two drugs targeting highly distinct molecules but achieving a quite similar immunosuppressive function as we will see below on in this paragraph.

The first approval concerns rheumatoid arthritis in 2006 and came from studies testing a cytotoxic chimeric antibody, rituximab, directed against a ubiquitous receptor expressed at the surface of B-lymphocytes in patients suffering from B-cell lymphoma. The drug was found highly active as expected, but most importantly for our present consideration a case report was published showing benefits also observed at the autoimmune level in a patient co-suffering from rheumatoid arthritis [23]. Hence, a new therapeutic way in autoimmunity was coined, the B-cell depletion. This approval was extended to pemphigus vulgaris in 2018. The targeted molecule on B cells was the CD20 molecule. At that time, it was known that all mature B cells express CD20, but a physiological function was elusive. CD20 is a tetraspan membrane molecule. It is thought to play a role in signaling own to its association with the BCR. There is no ligand described so far. The function of CD20 appears rather discrete and/ or redundant since no gross alteration of B-cell responses was observed in CD20-deficient animals [24]. In the human system, deficient patients mount impaired T-independent antibody responses [25]. Ocrelizumab, the second-generation humanized anti-CD20 was approved for multiple sclerosis in 2017. In June 2020, one could count not less than 14 other autoimmune diseases tested with an anti-CD20 according to clinicaltrials.gov. This includes systemic lupus erythematosus, systemic sclerosis, vasculitis, hemolytic anemia, membranous nephropathy, Grave's disease, T1 diabetes, IgA nephropathy, neuromyelitis optica, Stiff Person syndrome, thrombocytopenia, polyangitis, Sjögren's syndrome, and autoimmune encephalitis. In addition to ocrelizumab, other humanized anti-CD20, veltuzumab, ocaratuzumab (mutated for an improved Fc receptor binding) and obinutuzumab (glycoengineered to remove fucose residues) have been developed. A fully human anti-CD20, ofatumumab, also exists. Taken together, a large panel of compounds is nowadays available to target CD20 in autoimmunity.

The second approval concerns systemic lupus erythematosus in 2011 and is based on an antagonist antibody, belimumab, directed against the B-cell activation factor from the TNF superfamily (BAFF). BAFF is one of the latest identified members of this superfamily, TNFSF13b [26]. Precisely, BAFF acts on B-cells extramedullary at their last immature stage, the transitional one, to provide a survival signal enabling them to reach their final mature stage. It does so by stimulating BAFF-R [27]. Note that BAFF shares two common receptors with the APRIL molecule defined above, TACI and BCMA [28]. However, these latter receptors are not involved in this process. BAFF-deficient animals gave stricking phenotype with the almost complete disappearance of the mature B-cell pool. Such a result has been the proof of concept to design a BAFF antagonism in the B-cell depletion era. In June 2020, one could count not less than eight other autoimmune diseases tested with belimumab according to clinicaltrials.gov. This includes vasculitis, polyangitis, membranous nephropathy, systemic sclerosis, myositis, Sjögren's syndrome, rheumatoid arthritis, thrombocytopenia, and Grave's disease. Another humanized BAFF, tabalumab, is also under development.

One important concern regarding CD20 and BAFF targeting in autoimmunity is their lack of action on established plasmocytes. Indeed, both CD20 and BAFF-R expressions are lost upon differentiation of B cells into plasmocytes. As described previously, BAFF has two other receptors, TACI and BCMA, in addition to BAFF-R. TACI is only expressed by a fraction of plasmocytes, while BCMA is ubiquitous. This render BAFF antagonism potentially efficient to target plasmocytes. However, this has not been observed experimentally [29]. The latter observation is due to the low affinity reported for BAFF with BCMA [30]. Taken together, these two treatments deplete patients' pool of mature B cells, impairing the generation of post-diagnostic new plasmocytes from mature B-cell precursors, but leaving untouched established plasmocytes. There is no doubt that these treatments show a great efficacy, and are definitely part of the therapeutic revolution that is currently ongoing in autoimmunity. They led to two new and essential non-overlapping concepts in autoimmunity. The first one is that autoimmune diseases triggered by pathogenic antibodies may be fueled in a chronic manner by constantly generated antibody-secreting cells. The second one is that B cells may play a significant role by their ability to mediate a non-antibody-secreting function such as the secretion of inflammatory cytokines and/or the presentation of autoantigens to T cells [31]. Nevertheless, a burning question remains, what is going on with the established plasmocytes secreting pathogenic antibodies left in patients upon treatment. As a relevant example, we are providing evidences that plasmocytes infiltrating an autoimmune tissue, the liver of autoimmune hepatitis, and the thyroid of an Hashimoto disease are not susceptible to these two treatments own to their lack of CD20 and BAFFR (Fig. 1).

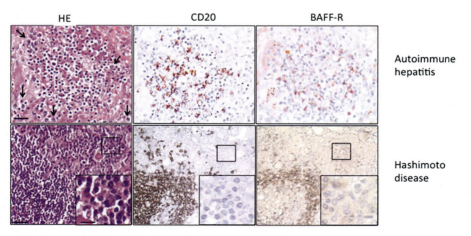

FIG. 1 Expression of CD20 and BAFF-R in plasmocytes infiltrating autoimmune organs. Serial sections of an autoimmune liver (upper panel) and an autoimmune thyroid (bottom panel) were stained with hematoxilin-eosin (HE), anti-CD20, and anti-BAFF-R by immunohistochemistry. Arrows in the upper panel show plasmocytes. Scale bar: 20 μm. Box and insert in the bottom panel show a regions of extrafollicular plasmocyte accumulation. Scale bar: 5 μm for inserts.

4 Drugs in the pipeline

B-cell depletion has demonstrated a clear efficacy and is at the origin of many trials in autoimmunity. In addition to the extensive list of autoimmune diseases tested with anti-CD20 and anti-BAFF antibodies, new targets are also currently tested/developed. Other surface receptors ubiquitously expressed at the surface of mature B cells have been identified. The depleting antibody inebilizumab and the nondepleting antibody epratuzumab, have been generated against CD19 and CD22, respectively [32,33]. CD19 is a molecule from the immunoglobulin superfamily [34]. It is part of the BCR complex at the surface of B cells, associating with the other coreceptors CD21 and CD81 and contributing to B-cell signaling. CD19-deficient mice showed impaired B-cell responses. Patients deficient for CD19 suffer from antibody paucity. CD22 is part of the family of sialic acid-recognizing Ig superfamily lectins [35]. Epratuzumab induces only a modest depletion of B cells. However, it potently inhibits B-cell activation due to the fact that CD22 is an inhibitory receptor containing in its cytoplasmic tail an immunoreceptor tyrosine-based inhibition motif. Genetically deficient animals for CD22 harbor an upregulation of serum IgM and in some case of autoantibodies. BAFF-R is also targeted with the depleting antibody ianalumab [36]. BAFF-R is the only BAFF receptor on mature naive B cells, and belongs to the TNF superfamily [37]. BAFF-R transduces a key late survival signal to immature B cells. BAFF-R deficient animals display a profound alteration in their peripheral pool of mature B cells. A similar phenotype was observed in deficient patients. Another compound targeting BAFF, atacicept, is also currently tested in advanced clinical trials [38]. Atacicept is a solubilized form of the common BAFF/APRIL receptor, TACI. Due to the APRIL specificity, atacicept is able to deplete established plasmocytes. These have been demonstrated in animal models [39]. Two antagonist antibodies directed against APRIL have also been generated [40,41]. These reagents have not yet been tested in autoimmune diseases, but one of them is tested in IgA nephropathy, a syndrome also driven by an aberrant production of antibodies. Finally, bortezomib, a proteasome inhibitor used to treat multiple myeloma is also tested in autoimmunity. Proteasome inhibition leads to plasmocyte apoptosis by the lethal accumulation of unfolded proteins mostly constituted by immunoglobulins.

Among this list of new drugs in clinical trials, what are the best candidates to target plasmocytes? As stated above, CD20 expression is lost during plasmocyte differentiation. Gradual decrease of CD20 starts at the plasmablast stage, so that these cells residing in secondary lymphoid organs during their genesis and circulating in the blood harbors an intermediate level of CD20 expression [42]. In the bone marrow, all antibody-producing cells are CD20 negative. The latter is also true in the gut. CD19 bears the advantage to be lost after CD20 during plasmocyte differentiation. Hence, there is a fraction of antibody-secreting cells in bone marrow that still expresses CD19, as well as in the gut. An extensive literature exists on this issue. Some authors have reported that the CD19$^-$ cells are the major fraction of antibody-secreting cells in the human bone marrow [43]. Detailed analysis in the mouse system revealed that CD19$^+$ antibody-secreting cells in the bone marrow harbors signs of immaturity with a higher expression of MHC class II and lower expression of the transcription factor Blimp-1. Hence, it is thought that CD19$^+$ cells represent an intermediate stage before terminal differentiation in long-lived cells [44]. CD22 pattern of expression during B-cell differentiation mirrors that of CD20 [45]. BAFF-R is also lost upon differentiation and found absent in bone marrow antibody-producing cells [46]. At variance, atacicept is clearly a good candidate, and may present the advantage to also impair the inflammatory/antigen presentation action of B cells (if needed) by its action on BAFF. Bortezomib is also a very good one. It has been shown to efficiently deplete plasmocytes in an animal model [47]. Time is needed to evaluate this promising reagents in autoimmunity. Bortezomib is the first molecule to make the jump from the multiple myeloma hemato-oncology field to the autoimmunity one. Very certainly it will not be the only one. Indeed, amazing progresses have recently been achieved in the specific field of multiple myeloma, a still incurable neoplasm, with the identification of surface receptors targeted by depleting compounds. These include anti-CD38 with daratumumab, anti-SLAM-F7 (originally called CS-1 and known as CD319) with elotuzumab and anti-BCMA with belantamab. These approaches are active against multiple myeloma tumor cells, and should therefore also be efficient for autoimmune diseases triggered by healthy plasmocytes. Some of these antibodies have been further developed as chimeric antigen receptors expressed at the surface of transduced T cells infused to patients. As of today, CAR-BCMA T cells appears to be extremely effective in multiple myeloma [48]. One may imagine a CAR-T cell approach applied to autoimmune patients in the future. Regarding the plasmocyte selectivity of these targets, BCMA is definitely the best candidate own to its ubiquitous and highly restricted expression. CD38 is less restricted with a wide expression on hematopoietic as well as non-hematopoietic cells. The expression of SLAM-F7 is less known, but it is at least expressed by NK cells.

Could we imagine new targets in addition to the ones discussed above? As stated above, plasmablasts are short-lived and need to find a survival niche. Homing to niches is driven by identified chemokines, and one may wish to target these chemokines to avoid long-term plasmocyte establishment. CXCR4 antagonist compounds have been generated own to its function as a coreceptor for the human immunodeficiency virus and its role in the metastasis of several solid tumors. These antagonists have been tested in animal models of autoimmunity [49]. However, the pleiotropic function of this chemokine receptor in immunity and hematopoiesis may constitute a chief barrier to translate it to patients. The existing antagonist of CXCR3 has also been tested in animal models of autoimmunity [50].

Survival factors produced by plasmocyte-specific niches are also quite well known. However, redundancy will clearly constitute a chief barrier. One way to circumvent this problem could be by targeting their common coreceptor, the HSPG CD138. According to the ubiquitous expression on plasmocytes, CD138 may be viewed as an ideal target. Drugs targeting CD138 have been designed for the purpose of multiple myeloma treatment [51]. Rationales differ in oncology and autoimmunity. Cancer treatments due to the high lethality associated with these diseases may tolerate adverse events. This is not the case in autoimmunity. In the case of CD138, it is highly unlikely that drugs targeting this molecule will be applied to autoimmune patients given its known non-plasmocyte expression pattern. Indeed, this HSPG is expressed in vital organs such as the liver [52]. Nevertheless, CD138 might still be valuable to target plasmocytes in the case one considers posttranslational modifications occurring on its heparan sulfate chain. One may even think of using heparin, a low-molecular weight soluble HSPG or a derivative, as an antagonist of plasmocyte survival factors binding CD138. Such an approach has already been assessed in oncology [53]. Furthermore, heparan sulfate chains associated to the proteoglycan protein core of HSPG are variable according to their pattern of sulfation, and this variation is cell type-specific according to the pattern of expression of sulfotransferases in a given cell [54]. We have even observed in the laboratory that the heparan sulfate motif varies according to the organ homing plasmocytes (unpublished data). In consequence, one may imagine finding organ-specific targets at the surface of plasmocytes. Such target will constitute a quite ideal treatment; specific to a single autoimmune disease, if one considers the targeting of plasmocytes frequently infiltrating the autoimmune tissue (see below).

Autologous hematopoietic stem cell transplantation following a lymphoablative regimen is considered in the treatment of refractory autoimmunity [55]. Such an approach has the advantage to wipe out all precursors of pathogenic immune cells that still reside in the patient. Aside from such a drastic treatment, specific removal of plasmocytes including the "bad" autoimmune ones might be possible by new vaccinations applied to patients. Indeed, animal models have clearly highlighted the fact that plasmocyte establishment in the bone marrow is reversible under the dominance of a competitive regulation process. Hence, patient vaccinations should eliminate "bad" plasmocytes with newly generated ones with, in addition, the advantage that these new cells will be directed against common human pathogens.

5 Autoimmune diseases that may benefit from plasmocyte targeting

Most if not all autoimmune diseases are associated with the presence of circulating auto-antibodies. These autoantibodies are directed against multiple self-components. One may distinguish two kinds of autoantibodies. The first kind is considered as a consequence of the autoimmune attack. This includes all antibodies directed against intracellular components, such as cytoplasmic/mitochondrial/nuclear proteins and DNA. These antibodies are thought to arise after an aberrant induction of host cell death, exposing new antigens that the immune system considers as nonself. Systemic lupus erythematous with its associated high cell death is clearly a relevant example. Indeed, all autoantibodies found in lupus patients are directed against nuclear antigens. Such autoantibodies are thought to exacerbate the disease by increasing the inflammation in the tissue(s) hosting cell death. There is no reason to target plasmocytes against these autoantigens, since new cells with an identical reactivity will be spontaneously regenerated. The autoimmune diseases that may benefit from plasmocyte targeting are diseases harboring autoantibodies directed against an antigen exposed at the cell surface, even transiently. Such antibodies may react with viable cells and initiate the disease, either by inducing antibody-dependent cellular and complement-dependent cytotoxicities or by interfering in an agonist and/or antagonist manner with the function of a key receptor for the physiological function of an organ. The best proof for the pathogenic property of these antibodies has been the passive transfer in animals followed by a rapid induction of the disease. Such proof has been obtained with cytotoxic antibodies and agonist/antagonist antibodies. Table 1 is giving a list of autoimmune diseases harboring a common autoantibody directed against a cell surface antigen. For some of these antibodies, pathogenicity has been demonstrated in an animal model by passive transfer. The infiltration of plasmocytes in the autoimmune tissue is indicated together with the presence of ectopic germinal centers. This is giving an idea on the putative location of pathogenic plasmocytes in the diseases. It is thought that patients also harbor medullary plasmocytes.

This table is telling us that autoimmune diseases associated to a pathogenic autoantibody are not rare. In most of the cases antibody-secreting cells localizes in the bone marrow as well

9. Plasmocyte depletion in autoimmune diseases

TABLE 1 List of the autoimmune diseases that may benefit from plasmocyte targeting.

Disease	PC Infiltration	Cell surface autoantigen	Host cell targeted
Autoimmune hepatitis	Yes[a]	Asialoglycoprotein	Hepatocyte
Rheumatoid arthritis	Yes[a]	Glucose-6-phosphate isomerase[b]	Synoviocyte
Sjögren disease	Yes[a]	Aquaporin-5	Acinar cell
Multiple sclerosis	Yes[a]	Myelin oligodendrocyte glycoprotein	Oligodendrocyte
Neuromyelitis optica	Yes[a]	Aquaporin 4[b]	Astrocyte
Autoimmune encephalitis	Yes	N-methyl D-aspartate receptor[b]	Neuron
Graves' disease	No	Thyroid-stimulating receptor[b]	Thyrocyte
Hashimoto disease	Yes[a]	Thyroglobulin[b]	Thyrocyte
Pemphigus vulgaris	Yes[a]	Desmoglein[b]	Keratinocyte
Myasthenia gravis	No	Acetylcholine receptor[b]	Myocyte

[a] Indicates presence of ectopic GCs in some patients.
[b] Indicates demonstration of pathogenicity upon passive transfer in an animal model.

as the autoimmune tissue. Also, a local generation of these cells may occur own to the presence of ectopic germinal centers, in addition to the one occurring in the draining lymph node. All these diseases may well benefit from a treatment targeting plasmocytes.

6 Conclusion

We have entered a new era regarding autoimmunity treatment with the introduction of immune-specific compounds that are timely replacing nonspecific immunosuppressive drugs applied for decades to patients. This revolution also concerns the humoral immunity with a wave of compounds under the general name of B-cell depletion agents. Two of these compounds have been approved after convincing results in advanced clinical trials, and now constitute either a first line add-on treatment (anti-BAFF in systemic lupus erythematous) or part of the therapeutic option (anti-CD20 in multiple sclerosis). New drugs showing promising effects in clinical trials are also in the pipeline. However, and quite unexpectedly, none of these drugs directly target the effector cell of the humoral immunity, the plasmocyte. Plasmocyte targeting still constitutes an actual challenge, especially for autoimmune diseases initially triggered by an autoantibody. One aim of this chapter was to list targets that may be at the basis of a plasmocyte-depletion treatment. Hopefully, such targets have already been identified. As of today, BCMA according to its highly specific expression pattern is thought to be the most promising one. Ideally, one may even want to target plasmocytes in an organ-specific manner to elaborate treatments specific of a single disease. In this latter situation, posttranslational modifications of the CD138 molecules exposed at the surface of plasmocytes should be scrutinized.

References

[1] J.L. Eddy, K. Krukowski, L. Janusek, H.L. Mathews, Glucocorticoids regulate natural killer cell function epigenetically, Cell. Immunol. 290 (1) (2014) 120–130.

[2] I.M. Mumtaz, B.F. Hoyer, D. Panne, K. Moser, O. Winter, Q.Y. Cheng, et al., Bone marrow of NZB/W mice is the major site for plasma cells resistant to dexamethasone and cyclophosphamide: implications for the treatment of autoimmunity, J. Autoimmun. 39 (3) (2012) 180–188.

[3] B.F. Hoyer, K. Moser, A.E. Hauser, A. Peddinghaus, C. Voigt, D. Eilat, et al., Short-lived plasmablasts and long-lived plasma cells contribute to chronic humoral autoimmunity in NZB/W mice, J. Exp. Med. 199 (11) (2004) 1577–1584.

[4] J.G. Cyster, Homing of antibody secreting cells, Immunol. Rev. 194 (2003) 48–60.

[5] S. Lacotte, M. Decossas, C. Le Coz, S. Brun, S. Muller, H. Dumortier, Early differentiated CD138(high) MHCII+ IgG+ plasma cells express CXCR3 and localize into inflamed kidneys of lupus mice, PLoS One 8 (3) (2013), e58140.

[6] S. Zehentmeier, K. Roth, Z. Cseresnyes, Ö. Sercan, K. Horn, R.A. Niesner, et al., Static and dynamic components synergize to form a stable survival niche for bone marrow plasma cells, Eur. J. Immunol. 44 (8) (2014) 2306–2317.

[7] M. Hahne, T. Kataoka, M. Schröter, K. Hofmann, M. Irmler, J.L. Bodmer, et al., APRIL, a new ligand of the tumor necrosis factor family, stimulates tumor cell growth, J. Exp. Med. 188 (6) (1998) 1185–1190.

[8] O. Winter, K. Moser, E. Mohr, D. Zotos, H. Kaminski, M. Szyska, et al., Megakaryocytes constitute a functional component of a plasma cell niche in the bone marrow, Blood 116 (11) (2010) 1867–1875.

[9] V.T. Chu, A. Fröhlich, G. Steinhauser, T. Scheel, T. Roch, S. Fillatreau, et al., Eosinophils are required for the maintenance of plasma cells in the bone marrow, Nat. Immunol. 12 (2) (2011) 151–159.

[10] T. Matthes, I. Dunand-Sauthier, M.L. Santiago-Raber, K.H. Krause, O. Donze, J. Passweg, et al., Production of the plasma-cell survival factor a proliferation-inducing ligand (APRIL) peaks in myeloid precursor cells from human bone marrow, Blood 118 (7) (2011) 1838–1844. [Internet]. Disponible sur http://www.ncbi.nlm.nih.gov/pubmed/21642598.

[11] M. Delehedde, M. Lyon, N. Sergeant, H. Rahmoune, D.G. Fernig, Proteoglycans: pericellular and cell surface multireceptors that integrate external stimuli in the mammary gland, J. Mammary Gland Biol. Neoplasia 6 (3) (2001) 253–273.

[12] K. Ingold, A. Zumsteg, A. Tardivel, B. Huard, Q.G. Steiner, T.G. Cachero, et al., Identification of proteoglycans as the APRIL-specific binding partners, J. Exp. Med. 201 (9) (2005) 1375–1383. [Internet]. Disponible sur http://www.ncbi.nlm.nih.gov/pubmed/15851487.

[13] C. Bret, D. Hose, T. Reme, A.-C. Sprynski, K. Mahtouk, J.-F. Schved, et al., Expression of genes encoding for proteins involved in heparan sulphate and chondroitin sulphate chain synthesis and modification in normal and malignant plasma cells, Br. J. Haematol. 145 (3) (2009) 350–368.

[14] J. Wijdenes, W.C. Vooijs, C. Clément, J. Post, F. Morard, N. Vita, et al., A plasmocyte selective monoclonal antibody (B-B4) recognizes syndecan-1, Br. J. Haematol. 94 (2) (1996) 318–323.

[15] T. Höfer, G. Muehlinghaus, K. Moser, T. Yoshida, H.E. Mei, K. Hebel, et al., Adaptation of humoral memory, Immunol. Rev. 211 (2006) 295–302.

[16] I. Chernova, D.D. Jones, J.R. Wilmore, A. Bortnick, M. Yucel, U. Hershberg, et al., Lasting antibody responses are mediated by a combination of newly formed and established bone marrow plasma cells drawn from clonally distinct precursors, J. Immunol. 193 (10) (2014) 4971–4979.

[17] T. Slocombe, S. Brown, K. Miles, M. Gray, T.A. Barr, D. Gray, Plasma cell homeostasis: the effects of chronic antigen stimulation and inflammation, J. Immunol. 191 (6) (2013) 3128–3138.

[18] O.J.B. Landsverk, O. Snir, R.B. Casado, L. Richter, J.E. Mold, P. Réu, et al., Antibody-secreting plasma cells persist for decades in human intestine, J. Exp. Med. 214 (2) (2017) 309–317.

[19] K. Pollok, R. Mothes, C. Ulbricht, A. Liebheit, J.D. Gerken, S. Uhlmann, et al., The chronically inflamed central nervous system provides niches for long-lived plasma cells, Acta Neuropathol. Commun. 5 (1) (2017) 88.

[20] N. Chihara, T. Aranami, S. Oki, T. Matsuoka, M. Nakamura, H. Kishida, et al., Plasmablasts as migratory IgG-producing cells in the pathogenesis of neuromyelitis optica, PLoS One 8 (12) (2013), e83036.

[21] J.H. Fritz, O.L. Rojas, N. Simard, D.D. McCarthy, S. Hapfelmeier, S. Rubino, et al., Acquisition of a multifunctional IgA+ plasma cell phenotype in the gut, Nature 481 (7380) (2011) 199–203.

[22] C. Cerqueira, B. Manfroi, S. Fillatreau, IL-10-producing regulatory B cells and plasmocytes: molecular mechanisms and disease relevance, Semin. Immunol. 44 (2019) 101323.

[23] A. Protheroe, J.C. Edwards, A. Simmons, K. Maclennan, P. Selby, Remission of inflammatory arthropathy in association with anti-CD20 therapy for non-Hodgkin's lymphoma, Rheumatology (Oxford) 38 (11) (1999) 1150–1152.

[24] J. Uchida, Y. Lee, M. Hasegawa, Y. Liang, A. Bradney, J.A. Oliver, et al., Mouse CD20 expression and function, Int. Immunol. 16 (1) (2004) 119–129.

[25] T.W. Kuijpers, R.J. Bende, P.A. Baars, A. Grummels, I.A.M. Derks, K.M. Dolman, et al., CD20 deficiency in humans results in impaired T cell-independent antibody responses, J. Clin. Invest. 120 (1) (2010) 214–222.

[26] P. Schneider, F. MacKay, V. Steiner, K. Hofmann, J.L. Bodmer, N. Holler, et al., BAFF, a novel ligand of the tumor necrosis factor family, stimulates B cell growth, J. Exp. Med. 189 (11) (1999) 1747–1756.

[27] J.S. Thompson, S.A. Bixler, F. Qian, K. Vora, M.L. Scott, T.G. Cachero, et al., BAFF-R, a newly identified TNF receptor that specifically interacts with BAFF, Science 293 (5537) (2001) 2108–2111. [Internet]. Disponible sur http://www.ncbi.nlm.nih.gov/pubmed/11509692.

[28] C. Bossen, P. Schneider, BAFF, APRIL and their receptors: structure, function and signaling, Semin. Immunol. 18 (5) (2006) 263–275.

[29] C. Bossen, T.G. Cachero, A. Tardivel, K. Ingold, L. Willen, M. Dobles, et al., TACI, unlike BAFF-R, is solely activated by oligomeric BAFF and APRIL to support survival of activated B cells and plasmablasts, Blood 111 (3) (2008) 1004–1012.

[30] E.S. Day, T.G. Cachero, F. Qian, Y. Sun, D. Wen, M. Pelletier, et al., Selectivity of BAFF/BLyS and APRIL for binding to the TNF family receptors BAFFR/BR3 and BCMA, Biochemistry 44 (6) (2005) 1919–1931.

[31] A. Getahun, J.C. Cambier, Non-antibody-secreting functions of B cells and their contribution to autoimmune disease, Annu. Rev. Cell Dev. Biol. 35 (2019) 337–356.

[32] F. Paul, O. Murphy, S. Pardo, M. Levy, Investigational drugs in development to prevent neuromyelitis optica relapses, Expert Opin. Investig. Drugs 27 (3) (2018) 265–271.

[33] D. Geh, C. Gordon, Epratuzumab for the treatment of systemic lupus erythematosus, Expert. Rev. Clin. Immunol. 14 (4) (2018) 245–258.

[34] T.F. Tedder, CD19: a promising B cell target for rheumatoid arthritis, Nat. Rev. Rheumatol. 5 (10) (2009) 572–577.

[35] V.S. Mahajan, S. Pillai, Sialic acids and autoimmune disease, Immunol. Rev. 269 (1) (2016) 145–161.

[36] T. Dörner, M.G. Posch, Y. Li, O. Petricoul, M. Cabanski, J.M. Milojevic, et al., Treatment of primary Sjögren's syndrome with ianalumab (VAY736) targeting B cells by BAFF receptor blockade coupled with enhanced, antibody-dependent cellular cytotoxicity, Ann. Rheum. Dis. 78 (5) (2019) 641–647.

[37] C.R. Smulski, H. Eibel, BAFF and BAFF-receptor in B cell selection and survival, Front. Immunol. 9 (2018) 2285.

[38] E. Samy, S. Wax, B. Huard, H. Hess, P. Schneider, Targeting BAFF and APRIL in systemic lupus erythematosus and other antibody-associated diseases, Int. Rev. Immunol. 36 (1) (2017) 3–19.

[39] P. Haselmayer, M. Vigolo, J. Nys, P. Schneider, H. Hess, A mouse model of systemic lupus erythematosus responds better to soluble TACI than to soluble BAFFR, correlating with depletion of plasma cells, Eur. J. Immunol. 47 (6) (2017) 1075–1085.

[40] M. Guadagnoli, F.C. Kimberley, U. Phan, K. Cameron, P.M. Vink, H. Rodermond, et al., Development and characterization of APRIL antagonistic monoclonal antibodies for treatment of B-cell lymphomas, Blood 117 (25) (2011) 6856–6865.

[41] J.R. Myette, T. Kano, H. Suzuki, S.E. Sloan, K.J. Szretter, B. Ramakrishnan, et al., A proliferation inducing ligand (APRIL) targeted antibody is a safe and effective treatment of murine IgA nephropathy, Kidney Int. 96 (1) (2019) 104–116.

[42] H.E. Mei, S. Schmidt, T. Dörner, Rationale of anti-CD19 immunotherapy: an option to target autoreactive plasma cells in autoimmunity, Arthritis Res. Ther. 14 (Suppl. 5) (2012) S1.

[43] D.C. Nguyen, C.J. Joyner, I. Sanz, F.E.-H. Lee, Factors affecting early antibody secreting cell maturation into long-lived plasma cells, Front. Immunol. 10 (2019) 2138.

[44] A. Kallies, J. Hasbold, D.M. Tarlinton, W. Dietrich, L.M. Corcoran, P.D. Hodgkin, et al., Plasma cell ontogeny defined by quantitative changes in blimp-1 expression, J. Exp. Med. 200 (8) (2004) 967–977.

[45] F. Hiepe, A. Radbruch, Plasma cells as an innovative target in autoimmune disease with renal manifestations, Nat. Rev. Nephrol. 12 (4) (2016) 232–240.

[46] J.R. Darce, B.K. Arendt, X. Wu, D.F. Jelinek, Regulated expression of BAFF-binding receptors during human B cell differentiation, J. Immunol. 179 (11) (2007) 7276–7286.

[47] T. Alexander, Q. Cheng, J. Klotsche, L. Khodadadi, A. Waka, R. Biesen, et al., Proteasome inhibition with bortezomib induces a therapeutically relevant depletion of plasma cells in SLE but does not target their precursors, Eur. J. Immunol. 48 (9) (2018) 1573–1579.

[48] M. D'Agostino, N. Raje, Anti-BCMA CAR T-cell therapy in multiple myeloma: can we do better? Leukemia 34 (1) (2020) 21–34.

[49] E.M. García-Cuesta, C.A. Santiago, J. Vallejo-Díaz, Y. Juarranz, J.M. Rodríguez-Frade, M. Mellado, The role of the CXCL12/CXCR4/ACKR3 axis in autoimmune diseases, Front. Endocrinol. (Lausanne) 10 (2019) 585.

[50] M. Metzemaekers, V. Vanheule, R. Janssens, S. Struyf, P. Proost, Overview of the mechanisms that may contribute to the non-redundant activities of interferon-inducible CXC chemokine receptor 3 ligands, Front. Immunol. 8 (2017) 1970.

[51] K.C. Anderson, The 39th David A. Karnofsky Lecture: bench-to-bedside translation of targeted therapies in multiple myeloma, J. Clin. Oncol. 30 (4) (2012) 445–452.

[52] K.I. Stanford, J.R. Bishop, E.M. Foley, J.C. Gonzales, I.R. Niesman, J.L. Witztum, et al., Syndecan-1 is the primary heparan sulfate proteoglycan mediating hepatic clearance of triglyceride-rich lipoproteins in mice, J. Clin. Invest. 119 (11) (2009) 3236–3245.

[53] B. Casu, I. Vlodavsky, R.D. Sanderson, Non-anticoagulant heparins and inhibition of cancer, Pathophysiol. Haemost. Thromb. 36 (3–4) (2008) 195–203.

[54] M. Kusche-Gullberg, L. Kjellén, Sulfotransferases in glycosaminoglycan biosynthesis, Curr. Opin. Struct. Biol. 13 (5) (2003) 605–611.

[55] S.-A. Ng, K.M. Sullivan, Application of stem cell transplantation in autoimmune diseases, Curr. Opin. Hematol. 26 (6) (2019) 392–398.

CHAPTER

10

Biological aging and autoimmunity

Mustafa Erinç Sitar[a,b,]*

[a]Faculty of Medicine, Department of Clinical Biochemistry, Maltepe University, Istanbul, Turkey
[b]Maltepe University Experimental Animals Application and Research Center, Istanbul, Turkey
*Corresponding author

Abstract

All of the functional negative changes that occur in the organism during their lifespan are called "aging." This phenomenon is a problem as old as the human history. Academicians and authorities of the societies tried to solve the problem on behalf of humanity. Although a lot of information has been obtained about it, not all of its biological mechanisms have been explained. During this process, the changes that occur in the body can be considered holistically or separately. Our immune system, both as a single system and together with other systems like neuroendocrine system, is either directly affected by aging or directly affects aging. Many changes occur, such as elevation of clonal T-cell subsets, postpuberty thymus involution, decline of the ability to differentiate between self and nonself, alteration of the cytokine profile with a tendency to proinflammatory direction, and change in the expression of cell surface receptors. Changes that occur in human immune system, which is also called immunocenescence, are directly associated with the increased risk of autoimmune diseases and malignancies. The procedures that can be done to ensure healthy aging, prevent autoimmune diseases, and decrease the cancer risk and prolong longevity are hidden in these mechanisms.

Keywords

Adaptive Immunity, Aging, Autoimmune diseases, Inflammaging, Immunosenescence, Innate immunity

1 Introduction

"When do we start to age? Can we stop aging and reverse it? Is aging a disease or a physiological process?" "Do we have to get old?" "What are the individual or societal benefits of aging?"; Questions like these have always been asked and their answers sought in the world of academia and literature throughout history. According to the data from the WHO (World Health Organization), it is stated that 2 billion people will be over 60 years old in the 2050s, and approximately 80% of elderly people will live in low- or middle-income countries [1]. In addition to low birth rates, easier and higher access to health services and low death rates also support these statistics. Maximum lifespan, which is the highest number of years that a human being can reach, is approximately 122 years and it has not changed during recent centuries [2]. However, it is undeniable that life span mean of almost every country is rising and this issue, which is named the "Silver Tsunami," will have profound effects on the health systems, general insurances, pension structures, financial status, and social lives. Achieving a healthy aging, developing technologies for high-quality self-care in the Silver Tsunami, adaptation to changing business life for elderly people who continue to work, maintaining the comfortable and independent lives of the societies' senior citizens, and the retirement issue are all of the existing concerns associated with aging.

First, it is necessary to clearly define the problem to be able to deal with it. Epidemiologists classify aging into three categories: young-aged period between 65 and 74 years old, middle-aged period between 75 and 84 years old, and advanced-aged period over the age of 85 [3, 4]. Indeed, aging begins at the first second of life at birth and ends with death. However, although those calendar-based definitions are necessary, they are not sufficient to explain biological and physiological processes. Aging is all of the changes that emerge at the molecular level during the life and affect all the cellular systems, which are irreversible and unavoidable. Those changes can affect the organism as a whole and lead to increasing risk of diseases like Alzheimer's, Parkinson, Type 2 diabetes mellitus, coronary heart disease, stroke, cataract, osteoporosis, osteoarthritis, malignancies and also susceptibility to infections with rising mortality and morbidity due to ongoing functional and cognitive losses [5–8]. These diseases do not appear suddenly in every person like the days marked on the calendar at the same age. It would be superficial to explain the aging phenomenon only chronologically with regard to the passing of the calendar days, since biological aging and chronological aging are two distinct concepts. This is quite logical in today's world as we move towards the world of "personalized medicine" [6]. Due to the different mitotic activities, molecular properties, environmental and epigenetic factors, biological aging rates differ even in different organs and tissues of a single organism [9] and the immune system is not an exception to this undesirable situation. Aseptic chronic inflammation state is called inflammaging or immunosenescence. Decreased responsiveness to vaccines, elevated susceptibility to serious infections, increased risk of autoimmunity, diminished ability to distinguish between self and nonself, and increased incidence of chronic inflammatory diseases and tumors are the result of immunosenescence [10, 11]. In this chapter, immunosenescence, autoimmune diseases, fundamental changes of cellular aging, age-related clinical manifestations, and the epidemiology of autoimmune diseases in elderly individuals will be discussed.

2 Immunosenescence

Organisms are constantly exposed to invader infectious agents and in most cases can resist infections successfully. It is the individual's immune system that provides defense mechanisms against these infectious agents and against the body's mutated or malignant self-cells [12]. Our immune system is divided into two compartments: (I) innate/natural immunity, which is independent of antigen and cannot create long-term memory and (II) protective/adaptive immunity, which provides antigen-specific and long-term protection against repetitive exposures. Indeed, natural/innate immunity is a strong early, first line warning, and active defense system. Many infectious agents are immediately taken under control by the innate immunity, thus paving the way for the acquired immunity to operate immune reactions for a longer time and more effectively [13]. Although these two systems seem to be separate, there are also important functions that need to be done collaboratively such as antigen presentation. Here are the changes that occur with aging in the elements of the innate immunity, listed below:

(a) In the skin, epidermis becomes thinner, cell turnover slows down, barrier function of the skin and its resistance weaken [14].

(b) The frequency of mucociliary beats is decreased and susceptibility to pneumonia increases [15].

(c) Attenuation of neutrophil phagocytosis and production of reactive oxygen species [16, 17].

(d) Adverse effect on macrophage functions such as release of proinflammatory mediators, CD14 expression, Toll-like receptor (TLR) activation, and antigen presentation [18, 19].

(e) Decreased proliferation and cytotoxicity, but increased in the quantity of natural killer (NK) cells [20].

(f) Low IgE concentration and decreased chemotaxis of eosinophils [21].

(g) Decrease in the capacity of antigen presenting dendritic cells (DCs) to present their antigens properly to CD4$^+$ and CD8$^+$ T cells [22].

When it comes to changes in the adaptive immunity through aging:

(a) In cellular immunity, turnover rates of T cells diminish dramatically, IL-2 synthesis and its receptor expression decreases, naïve T cell number decreases while memory T cells increase in quantity clonally [11, 23–25].

(b) In humoral immunity, naïve B cell volume decreases but memory B cells increase along with alterations in concentration and affinity of immunoglobulin types [23, 24, 26].

(c) Thymus gradually becomes smaller in size, fat tissue replaces it, and the gland loses its endocrine features [27].

Furthermore, continuous antigenic stimulation, T cell subset changes, metabolic dysregulations, and telomere shortening are the contributors of aging in the immune system [28]. Taken together, a better understanding of immune dysfunctions that occur in old ages, called immunocenescence, may be the key to reach a successful aging in the Silver Tsunami. Slowing down, preventing, or even reversing all these changes stands in front of us as therapeutic aims.

3 Immune and autoimmune theories of aging

Roy L. Walford put forward the immunologic theory of aging in the late 1960s [27]. Walford stated that the immune system, which is beneficial and protective for human in the reproductive periods, becomes the main cause of tissue damage in old ages. According to this theory, the whole process was pictured. Immune system, following a time pattern, reaches its peak function at puberty and gradually declines later [29]. If the body cannot protect itself from potential dangers, death is inevitable due to age-related maladies. Hallmarks of the "Immunological Theory of Aging" are deleterious changes in the whole immune system, development of an unbalanced chronic inflammation with aging (also called inflammaging), and the inability to defend the body against invaders. In other words, aging immune system can contribute to Weismann's "Wear and Tear Theory of Aging," which he put forward at the end of the 1800s [30]. This old but well-established theory defined aging as an accumulation of errors. Accretion of damages by everyday errors will eventually overcome the capacity to work properly and senescence will prevail [31]. The elements of the immune system gradually begin to wear out as they face every day's stresses. Therefore, immunosenescence contributes to some serious burdens to the aging process by adding such errors. There is a quite good example of this aforementioned issue. While the cells of the innate immune system kill bacteria and viruses, they produce reactive oxygen and nitrogen species by the mechanism called respiratory burst. If organelle barriers and antioxidants were not present, this could be quite harmful to the host itself [32]. Age-related reduction in the respiratory burst is unavoidable [33]. The harmful factors that are produced during dysfunctional respiratory burst can directly cause aging.

In gerontology society, there is another view for the relationship between aging theories and immunity. When we come to this second view, "Autoimmunity Theory of Aging," which states losing capability of separating foreign factors from self-owned entities is the matter [28]. It is a fact that as people get older, the amount of antibodies that cannot distinguish self from nonself increases [27]. Different mechanisms are involved in the induction of autoimmunity during aging. For instance, thymus involution, dominance of a different cytokine profile that causes chronic inflammation, low rate of programmed T cell death, reduction in naïve T cells, and the presence of higher number of memory cells are of the implicated mechanisms [34–36]. Increasing immunogenetic diversity of cells as the organism ages is another culprit as well [5]. Accumulated DNA damages in nuclei of immune cells, rescheduling of metabolism and inducing cell-specific sustained distress signals contribute to long-standing immunogenic diversity [37]. In general, even if the antibodies produced with aging increase, as long as the immune tolerance functions, it might cause no serious complication [36]. However, throughout the aging process, the capability of T and B cells in mediating immune response decreases while the frequency of autoreactive cells increases. When the immune system fails to preserve certain checkpoints, tolerance mechanisms will not be successful and age-related clinical problems, including autoimmunity, will arise [35, 38]. Increased prevalence of autoimmune diseases in the elderly and the low rate of response to ordinary antigenic stimuli can be seen as the main results of this phenomenon.

4 Autoimmune diseases, cancer, and their relations with aging

Malignancies, autoimmune diseases, and aging can be consequences of similar mechanisms. Considering possible pathophysiological associations between aforementioned conditions, elucidation of the underlying mechanisms is of interest. If human antibodies attack their own components rather than foreign invaders, the situation can damage healthy tissues, which is called "autoimmune diseases." It is a fact that inflammation secondary to a prolonged illness lasts for a long time and immune balance is disrupted, therefore, the body ages during this time. Clinical presentation, response to therapeutic agents, and the progression process of autoimmune diseases are quite different in elderly compared to their younger individuals

(Table 1). Almost every autoimmune disease disproportionately affects the female sex [72]. However, there are remarkable differences in some of the autoimmune diseases concerning the age and sex differences. Difference in male-to-female ratio closes with old age for systemic lupus erythematosus (SLE); sarcoidosis and Sjögren's disease are becoming more common in elderly women; and the evidence on rheumatoid arthritis, Wegener granulomatosis, primary biliary cirrhosis and giant cell arteritis that are more common in elderly, are of the most striking examples [72] (Table 1). Different concentrations and actions of reproductive hormones at different levels of menstrual cycle and reproductive phases of the women including pregnancy and menopause, higher quantities of mutations originating from X chromosome, and variable duration of exposure to environmental risk factors can be attributed to the different prevalence of autoimmune diseases between male and female and in different age groups [73]. The reasons why women in societies living in the same country and environmental factors live longer than men can be examined based on this neuroendocrine and immunological connection as well. The dramatic differences observed in old age due to gender in relation to its biomedical significance in medical literature have not been widely investigated and still awaits access to light [74].

TABLE 1   The most important and common autoimmune diseases, their epidemiological data related to aging and their general clinical course for the old-aged patients.

Autoimmune diseases	Age related epidemiological changes	Clinical course of the disease for the elderly	References
Primary biliary cirrhosis	Markedly increased prevalence rate seen in older individuals	Very similar laboratory results and treatment options on both young and elderly patients	[39, 40]
Systemic lupus erythematosus	Female/male gender ratio and higher frequency of non-Caucasian patients decline with increasing age	Late-onset disease has milder and more disguise presentation	[41–44]
Rheumatoid arthritis	The disease occurs at the same rate in both genders	Acute initiation pattern in the old population rather than slow onset in the younger patients	[45]
Polyarteritis nodosa	More common in males in the elderly	Broad spectrum from cutaneous involvement to severe systemic involvement in the elderly	[46]
Churg–Strauss vasculitis	Rising frequency in elderly case reports of Churg–Strauss vasculitis is reported	Elderly are more prone to have complications and gastrointestinal involvement during the course of the disease	[47]
Wegener's Granulomatosis	Total occurrence of complications is similar in all age groups including senior citizens	Central nervous system involvement and renal failure are more common in the elderly	[48]
Takayasu's vasculitis	Less than 20% of cases begin after the age of 50	Difficult differential diagnosis with giant cell arteritis for elderly male patients	[49]

Continued

10. Biological aging and autoimmunity

TABLE 1 The most important and common autoimmune diseases, their epidemiological data related to aging and their general clinical course for the old-aged patients—cont'd

Autoimmune diseases	Age related epidemiological changes	Clinical course of the disease for the elderly	References
Polymyalgia rheumatic	It is more common in elderly citizens and it is rare to be diagnosed under the age of 50	The disease usually relapses despite appropriate treatment	[50]
Giant cell arteritis (temporal arteritis)	Increased peak age of onset for the elderly as a striking feature	It is a disease that is almost entirely seen in the elderly, needs therapy for a long time and evaluation of glucocorticoid adverse reactions	[39, 51]
Behçet's disease	Onset of the disorder is very rare and unusual in geriatric ages	Both Behçet's disease and myelodysplastic syndrome in the same person is a quite common presentation of this disease for the elderly population	[52]
Psoriasis	The incidence of the disease is higher in patients in their 60s for the current world	Associated with another serious autoimmune disease of the elderly, "bullous pemphigoid"	[53, 54]
Sjögren's syndrome	It is significantly more common in women around the age of 50	Sensitivity of serological tests in the diagnosis of the disease decreases in elderly	[55]
Inflammatory bowel diseases (Chron's and ulcerative colitis)	Approximately one out of every three inflammatory bowel patients either enter the geriatric age while the disease continues or they directly get these diseases in their geriatric ages	Clinical courses are entirely vague and different in elderly onset and younger onset patients	[56]
Coeliac disease	Formerly known as pediatric or early adulthood disease, now one out of every four patients diagnosed with Coeliac in developed countries is in their 60s or more	High tendency to autoimmune disorders and cancer in the elderly and one of the most common cause of malabsorption after the sixth decade	[57, 58]
Multiple sclerosis	The proportion of patients who take their first diagnosis as multiple sclerosis at geriatric age is approximately 10% of all multiple sclerosis patients	Late diagnosis in advanced ages may indicate a poor prognosis	[59, 60]
Graves' disease	In the elderly population, this disease is significantly more common in women	Clinical onset in the elderly can be elusive and vague, for example atrial fibrillation may be the primary onset	[61, 62]
Hashimoto thyroiditis	It is the most common hormonal disorder in the elderly, and women are at greater risk	Hypothyroidism is related with high death rate	[63, 64]
Pernicious anemia	It is one of the most frequent cause of cobalamin deficiency, affecting nearly one in every 20 elderly	There is a certain increased risk for many types of cancer, especially gastric type	[65, 66]

198

TABLE 1 The most important and common autoimmune diseases, their epidemiological data related to aging and their general clinical course for the old-aged patients—cont'd

Autoimmune diseases	Age related epidemiological changes	Clinical course of the disease for the elderly	References
Systemic sclerosis	It is significantly more common in women	The elderly have a mortality risk of over 50% within 2 years after diagnosis	[67]
Sarcoidosis	It is more common in elderly women at a rate of three-fourth as in the young patient group	Imaging techniques in the elderly show more advanced disease and remission is much less common	[68]
Primary idiopathic thrombocytopenic purpura	There are two peaks at different ages in general population, one during childhood and one during geriatric period	Complications such as hemorrhage and thrombosis are much more common due to both natural age related and disease-related issues compared to young people	[69]
Myasthenia gravis	While the male/female ratio is close to one in the young-aged period, the male dominance becomes more pronounced in the middle- and advanced-aged periods	Prognosis is good generally but remission rate is low	[70]
Ankylosing spondylitis	Late onset diagnosed patient ratio is increasing due to general increase in average life expectancy and enriched diagnostic modalities	Analytical parameters such as erythrocyte sedimentation rate (ESR) and c reactive protein (CRP), which are usually at normal levels in young patients, are significantly higher in those diagnosed in the geriatric period	[71]

Aging is recognized as the most important and leading risk factor for cancer development. Almost half of cancer patients are geriatric patients. [75]. In the basic immune system physiology, NK cells and cytotoxic $CD8^+$ T cell precisely inspect other cells to prevent cancer cell formation [76, 77]. If these cancer surveillance mechanisms suppressed, malignancies occur. Supporting examples are the marked increase in the risk of Kaposi's sarcoma and lymphoma in HIV (human immunodeficiency virus) infected patients, and solid organ tumors that are a possible complication following immunosuppressive therapy in organ transplant patients [78, 79]. Meanwhile, long-term inflammation and initiation of autoimmunity are detectable in newly diagnosed cancer patients [80]. Chronic immune stimulations, oxidative stress, imbalance in immune mediator molecules, mutations, and different environmental stimuli contribute to the risk of tumor formation in the autoimmune diseases [81, 82]. Systemic lupus erythematosus (SLE), scleroderma, multiple sclerosis, celiac disease, Crohn's disease, Graves' disease, Hashimoto's thyroiditis, pernicious anemia, and psoriasis are autoimmune diseases that are associated with the risk of cancer development. Among these, celiac disease and inflammatory bowel diseases are at the forefront in relation to cancer incidents, in particular gastrointestinal cancers and non-Hodgkin's lymphoma (NHL) [80, 83–87]. In some autoimmune diseases such as myasthenia gravis, the incidence of cancer is so high that it is recommended in guidelines to start tumor investigation immediately when the disease is diagnosed [88, 89].

5 Conclusion

Aging is a difficult, complicated, and unavoidable period of human life. For the time, it cannot be cured at all but can be managed to be healthier. Although the aging of the human, the aging of the immune system, and risk of autoimmune diseases are compared to a complex intertwined tangle, they are all like a well-woven spider web. Considering the complexity of the immune system, its association with other physiologic systems in the process of aging is undeniable. In addition to genetic factors, environmental factors such as exposure to oxidative damage, sunlight, nutrition and diet, lifestyle of individuals, physical activity in contrast to sedentary life, and geography-related matters, all play an important role in age-related changes.

Even there are still unexplained relationships between autoimmunity pattern alteration during aging, malignancies, and molecular mechanisms of aging itself, we claim that it might be possible to increase the longevity. In order to achieve this goal, gerontologists should conduct more studies regarding the most important issues in this field such as (i) patients with rare diseases related to aging like progeria are also known also as "premature aging"; (ii) twins having the same genome but living in different environments could experience different longevity; (iii) physiology of people in their centenarians; and (iv) big data mining and bioinformatics from previous health archives. Therefore, by investigating these issues our horizons will expand and our perspective on aging will increase.

References

[1] WHO, Ageing and Health, 2018. 5 February 2018.
[2] J. Miquel, An update of the oxidation-inflammation theory of aging: the involvement of the immune system in oxi-inflamm-aging, Curr. Pharm. Des. 15 (26) (2009) 3003–3026.
[3] WHO Scientific Group on the Epidemiology of Aging, The Uses of Epidemiology in the Study of the Elderly, World Health Organization, 1984.
[4] T. Beğer, H. Yavuzer, Yaşlılık ve yaşlılık epidemiyolojisi, Klinik gelişim 25 (3) (2012) 1–3.
[5] M.E. Sitar, et al., Current aspects of ageing theories and classification according to mechanisms, Turk. J. Geriatri. 16 (3) (2013) 339–346.
[6] C.L. Fasching, Telomere length measurement as a clinical biomarker of aging and disease, Crit. Rev. Clin. Lab. Sci. 55 (7) (2018) 443–465.
[7] T. Fulop, et al., Aging, frailty and age-related diseases, Biogerontology 11 (5) (2010) 547–563.
[8] M. Michaud, et al., Proinflammatory cytokines, aging, and age-related diseases, J. Am. Med. Dir. Assoc. 14 (12) (2013) 877–882.
[9] S. Aydin, et al., Galactose-induced aging model in rat testicular tissue, J. Coll. Physicians Surg. Pak. 28 (7) (2018) 501–504.
[10] A.A. Sadighi Akha, Aging and the immune system: an overview, J. Immunol. Methods 463 (2018) 21–26.
[11] M. Prelog, Aging of the immune system: a risk factor for autoimmunity? Autoimmun. Rev. 5 (2) (2006) 136–139.
[12] G. Mayer, in: R.C. Hunt (Ed.), Natural Nonspesific Immunity in Microbiology and Immunology On-Line, University of South Carolina, School of Medicine, 2015.
[13] A.K. Abbas, et al., Temel immünoloji: immün sistemin işlev ve bozuklukları, Medikal Yayıncılık, 2007.
[14] S. Laube, Skin infections and ageing, Ageing Res. Rev. 3 (1) (2004) 69–89.
[15] K.L. Bailey, et al., Aging causes a slowing in ciliary beat frequency, mediated by PKCε, Am. J. Phys. Lung Cell. Mol. Phys. 306 (6) (2014) L584–L589.
[16] C. Tortorella, et al., Age-related impairment of GM-CSF-induced signalling in neutrophils: role of SHP-1 and SOCS proteins, Ageing Res. Rev. 6 (2) (2007) 81–93.
[17] C.F. Fortin, et al., Aging and neutrophils: there is still much to do, Rejuvenation Res. 11 (5) (2008) 873–882.

[18] C. Sebastián, et al., MacrophAging: a cellular and molecular review, Immunobiology 210 (2–4) (2005) 121–126.

[19] A.C. Shaw, et al., Aging of the innate immune system, Curr. Opin. Immunol. 22 (4) (2010) 507–513.

[20] Y. Zhang, et al., In vivo kinetics of human natural killer cells: the effects of ageing and acute and chronic viral infection, Immunology 121 (2) (2007) 258–265.

[21] T. Yagi, et al., Failure of aged rats to accumulate eosinophils in allergic inflammation of the airway, J. Allergy Clin. Immunol. 99 (1) (1997) 38–47.

[22] T. Fulop, et al., On the immunological theory of aging. Aging: facts and theories, in: Interdisciplinary Topics in Gerontology, Karger, Basel, 2014, pp. 163–176.

[23] A. Moskalev, I. Stambler, C. Caruso, Innate and adaptive immunity in aging and longevity: the foundation of resilience, Aging Dis. 11 (6) (2020) 1363.

[24] A. Aiello, et al., Immunosenescence and its hallmarks: how to oppose aging strategically? A review of potential options for therapeutic intervention, Front. Immunol. 10 (2019) 2247.

[25] R.L. Whisler, L. Beiqing, M. Chen, Age-related decreases in IL-2 production by human T cells are associated with impaired activation of nuclear transcriptional factors AP-1 and NF-AT, Cell. Immunol. 169 (2) (1996) 185–195.

[26] L. Müller, S. Di Benedetto, G. Pawelec, The immune system and its dysregulation with aging, Subcell. Biochem. 91 (2019) 21–43.

[27] J. Diggs, Autoimmune theory of aging, in: Encyclopedia of Aging and Public Health, Springer US, Boston, MA, 2008, pp. 143–144.

[28] C. Castelo-Branco, I. Soveral, The immune system and aging: a review, Gynecol. Endocrinol. 30 (1) (2014) 16–22.

[29] K. Jin, Modern biological theories of aging, Aging Dis. 1 (2) (2010) 72.

[30] J. Miquel, J.E. Fleming, Testing ageing theories, in: Drosophila as a Model Organism for Ageing Studies, Springer, 1988, pp. 17–29.

[31] A. De, C. Ghosh, Basics of Aging Theories and Disease Related Aging—An Overview, Pharma News, 2021.

[32] C.E. Finch, et al., Cell resilience in species life spans: a link to inflammation? Aging Cell 9 (4) (2010) 519–526.

[33] G. Di Lorenzo, et al., Granulocyte and natural killer activity in the elderly, Mech. Ageing Dev. 108 (1) (1999) 25–38.

[34] E. Boren, M.E. Gershwin, Inflammaging: autoimmunity, and the immune-risk phenotype, Autoimmun. Rev. 3 (5) (2004) 401–406.

[35] S. Stacy, et al., Immunological memory and late onset autoimmunity, Mech. Ageing Dev. 123 (8) (2002) 975–985.

[36] H.-C. Hsu, J.D. Mountz, Origin of late-onset autoimmune disease, Immunol. Allergy Clin. North Am. 23 (1) (2003) 65–82.

[37] C.M. Weyand, J.J. Goronzy, Aging of the immune system. Mechanisms and therapeutic targets, Ann. Am. Thorac. Soc. 13 Suppl 5 (Suppl. 5) (2016) S422–S428.

[38] J.J. Goronzy, C.M. Weyand, Immune aging and autoimmunity, Cell. Mol. Life Sci. 69 (10) (2012) 1615–1623.

[39] A. Watad, et al., Autoimmunity in the elderly: insights from basic science and clinics—a mini-review, Gerontology 63 (6) (2017) 515–523.

[40] K. Tajiri, Y. Shimizu, Liver diseases in the elderly, in: Liver Pathophysiology, Elsevier, 2017, pp. 331–339.

[41] G. Montoya-Ortiz, Immunosenescence, aging, and systemic lupus erythematous, Autoimmune Dis. 2013 (2013) 267078.

[42] S. Lalani, J. Pope, C. PESCHKEN, Clinical features and prognosis of late-onset systemic lupus erythematosus: results from the 1000 faces of lupus study, J. Rheumatol. 37 (1) (2010) 38–44.

[43] S. Pu, et al., The clinical features and prognosis of lupus with disease onset at age 65 and older, Lupus 9 (2) (2000) 96–100.

[44] H. Peleg, O.E. Tayer-Shifman, Systemic lupus erythematosus in geriatrics, in: Rheumatic Disease in Geriatrics, Springer, 2020, pp. 201–205.

[45] Y. Yazici, S.A. Paget, Elderly-onset rheumatoid arthritis, Rheum. Dis. Clin. N. Am. 26 (3) (2000) 517–526.

[46] A. Awisat, Approach to a geriatric patient with suspected vasculitis, in: Rheumatic Disease in Geriatrics, Springer, 2020, pp. 375–379.

[47] M. Uchiyama, et al., Elderly cases of Churg–Strauss syndrome: case report and review of Japanese cases, J. Dermatol. 39 (1) (2012) 76–79.

[48] S.S. Krafcik, et al., Wegener's granulomatosis in the elderly, Chest 109 (2) (1996) 430–437.

[49] F. Onen, N. Akkoc, Epidemiology of Takayasu arteritis, Presse Med. 46 (7–8) (2017) e197–e203.

10. Biological aging and autoimmunity

[50] M.A. González-Gay, E.L. Matteson, S. Castañeda, Polymyalgia rheumatica, Lancet 390 (10103) (2017) 1700–1712.
[51] A. Awisat, R. Luqmani, Giant cell arteritis, in: Rheumatic Disease in Geriatrics, Springer, 2020, pp. 281–291.
[52] M. Brodavka, M. Lidar, Autoinflammatory diseases in the geriatric population, in: Rheumatic Disease in Geriatrics, Springer, 2020, pp. 319–331.
[53] A. Wilczek, M. Sticherling, Concomitant psoriasis and bullous pemphigoid: coincidence or pathogenic relationship? Int. J. Dermatol. 45 (11) (2006) 1353–1357.
[54] N. Balato, et al., Managing moderate-to-severe psoriasis in the elderly, Drugs Aging 31 (4) (2014) 233–238.
[55] A.N. Baer, B. Walitt, Sjögren syndrome and other causes of sicca in older adults, Rheum. Dis. Clin. N. Am. 44 (3) (2018) 419.
[56] S. Taleban, et al., Inflammatory bowel disease and the elderly: a review, J. Crohn's Colitis 9 (6) (2015) 507–515.
[57] H.J. Freeman, Adult celiac disease in the elderly, World J Gastroenterol 14 (45) (2008) 6911.
[58] P.R. Holt, Diarrhea and malabsorption in the elderly, Gastroenterol. Clin. N. Am. 30 (2) (2001) 427–444.
[59] H.J. Bauer, F. Hanfeld, Multiple sclerosis: its impact from childhood to old age, Major Probl. Neurol. 26 (1993) 177.
[60] A. Awad, O. Stüve, Multiple sclerosis in the elderly patient, Drugs Aging 27 (4) (2010) 283–294.
[61] S. Morganti, et al., Thyroid disease in the elderly: sex-related differences in clinical expression, J. Endocrinol. Invest. 28 (11 Suppl. Proceedings) (2005) 101–104.
[62] B. Pokhrel, K. Bhusal, Graves Disease, StatPearls, 2020 (Internet).
[63] J.G. Hollowell, et al., Serum TSH, T4, and thyroid antibodies in the United States population (1988 to 1994): National Health and nutrition examination survey (NHANES III), J. Clin. Endocrinol. Metabol. 87 (2) (2002) 489–499.
[64] V. Calsolaro, et al., Overt and subclinical hypothyroidism in the elderly: when to treat? Front. Endocrinol. 10 (2019) 177.
[65] G. Murphy, et al., Cancer risk after pernicious anemia in the US elderly population, Clin. Gastroenterol. Hepatol. 13 (13) (2015) 2282–2289.e4.
[66] E. Andrès, et al., Vitamin B12 (cobalamin) deficiency in elderly patients, CMAJ 171 (3) (2004) 251–259.
[67] L. Czirjak, Z. Nagy, G. Szegedi, Systemic sclerosis in the elderly, Clin. Rheumatol. 11 (4) (1992) 483–485.
[68] M. Rubio-Rivas, X. Corbella, J. Mañá, Elderly sarcoidosis: a comparative study from a 42-year single-centre experience, Respir. Med. 152 (2019) 1–6.
[69] G. Moulis, et al., Epidemiology of incident immune thrombocytopenia: a nationwide population-based study in France, Blood 124 (22) (2014) 3308–3315.
[70] J.A. Aarli, Myasthenia gravis in the elderly: is it different? Ann. N. Y. Acad. Sci. 1132 (1) (2008) 238–243.
[71] É. Toussirot, Late-onset ankylosing spondylitis and spondylarthritis, Drugs Aging 27 (7) (2010) 523–531.
[72] G.S. Cooper, B.C. Stroehla, The epidemiology of autoimmune diseases, Autoimmun. Rev. 2 (3) (2003) 119–125.
[73] J. Chubak, S.S. Tworoger, Y. Yasui, C.M. Ulrich, F.Z. Stanczyk, A. McTiernan, Associations between reproductive and menstrual factors and postmenopausal sex hormone concentrations, Cancer Epidemiol. Biomarkers Prev. 13 (8) (2004) 1296 -1301.
[74] R. Ostan, et al., Gender, aging and longevity in humans: an update of an intriguing/neglected scenario paving the way to a gender-specific medicine, Clin. Sci. (Lond.) 130 (19) (2016) 1711–1725.
[75] X. Zhang, et al., The biology of aging and cancer: frailty, inflammation, and immunity, Cancer J. 23 (4) (2017) 201–205.
[76] L. Naldi, Malignancy concerns with psoriasis treatments using phototherapy, methotrexate, cyclosporin, and biologics: facts and controversies, Clin. Dermatol. 28 (1) (2010) 88–92.
[77] S.M. Candeias, U.S. Gaipl, The immune system in cancer prevention, development and therapy, AntiCancer Agents Med. Chem. 16 (1) (2016) 101–107.
[78] G. Barbaro, G. Barbarini, HIV infection and cancer in the era of highly active antiretroviral therapy, Oncol. Rep. 17 (5) (2007) 1121–1126.
[79] E.A. Engels, et al., Spectrum of cancer risk among US solid organ transplant recipients, JAMA 306 (17) (2011) 1891–1901.
[80] A.L. Franks, J.E. Slansky, Multiple associations between a broad spectrum of autoimmune diseases, chronic inflammatory diseases and cancer, Anticancer Res. 32 (4) (2012) 1119–1136.
[81] D.T. Alexandrescu, et al., On the missing link between inflammation and cancer, Dermatol. Online J. 17 (1) (2011) 10.
[82] S.I. Grivennikov, F.R. Greten, M. Karin, Immunity, inflammation, and cancer, Cell 140 (6) (2010) 883–899.

[83] T. Mizushima, et al., Malignancy in Crohn's disease: incidence and clinical characteristics in Japan, Digestion 81 (4) (2010) 265–270.

[84] J. Askling, et al., Cancer incidence in a population-based cohort of individuals hospitalized with celiac disease or dermatitis herpetiformis, Gastroenterology 123 (5) (2002) 1428–1435.

[85] K. Hemminki, et al., Cancer risks in ulcerative colitis patients, Int. J. Cancer 123 (6) (2008) 1417–1421.

[86] M.J. Goldacre, et al., Cancer in patients with ulcerative colitis, Crohn's disease and coeliac disease: record linkage study, Eur. J. Gastroenterol. Hepatol. 20 (4) (2008) 297–304.

[87] K. Hemminki, et al., Cancer risks in Crohn disease patients, Ann. Oncol. 20 (3) (2009) 574–580.

[88] M.J. Titulaer, et al., Screening for small-cell lung cancer: a follow-up study of patients with Lambert-Eaton myasthenic syndrome, J. Clin. Oncol. 26 (26) (2008) 4276–4281.

[89] M. Hartert, et al., A follicular dendritic cell sarcoma of the mediastinum with immature T cells and association with myasthenia gravis, Am. J. Surg. Pathol. 34 (5) (2010) 742–745.

CHAPTER

11

Efficacy and safety of immune checkpoint inhibitors and cytokine therapy in autoimmune diseases

Reyhaneh Sabourian[a,b], Seyedeh Zohreh Mirjalili[a,b], and Nima Rezaei[b,c,d,]*

[a]Department of Drug and Food Control, Faculty of Pharmacy, Tehran University of Medical Sciences, Tehran, Iran [b]Network of Immunity in Infection, Malignancy and Autoimmunity (NIIMA), Universal Scientific Education and Research Network (USERN), Tehran, Iran [c]Research Center for Immunodeficiencies, Children's Medical Center, Tehran University of Medical Sciences, Tehran, Iran [d]Department of Immunology, School of Medicine, Tehran University of Medical Sciences, Tehran, Iran

*Corresponding author

Abstract

Immune checkpoint and cytokine inhibitors are being employed in different conditions including prevention of organ transplant rejection and autoimmune diseases such as rheumatoid arthritis and systemic lupus erythematosus, especially in patients who are refractory to disease-modifying antirheumatic drugs (DMARDs). On the other hand, some potential risks of these agents have to be taken into account: (i) immune responses such as anaphylactic reaction and generation of antibodies against the therapeutic agents, (ii) organ-specific adverse events, and (iii) increase risk of infections and malignancies. In this chapter, clinical trials in phase I/II/III on the safety and efficacy of some immune checkpoint and cytokine inhibitors for the treatment of autoimmune diseases and organ transplant rejection are reviewed.

Keywords

Efficacy, Safety, Immune checkpoint inhibitor, Cytokine, Autoimmune diseases

1 Introduction

During an autoimmune disease, immunoglobulins (Ig) and other components of the immune system attack healthy cells instead of alien matters, which lead to inflammation in the affected tissue. These disorders can influence any part of the patient' body, including blood, skin, and gastrointestinal system [1]. There are more than 80 known autoimmune diseases, such as systemic lupus erythematosus (SLE), rheumatoid arthritis (RA), plaque psoriasis (PP), multiple sclerosis (MS), inflammatory bowel disease (IBD), and type 1 diabetes mellitus (T1DM) [2].

Since the first reports of the production of monoclonal antibodies (mAbs) by Kohler et al. who had applied a technology of hybridoma [3], mAbs have made a phenomenal revolution from investigational molecules to potent medicines. Autoimmune diseases are one of the fields that profited the most from the mentioned novel therapies that remarkably influence the quality of patient care. mAbs specifically identify unique epitopes and effectively attack their targets [4]. Cytokines are a broad group of small proteins that contribute to different immune responses [5]. These molecules are classified by their structure, mechanism of action, or their producer cells [6].

A huge category of autoimmune diseases' therapies consists of cytokine inhibitors that are administrated alone or in combination with different classes of immunosuppressive drugs. These therapies have been demonstrated to be reasonably efficient. Some cytokines have been represented as considerable targets for the treatment or control of autoimmune diseases such as tumor necrosis factor-α (TNF-α) and different interleukins (IL) [7]. Despite the presence of more than 90 cytokines and their crucial role in the regulation of autoimmune responses, not all of them are promising targets for the treatment of autoimmune disease [8]. This chapter focuses on the most effective treatment targets including tumor necrosis factor α (TNF-α), interleukin-6 (IL-6), IL-17, and IL-23 and discusses their safety and efficacy attributes.

Immune checkpoint inhibitors (ICIs) have been investigated in several studies for different types of melanoma and solid tumors [9, 10]. These compounds potentially target cytotoxic T-lymphocyte-associated antigen-4 (CTLA-4), programmed cell death 1 (PD-1), and programmed cell death-ligand 1 (PD-L1).

All of the above-mentioned treatments are possible through a mAb or some fractions of it. This chapter has collected different kinds of therapies for autoimmune diseases with a focus on safety and efficacy of these agents.

2 Immunogenicity of mAbs and its effect on efficacy and safety

The adverse immune reactions, which is attributed to the immunogenicity of the therapeutic agents, lead to the generation of antidrug antibodies (ADAs) that are responsible for increased clearance of the therapeutic mAb and safety complications of the treatment. There are four major types of mAbs, known as murine, chimeric, humanized, and fully human antibodies. As well, immune response against mAbs progressively reduced from mouse to chimeric to humanize and then to fully human mAbs [11].

As mentioned before, immunogenicity may have negative effect on the efficacy and safety of mAbs. Therefore, the potential of immunogenicity of every novel therapeutic antibody have to be carefully investigated. Currently, common mAbs that are used in autoimmune diseases target several molecules such as cytokines and immune checkpoints.

3 Inflammatory cytokine inhibition in autoimmune diseases

TNF-α, IL-6, IL-17, and IL-23 are critical cytokines in immune system pathways and dysregulation in these pathways lead to autoimmune reactions and development of autoimmune diseases including rheumatoid arthritis (RA), inflammatory bowel disease (IBD), and psoriasis [8].

3.1 Anti-TNF-α

TNF-α is the most known and clinically targeted cytokine [8]. Anti-TNF-α agents are important drugs in several inflammatory diseases such as psoriatic arthritis (PSA), rheumatoid arthritis (RA), juvenile idiopathic arthritis (JIA), inflammatory bowel disease (IBD), ankylosing spondylitis (AS), and refractory uveitis. This category of drugs consists of infliximab, adalimumab, etanercept, and recently approved golimumab and certolizumab pegol. Besides increased susceptibility to infections, immunogenicity is the most important adverse effect (AE) of these drugs [12].

3.1.1 Infliximab

Infliximab is a chimeric monoclonal antibody and capable of mediating immune-related adverse events (irAEs). It is the best-known drug in its category and has the US Food and Drug Administration (US FDA) approval for a number of autoimmune diseases (Table 1). In a prospective study, the efficacy of infliximab in refractory uveitis was evaluated. It was effective in most of the patients and tolerable during the 50 weeks period of the study. Despite obvious benefit in some patients, the frequency of serious toxic effects was surprisingly high [13]. However, in another study, it was safe and efficient in refractory uveitis associated with Behcet's disease [14]. These results were then confirmed by an open-labeled trial [15]. Safety and efficacy of infliximab and adalimumab were assessed during a 1-year follow-up study on refractory uveitis due to JIA. Both of the drugs were safe and effective in addition to a higher efficacy that was observed for adalimumab [16]. In a retrospective study, most of the patients (%85) were improved after infliximab therapy and only 15% of patients experienced lack of efficacy or side effects [26].

In addition to uveitis, safety and efficacy of infliximab have been evaluated in patients with active SLE. It was effective and led to improvement in disease parameters without significant AEs [17, 18]. In two different case reports, infliximab therapy in patients under the traditional SLE therapies led to a reduction in the dosage of other administered drugs along with the signs of remission in disease parameters [27, 28].

A study was performed to investigate the efficacy and safety of infliximab in AS patients. This multicenter study confirmed improvement of patients along with mild to moderate AE [19, 20]. Long-term discontinuation of infliximab therapy in AS patients and its readministration showed local infections in only one patient and was safe and efficient in the rest of the patients [29].

Although infliximab is not formally approved by the US FDA for JIA, intra-articular injection of infliximab in JIA patients with temporomandibular joint arthritis was evaluated. Without special AEs, infliximab decreased disease progression and represented promising responses [30], and intravenous infusion of infliximab in addition to methotrexate (MTX) turned to be safe and effective [21, 31]. Moreover, inflammatory mediators including serum IL-6, soluble adhesion molecules, and myeloperoxidase were decreased in JIA patients after infliximab therapy [22].

TABLE 1   Summary of some studies on safety and efficacy of infliximab.

Indication	Dose (mg)	Size patient group	Duration of study	Primary endpoint	Met primary endpoint?	Number of patients with serious AEs	Refs.
Uveitis[a]	3–5 mg/kg at W 0, 2, 6, 14 then every 8 W	23	50 W	Criteria for clinical assessment at W 10	Yes: 78% of treated patients improved	6 of 23 patients	[13]
	5 mg/kg at W 0, 2, 6 then every 8 W	6	3 Y	Criteria for clinical assessment at W 8	Yes: all patients had achieved improvement at W 8	0 of 6 patients	[14]
	5 mg/kg at W 0, 2, 6 then every 8 W	10	3 Y	Criteria for clinical assessment during follow-up period	There was a remarkable improvement in visual acuity with no significant adverse reaction	0 of 10 patients	[15]
	INF; 5 mg/kg IV inf (0, 2, 6, 12 then every 8 W), ADA; 1 mg/kg every 2 W SC (max 40 mg)	91	1 Y	Changes in uveitis course and in number of ocular complications	Remission in 55.3% of 91 patients; INF 42.8% vs ADA 67.4%, $P = .025$	0 of 91 patients	[16]
SLE	3 mg/kg at W 0,2 6 then every 8 W, control	27	24 W	SF-36, PGA, SLEDAI, SLICC/ACR-DI at W 24	Yes: only SLEDAI (28 points) vs control (13 points, $P = .035$)	0 of 27 patients	[17]
	300 mg (at W 0, 2, 6, 10)	6	52 W	SLEDAI and SIS at W 10	Yes: SLEDAI, 9 vs 5 at baseline $P < .002$; SIS, 10 vs 6 at baseline $P < .001$	0 of 6 patients	[18]
AS	5 mg/kg IV inf (at W 0, 2, 6, 12, 18), PBO	357	24 W	ASAS20 at W 24	Yes: 5 mg/kg (61.2%) vs PBO (19.2%, $P < .001$)	5 mg/kg (7 of 202 patients) vs PBO (2 of 75 patients)	[19]
	5 mg/kg after starting dose every 6 W, PBO for 24 W then 5 mg/kg every 6 W	279	2 Y	ASAS20 at W 102	Yes: 5 mg/kg (73.9%) vs PBO to 5 mg/kg (72.1%)	Combined (5 of 275 patients)	[20]
	3 mg/kg at W 0, 2, 6 then every 8 W	24	2 Y	28-joint count	Yes: after 1 Y (0), 6 M (0), 2 W (2) vs baseline (6, $P < .05$)	0 of 24 patients	[21]
	3 mg/kg at W 0, 2, 6 then every 6 W	8	24 W	Number of active joints and levels of CRP, IL-6, MPO, sICAM-1 at W 6	Number of active joints (16 to 4, $P < .01$), CRP (31 to 8 $P < .001$), IL-6 (14.6 to 7.6 $P < .05$), MPO (584 to 374, $P < .05$), sICAM-1 (145 to 129, $P < .001$) from W 0 to W 6	–	[22]

CD	Induction: 5 mg/kg (W 0, 2, 6) Maintenance: 5 mg/kg every 8 W, 5 mg/kg every 12 W	112	54 W	PCDAI > 15, PCDAI < 10 at W 10, 54	Yes: W 10 (95%, 58.9%) W 54 every 8 W (63%, 55.8%, $P = .002$) vs W 54 every 12 W (33%, 23.5%, $P < .001$)	W 10 (7 of 9 patients) W 54 (15 of 103 patients)	[23]
	5 mg/kg every 8 and 12 W, 10 mg/kg every 8 W	60	3 Y	PGA	80% at Y 3 having no to mild disease	6 of 60 patients	[24]
PP	10 mg/kg, 5 mg/kg, PBO (W 0, 2, 6)	33	10 W	Proportion of patients with good and clear at PGA scale at W 10	10 mg/kg (91%), 5 mg/kg (82%), PBO (18%, $P = .0019$ and $P = .0089$ respectively)	0 of 33 patients	[25]

Abbreviations: *AE*, adverse events; *W*, week; *INF*, infliximab; *ADA*, adalimumab; *IV inf*, intravenous infusion; *SC*, subcutaneous; *SF-36*, 36-item short-form health survey; *PGA*, patient global assessment; *SLEDAI*, systemic lupus erythematosus disease activity index; *SLICC/ACR-DI*, Systemic Lupus International Collaborating Clinics/American College of Rheumatology Damage Index for Systemic Lupus Erythematosus; *SIS*, systemic lupus erythematosus index score; *AS*, ankylosing spondylitis; *ASAS20*, 20% improvement response according to the Assessment in Ankylosing Spondylitis International Working Group criteria; *CRP*, C-reactive protein (mg/L); *IL*, interleukin (pg/mL); *MPO*, myeloperoxidase (ng/mL); *sICAM-1*, soluble intercellular adhesion molecule 1 (ng/mL); *CD*, Crohn's disease; *PCDAI > 15*, clinical response (decrease from baseline in the Pediatric Crohn's Disease Activity Index PCDAI score > 15 points; total score < 30); *PCDAI < 10*, clinical remission (PCDAI score < 10 points); *PGA*, score on the physician's global assessment.
[a] *Autoimmune-associated uveitis.*

In a randomized, multicenter, open-label study, safety and efficacy of induction and maintenance therapy of infliximab in pediatric Crohn's disease (CD) were evaluated. Eight- and twelve-weeks dosing intervals of infliximab was compared, in which eight-weeks dosing interval represented better results and was the superior regimen. Rate of adverse effects was higher in eight-weeks-interval but in serious adverse effects both regimens were the same [23]. The mentioned study was continued for 3 years more to evaluate the long-term efficacy and safety of infliximab in pediatrics with CD. It was well-tolerated and efficient in extended treatment period. In 10% of patients, serious AEs including thyroid and intra-abdominal abscesses and upper respiratory infections was observed [24]. Lack of efficacy of infliximab in CD can be because of the low-dose regimen. Therefore, Hendler et al. evaluated the effect of high-dose infliximab therapy that was associated with more serious side effects in patients [32]. Moreover, infliximab is an efficient drug in plaque psoriatic patients, with high efficacy and no serious AEs [25].

3.1.2 *Adalimumab*

Adalimumab (ADA) is a TNF-α inhibitor with different indications including PP, PsA, JIA, CD, ulcerative colitis (UC), uveitis, hidradenitis suppurativa, AS, and RA. The most prevalent AEs of the adalimumab are infection, antibody development, positive antinuclear antibodies (ANA) titer, injection site reaction, increased creatine phosphokinase, upper respiratory tract infection, skin rash, headache, and sinusitis [33] (Table 2). It was safe and effective in etanercept-treated PP patients with inadequate response to treatment. No serious AEs was observed during therapy and most recorded AEs were infections [34]. In a multicenter open-labeled study, efficacy of adalimumab was examined in adult Japanese psoriatic patients. Only expected AEs were reported and infections were the most prevalent AEs [35]. Nonresponsive PsA patients to disease-modifying antirheumatic drugs (DMARDs) significantly improved after ADA therapy in a double-blinded study and the frequency of AEs were similar to the placebo group [36]. In two studies, in which the efficacy and safety of ADA were compared with infliximab in JIA-associated uveitis, ADA has shown better remission and lower number of new ocular complications than infliximab, without any serious AE [37]. In the other study in patients aged 2 to 4 years, ADA and etanercept have shown an acceptable efficacy, but ADA has caused a slightly higher infection rate. Moreover, four serious AEs were reported [38]. In addition, ADA is a good and efficient option for Crohn's disease (CD) therapy but the AEs caused cessation of treatment [48]. At week 12, a good remission rate was reported for adalimumab in the treatment of CD, but surgery was still necessary for some patients [39]. Administration of adalimumab has caused early remission in patients who had poor response with corticosteroids and/or immunosuppressive therapy for UC [40]. One-year ADA therapy has demonstrated good risk to benefit profile in UC [41]. Furthermore, ADA was revealed as a safe and effective option in treating patients with refractory uveitis [42]. It could control uveitis with the least corticosteroid support and caused reasonable improvement of the signs of the disease [49]. ADA has shown a good safety and efficacy profile for treating hidradenitis suppurativa [43]. Significant remission has been shown by adalimumab therapy after 2 months but recurrence was seen 11 weeks after the cessation [44]. In a cohort study, adalimumab therapy has shown efficacy in AS patients [45]. Adalimumab has demonstrated a noticeable consistent remission in AS patients with poor response to NSAID therapy [46]. RA patients with failed DMARD therapy have gained rapid, noticeable, and maintained response to adalimumab monotherapy [47].

TABLE 2 Summary of some studies on safety and efficacy of adalimumab.

Indication	Dose (mg)	Size patient group	Duration of study	Primary endpoint	Met primary endpoint?	Number of patients with serious AEs	Refs.
PP	40 mg every 2 W	85	24 W	PGA score 0 or 1 at W 12	Yes: 34% vs baseline	No serious AEs	[34]
Psoriasis	80 mg then 40 mg every 2 W	731	24 W	PASI 75/90, DLQI at W 16	Yes: $P < .0001$ for all	24 of 731 patients	[35]
PsA	DB: 40 mg every 2 W, PBO; OL: 40 mg every 2 W	100	24 W	ACR20 at W 12	Yes: 40 mg (39%) vs PBO (16%, $P = .012$)	DB: 40 mg (1 of 51 patients) vs PBO (2 of 49 patients) OL: 3 of 97 patients	[36]
JIA	ADA 1 mg/kg (max 40 mg) SC every 2 W, INF 5 mg/kg IV inf at 0, 2, 6, 12 W, and then continued every 6–8 W	154	24 M	Absence of flare for >6 M	Yes: ADA (60.0%) vs INF (20.3%, $P < .001$)	No serious AEs	[37]
	ADA, etanercept as registered	85	24 M	JADAS-MDA at 6, 12, 24 M and PedACR 50/70/90 at 24 M	JADAS-MDA; etanercept 55/58/58% vs ADA 50/71/66% PedACR 50/70/90; etanercept 64/54/41% vs ADA 56/33/22%	Etanercept (3 of 74 patients) vs ADA (1 of 11)	[38]
CD	As registered	103	12 M	CR-70	CR-70 was 68.7%, 74.5% and 88.4% after week 4, 8 and 12 of treatment, respectively	6.3% of the patients	[39]
UC	80/40 (80 mg at W 0, then 40 mg every 2 W), 160/80 (160/80 mg at w 0, 2 then 40 mg every 2 W), PBO	273	52 W	Response at W 8	Yes: 80/40 (43%), 160/80, (50%) vs PBO, (35%, $P = .044$ for 160/80)	ADA (33 of 177 patients) vs PBO (14 of 96 patients)	[40]
	ADA 160 mg at W 0 and then 80 mg at W 2	73	52 W	Clinical response at W 12	Yes: 75.3% of the patients showed short-term clinical response at week 12	No serious AEs	[41]
Uveitis	40 mg SC every 2 W	31	50 W	Clinical response at W 10	Yes: 68% of patients	2 of 31 patients	[42]

Continued

TABLE 2 Summary of some studies on safety and efficacy of adalimumab—cont'd

Indication	Dose (mg)	Size patient group	Duration of study	Primary endpoint	Met primary endpoint?	Number of patients with serious AEs	Refs.
HS	40 mg every W	151	168 W	HiSCR at W 12	Yes: 52.3% that maintained through W 168	12 of 88 patients	[43]
	80 mg at W 0 then 40 mg every W	15	48 W	Sartorius score at W 12	Yes: 38.6 vs 16.5 baseline ($P = .001$)	No serious AEs	[44]
AS	40 mg every 2 W	1250	20 W	BASDAI 50, ASAS40, ASAS partial remission at W 12	Yes: BASDAI 50 (57.2%), ASAS40 (53.7%), ASAS partial remission (27.7%)	43 of 1250 patients	[45]
	40 mg SC every 2 W, PBO	315	24 W	ASAS20 at W 12	Yes: 40 mg (58.2%) vs PBO (20.6%, $P < .001$)	40 mg (6 of 208 patients) vs PBO (3 of 107 patients)	[46]
RA	20 mg every 2 W, 20 mg every W, 40 mg every 2 W, 40 mg every W, PBO	544	26 W	ACR20 at W 26	20 mg every 2 W (35.8%), 20 mg every W (39.3%), 40 mg every 2 W (46.0%), 40 mg every W (53.4%) vs PBO (19.1%, $P \leq .01$ for all)	ADA (53 of 434 patients) vs PBO (16 of 110 patients)	[47]

Abbreviations: *AE*, adverse events; *PP*, plaque psoriasis; *W*, week; *PGA score 0 or 1*, physician global assessment clear or almost clear; *PASI 75/90*, proportion of patients with 75% or 90% improvement in Psoriasis Area and Severity Index; *DLQI*, Dermatology Life Quality Index; *PsA*, psoriatic arthritis; *DB*, double-blind period; *PBO*, placebo; *OL*, open-label period; *ACR20*, 20% improvement according to the American College of Rheumatology core criteria; *JIA*, juvenile idiopathic arthritis; *INF*, infliximab; *IV inf*, intravenous infusion; *ADA*, adalimumab; *SC*, subcutaneous; *M*, month; *JADAS-MDA*, Juvenile Arthritis Disease Activity Score minimal disease activity; *PedACR50/70/90*, 50/70/90% improvement according to the pediatric American College of Rheumatology core criteria; *CD*, Crohn's disease; *CR-70*, Crohn's Disease Activity Index decrease by 70 points; *UC*, ulcerative colitis; *HS*, hidradenitis suppurativa/acne inversa; *HiSCR*, hidradenitis suppurativa clinical response; *AS*, ankylosing spondylitis; *ASAS40 or 20*, 40% or 20% improvement response according to the Assessment in Ankylosing Spondylitis International Working Group criteria; *BASDAI50*, 50% improvement in the Bath AS Disease Activity Index; *ACR20*, proportion of patients achieving American College of Rheumatology 20% improvement.

3.1.3 Golimumab

Golimumab is a fully human mAb, a TNF-α inhibitor approved by the FDA for the treatment of AS, PsA, RA, spondyloarthritis, and UC [137]. Noticeable improvement of the signs of AS patients with golimumab was concluded from a phase III, placebo-controlled study [50]. The other study demonstrated a significant development of physical function over 52 weeks in AS patients without unpredicted safety problems [51]. IV administration of golimumab has shown noticeable reduction in the signs of PsA up to week 24 with same AEs as other anti-TNF agents [52]. Subcutaneous administration of golimumab have demonstrated sustained clinical efficacy in a long-term study [53]. A combination regimen of IV golimumab and MTX have shown similar medical efficacy in RA patients of more than 65 years of age or under 65 years old. However, more serious infections was reported in elderly patients [54]. Furthermore, it was established that concomitant use of corticosteroids and NSAIDs can be reduced with golimumab therapy in RA patients [55]. Administration of subcutaneous golimumab has shown satisfactory safety and efficacy profile in spondyloarthritis [56]. Favorable risk to benefit profile has been seen for golimumab in UC patients [57]. In addition, results of a 6-month study have shown safety and efficacy of golimumab for causing sustained improvement in UC outpatients [58] (Table 3).

3.1.4 Certolizumab pegol

Certolizumab pegol is a pegylated antigen-binding section of a recombinant human mAb. It is a TNF-α inhibitor for treating the symptoms CD, RA, PsA, AS, and PP [138]. According to a 7-year clinical study, well tolerability and some cases of maintaining remission have been seen in certolizumab pegol (CZP) therapy in CD patients [59]. In addition, continuous treatment was more effective than interrupted therapy [60]. Both CZP and CZP plus MTX regimens demonstrated a suitable safety profile over 7 years with a proper effectiveness in RA patients [61]. Addition of CZP to nonbiologic DMARDs is an effective choice in RA, but CZP should not be withdrawn in cases of recovery [62]. CZP therapy in PsA patients has shown long-term efficacy that was consistent over 4 years [139]. Independent to previous anti-TNF therapy, rapid remission was observed with CZP therapy in PsA patients [63]. After 1 week, a rapid remission was observed with CZP therapy in AS patients [64]. In addition, CZP have demonstrated noticeable improvement up to 16 weeks in psoriasis patients either with or without previous biologic therapy [65]. All endpoints were significantly greater in improving psoriasis symptoms for certolizumab versus placebo. Administration of 400 mg certolizumab has shown a better response than 200 mg dosing and similar to etanercept response in psoriasis patients [66] (Table 4).

3.1.5 Etanercept

Etanercept is a TNF blocker that comprises two p75 TNF receptors bonded to the fragment crystallizable (Fc) region of human IgG. It is approved in adults to prevent joint damage caused by RA, PsA, and AS. Etanercept is also used to treat PP patients (4 years and older) and JIA patients (2 years and older) [140]. Etanercept have shown a satisfactory safety and efficacy profile with reducing serious infections' rate in RA patients through a 5-year period [67]. In another study, etanercept have shown constant efficacy over 10 years in both early and long-lasting RA patients [68]. Subcutaneous administration of etanercept have demonstrated remission in PsA patients and was well tolerated [69]. In addition, it showed superior efficacy

TABLE 3 Summary of some studies on safety and efficacy of golimumab.

Indication	Dose (mg)	Size patient group	Duration of study	Primary endpoint	Met primary endpoint?	Number of patients with serious AEs	Refs.
AS	2 mg/kg IV inf at W 0, 4, 12 then every 8 W, PBO with crossover to GOL at W 16	208	28 W	ASAS20 at W 16	Yes: 2 mg/kg (73.3%) vs PBO (26.2%, $P < .001$)	GOL (2 of 105 patients) vs PBO (2 of 105 patients)	[50]
	50 mg SC at W 0 to 48, PBO at W 0 to 20 followed by GOL 50 mg from W 24 to 48; both every 4 W	213	56 W	ASAS20 at W 14	Yes: GOL (49.1%) vs PBO (24.8%, $P < .001$)	GOL (1 of 108 patients) vs PBO (0 of 105 patients)	[51]
PsA	2 mg/kg IV at W 0, 4, 12, 20, PBO	480	24 W	ACR20 at W 14	Yes: GOL (75.1%) vs PBO (21.8%, $P < .001$)	GOL (7 of 240 patients) vs PBO (8 of 239 patients)	[52]
	50 mg or 100 mg SC every 4 W, PBO	405	268 W	ACR20, DAS28-CRP, PASI50 at W 256	No: ACR20: 100 mg (69.9%), 50 mg (65.8%) vs PBO (62.8%); DAS28-CRP: 100 mg (84.9%), 50 mg (83.6%) vs PBO (75.2%); PASI50: 100 mg (88%), 50 mg (78.9%) vs PBO (79.7%)	100 mg (25 of 146 patients) vs 50 mg (29 of 146 patients)	[53]
RA	2 mg/kg IV at W 0, 4 then every 8 W to W 100, PBO	592	112 W	ACR20 at W 24	No: GOL for patients <65 Y (61.6%) vs PBO (31.3%, $P < .001$) and those ≥65 Y (69.5%) vs PBO (33.3%; $P < .01$)	Patients <65 Y (90 of 508) vs patients ≥65 Y (19 of 76)	[54]
	MTX (G1), GOL 100 mg (G2), GOL 50 mg + MTX (G3), GOL 100 mg + MTX (G4)	444	268 W	ACR20 at W 256	No: G1 (60.2%), G2 (60.9%), G3 (69.7%), G4 (64.0%)	172 of 444 patients	[55]
SpA	50 mg SC every 4 W, PBO	197	16 W	ASAS20 at W 16	Yes: 50 mg (71.1%) vs PBO (40.0%, $P < .0001$)	50 mg (1 of 97 patients) vs PBO (2 of 100 patients)	[56]
UC	100 mg SC every 4 W, PBO	144	54 W	Clinical response at W 54	Yes: 100 mg (56.3%) vs PBO (19.4%)	100 mg (1 of 32 patients) vs PBO (4 of 31 patients)	[57]
	200 mg at W 0, 100 mg at W 2 then 100 or 50 mg at W 6 and then every 4 W	93	6 M	Clinical remission at 6-month follow-up	Clinical remission was achieved in 36.5% of patients	–	[58]

Abbreviations: *AE*, adverse events; *AS*, ankylosing spondylitis; *IV inf*, intravenous infusion; *W*, week; *PBO*, placebo; *GOL*, golimumab; *ASAS20*, 20% improvement response according to the Assessment in Ankylosing Spondylitis International Working Group criteria; *PsA*, psoriatic arthritis; *ACR20*, 20% improvement according to the American College of Rheumatology core criteria; *DAS28-CRP*, Disease Activity Score based on 28 joints using C-reactive protein; *PASI50*, proportion of patients with 50% improvement in Psoriasis Area and Severity Index; *RA*, rheumatoid arthritis; *Y*, year; *MTX*, methotrexate; *SpA*, spondyloarthritis; *UC*, ulcerative colitis; *M*, month.

TABLE 4 Summary of some studies on safety and efficacy of certolizumab pegol.

Indication	Dose (mg)	Size patient group	Duration of study	Primary endpoint	Met primary endpoint?	Number of patients with serious AEs	Refs.
CD	400 mg every 4 W	595	7 Y	Assessment of the safety	Safety profile is consistent with the placebo-controlled short-term studies	240 of 595 patients	[59]
	400 mg every 4 W (continuous), PBO (drug-interruption)	668	18 M	Clinical response at W 26	Continuous (56.3%) vs PBO (37.6%)	Continuous (27 of 141 patients) vs PBO (17 of 100 patients)	[60]
RA	400 mg SC every 4 W with or without MTX	427	304 W	ACR20/50/70 at W 24	CZP + MTX (51.2/18.4/0%) vs CZP (52.7/27.3/7.3%)	25.2 per patient-year	[61]
	400 mg at W 0, 2, 4 then 200 mg every 2 W, PBO	194	52 W	CDAI at W 20 and 24	Yes: W 20 (18.8%) vs PBO (6.1%, $P \leq .05$); W 24 (63.0%) vs PBO (29.7%, $P < .001$)	CZP (5 of 96 patients) vs PBO (7 of 98 patients)	[62]
PsA	200 mg every 2 W, 400 mg every 4 W, PBO	368	24 W	ACR20 at W 12	Yes: 200 mg (58.0%) and 400 mg (51.9%) vs PBO (24.3%, $P < .001$)	200 mg (8 of 138 patients), 400 mg (13 of 135 patients) vs PBO (6 of 136 patients)	[63]
AS	200 mg every 2 W, 400 mg every 4 W, PBO	325	24 W	ASAS20 at W 12	Yes: 200 mg (57.7%) and 400 mg (63.6%) vs PBO (38.3%, $P < .004$)	200 mg (4 of 111 patients), 400 mg (7 of 107 patients) vs PBO (5 of 107 patients)	[64]
PP	200 mg every 2 W, 400 mg every 4 W, PBO	850	16 W	PASI75 and PGA 0/1 at W 16	Yes: PASI75: 400 mg (80.1%), 200 mg (74.5%) vs PBO (7.5%, $P < .0001$) Yes: PGA 0/1: 400 mg (63.7%), 200 mg (54.6%) vs PBO (2.8%, $P < .0001$)	200 mg (5 of 350 patients), 400 mg (16 of 342 patients) vs PBO (7 of 157 patients)	[65]
	CZP 400 mg every 2 W, CZP 200 mg every 2 W, PBO, ETN 50 mg twice every W	559	48 W	PASI75 at W 12	Yes: CZP 200 mg (61.3%), CZP 400 mg (66.7%) vs PBO (5%, $P < .0001$)	200 mg (1 of 165 patients), 400 mg (4 of 167 patients) vs ETN (1 of 168 patients) vs PBO (5 of 57 patients)	[66]

Abbreviations: *AE*, adverse events; *CD*, Crohn's disease; *W*, week; *Y*, year; *PBO*, placebo; *M*, month; *RA*, rheumatoid arthritis; *SC*, subcutaneous; *MTX*, methotrexate; *PsA*, psoriatic arthritis; *ACR20//50/70*, 20/50/70% improvement according to the American College of Rheumatology core criteria; *CZP*, certolizumab pegol; *CDAI*, Clinical Disease Activity Index; *mTSS*, modified Total Sharp Score change from baseline; *AS*, ankylosing spondylitis; *ASAS20*, 20% improvement response according to the Assessment in Ankylosing Spondylitis International Working Group criteria; *PP*, plaque psoriasis; *PASI75*, proportion of patients with 75% improvement in Psoriasis Area and Severity Index; *PGA 0/1*, physician global assessment clear or almost clear; *ETN*, etanercept.

than sulfasalazine in the remission of AS patients after 2 weeks of treatment [70]. Moreover, constant efficacy in AS patients over 192 weeks without defining any deaths was observed [71]. Children and adolescents with PP who continued etanercept therapy for 264 weeks have shown persistent efficacy without any unpredicted AEs [72] (Table 5).

3.2 Interleukin-6

Similar to TNF-α, IL-6 is an important cytokine in inflammatory pathways in many diseases such as T1DM, SLE, and RA. The first approved agent in this category was tocilizumab for the treatment of RA [141].

3.2.1 *Tocilizumab*

Tocilizumab is an anti-IL-6 receptor antagonist mAb of IgG1 subclass and has been widely studied in RA (Table 6). Moreover, it has the US FDA approval for the treatment of systemic JIA, polyarticular JIA, giant cell arthritis, and chimeric antigen receptor (CAR) T-cell-Induced severe or life-threatening cytokine release syndrome [141]. Its long-term safety and efficacy as monotherapy in RA patients was first demonstrated in STREAM study, a 3-month randomized trial followed by a 5-year extension study to evaluate the long-term effects of this drug [73]. Tocilizumab therapy reduced the need for corticosteroid in 88.6% of patients and 31.8% of the patients discontinued corticosteroid therapy. After 5 years of follow-up, one patient demonstrated serious infections, which developed antitocilizumab antibodies in the first 3 months of treatment, while there were not any reported tuberculosis or systemic opportunistic infections in other patients. From 94 patients who finished the study, four cases of malignancies were detected. Therefore, much longer studies are required [73]. Subcutaneous (SC) administration of tocilizumab led to similar AEs as the intravenous (IV) administration [74, 142]. In addition, it was efficient in combination with DMARD in patients with moderate to severe RA cases [75]. Injection site reaction occurred in 13% of patients and nasopharyngitis was the most frequent AE in these patients [142]. Moreover, in patients with inadequate response to the administration of tocilizumab with other intervals, decreasing the administration intervals to 1 week led to a sufficient response with similar AEs [76].

Polyarticular JIA patients benefited from tocilizumab therapy after inadequate response to MTX. Different predictable mild AEs were observed in addition to serious AEs (pneumonia and gastroenteritis) in 4 of 19 patients [77]. Withdrawal effect of tocilizumab was investigated in a three-phase study. Patients with response to 24-week treatment in part one, entered the phase two and divided in a 1:1 ratio to placebo and tocilizumab groups. JIA flare incidence rate was higher in the placebo group (48.1% versus 25.6%). Observed safety profile in polyarticular JIA patients was similar to that seen in RA adult patients and infection was the most-common serious AEs [78]. Since JIA patients are at the risk of uveitis, safety and efficacy of tocilizumab in anti-TNF-α treated patients with refractory uveitis was studied for the first time by Ramanan et al., however, further studies are necessary to determine the efficacy of tocilizumab in these cases [79].

Previous studies demonstrated that IL-6 is elevated in SLE patients. In a phase I dose-response clinical study, it was reported that three doses of tocilizumab resulted in a dose-related decrease in the neutrophil count. Although, 68% of patients reported AEs, most of them were mild-to-moderate infections and easily tolerated by patients. Only one patient stopped

TABLE 5 Summary of some studies on safety and efficacy of etanercept.

Indication	Dose (mg)	Size patient group	Duration of study	Primary endpoint	Met primary endpoint?	Number of patients with serious AEs	Refs.
RA	ETN 25 mg SC twice every W	549	5 Y	ACR20/50/70 at Y5	Yes: 78%, 51%, and 32%, respectively	130 of 549 patients	[67]
	ETN 25 mg SC twice every W	1272	10 Y	Long-term safety evaluation	Five opportunistic infections; Occurrence of all malignancies similar to that expected in the general population; Occurrence of lymphomas higher than expected in the general population	Early RA: (0.12 per patient-year), Longstanding RA: ETN (0.18)	[68]
PsA	25 mg SC twice every W, PBO	205	48 W	ACR20 at W 12	Yes: 25 mg (59%) vs PBO (15%, $P < .0001$)	25 mg (4 of 101 patients), PBO (4 of 104 patients)	[69]
AS	50 mg ETN SC every W, SSZ 3 mg/day	566	16 W	ASAS20 at W 16	Yes: ETN (75.9%) vs SSZ (52.9%, $P < .0001$)	ETN (7 of 379 patients), SSZ (4 of 187 patients)	[70]
	50 mg every W	277	192 W	ASAS20 at W 96, 192	W 96 (71%) and W 196 (81%)	33 of 257 patients	[71]
PP	8 mg/kg (max 50 mg) every W	211	264 W	PASI75/90 at W 96	PASI75 (60% to 70%), PASI90 (30% to 40%)	7 of 211 patients	[72]

Abbreviations: *AE*, adverse events; *RA*, rheumatoid arthritis; *ACR20//50/70*, 20/50/70% improvement according to the American College of Rheumatology core criteria; *ETN*, etanercept; *SC*, subcutaneous, *W*, week; *Y*, year; *PsA*, psoriatic arthritis; *PBO*, placebo; *AS*, ankylosing spondylitis; *ACR20*, proportion of patients achieving American College of Rheumatology 20% improvement; *SSZ*, sulfasalazine; *ASAS20*, 20% improvement response according to the Assessment in Ankylosing Spondylitis International Working Group criteria; *PP*, plaque psoriasis; *PASI75/90*, proportion of patients with 75% or 90% improvement in Psoriasis Area and Severity Index.

TABLE 6 Summary of some studies on safety and efficacy of tocilizumab.

Indication	Dose (mg)	Size patient group	Duration of study	Primary endpoint	Met primary endpoint?	Number of patients with serious AEs	Refs.
RA	8 mg/kg every 4 weeks	143	5 Y	ACR 20/50/70 at Y5	Yes: ACR 20 (84%), ACR 50 (69.1%), ACR 70 (43.6%)	77 of 143 patients	[73]
	SC 162 mg every 2 weeks, IV 8 mg/kg every 4 weeks	319	2 Y	ACR 20 at W 24	Yes: SC (79.2%) vs IV (88.5%)	SC (6 of 173 patients), IV (10 of 173 patients)	[74]
	SC 162 mg weekly, IV 8 mg/kg every 4 weeks	1262	24 W	ACR 20 at W 24	Yes: SC (69.4%) vs IV (73.4%)	SC (34 of 631 patients), IV (43 of 631 patients)	[75]
	SC 162 mg weekly, SC 162 mg every 2 weeks	42	52 W	DAS28-ESR at W 12	Yes:	8 of 42 patients	[76]
pJIA	8 mg/kg every 4 weeks	19	48 W	ACR Pedi 30 at W 12	Yes: ACR Pedi 30 (94.7%)	4 of 19 patients	[77]
	8 or 10 mg/kg every 4 weeks, PBO	188	40 W	JIA flare at W 40	Yes: 8 or 10 mg/kg (25.6%) vs PBO (48.1%, $P = .0024$)	17 of 188 patients	[78]
Uveitis[a]	162 mg SC every 2 or 3 weeks	22	36 W	Treatment response at W 12	–	–	[79]
SLE	2 mg/kg, 4 mg/kg, 8 mg/kg IV every other W for 12 W	16	20 W	SLAM at week 14	Yes: significant decrease in score ($P = .002$)	1 of 16 patients	[80]
SSc	DB: 162 mg SC weekly, PBO for 48 W, OL: 162 mg SC weekly for both	87	96 W	mRSS at week 48	No: 162 mg (−5.6) vs PBO (−3.1)	DB: 162 mg (14 of 43 patients) vs PBO (16 of 44 patients) OL: 11 of 61 patients	[81]
NMOSD	TCZ 8 mg/kg IV every 4 W, Aza 2–3 mg/kg oral per day	118	90 W	Median time to first relapse	Yes: TCZ 78.9 W vs Aza 56.7 W, $P = .0026$	TCZ (6 of 59 patients) vs Aza (11 of 59 patients)	[82]

Abbreviations: *AE*, adverse events; *RA*, rheumatoid arthritis; *Y*, year; *ACR20/50/70*, proportion of American College of Rheumatology 20/50/70 score; *SC*, subcutaneous; *IV*, intravenous; *W*, week; *DAS28-ESR*, Disease Activity Score based on 28 joints using erythrocyte sedimentation rate; *ACR Pedi 30*, more than 30% improvement in American College of Rheumatology Pediatric score; *JIA flare*, proportion of patients in whom a JIA-flare occurred; *SLAM*, Systemic Lupus Activity Measure; *DB*, Double-blind period; *OL*, open-label period; *mRSS*, modified Rodnan Skin Score; *TCZ*, tocilizumab; *Aza*, azathioprine.
[a] *JIA-associated Uveitis.*

the treatment because of neutropenia [80]. In a case report, a patient with the history of RA that was complicated with SLE was treated with tocilizumab in combination with tacrolimus, which resulted in complete remission of RA and decreased serological SLE markers [143].

Systemic sclerosis (SSc) is a rare autoimmune disorder that is distinguished by fibrosis, inflammation, and microvascular damage of several organs [144]. While observing severe AEs were more common in the tocilizumab group, it was associated with improvement in the lung and skin fibrosis in addition to the physical improvement. Hence, tocilizumab could be a promising option in SSc patients [81].

Most recently, a randomized multicenter phase II study evaluated safety and efficacy of tocilizumab compared to azathioprine in neuromyelitis optica spectrum disorder (NMOSD), a severe deliberating rare autoimmune disorder of the CNS. In NMOSD, decreased frequency of the relapses, which can lead to the reduction of patients' disability, was observed in tocilizumab-treated patients [82].

3.2.2 *Sarilumab*

Sarilumab is a new antagonist of IL-6 receptor, which inhibits both soluble- and membrane-bound IL-6 receptors that is successfully approved by the US FDA for RA as monotherapy or in combination with nonbiologic DMARDs [145] (Table 7). Safety and efficacy of sarilumab in MTX irresponsive RA patients were evaluated in investigations conducted by Genovese et al., in which two doses (150 and 200 mg) of sarilumab were administered every 2 weeks in addition to MTX treatment. Patients undergoing initial treatment with 200 mg sarilumab showed the best radiographic outcomes [83]. However, in cases with serious AEs, dose reduction to 150 mg potentially diminished the AEs [84]. The most frequent AEs were neutropenia, injection site erythema, elevated alanine aminotransferase (ALT), and upper respiratory tract infections [84]. Long-term safety and efficacy of sarilumab were demonstrated by 5 years of sarilumab treatment [146]. In the MONARCH, a phase III double-blind study, patients divided into two groups receiving adalimumab or sarilumab for 24 weeks. Sarilumab was superior in improving the disease symptoms and physical activity [85]. Then in the open-labeled phase, all the patients received sarilumab and safety of switching from adalimumab to sarilumab was investigated. Switched patients represented no safety issue and disease was attenuated in several patients [147]. Data obtained from two studies were matched together to compare the safety and tolerability of sarilumab and tocilizumab. Incidence of serious AEs were not clinically significant for sarilumab and tocilizumab groups [148]. Dose-finding, safety, and efficacy study for sarilumab in polyarticular JIA patients demonstrated no serious AE and suggested a similar dose as the adult RA dose regimen [86]. Moreover, evidence suggests posterior segment noninfectious uveitis (NIU) patients might benefit from sarilumab SC therapy, although further large-scale studies are required. The most common ocular AEs were uveitis and retinal infiltration, whereas cough and headache were the most frequent nonocular AEs [87].

3.2.3 *Sirukumab*

Sirukumab is a human monoclonal antibody that blocks circulating IL-6. Janssen Biotech, Inc. introduced Sirukumab and sought out a biologic license application. They failed to receive the US FDA approval because further clinical data was needed to evaluate the safety of Sirukumab in RA [149]. It is now under review by health authorities in Japan and Europe [149].

TABLE 7 Summary of some studies on safety and efficacy of sarilumab.

Indication	Dose (mg)	Size patient group	Duration of study	Primary endpoint	Met primary endpoint?	Number of patients with serious AEs	Refs.
RA	DB: 150 mg, 200 mg, PBO SC every 2 W OL: 200 mg SC every 2 W	1197	2 Y	ACR20 at W 24 HAQ-DI at W 16 AHS at W 52	Yes: 150 mg (ACR20, 58%; HAQ-DI, −0.53; SHS, 0.90), 200 mg (ACR20, 66.4%; HAQ-DI, −0.55; SHS 0.25) vs PBO (ACR20, 33.4%; HAQ-DI, −0.29; SHS 2.78, $P < .0001$ for all)	DB: 150 mg (38 of 431 patients), 200 mg (38 of 424 patients) vs PBO (23 of 427 patients) OL: 29 of 284 patients	[83, 84]
	SARI 200 mg SC every 2 W, ADA 40 mg every 2 W	369	24 W	DAS28-ESR at W 24	Yes: SARI (−3.28) vs IV (−2.20), $P < .0001$	SARI (9 of 184 patients), ADA (12 of 185 patients)	[85]
pJIA	2–2.5 mg/kg every 2 W, 3–4 mg/kg every 2 W, 2–2.5 mg/kg every W	42	12 W	Pharmacokinetic	Yes: This dose was comparable with corresponding adult dose	0 of 42 patients	[86]
NIU	200 mg SC every 2 weeks, PBO	58	16 W	VH or systemic corticosteroid at W 16	No: 200 mg (46.1%) vs PBO (30.0%, $P = .2354$)	200 mg (2 of 38 patients) vs PBO (1 of 20 patients)	[87]

Abbreviations: *AE*, adverse events; *RA*, rheumatoid arthritis; *PBO*, placebo; *W*, week; *DB*, double-blind period; *OL*, open-label period; *Y*, year; *ACR20*, proportion of patients achieving American College of Rheumatology 20% improvement; *HAQ-DI*, change from baseline in the Health Assessment Questionnaire disability index; *SHS*, change from baseline in the modified Sharp/van der Heijde score of radiographic damage; *SARI*, sarilumab; *ADA*, adalimumab; *DAS28-ESR*, Disease Activity Score based on 28 joints using erythrocyte sedimentation rate; 2-step reduction in vitreous haze (VH) on the Miami scale or with a reduction of systemic corticosteroids (prednisolone or equivalent) to a dose of <10 mg/day.

In lupus nephritis (LN), levels of IL-6 increases and theoretically sirukumab, an IL-6 receptor antagonist, can be efficient (Table 8). In a phase II clinical trial, efficacy and safety of sirukumab were evaluated in LN patients who were refractory to DMARD and/or corticosteroid therapy. In the treatment group, the primary endpoint was not improved. However, it was worsened in the placebo group. Five of 19 patients from the treatment group discontinued therapy because of serious AEs including elevated liver enzymes, anaphylactic reaction, pneumonia, exacerbation of LN, and neutropenia [88].

In spite of LN, sirukumab is widely investigated in RA. In a two-phase randomized crossover study with the aims of proof of concept and dose-finding, Sirukumab therapy improved disease parameters in patients with active RA despite the MTX therapy [89]. In SIRROUND-D, a phase III study in DMARDs refractory patients, sirukumab efficacy was demonstrated by expected AEs including elevated liver enzymes, infections, and injection site reactions [90]. In the subgroup analysis of Japanese patients of SIRROUND-D study, the effectiveness was confirmed and no safety signal was observed [150, 151].

3.3 Interleukin-17

T helper 17 cell produces IL-17 (also known as IL-17A) after activation with IL-23, a proinflammatory cytokine. Activation of IL-17 signaling pathway is frequently detected in the pathogenesis of autoimmune diseases such as psoriasis [152].

3.3.1 *Secukinumab*

Secukinumab is a fully human IgG1k monoclonal antibody that directly inhibits IL-17. It has been widely used for the treatment of AS, PsA, and PP [153] (Table 9). In a phase II clinical study, efficacy of secukinumab in active AS patients was evaluated in comparison with the placebo group. It was well-tolerated with only one serious AE (infection) in addition to meet primary endpoint in 59% of the treatment group versus 24% in the placebo group [91]. Secukinumab significantly provided fast and sustained improvement with expected and not-dose-related AEs [92]. Effect of loading dose on the efficacy of treatment was investigated, but treatment was not along with significant improvement because of the high response in the placebo group [93].

In a regimen-finding study of secukinumab in PP patients, three different dose intervals were evaluated in front of placebo. Early and monthly treatment led to an effective treatment with no clinically significant AEs, although evaluation of the long-term safety requires more investigations [94]. In place of dose-finding, another phase II study was conducted that revealed secukinumab was efficient in two doses. However, after treatment during the follow-up period, the amount of primary endpoint gradually decreased in treated patients [95]. Secukinumab administration by auto-injector enables patients to easily use the drug and manage their disease, so its efficacy and tolerability using these devices was observed [96]. In addition, secukinumab was superior to ustekinumab with a similar safety profile [97]. In a prospective real-life study, secukinumab efficacy was the same as the results of phase III clinical trials and with 95% of patients' adherence [98].

In addition to the above-mentioned indications, secukinumab in PsA was also evaluated. Although the primary endpoint was not met, some benefits were seen in the treatment group [99]. This efficacy was confirmed in a phase III clinical study by 150 and 300 mg treatment with secukinumab [100]. The observed efficacy was constant in extension period of study [154].

TABLE 8 Summary of some studies on safety and efficacy of sirukumab.

Indication	Dose (mg)	Size patient group	Duration of study	Primary endpoint	Met primary endpoint?	Number of patients with serious AEs	Refs.
LN	10 mg/kg IV every 4 W, PBO	25	24 W	Proteinuria% at W 24[a]	No: 10 mg/kg (0%) vs PBO (−0.43%)	10 mg/kg (10 of 21 patients) vs PBO (0 of 4 patients)	[88]
RA	100 mg every 2 W, 100, 50, 25 mg every 4 W, PBO	151	38 W	ACR50 at W 24	Yes: Only 100 mg every 2 W (26.7%) vs PBO (3.3%, $P = .026$)	Sirukumab (11 of 121 patients) vs PBO (4 of 30 patients)[b]	[89]
	100 mg every 2 W, 50 mg every 4 W SC, PBO	1670	52 W	ACR 20 at W 16 SHS at W 52	Yes: ACR 20; 100 mg (53.5%), 50 mg (54.8%) vs PBO (26.4%, $P < .001$) Yes: SHS; 100 mg (0.46), 50 mg (0.5) vs PBO (3.692, $P < .001$)	Sirukumab (138 of 1325 patients) vs PBO (38 of 556 patients)	[90]

Abbreviations: *AE*, adverse events; *LN*, lupus nephritis; *IV*, intravenous; *W*, week; *PBO*, placebo; *RA*, rheumatoid arthritis; *ACR50*, proportion of patients achieving American College of Rheumatology 50% improvement; *ACR20*, proportion of patients achieving American College of Rheumatology 20% improvement; *SHS*, change from baseline in the modified Sharp/van der Heijde score.

[a] *Median percentage reduction in proteinuria from baseline.*
[b] *Information of the part B (dose-finding) is included.*

TABLE 9 Summary of some studies on safety and efficacy of secukinumab.

Indication	Dose (mg)	Size patient group	Duration of study	Primary endpoint	Met primary endpoint?	Number of patients with serious AEs	Refs.
AS	10 mg/kg, PBO twice IV 3 W apart	37	28 W	ASAS20 at W 6	Yes: 10 mg/kg (59%) vs PBO (24%)	1 of 24 patients	[91]
	150, 300, PBO SC 4 W apart after IV loading	226	52 W	ASAS20 at W 6	Yes: 300 mg (60.5%, $P < .01$), 150 mg (58.1%, $P < .05$) vs PBO (36.8%)	1 of 150 patients vs PBO (1 of 75) then 12 of 223	[92]
	150 (with and without IV loading) SC W 0, 1, 2, 3 and 4 then 4 weeks apart, PBO	350	104 W	ASAS20 at W 6	NO: 150 mg + 150 mg IV loading (59.5%), 150 mg (61.5%) vs PBO (47%)	4 of 233 patients, PBO (4 of 117)	[93]
PP	150 mg single (0 W), early (0, 1, 2, 4 W), monthly (0, 4, 8 W), PBO	404	44 W	PASI75 at W 12	Yes: for early (54.5%), monthly (42.0%) vs PBO (1.5%, $P < .001$) No: single (10.6, $P = .225$)	12 of 337 patients, PBO (1 of 67)	[94]
	25 mg (0 W), 25, 75, 150 mg (0, 4, 8 W), PBO	125	36 W	PASI75 at W 12	Yes: 75 mg (57%), 150 mg (82%) vs PBO (9%, $P < .001$, $P = .002$)	3 of 103 patients, PBO (2 of 22)	[95]
	150 mg, 300 mg, PBO SC by pen (0, 1, 2, 3, 4 W then every 4 W)	220	208 W	PASI75 and IGA mod 2011 0/1 at W 12	Yes: 150 mg (71.7%, 53.3%), 300 mg (86.7%, 73.3%) vs PBO (3.3%, 0%, $P < .0001$ for all)	4 of 121 patients, PBO (1 of 61)	[96]
	300 mg SC by pen (0, 1, 2, 3, 4 W then every 4 W) vs ustekinumab as labeled	676	52 W	PASI90 at W 16	Yes: 300 mg secukinumab (79.0%) vs ustekinumab (57.6%, $P < .0001$)	3 of 335 for patients both	[97]
	300 mg SC by pen (0, 1, 2, 3, 4 W then every 4 W)	158	52 W	PASI75 and PASI90 at 4, 12, 24, 52 W	Yes: PASI 75 (57%, 83.3%, 89%, 78.5%), PASI 90 (27.8%, 62%, 64.6%, 63.2%), respectively	No serious AEs	[98]
PsA	10 mg/kg IV 3 W apart	42	24 W	ACR20 at W 6	No: 10 mg/kg (39%) vs PBO (23%, $P = .27$)	4 of 28 patients, PBO (1 of 17)	[99]
	75 mg, 150 mg, 300 mg PBO SC (0, 1, 2, 3, 4 W then every 4 W)	397	52 W	ACR20 at W 24	Yes: 150 mg (51%), 300 mg (54%), 75 mg (29.3%) vs PBO (15.3%, $P < .0001$, $P = .0399$)	10 of 299 patients, PBO (2 of 98)	[100]

Abbreviations: *AE*, adverse events; *AS*, ankylosing spondylitis; *PBO*, placebo; *IV*, intravenous; *W*, week; *ASAS20*, 20% Assessment of SpondyloArthritis international Society; *PP*, plaque psoriasis; *PASI75/90*, 75% or 90% improvement Psoriasis Area and Severity Index; *PsA*, psoriatic arthritis; *ACR20*, proportion of American College of Rheumatology 20.

3.3.2 *Ixekizumab*

Ixekizumab is a humanized IgG4 mAb that interacts with IL-17 and is effective in reducing inflammation in autoimmune diseases [101] (Table 10). Patients with moderate-to-severe PP had benefits from ixekizumab treatment that sustained for 20 weeks. Patients did not have any serious AEs and treatment-related AEs were not significantly different in the placebo group [101]. After a 12-week treatment-free period, long-term safety and efficacy of ixekizumab were confirmed in an open-labeled extension study. Because no placebo group was continued in this study, it was not possible to compare the obtained safety or efficacy results [102]. In two independent phase III randomized trials, UNCOVER-2 and UNCOVER-3, patients randomized in four groups including placebo, etanercept, and ixekizumab (in two dosing intervals). In both studies, ixekizumab had superior efficacy than placebo and even than etanercept, with expected AEs. Therefore, it proved ixekizumab as a biologic treatment option in psoriasis [103]. In a head-to-head trial, efficacy and safety of ixekizumab and ustekinumab were compared. Although ixekizumab was associated with more frequent injection site reactions and severe AEs, it showed a better efficacy [104].

In a phase III active controlled study, safety and efficacy of ixekizumab was investigated in AS patients. In this study, in addition to placebo and ixekizumab, adalimumab was on the arms of study as the reference drug. Ixekizumab was superior to the reference drug with similar safety profile [105]. Unlike the previous study, AS patients with inadequate response or intolerance for TNF-α were included in a phase III study. Significant and fast improvement achieved in this study suggests ixekizumab as an efficient therapeutic agent in TNF-α unresponsive patients [106].

PsA patients who were irresponsive or intolerant to TNF-α inhibitors, in a phase III trial, showed acceptable response to the ixekizumab treatment. In this study, 80 mg ixekizumab was administered every 2 or 4 weeks. In every 4 weeks administration, higher efficacy in primary endpoint was provided in addition to lesser serious AEs compared to every 2-weeks dosing interval [107]. This efficacy was sustained in the extension period of the study [108].

3.3.3 *Brodalumab*

Brodalumab is a human IgG2 mAb that antagonizes IL-17RA so blocks the activity of IL-17A, IL-17E (also known as IL-25), IL-17F, and IL-17A/F heterodimer [109]. The role of IL-17A, IL-17C, and IL-17F were established in the pathogenesis of PP (Table 11). In a dose-finding study of brodalumab in moderate to severe PP, patients randomized to four different doses and placebo groups. In this phase II clinical trial, a dose-related response was observed and the efficacy of the treatment versus placebo was confirmed [109]. One dose of brodalumab from a previous study was selected and used in an extension study, which demonstrated the long-term safety and efficacy in PP patients [110]. In addition, as PP is a chronic disease, treatment should be safe and efficient for a life-long period. Brodalumab represented constant efficacy during 5 years of treatment without inducing new safety concerns and improved the quality of life of the PP patients [111]. Moreover, PP patients that failed to treat by IL-17 antagonist agents, particularly secukinumab, responded to the switch of the treatment to brodalumab and only minor AEs were observed in a retrospective study [112].

TABLE 10 Summary of some studies on safety and efficacy of ixekizumab.

Indication	Dose (mg)	Size patient group	Duration of study	Primary endpoint	Met primary endpoint?	Number of patients with serious AEs	Refs.
PP	10, 25, 75, 150 mg, PBO SC (0, 2, 4, 8, 12, 16 W)	142	20 W	PASI75 at W 12	Yes: 25 mg (76.7%), 75 mg (82.8%), 150 mg (82.1%) vs PBO (7.7%, $P < .001$ for all)	No serious AEs	[101]
	120 mg SC every 4 W after 10, 25, 75, 150 mg, PBO SC (0, 2, 4, 8, 12, 16 W)	120	52 W	PASI75 at W 52	Yes: 120 mg (77%)	10 of 120 patients	[102]
	80 mg every 2 W, 80 mg 4 W, SC after 160 mg starting dose, ETN 50 mg twice every W, PBO	1224	12 W	PASI75 at W 12	Yes: 80 mg Q2W (89.7%), 80 mg Q4W (77.5%), ETN (41.6%), PBO (2.4%, $P < .0001$ for all)	ETN (14 of 739 patients), 80 mg Q2W (14 of 734 patients), 80 mg Q4W (14 of 729 patients), PBO (7 of 360)	[103]
		1346			Yes: 80 mg Q2W (87.3%), 80 mg Q4W (84.2%), ETN (53.4%), PBO (7.3%, $P < .0001$ for all)		
	IXE 80 mg SC Q2W for 12 W then Q4W, ustekinumab as labeled (0, 4, 16, 28, 48 W)	302	52 W	PASI90 at W 12	Yes: IXE (72.8%), ustekinumab (42.2%, $P < .001$)	IXE (9 of 135 patients), ustekinumab (6 of 166 patients)	[104]
AS	80 mg IXE, 40 mg ADA, PBO SC IXE every 2 or 4 W	341	16 W	ASAS40 at W 16	Yes: IXE Q2W (52%), IXE Q4W (48%) vs PBO (24%, $P < .001$)	2 of 164 patients, PBO (0 of 87)	[105]
	80 mg IXE, PBO SC IXE every 2 or 4 W after 80 mg or 160 mg starting dose	316	16 W	ASAS40 at W 16	Yes: IXE Q2W (30.6%), IXE Q4W (25.4%) vs PBO (12.5%, $P = .003$, $P = .017$)	7 of 212 patients vs PBO (5 of 104)	[106]
PsA	80 mg Q2W, 80 mg Q4W, SC after 160 mg starting dose, PBO	363	24 W	ACR20 at W 24	Yes: 80 mg Q2W (48%), 80 mg Q4W (53%) vs PBO (20%, $P < .0001$ for both)	80 mg Q2W (8 of 123 patients) 80 mg Q4W (3 of 122 patients), PBO (4 of 118)	[107]
	80 mg Q2W, 80 mg Q4W, SC after 160 mg starting dose	310	52 W	ACR 0 at W 52	Yes: 80 mg Q2W (51%), 80 mg Q4W (61%)	15 of 228 patients	[108]

Abbreviations: *AE*, adverse events; *PP*, plaque psoriasis; *PBO*, placebo; *SC*, subcutaneous; *W*, week; *PASI 75*, 75% improvement Psoriasis Area and Severity Index; *Q2W*, every 2 weeks; *Q4W*, every 4 weeks; *ETN*, etanercept; *IXE*, ixekizumab; *PASI 90*, 90% improvement Psoriasis Area and Severity Index; *AS*, ankylosing spondylitis; *ADA*, adalimumab; *ASAS40*, 40% Assessment of SpondyloArthritis international Society; *PsA*, psoriatic arthritis; *ACR 20*, proportion of American College of Rheumatology 20.

TABLE 11 Summary of some studies on safety and efficacy of brodalumab.

Indication	Dose (mg)	Size patient group	Duration of study	Primary endpoint	Met primary endpoint?	Number of patients with serious AEs	Refs.
PP	70 mg, 140 mg, 210 mg SC (0, 1, 2, 4, 6, 8, 10 W), 280 mg (monthly), PBO	198	12 W	PASI score at W 12	Yes: 70 mg (45%), 140 mg (85.9%), 210 mg (86.3%), 280 mg (76%) vs PBO (16%, $P < .001$ for all)	12 of 337 patients, PBO (1 of 67)	[109]
	210 mg SC every 2 W	181	120 W	sPGA score 0/1	Yes: sPGA score 0/1 (72% at W 120) vs (90% at W 12)	15 of 181 patients	[110]
	210 mg SC every 2 W	181	240 W	sPGA score 0/1	Yes: sPGA score 0/1 (77.3% at W 240) vs (90.3% at W 12)	40 of 181 patients	[111]
	210 mg SC (0, 1, 2 W then every 2 W)	23	24 W	PASI75 at week 12	Yes: 210 mg (47.8%)	0 of 23 patients	[112]

Abbreviations: *AE*, adverse events; *PP*, plaque psoriasis; *PBO*, placebo; *SC*, subcutaneous; *W*, week; *PASI score*, mean percentage improvements in the PASI score; *sPGA score 0/1*, static physician global assessment clear/almost clear of psoriasis; *PASI 75*, 75% improvement Psoriasis Area and Severity Index.

3.4 Interleukin-23

IL-23 is a proinflammatory cytokine that can be targeted in many autoimmune diseases because of its effect on immune responses. Indeed, autoimmunity could be controlled by preventing IL-23 signaling [155].

3.4.1 *Ustekinumab*

Ustekinumab is a fully human mAb that avoids the interface of IL-12 and IL-23 attaching to its receptor and blocks inflammatory pathways. Ustekinumab is used to treat plaque psoriasis in adults and children who are at least 12 years old. It is also used to treat PsA in adults, and is sometimes prescribed with MTX. Ustekinumab is also used in adults to treat moderately to severely active CD or UC [156]. Ustekinumab have shown constant efficacy over 1 year in patients with plaque psoriasis [113]. Ustekinumab can be effective for PsA patients who had failure in TNF-inhibitors therapy [114]. In a placebo-controlled phase III study, ustekinumab have demonstrated maintained efficacy for 2-year in PsA patients [115]. Administration of subcutaneous ustekinumab in patients with CD have shown safety and maintained efficacy up to 92 weeks [116]. In addition, it has shown noticeable efficacy at week 4–6 in CD patients with previous infliximab therapy [117]. Good remission rate and safety was reported for ustekinumab in treatment-refractory patients with UC [118]. It has shown better efficacy than placebo with maintaining remission in ulcerative colitis patients [119] (Table 12).

3.4.2 *Guselkumab*

Guselkumab is an anti-IL-23 p19 human IgG1 mAb. It is a member of the interleukin inhibitors and is used to treat PP and Psoriasis [157] (Table 13). Patients with PP and poor response to ustekinumab treatment have shown good response to guselkumab therapy [120]. However, guselkumab had a weaker effect in contrast to ixekizumab for plaque psoriasis [121]. Furthermore, existing evidence presents well tolerability and maintaining response of guselkumab without any deaths or serious AEs in patients with plaque psoriasis [122]. Guselkumab have shown superior efficacy than adalimumab up to 48 weeks in the treatment of moderate to severe psoriasis [123]. Subcutaneous injection of guselkumab has caused remission through 44 weeks in patients with psoriatic arthritis [124].

3.4.3 *Tildrakizumab*

Tildrakizumab is a humanized IgG1 mAb against p19-subunit of IL-23A that has the US FDA approval for plaque psoriasis treatment. Tildrakizumab reduces the effects of the substances in the body that can cause inflammation. Moreover, it is used to treat moderate-to-severe psoriasis in adults [158]. Tildrakizumab therapy has shown a good risk to benefit profile during 3 years in psoriasis patients with partial response or no response to etanercept [125]. In addition, tildrakizumab has demonstrated continued 1-year efficacy that was preserved after 20 weeks of treatment cessation in patients with plaque psoriasis [126] (Table 14).

3.4.4 *Risankizumab*

Risankizumab is an anti-IL-23p19 humanized IgG1 mAb that is approved for treating moderate-to-severe psoriasis in adults [159]. Continuous treatment with risankizumab

TABLE 12 Summary of some studies on safety and efficacy of ustekinumab.

Indication	Dose (mg)	Size patient group	Duration of study	Primary end-point	Met primary endpoint?	Number of patients with serious AEs	Refs.
PP	45 mg (Patients ≤100 kg), 90 mg (patients >100 kg)	489	52 W	PASI75 at W 12	Outcomes were similar between treatment arms	45 mg (9.4[a]), 90 mg (10.5[a])	[113]
PsA	45 mg (patients ≤100 kg), 90 mg (patients >100 kg) at W 0, 4 then every 12 W	65	24 M	MDA at M 6	30.7%	No serious AEs	[114]
	45 mg, 90 mg SC, PBO at W 0, 4 then every 12 W	615	108 W	BASDAI20/50/70, ASDAS-CRP at W 24	Yes: BASDAI20/50/70 (54.8/29.3/15.3% vs baseline 32.9/11.4/0%, $P \leq .002$); ASDAS-CRP (27.8% vs 3.9%, $P < .001$)	UST (2 of 164 patients) vs PBO (2 of 92)	[115]
CD	90 mg every 8 W, 90 mg every 12 W, PBO	718	96 W	Median CDAI score at W 44	90 mg every 12 W (95.5), 90 mg every 8 W (70.5) vs PBO (96)	UST (18.82[a]) vs PBO (19.24[a])	[116]
	PBO at W 0–3 then 90 mg UST SC at W 8–11, PBO at W 0 then 4.5 mg/kg UST IV at W 8 both with crossover	131	28 W	70 point reduction in CDAI score at W 8	No: UST (49%) vs PBO (40%, $P = .34$)	UST (2 of 52 patients) vs PBO (3 of 52)	[117]
UC	90 mg SC Q8W after 6 mg/kg IV	19	50 W	Clinical remission at 1, 3, 6, 9 and 12 M	37%, 58%, 58%, 53% and 53% of patients, respectively	No serious AEs	[118]
	90 mg SC Q12W, 90 mg SC Q8W after 130 mg IV induction, PBO	961	52 W	Clinical remission at W 44	Yes: Q12W (38.4%), Q8W (43.8%) vs PBO (24.0%, $P = .002, P < .001$)	Q12W (13 OF 172), Q8W (15 of 176) vs PBO (17 of 175)	[119]

Abbreviations: *AE*, adverse events; *PP*, plaque psoriasis; *W*, week; *PASI75*, proportion of patients with 75% improvement in Psoriasis Area and Severity Index; *PsA*, psoriatic arthritis; *MDA*, minimal disease activity; *M*, month; *SC*, subcutaneous; *BASDAI2050/70*, 20/50/70% improvement in Bath Ankylosing Spondylitis Disease Activity Index; *ASDAS-CRP*, Ankylosing Spondylitis Disease Activity Score employing C reactive protein; *UST*, ustekinumab; *CD*, Crohn's disease; *Q*, every; *CDAI*, Clinical Disease Activity Index; *UC*, ulcerative colitis; *IV*, intravenous.

[a] *Rate per 100 patient-year.*

TABLE 13 Summary of some studies on safety and efficacy of guselkumab.

Indication	Dose (mg)	Size patient group	Duration of study	Primary endpoint	Met primary endpoint?	Number of patients with serious AEs	Refs.
PP	Guselkumab 100 mg at W 16, 20 then every 8 W, UST (45 or 90 mg every 12 W)	871	60 W	IGA 0/1, at least a two-grade improvement at W 28–40	Yes: IGA 0/1: Guselkumab (1.5) vs UST (0.7, $P < .001$); Two-grade improvement at W 28: guselkumab (31.1%) vs UST (14.3%, $P = .001$)	Guselkumab (9 of 135 patients) vs UST (20 of 585)	[120]
	Guselkumab 100 mg SC at W 0, 4, 12, IXE 160 mg SC at W 0 then 80 mg every 2 W to 12	1027	24 W	PASI100 at W 12	Guselkumab (25%) vs IXE (41%, $P < .001$)	Guselkumab (13 of 506 patients), IXE (16 of 519)	[121]
	Guselkumab SC 10 mg, 30 mg, 100 mg, 300 mg, PBO	24	24 W	PASI score[a] at W 16	Yes: 10 mg (63%), 30 mg (91%), 100 mg (87%) and 300 mg (91%) vs PBO (5%)	No serious AEs	[122]
Psoriasis	Guselkumab 100 mg at W 0, 4 then every 8 W, PBO, ADA 80 mg at W 0, 40 mg at W 1 then 40 mg every 2 W	837	48 W	IGA 0/1, PASI90 at W 16	Yes: IGA 0/1: Guselkumab (85.1%) vs PBO (6.9%, $P < .001$) Guselkumab (85.1%) vs ADA (65.9%) Yes: PASI90: Guselkumab (73.3%) vs PBO (2.9%, $P < .001$); Guselkumab (73.3%) vs ADA (49.7%)	Guselkumab (16 of 329 patients), ADA (15 OF 333 patients) vs PBO (3 of 174)	[123]
PsA	Guselkumab 100 mg at W 0, 4 then every 8 W, PBO; with cross-over	149	56 W	ACR20 at W 24	Yes: guselkumab (58%) vs PBO (18%, $P < .0001$)	Guselkumab (6 of 100 patients), PBO (1 of 49)	[124]

Abbreviations: *AE*, adverse events; *PP*, plaque psoriasis; *W*, week; *IGA 0/1*, Investigator's Global Assessment clear/minimal; *SC*, subcutaneous; *UST*, ustekinumab; *IXE*, ixekizumab; *PASI100*, proportion of patients with 100% improvement in Psoriasis Area and Severity Index; *PBO*, placebo; *ADA*, adalimumab; *PASI90*, proportion of patients with 90% improvement in Psoriasis Area and Severity Index; *PsA*, psoriatic arthritis; *ACR20*, proportion of American College of Rheumatology 20.
[a] *The median per cent improvement from baseline in PASI score.*

TABLE 14 Summary of some studies on safety and efficacy of tildrakizumab.

Indication	Dose (mg)	Size patient group	Duration of study	Primary endpoint	Met primary endpoint?	Number of patients with serious AEs	Refs.
Psoriasis	200 mg, 100 mg SC	1551	148 W	PASI75/90/100 at W 148	200 mg (80.2/59.9/32.6%), 100 mg (72.6/53.8/28.9%) PASI75/90/100, respectively	100 mg (5.86[a]), 200 mg (5.47[a])	[125]
PP	5, 25, 100, 200 mg SC at W 0 and 4 then every 12 W, PBO	355	72 W	PASI75 at W 16	Yes: 5 mg (33.3%), 25 mg (64.4%), 100 mg (66.3%), 200 mg (74.4%) vs PBO (4.4%, $P \leq .001$)	5 mg (0 of 13), 25 mg (5 of 94), 100 mg (6 of 153), PBO (0 of 45)	[126]

Abbreviations: *AE*, adverse events; *SC*, subcutaneous; *W*, week; *PASI75/90/100*, proportion of patients with 75/90/100% improvement in Psoriasis Area and Severity Index; *PP*, plaque psoriasis; *PBO*, placebo.

[a] *Events per 100 patient-years of exposure.*

has demonstrated better efficacy than withdrawing regimen to placebo at week 52 and 104 in PP patients [127]. Risankizumab has shown similar efficacy to secukinumab at week 16, but it had better efficacy than secukinumab after week 52 of PP treatment [128]. Risankizumab can show good efficacy without any unexpected AE in the treatment of PP [129] (Table 15).

4 ICIs in autoimmune disease

CTLA-4 is a receptor protein and functions as an immune checkpoint that down regulates T-cell-mediated pathways [160]. It has a negative regulatory effect on T-cell-dependent immune responses; therefore, agonists of this receptor can down-regulate the immune system and can be advantageous in autoimmune diseases. Autoimmune responses in animals with mutation and polymorphism in CTLA-4 genes suggest that CTLA-4 is responsible for autoimmune diseases [161].

Antagonists of CTLA-4 made an interesting field of study for cancer treatments. These antibodies indirectly modulate T-cell-mediated pathways. Ipilimumab is an anti-CTLA-4 monoclonal antibody that inhibits immune system tolerance to tumors.

4.1 Abatacept

Abatacept (CTLA-4-Ig) is a fusion protein of CTLA-4 and Fc region of the human IgG1 and acts as a selective costimulation blocker ensued to T-cell-activation inhibition. The US FDA approved it for PsA, RA, and JIA [162]. Moreover, it is under investigation for efficacy and safety evaluation for other autoimmune diseases including Relapsing remitting multiple sclerosis (RRMS) and T1DM (Table 16).

Efficacy of abatacept in PsA was evaluated in a phase III double-blinded placebo controlled study. There was significant efficacy after the treatment and the beneficial effects were maintained for 52 weeks. Besides, it was tolerated without any safety signal. Only one patient had severe AE (pneumonia) that caused treatment cessation. However, this patient had a history of smoking and chronic obstructive pulmonary disease (COPD) [130]. The long-term safety profile and efficacy of abatacept in RA patients were evaluated in a 6-month double-blinded study extended open-labeled for 5 years. This study indicated that patients without adequate response to methotrexate therapy showed consistent improvement by abatacept treatment [131, 132]. Additionally, abatacept is efficient in JIA patients without adequate response to DMARD and anti-TNF-α therapies, even in patients who were not responsive during the initial 4-month treatment by abatacept. Production of antiabatacept antibodies was not correlated to its efficacy or safety concerns [133]. Number of patients with antibody development and with severe AEs did not increase by continuing the treatment for 7 years [163].

Genetic studies revealed the association of CTLA-4 gene polymorphism with increased susceptibility to MS [164]. RRMS patients in a phase 1 clinical trial were evaluated after CTLA-4-Ig (abatacept) therapy, which showed efficacy of the abatacept in inflammatory diseases [134]. While a phase II double-blinded multicenter study on abatacept, reported no significant efficacy in RRMS patients [135].

TABLE 15 Summary of some studies on safety and efficacy of risankizumab.

Indication	Dose (mg)	Size patient group	Duration of study	Primary endpoint	Met primary endpoint?	Number of patients with serious AEs	Refs.
PP	150 mg SC at W 0, 4, 16 then every 12 W, PBO	507	104 W	PASI90 and sPGA 0/1 at W 16.	Yes: PASI90: 150 mg (73.2%) vs PBO (2.0%); sPGA 0/1: 150 mg (83.5%) vs PBO (7.0%, $P < .001$ for both)	150 mg (7 of 407 patients), PBO (4 of 100)	[127]
	Risankizumab 150 mg, secukinumab 300 mg	327	88 W	PASI90 at W 16, 52	No: W 16: Risankizumab (73.8%), secukinumab (65.6%) Yes: W 52: Risankizumab (86.6%) secukinumab (57.1%, $P < .001$)	Risankizumab (9 of 164 patients), secukinumab (6 of 163)	[128]
	75 mg, 150 mg at W 0, 4, 16, 28 and 40, PBO with cross-over	171	52 W	PASI90 at W 16	Yes: 75 mg (76%), 150 mg (75%) vs PBO (2%, $P < .001$)	75 mg (2 of 58 patients), 150 mg (2 of 55) vs PBO (1 of 58)	[129]

Abbreviations: *AE*, adverse events; *PP*, plaque psoriasis; *SC*, subcutaneous; *PBO*, placebo; *W*, week; *PASI90*, proportion of patients with 90% improvement in Psoriasis Area and Severity Index; *sPGA 0/1*, static physician global assessment clear or almost clear.

TABLE 16 Summary of some studies on safety and efficacy of abatacept.

Indication	Dose (mg)	Size patient group	Duration of study	Primary endpoint	Met primary endpoint?	Number of patients with serious AEs	Refs.
PsA	125 mg SC, PBO	424	52 W	ACR20 at W 24	Yes: 125 mg (39.4%) vs PBO (22.3%, $P < .001$)	125 mg (6 of 213 patients) vs PBO (9 of 211)	[130]
RA	DB: SC 125 mg every W after 10 mg/kg IV inf, IV 10 mg/kg on days 1,15,29 then every 4 W	1457	6 M	ACR20 at M 6	Yes: SC (76%), IV (75.8%), no inferiority of SC	SC (31 of 736 patients), IV (35 of 721)	[131]
	OL: SC 125 mg every W	1373	5 Y	AE of special interest	Infection (38.6[a]), serious infection (1.68[a]), malignancies (1.09[a]), autoimmune disorders (1.33[a])	353 of 1373 patients	[132]
JIA	10 mg/kg IV every 4 W	153	21 M	ACR Pedi 30/50/70/90/100	Yes: 90/8/75/57/39% improvement	14 of 153 patients	[133]
RRMS	2, 10, 20, 35 mg/kg IV inf	16	3 M	MBP proliferation at M 2	Reduction was observed	No serious AEs	[134]
RRMS	500/mg g IV inf every 4 W, PBO	65	52 W	Mean n of lesions[b] every 4 W	No: abatacept (0.43), PBO (1.66, $P = .87$)	Abatacept (2 of 44 patients) vs PBO (0 of 21)	[135]
T1D	10 mg/kg (max 1 g) on days 1, 14, 28 then every M, PBO	112	2 Y	Adjusted C-peptide AUC at Y 2	Yes: abatacept (0.378 nmol/L), PBO (0.238 nmol/L, $P = .0029$)	–	[136]

Abbreviations: *AE*, adverse events; *PsA*, psoriatic arthritis; *SC*, subcutaneous; *PBO*, placebo; *W*, week; *ACR20*, proportion of American College of Rheumatology 20; *RA*, rheumatoid arthritis; *DB*, double-blind period; *OL*, open-label period; *IV inf*, intravenous infusion; *M*, month; *ACR Pedi 30/50/70/90/100*, ACR Pediatric 30 (Pedi 30), Pedi 50, Pedi 70, Pedi 90, and Pedi 100 criteria for improvement; *RRMS*, relapsing remitting multiple sclerosis; *MBP*, myelin basic protein; *T1D*, type 1 diabetes mellitus.
[a] *Events per 100 patient-years of exposure.*
[b] *Mean number of new gadolinium-enhancing (Gd +) lesions on MRI imaging.*

Because T1DM is related to T-cell activation, modulators of T-cell activation such as abatacept can have promising effects in disease control. Abatacept therapy in recent onset T1DM patients slowed down the reduction of β-cells' function during the treatment period and decreased HbA1c level. There was no serious AEs and infusion site reaction was the most-observed AE [136]. Persistence of the effect of 2-year abatacept therapy in early onset T1DM patients was assessed by a 1-year off-treatment period, that the beneficial effects such as slowing the reduction in β-cell function was observed [165].

4.2 Belatacept

Belatacept is another CTLA-4-Ig and approved by the US FDA for kidney transplant [166]. Actually, the immune system is responsible for organ graft loss and down-regulation of T-cell-mediated immune pathways by CTLA-4 agonists might be a solution for this problem. Although calcineurin inhibitors including cyclosporine prevent acute organ rejection during the first year of therapy, it is associated with several AEs such as renal and cardiovascular toxicities during the long-term administration. In this situation, selective CTLA-4-Ig, belatacept, can be used instead of toxic drugs. It is not superior to cyclosporine in prevention of acute rejection in the first year of treatment; however, it can preserve the renal function and reduce nephropathy [167]. This study was extended for long-term safety evaluation of belatacept for 5 years. Beneficial effects of belatacept such as increased glomerular filtration rate (GFR) were observed. Safety evaluations demonstrate lower incidence of severe AEs in belatacept-treated groups but in both groups the frequency of detected malignancies was similar [168]. Posttransplant proliferative disorder was more frequent in belatacept-treated patients versus cyclosporine therapy [169]. In BENEFIT a phase III randomized clinical trial by 686 patients on the efficacy of belatacept, acute rejection of kidney transplant was unexpectedly higher than cyclosporine-treated group [169]. Extended follow up to 7 years after kidney transplant revealed an increase in mean estimated GFR from for both of the studied belatacept regimens, while it decreased in the cyclosporine regimen. In addition, the rate of death due to organ rejection after 7 years were obviously lower for belatacept [170]. Despite the promising features, more acute rejections with belatacept hinder its widespread use. In a belatacept-based immunosuppression regimen with rabbit antithymocyte globulin (rATG) induction and maintenance by everolimus was suggested to maintain the excellent GFR with low acute rejection rate [171].

5 Conclusion

Autoimmune diseases are deliberating and hard to manage. Because of the requirement of life-long treatment, traditional treatments for autoimmune diseases lead to several treatment-associated AEs.

In this condition, biologic drugs despite coexisting common AEs including injection side reaction, antidrug antibody production, and infections can be promising alternative treatment options. When we look closely at the approved indications of these drugs, they are often used in circumstances where there is inadequate response to the previous drugs. In conditions that there is not any efficient treatment, DMARD refractory RA patients for instance, common AEs of biologic drugs might be tolerable. However, further investigations to diminish these AEs are important to increase these patients' quality of life. In fact, this goal could be achieved, when the treatment is not associated with a life-threatening complication by balancing the efficacy and safety of the drug.

References

[1] M. Luan, et al., The shared and specific mechanism of four autoimmune diseases, Oncotarget 8 (65) (2017) 108355.

[2] M. Böhm, et al., New insight into immunosuppression and treatment of autoimmune diseases, Clin. Exp. Rheumatol. 24 (1 Suppl. 40) (2006) S67–S71.

[3] G. Köhler, C. Milstein, Continuous cultures of fused cells secreting antibody of predefined specificity, Nature 256 (5517) (1975) 495–497.

[4] L.B. Nicholson, The immune system, Essays Biochem. 60 (3) (2016) 275–301.

[5] M. Feldmann, F.M. Brennan, R. Maini, Cytokines in autoimmune disorders, Int. Rev. Immunol. 17 (1–4) (1998) 217–228.

[6] B.P.K. CynthiaKassab, H. Caruso, S. Al Enazy, A.B. Heimberger, Chapter 15—Immunomodulatory methods, in: Nervous System Drug Delivery, Principles and Practice, Academic Press, 2019.

[7] I. Astrakhantseva, et al., Modern anti-cytokine therapy of autoimmune diseases, Biochemistry (Moscow) 79 (12) (2014) 1308–1321.

[8] Y. Lai, C. Dong, Therapeutic antibodies that target inflammatory cytokines in autoimmune diseases, Int. immunol. 28 (4) (2016) 181–188.

[9] K. Madden, M.K. Kasler, Immune checkpoint inhibitors in lung cancer and melanoma, Semin. Oncol. Nurs. 35 (5) (2019) 150932.

[10] K. Yang, et al., Retreatment with immune checkpoint inhibitors in solid tumors: a systematic review, Ther. Adv. Med. Oncol. 12 (2020). 1758835920975353.

[11] F.A. Harding, et al., The immunogenicity of humanized and fully human antibodies: residual immunogenicity resides in the CDR regions, In MAbs 2 (3) (2010) 256–265.

[12] O. Shovman, et al., Diverse patterns of anti-TNF-α-induced lupus: case series and review of the literature, Clin. Rheumatol. 37 (2) (2018) 563–568.

[13] E.B. Suhler, et al., A prospective trial of infliximab therapy for refractory uveitis: preliminary safety and efficacy outcomes, Arch. Ophthalmol. 123 (7) (2005) 903–912.

[14] A.M.A. El-Asrar, et al., Long-term safety and efficacy of infliximab therapy in refractory uveitis due to Behçet's disease, Int. Ophthalmol. 26 (3) (2005) 83–92.

[15] H. Al-Rayes, et al., Safety and efficacy of infliximab therapy in active Behcet's uveitis: an open-label trial, Rheumatol. Int. 29 (1) (2008) 53–57.

[16] M.E. Zannin, et al., Safety and efficacy of infliximab and adalimumab for refractory uveitis in juvenile idiopathic arthritis: 1-year followup data from the Italian Registry, J. Rheumatol. 40 (1) (2013) 74–79.

[17] S. Uppal, S. Hayat, R. Raghupathy, Efficacy and safety of infliximab in active SLE: a pilot study, Lupus 18 (8) (2009) 690–697.

[18] M. Aringer, et al., Safety and efficacy of tumor necrosis factor α blockade in systemic lupus erythematosus: an open-label study, Arthritis Rheum. 50 (10) (2004) 3161–3169.

[19] D. van der Heijde, et al., Efficacy and safety of infliximab in patients with ankylosing spondylitis: results of a randomized, placebo-controlled trial (ASSERT), Arthritis Rheum. 52 (2) (2005) 582–591.

[20] J. Braun, et al., Efficacy and safety of infliximab in patients with ankylosing spondylitis over a two-year period, Arthritis Care Res. 59 (9) (2008) 1270–1278.

[21] V. Gerloni, et al., Efficacy of repeated intravenous infusions of an anti-tumor necrosis factor α monoclonal antibody, infliximab, in persistently active, refractory juvenile idiopathic arthritis: results of an open-label prospective study, Arthritis Rheum. 52 (2) (2005) 548–553.

[22] T. Levälampi, et al., Effects of infliximab on cytokines, myeloperoxidase, and soluble adhesion molecules in patients with juvenile idiopathic arthritis, Scand. J. Rheumatol. 36 (3) (2007) 189–193.

[23] J. Hyams, et al., Induction and maintenance infliximab therapy for the treatment of moderate-to-severe Crohn's disease in children, Gastroenterology 132 (3) (2007) 863–873.

[24] J. Hyams, et al., Safety and efficacy of maintenance infliximab therapy for moderate-to-severe Crohn's disease in children: REACH open-label extension, Curr. Med. Res. Opin. 27 (3) (2011) 651–662.

[25] U. Chaudhari, et al., Efficacy and safety of infliximab monotherapy for plaque-type psoriasis: a randomised trial, Lancet 357 (9271) (2001) 1842–1847.

[26] M. Takeuchi, et al., Evaluation of the long-term efficacy and safety of infliximab treatment for uveitis in Behçet's disease: a multicenter study, Ophthalmology 121 (10) (2014) 1877–1884.

[27] S.J. Hayat, et al., Safety and efficacy of infliximab in a patient with active WHO class IV lupus nephritis, Clin. Rheumatol. 26 (6) (2007) 973–975.

[28] S.J. Hayat, S.S. Uppal, Therapeutic efficacy and safety profile of infliximab in active systemic lupus erythematosus, Mod. Rheumatol. 17 (2) (2007) 174–177.

[29] X. Baraliakos, et al., Safety and efficacy of readministration of infliximab after longterm continuous therapy and withdrawal in patients with ankylosing spondylitis, J. Rheumatol. 34 (3) (2007) 510–515.

[30] M.L. Stoll, et al., Safety and efficacy of intra-articular infliximab therapy for treatment-resistant temporomandibular joint arthritis in children: a retrospective study, Rheumatology 52 (3) (2013) 554–559.

[31] J. Mallol, Therapeutic effects of the anti-tumor necrosis factor monoclonal antibody, infliximab, in four children with refractory juvenile idiopathic arthritis, Allergol. Immunopathol. 35 (2) (2007) 52–56.

[32] S.A. Hendler, et al., High-dose infliximab therapy in Crohn's disease: clinical experience, safety, and efficacy, J. Crohn's Colitis 9 (3) (2015) 266–275.

[33] Drug.com, Adalimumab, 2020, (cited 2020 8/2/202). Available from https://www.drugs.com/ppa/adalimumab.html.

[34] R. Bissonnette, et al., Efficacy and safety of adalimumab in patients with plaque psoriasis who have shown an unsatisfactory response to etanercept, J. Am. Acad. Dermatol. 63 (2) (2010) 228–234.

[35] A. Asahina, et al., Safety and efficacy of adalimumab treatment in Japanese patients with psoriasis: results of SALSA study, J. Dermatol. 43 (11) (2016) 1257–1266.

[36] M.C. Genovese, et al., Safety and efficacy of adalimumab in treatment of patients with psoriatic arthritis who had failed disease modifying antirheumatic drug therapy, J. Rheumatol. 34 (5) (2007) 1040–1050.

[37] V. Cecchin, et al., Longterm safety and efficacy of adalimumab and infliximab for uveitis associated with juvenile idiopathic arthritis, J. Rheumatol. 45 (8) (2018) 1167–1172.

[38] D. Windschall, G. Horneff, Safety and efficacy of etanercept and adalimumab in children aged 2 to 4 years with juvenile idiopathic arthritis, Clin. Rheumatol. 35 (12) (2016) 2925–2931.

[39] C.-W. Chang, et al., Safety and efficacy of adalimumab for patients with moderate to severe Crohn's disease: the Taiwan Society of Inflammatory Bowel Disease (TSIBD) Study, Intest. Res. 12 (4) (2014) 287.

[40] Y. Suzuki, et al., Efficacy and safety of adalimumab in Japanese patients with moderately to severely active ulcerative colitis, J. Gastroenterol. 49 (2) (2014) 283–294.

[41] A. Bálint, et al., Efficacy and safety of adalimumab in ulcerative colitis refractory to conventional therapy in routine clinical practice, J. Crohn's Colitis 10 (1) (2016) 26–30.

[42] E.B. Suhler, et al., Adalimumab therapy for refractory uveitis: results of a multicentre, open-label, prospective trial, Br. J. Ophthalmol. 97 (4) (2013) 481–486.

[43] C.C. Zouboulis, et al., Long-term adalimumab efficacy in patients with moderate-to-severe hidradenitis suppurativa/acne inversa: 3-year results of a phase 3 open-label extension study, J. Am. Acad. Dermatol. 80 (1) (2019) 60–69. e2.

[44] M. Christina Goussi, et al., A prospective open-label clinical trial of efficacy of the every week administration of adalimumab in the treatment of hidradenitis suppurativa, J. Drugs Dermatol. 11 (5) (2012) s15–s20.

[45] M. Rudwaleit, et al., Effectiveness, safety, and predictors of good clinical response in 1250 patients treated with adalimumab for active ankylosing spondylitis, J. Rheumatol. 36 (4) (2009) 801–808.

[46] D. van der Heijde, et al., Efficacy and safety of adalimumab in patients with ankylosing spondylitis: results of a multicenter, randomized, double-blind, placebo-controlled trial, Arthritis Rheum. 54 (7) (2006) 2136–2146.

[47] L. Van de Putte, et al., Efficacy and safety of adalimumab as monotherapy in patients with rheumatoid arthritis for whom previous disease modifying antirheumatic drug treatment has failed, Ann. Rheum. Dis. 63 (5) (2004) 508–516.

[48] A. Teriaky, et al., The safety and efficacy of adalimumab in patients with Crohn's disease: the experience of a single Canadian tertiary care centre, Scand. J. Gastroenterol. 49 (3) (2014) 280–286.

[49] E.B. Suhler, et al., Safety and efficacy of adalimumab in patients with noninfectious uveitis in an ongoing open-label study: VISUAL III, Ophthalmology 125 (7) (2018) 1075–1087.

[50] A. Deodhar, et al., Safety and efficacy of golimumab administered intravenously in adults with ankylosing spondylitis: results through week 28 of the GO-ALIVE study, J. Rheumatol. 45 (3) (2018) 341–348.

[51] C. Bao, et al., Safety and efficacy of golimumab in Chinese patients with active ankylosing spondylitis: 1-year results of a multicentre, randomized, double-blind, placebo-controlled phase III trial, Rheumatology 53 (9) (2014) 1654–1663.

[52] A. Kavanaugh, et al., Safety and efficacy of intravenous golimumab in patients with active psoriatic arthritis: results through week twenty-four of the GO-VIBRANT study, Arthritis Rheumatol. 69 (11) (2017) 2151–2161.

[53] A. Kavanaugh, et al., Clinical efficacy, radiographic and safety findings through 5 years of subcutaneous golimumab treatment in patients with active psoriatic arthritis: results from a long-term extension of a randomised, placebo-controlled trial (the GO-REVEAL study), Ann. Rheum. Dis. 73 (9) (2014) 1689–1694.

[54] J. Tesser, et al., Efficacy and safety of intravenous golimumab plus methotrexate in patients with rheumatoid arthritis aged <65 years and those ≥65 years of age, Arthritis Res. Ther. 21 (1) (2019) 190.

[55] E.C. Keystone, et al., Safety and efficacy of subcutaneous golimumab in patients with active rheumatoid arthritis despite methotrexate therapy: final 5-year results of the GO-FORWARD trial, J. Rheumatol. 43 (2) (2016) 298–306.

[56] J. Sieper, et al., A randomized, double-blind, placebo-controlled, sixteen-week study of subcutaneous golimumab in patients with active nonradiographic axial spondyloarthritis, Arthritis Rheumatol. 67 (10) (2015) 2702–2712.

[57] T. Hibi, et al., Efficacy and safety of golimumab 52-week maintenance therapy in Japanese patients with moderate to severely active ulcerative colitis: a phase 3, double-blind, randomized, placebo-controlled study-(PURSUIT-J study), J. Gastroenterol. 52 (10) (2017) 1101–1111.

[58] A. Tursi, et al., Effectiveness and safety of golimumab in treating outpatient ulcerative colitis: a real-life prospective, multicentre, observational study in primary inflammatory bowel diseases centers, J. Gastrointestin. Liver Dis. 26 (3) (2017).

[59] W. Sandborn, et al., Long-term safety and efficacy of certolizumab pegol in the treatment of Crohn's disease: 7-year results from the PREC i SE 3 study, Aliment. Pharmacol. Ther. 40 (8) (2014) 903–916.

[60] G.R. Lichtenstein, et al., Continuous therapy with certolizumab pegol maintains remission of patients with Crohn's disease for up to 18 months, Clin. Gastroenterol. Hepatol. 8 (7) (2010) 600–609.

[61] R. Fleischmann, et al., Long-term maintenance of certolizumab pegol safety and efficacy, in combination with methotrexate and as monotherapy, in rheumatoid arthritis patients, Rheumatol. Ther. 4 (1) (2017) 57–69.

[62] J.S. Smolen, et al., Certolizumab pegol in rheumatoid arthritis patients with low to moderate activity: the CERTAIN double-blind, randomised, placebo-controlled trial, Ann. Rheum. Dis. 74 (5) (2015) 843–850.

[63] P. Mease, et al., Effect of certolizumab pegol on signs and symptoms in patients with psoriatic arthritis: 24-week results of a Phase 3 double-blind randomised placebo-controlled study (RAPID-PsA), Ann. Rheum. Dis. 73 (1) (2014) 48–55.

[64] R. Landewé, et al., Efficacy of certolizumab pegol on signs and symptoms of axial spondyloarthritis including ankylosing spondylitis: 24-week results of a double-blind randomised placebo-controlled Phase 3 study, Ann. Rheum. Dis. 73 (1) (2014) 39–47.

[65] A. Blauvelt, et al., Certolizumab pegol for the treatment of patients with moderate-to-severe chronic plaque psoriasis: pooled analysis of week 16 data from three randomized controlled trials, J. Eur. Acad. Dermatol. Venereol. 33 (3) (2019) 546–552.

[66] M. Lebwohl, et al., Certolizumab pegol for the treatment of chronic plaque psoriasis: results through 48 weeks of a phase 3, multicenter, randomized, double-blind, etanercept-and placebo-controlled study (CIMPACT), J. Am. Acad. Dermatol. 79 (2) (2018) 266–276. e5.

[67] L. Klareskog, et al., Assessment of long-term safety and efficacy of etanercept in a 5-year extension study in patients with rheumatoid arthritis, Clin. Exp. Rheumatol. 29 (2) (2011) 238.

[68] M.E. Weinblatt, et al., Safety and efficacy of etanercept beyond 10 years of therapy in North American patients with early and longstanding rheumatoid arthritis, Arthritis Care Res. 63 (3) (2011) 373–382.

[69] P.J. Mease, et al., Etanercept treatment of psoriatic arthritis: safety, efficacy, and effect on disease progression, Arthritis Rheum. 50 (7) (2004) 2264–2272.

[70] J. Braun, et al., Clinical efficacy and safety of etanercept versus sulfasalazine in patients with ankylosing spondylitis: a randomized, double-blind trial, Arthritis Rheum. 63 (6) (2011) 1543–1551.

[71] J.C. Davis, et al., Efficacy and safety of up to 192 weeks of etanercept therapy in patients with ankylosing spondylitis, Ann. Rheum. Dis. 67 (3) (2008) 346–352.

11. Efficacy and safety of mAbs in autoimmune diseases

[72] A.S. Paller, et al., Long-term safety and efficacy of etanercept in children and adolescents with plaque psoriasis, J. Am. Acad. Dermatol. 74 (2) (2016) 280–287. e3.

[73] N. Nishimoto, et al., Long-term safety and efficacy of tocilizumab, an anti-IL-6 receptor monoclonal antibody, in monotherapy, in patients with rheumatoid arthritis (the STREAM study): evidence of safety and efficacy in a 5-year extension study, Ann. Rheum. Dis. 68 (10) (2009) 1580–1584.

[74] A. Ogata, et al., A phase 3 study of the efficacy and safety of subcutaneous versus intravenous tocilizumab monotherapy in patients with rheumatoid arthritis (MUSASHI), Arthritis Care Res. 66 (3) (2014) 344–354.

[75] G.R. Burmester, et al., A randomised, double-blind, parallel-group study of the safety and efficacy of subcutaneous tocilizumab versus intravenous tocilizumab in combination with traditional disease-modifying antirheumatic drugs in patients with moderate to severe rheumatoid arthritis (SUMMACTA study), Ann. Rheum. Dis. 73 (1) (2014) 69–74.

[76] A. Ogata, Y. Tanaka, T. Ishii, M. Kaneko, H. Miwa, S. Ohsawa, R. Yamakawa, SHINOBI Study Group. Long-term safety and efficacy of weekly subcutaneous tocilizumab monotherapy in patients with rheumatoid arthritis who had an inadequate response to subcutaneous tocilizumab every other week: results from the open-label extension of the SHINOBI study, Mod. Rheumatol. 29 (5) (2019) 767–774.

[77] T. Imagawa, et al., Safety and efficacy of tocilizumab, an anti-IL-6-receptor monoclonal antibody, in patients with polyarticular-course juvenile idiopathic arthritis, Mod. Rheumatol. 22 (1) (2012) 109–115.

[78] H.I. Brunner, et al., Efficacy and safety of tocilizumab in patients with polyarticular-course juvenile idiopathic arthritis: results from a phase 3, randomised, double-blind withdrawal trial, Ann. Rheum. Dis. 74 (6) (2015) 1110–1117.

[79] A.V. Ramanan, et al., A phase II trial protocol of Tocilizumab in anti-TNF refractory patients with JIA-associated uveitis (the APTITUDE trial), BMC Rheumatol. 2 (1) (2018) 4.

[80] G.G. Illei, et al., Tocilizumab in systemic lupus erythematosus: data on safety, preliminary efficacy, and impact on circulating plasma cells from an open-label phase I dosage-escalation study, Arthritis Rheum. 62 (2) (2010) 542–552.

[81] D. Khanna, et al., Safety and efficacy of subcutaneous tocilizumab in systemic sclerosis: results from the open-label period of a phase II randomised controlled trial (faSScinate), Ann. Rheum. Dis. 77 (2) (2018) 212–220.

[82] C. Zhang, et al., Safety and efficacy of tocilizumab versus azathioprine in highly relapsing neuromyelitis optica spectrum disorder (TANGO): an open-label, multicentre, randomised, phase 2 trial, Lancet Neurol. 19 (5) (2020) 391–401.

[83] M.C. Genovese, et al., Sarilumab plus methotrexate in patients with active rheumatoid arthritis and inadequate response to methotrexate: results of a phase III study, Arthritis Rheumatol. 67 (6) (2015) 1424–1437.

[84] M.C. Genovese, et al., Two years of sarilumab in patients with rheumatoid arthritis and an inadequate response to MTX: safety, efficacy and radiographic outcomes, Rheumatology 57 (8) (2018) 1423–1431.

[85] G.R. Burmester, et al., Efficacy and safety of sarilumab monotherapy versus adalimumab monotherapy for the treatment of patients with active rheumatoid arthritis (MONARCH): a randomised, double-blind, parallel-group phase III trial, Ann. Rheum. Dis. 76 (5) (2017) 840–847.

[86] F. De Benedetti, et al., FRI0549 Sarilumab, a Human Monoclonal Antibody to the Interleukin-6 (IL-6) Receptor, in Polyarticular-Course Juvenile Idiopathic Arthritis (PCJIA): A 12-Week Multinational Open-Label Dose-Finding Study, BMJ Publishing Group Ltd, 2019.

[87] J. Heissigerová, et al., Efficacy and safety of sarilumab for the treatment of posterior segment noninfectious uveitis (SARIL-NIU):: the phase 2 SATURN study, Ophthalmology 126 (3) (2019) 428–437.

[88] B.H. Rovin, et al., A multicenter, randomized, double-blind, placebo-controlled study to evaluate the efficacy and safety of treatment with sirukumab (CNTO 136) in patients with active lupus nephritis, Arthritis Rheumatol. 68 (9) (2016) 2174–2183.

[89] J.S. Smolen, et al., Sirukumab, a human anti-interleukin-6 monoclonal antibody: a randomised, 2-part (proof-of-concept and dose-finding), phase II study in patients with active rheumatoid arthritis despite methotrexate therapy, Ann. Rheum. Dis. 73 (9) (2014) 1616–1625.

[90] T. Takeuchi, et al., Sirukumab for rheumatoid arthritis: the phase III SIRROUND-D study, Ann. Rheum. Dis. 76 (12) (2017) 2001–2008.

[91] D. Baeten, et al., Anti-interleukin-17A monoclonal antibody secukinumab in treatment of ankylosing spondylitis: a randomised, double-blind, placebo-controlled trial, Lancet 382 (9906) (2013) 1705–1713.

[92] K. Pavelka, et al., Efficacy, safety, and tolerability of secukinumab in patients with active ankylosing spondylitis: a randomized, double-blind phase 3 study, measure 3, Arthritis Res. Ther. 19 (1) (2017) 285.

[93] A.J. Kivitz, et al., Efficacy and safety of secukinumab 150 mg with and without loading regimen in ankylosing spondylitis: 104-week results from MEASURE 4 study, Rheumatol. Ther. 5 (2) (2018) 447–462.

[94] P. Rich, et al., Secukinumab induction and maintenance therapy in moderate-to-severe plaque psoriasis: a randomized, double-blind, placebo-controlled, phase II regimen-finding study, Br. J. Dermatol. 168 (2) (2013) 402–411.

[95] K. Papp, et al., Efficacy and safety of secukinumab in the treatment of moderate-to-severe plaque psoriasis: a randomized, double-blind, placebo-controlled phase II dose-ranging study, Br. J. Dermatol. 168 (2) (2013) 412–421.

[96] C. Paul, et al., Efficacy, safety and usability of secukinumab administration by autoinjector/pen in psoriasis: a randomized, controlled trial (JUNCTURE), J. Eur. Acad. Dermatol. Venereol. 29 (6) (2015) 1082–1090.

[97] D. Thaçi, et al., Secukinumab is superior to ustekinumab in clearing skin of subjects with moderate to severe plaque psoriasis: CLEAR, a randomized controlled trial, J. Am. Acad. Dermatol. 73 (3) (2015) 400–409.

[98] J.-M. Ortiz-Salvador, et al., A prospective multicenter study assessing effectiveness and safety of secukinumab in a real-life setting in 158 patients, J. Am. Acad. Dermatol. 81 (2) (2019) 427–432.

[99] I.B. McInnes, et al., Efficacy and safety of secukinumab, a fully human anti-interleukin-17A monoclonal antibody, in patients with moderate-to-severe psoriatic arthritis: a 24-week, randomised, double-blind, placebo-controlled, phase II proof-of-concept trial, Ann. Rheum. Dis. 73 (2) (2014) 349–356.

[100] I.B. McInnes, et al., Secukinumab, a human anti-interleukin-17A monoclonal antibody, in patients with psoriatic arthritis (FUTURE 2): a randomised, double-blind, placebo-controlled, phase 3 trial, Lancet 386 (9999) (2015) 1137–1146.

[101] C. Leonardi, et al., Anti-interleukin-17 monoclonal antibody ixekizumab in chronic plaque psoriasis, N. Engl. J. Med. 366 (13) (2012) 1190–1199.

[102] K.B. Gordon, et al., A 52-week, open-label study of the efficacy and safety of ixekizumab, an anti-interleukin-17A monoclonal antibody, in patients with chronic plaque psoriasis, J. Am. Acad. Dermatol. 71 (6) (2014) 1176–1182.

[103] C.E. Griffiths, et al., Comparison of ixekizumab with etanercept or placebo in moderate-to-severe psoriasis (UNCOVER-2 and UNCOVER-3): results from two phase 3 randomised trials, Lancet 386 (9993) (2015) 541–551.

[104] C. Paul, et al., Ixekizumab provides superior efficacy compared with ustekinumab over 52 weeks of treatment: results from IXORA-S, a phase 3 study, J. Am. Acad. Dermatol. 80 (1) (2019) 70–79. e3.

[105] D. van der Heijde, et al., Ixekizumab, an interleukin-17A antagonist in the treatment of ankylosing spondylitis or radiographic axial spondyloarthritis in patients previously untreated with biological disease-modifying anti-rheumatic drugs (COAST-V): 16 week results of a phase 3 randomised, double-blind, active-controlled and placebo-controlled trial, Lancet 392 (10163) (2018) 2441–2451.

[106] A. Deodhar, et al., Efficacy and safety of ixekizumab in the treatment of radiographic axial spondyloarthritis: sixteen-week results from a phase III randomized, double-blind, placebo-controlled trial in patients with prior inadequate response to or intolerance of tumor necrosis factor inhibitors, Arthritis Rheumatol. 71 (4) (2019) 599–611.

[107] P. Nash, et al., Ixekizumab for the treatment of patients with active psoriatic arthritis and an inadequate response to tumour necrosis factor inhibitors: results from the 24-week randomised, double-blind, placebo-controlled period of the SPIRIT-P2 phase 3 trial, Lancet 389 (10086) (2017) 2317–2327.

[108] M.C. Genovese, et al., Safety and efficacy of ixekizumab in patients with PsA and previous inadequate response to TNF inhibitors: week 52 results from SPIRIT-P2, Rheumatology 57 (11) (2018) 2001–2011.

[109] K.A. Papp, et al., Brodalumab, an anti-interleukin-17-receptor antibody for psoriasis, N. Engl. J. Med. 366 (13) (2012) 1181–1189.

[110] K. Papp, et al., Safety and efficacy of brodalumab for psoriasis after 120 weeks of treatment, J. Am. Acad. Dermatol. 71 (6) (2014) 1183–1190. e3.

[111] M.G. Lebwohl, et al., Efficacy, safety, and patient-reported outcomes in patients with moderate-to-severe plaque psoriasis treated with brodalumab for 5 years in a long-term, open-label, phase II study, Am. J. Clin. Dermatol. 20 (6) (2019) 863–871.

[112] C. Kromer, et al., Changing within the same class: efficacy of brodalumab in plaque psoriasis after treatment with an IL-17A blocker—a retrospective multicenter study, J. Dermatol. Treat. (2020) 1–5.

11. Efficacy and safety of mAbs in autoimmune diseases

[113] K. Reich, et al., One-year safety and efficacy of ustekinumab and results of dose adjustment after switching from inadequate methotrexate treatment: the TRANSIT randomized trial in moderate-to-severe plaque psoriasis, Br. J. Dermatol. 170 (2) (2014) 435–444.

[114] M.S. Chimenti, et al., Effectiveness and safety of ustekinumab in naive or TNF-inhibitors failure psoriatic arthritis patients: a 24-month prospective multicentric study, Clin. Rheumatol. 37 (2) (2018) 397–405.

[115] A. Kavanaugh, et al., Efficacy and safety of ustekinumab in psoriatic arthritis patients with peripheral arthritis and physician-reported spondylitis: post-hoc analyses from two phase III, multicentre, double-blind, placebo-controlled studies (PSUMMIT-1/PSUMMIT-2), Ann. Rheum. Dis. 75 (11) (2016) 1984–1988.

[116] W.J. Sandborn, et al., Long-term efficacy and safety of ustekinumab for Crohn's disease through the second year of therapy, Aliment. Pharmacol. Ther. 48 (1) (2018) 65–77.

[117] W.J. Sandborn, et al., A randomized trial of ustekinumab, a human interleukin-12/23 monoclonal antibody, in patients with moderate-to-severe Crohn's disease, Gastroenterology 135 (4) (2008) 1130–1141.

[118] T. Ochsenkühn, et al., Clinical outcomes with ustekinumab as rescue treatment in therapy-refractory or therapy-intolerant ulcerative colitis, 8 (1) (2020) 91–98.

[119] B.E. Sands, et al., Ustekinumab as induction and maintenance therapy for ulcerative colitis, N. Engl. J. Med. 381 (13) (2019) 1201–1214.

[120] R. Langley, et al., Efficacy and safety of guselkumab in patients with psoriasis who have an inadequate response to ustekinumab: results of the randomized, double-blind, phase III NAVIGATE trial, Br. J. Dermatol. 178 (1) (2018) 114–123.

[121] A. Blauvelt, et al., A head-to-head comparison of ixekizumab vs. guselkumab in patients with moderate-to-severe plaque psoriasis: 12-week efficacy, safety and speed of response from a randomized, double-blinded trial, Br. J. Dermatol. 182 (6) (2020) 1348–1358.

[122] O. Nemoto, et al., Safety and efficacy of guselkumab in Japanese patients with moderate-to-severe plaque psoriasis: a randomized, placebo-controlled, ascending-dose study, Br. J. Dermatol. 178 (3) (2018) 689–696.

[123] A. Blauvelt, et al., Efficacy and safety of guselkumab, an anti-interleukin-23 monoclonal antibody, compared with adalimumab for the continuous treatment of patients with moderate to severe psoriasis: results from the phase III, double-blinded, placebo-and active comparator–controlled VOYAGE 1 trial, J. Am. Acad. Dermatol. 76 (3) (2017) 405–417.

[124] A. Deodhar, et al., Efficacy and safety of guselkumab in patients with active psoriatic arthritis: a randomised, double-blind, placebo-controlled, phase 2 study, Lancet 391 (10136) (2018) 2213–2224.

[125] K. Reich, et al., Long-term efficacy and safety of tildrakizumab for moderate-to-severe psoriasis: pooled analyses of two randomized phase III clinical trials (re SURFACE 1 and re SURFACE 2) through 148 weeks, Br. J. Dermatol. 182 (3) (2020) 605–617.

[126] K. Papp, et al., Tildrakizumab (MK-3222), an anti-interleukin-23p19 monoclonal antibody, improves psoriasis in a phase IIb randomized placebo-controlled trial, Br. J. Dermatol. 173 (4) (2015) 930–939.

[127] A. Blauvelt, et al., Efficacy and safety of continuous risankizumab therapy vs treatment withdrawal in patients with moderate to severe plaque psoriasis: a phase 3 randomized clinical trial, JAMA Dermatol. 156 (6) (2020) 649–658.

[128] R.B. Warren, et al., Efficacy and safety of risankizumab vs. secukinumab in patients with moderate-to-severe plaque psoriasis (IMMerge): results from a phase III, randomized, open-label, efficacy–assessor-blinded clinical trial, Br. J. Dermatol 184 (1) (2021) 50–59.

[129] M. Ohtsuki, et al., Efficacy and safety of risankizumab in Japanese patients with moderate to severe plaque psoriasis: results from the Susta IMM phase 2/3 trial, J. Dermatol. 46 (8) (2019) 686–694.

[130] P.J. Mease, et al., Efficacy and safety of abatacept, a T-cell modulator, in a randomised, double-blind, placebo-controlled, phase III study in psoriatic arthritis, Ann. Rheum. Dis. 76 (9) (2017) 1550–1558.

[131] M.C. Genovese, et al., Subcutaneous abatacept versus intravenous abatacept: a phase IIIb noninferiority study in patients with an inadequate response to methotrexate, Arthritis Rheum. 63 (10) (2011) 2854–2864.

[132] M.C. Genovese, et al., Longterm safety and efficacy of subcutaneous abatacept in patients with rheumatoid arthritis: 5-year results from a phase IIIb trial, J. Rheumatol. 45 (8) (2018) 1085–1092.

[133] N. Ruperto, et al., Long-term safety and efficacy of abatacept in children with juvenile idiopathic arthritis, Arthritis Rheum. 62 (6) (2010) 1792–1802.

[134] V. Viglietta, et al., CTLA4Ig treatment in patients with multiple sclerosis: an open-label, phase 1 clinical trial, Neurology 71 (12) (2008) 917–924.

[135] S.J. Khoury, et al., ACCLAIM: a randomized trial of abatacept (CTLA4-Ig) for relapsing-remitting multiple sclerosis, Mult. Scler. J. 23 (5) (2017) 686–695.

[136] T. Orban, et al., Co-stimulation modulation with abatacept in patients with recent-onset type 1 diabetes: a randomised, double-blind, placebo-controlled trial, Lancet 378 (9789) (2011) 412–419.

[137] L.A. Raedler, Simponi aria (golimumab), the only fully human anti-TNF-α infused therapy, now approved for active psoriatic arthritis and for active ankylosing spondylitis, Ninth Annual Payers' Guide 11 (2018).

[138] E.D. Deeks, Certolizumab pegol: a review in inflammatory autoimmune diseases, BioDrugs 30 (6) (2016) 607–617.

[139] D. Van Der Heijde, et al., 4-year results from the RAPID-PsA phase 3 randomised placebo-controlled trial of certolizumab pegol in psoriatic arthritis, RMD Open 4 (1) (2018) e000582.

[140] A. Pan, V. Gerriets, Etanercept, in: StatPearls, StatPearls Publishing, 2020. [Internet] Updated. August 11.

[141] Drugs.com, Actemra Approval History, 2020, [cited 2020 8/11/2020]. Available from: https://www.drugs.com/history/actemra.html.

[142] A. Ogata, et al., Longterm safety and efficacy of subcutaneous tocilizumab monotherapy: results from the 2-year open-label extension of the MUSASHI study, J. Rheumatol. 42 (5) (2015) 799–809.

[143] K. Maeshima, et al., Successful tocilizumab and tacrolimus treatment in a patient with rheumatoid arthritis complicated by systemic lupus erythematosus, Lupus 21 (9) (2012) 1003–1006.

[144] C.P. Denton, D. Khanna, Systemic sclerosis, Lancet 390 (10103) (2017) 1685–1699.

[145] D. McCarty, A. Robinson, Efficacy and safety of sarilumab in patients with active rheumatoid arthritis, Ther. Adv. Musculoskelet. Dis. 10 (3) (2018) 61–67.

[146] M.C. Genovese, et al., Long-term safety and efficacy of sarilumab plus methotrexate on disease activity, physical function and radiographic progression: 5 years of sarilumab plus methotrexate treatment, RMD Open 5 (2) (2019) e000887.

[147] G.R. Burmester, et al., Safety and efficacy of switching from adalimumab to sarilumab in patients with rheumatoid arthritis in the ongoing MONARCH open-label extension, RMD Open 5 (2) (2019) e001017.

[148] P. Emery, et al., Safety and tolerability of subcutaneous sarilumab and intravenous tocilizumab in patients with rheumatoid arthritis, Rheumatology 58 (5) (2019) 849–858.

[149] Drugs.com, Janssen Receives Complete Response Letter From U.S. FDA for Sirukumab Biologics License Application, 2020, (cited 2020 8/6/2020). Available from: https://www.drugs.com/nda/plivensia_170922.html.

[150] T. Takeuchi, et al., Efficacy and safety of sirukumab in Japanese patients with moderate to severe rheumatoid arthritis inadequately controlled by disease modifying anti-rheumatic drugs: subgroup analysis of a phase 3 study, Mod. Rheumatol. 28 (6) (2018) 941–949.

[151] Y. Tanaka, et al., Efficacy and safety of sirukumab in Japanese patients with active rheumatoid arthritis who were refractory or intolerant to anti-tumor necrosis factor therapy: subgroup analysis of a randomized, double-blind, multicenter, phase 3 study (SIRROUND-T), Mod. Rheumatol. 29 (2) (2019) 306–313.

[152] N.C. Brembilla, L. Senra, W.-H. Boehncke, The IL-17 Family of Cytokines in Psoriasis: IL-17A and Beyond, Front. Immunol. 9, 2018, p. 1682.

[153] A. Deodhar, et al., Long-term safety of secukinumab in patients with moderate-to-severe plaque psoriasis, psoriatic arthritis, and ankylosing spondylitis: integrated pooled clinical trial and post-marketing surveillance data, Arthritis Res. Ther. 21 (1) (2019) 1–11.

[154] P.J. Mease, et al., Secukinumab in the treatment of psoriatic arthritis: efficacy and safety results through 3 years from the year 1 extension of the randomised phase III FUTURE 1 trial, RMD Open 4 (2) (2018) e000723.

[155] A.I.K. Abdo, G.J. Tye, Interleukin 23 and autoimmune diseases: current and possible future therapies, Inflamm. Res. 69 (5) (2020) 463–480.

[156] A. López-Ferrer, A. Laiz, L. Puig, The safety of ustekinumab for the treatment of psoriatic arthritis, Expert Opin. Drug Saf. 16 (6) (2017) 733–742.

[157] B. Olszewska, et al., Quo vadis, biological treatment for psoriasis and psoriatic arthritis? Adv. Dermatol. Allergol./Postepy Dermatol. Alergol. 35 (3) (2018) 231.

[158] A. Blauvelt, et al., Safety of tildrakizumab for moderate-to-severe plaque psoriasis: pooled analysis of three randomized controlled trials, Br. J. Dermatol. 179 (3) (2018) 615–622.

[159] V. Reddy, et al., Clinical evaluation of risankizumab-rzaa in the treatment of plaque psoriasis, J. Inflamm. Res. 13 (2020) 53.

[160] G. Herrero-Beaumont, M.J.M. Calatrava, S. Castañeda, Abatacept mechanism of action: concordance with its clinical profile, Reumatol. Clín. 8 (2) (2012) 78–83.

[161] A. Hosseini, et al., CTLA-4: from mechanism to autoimmune therapy, Int. Immunopharmacol. 80 (2020) 106221.

[162] Drug.com, Abatacept, 2020, 8/3/2020. Available from: https://www.drugs.com/ppa/abatacept.html.

[163] D.J. Lovell, et al., Long-term safety, efficacy, and quality of life in patients with juvenile idiopathic arthritis treated with intravenous abatacept for up to seven years, Arthritis Rheumatol. 67 (10) (2015) 2759–2770.

[164] E. Dinčić, et al., Association of polymorphisms in CTLA-4, IL-1ra and IL-1β genes with multiple sclerosis in Serbian population, J. Neuroimmunol. 177 (1–2) (2006) 146–150.

[165] T. Orban, et al., Costimulation modulation with abatacept in patients with recent-onset type 1 diabetes: follow-up 1 year after cessation of treatment, Diabetes Care 37 (4) (2014) 1069–1075.

[166] Drugs.com, Belatacept, 2020, (cited 2020 8/3/2020). Available from: https://www.drugs.com/ppa/belatacept.html.

[167] F. Vincenti, et al., Costimulation blockade with belatacept in renal transplantation, N. Engl. J. Med. 353 (8) (2005) 770–781.

[168] F. Vincenti, et al., Five-year safety and efficacy of belatacept in renal transplantation, J. Am. Soc. Nephrol. 21 (9) (2010) 1587–1596.

[169] F. Vincenti, et al., A phase III study of belatacept-based immunosuppression regimens versus cyclosporine in renal transplant recipients (BENEFIT study), Am. J. Transplant 10 (3) (2010) 535–546.

[170] F. Vincenti, et al., Belatacept and long-term outcomes in kidney transplantation, N. Engl. J. Med. 374 (4) (2016) 333–343.

[171] D. Wojciechowski, et al., Retrospective evaluation of the efficacy and safety of belatacept with thymoglobulin induction and maintenance everolimus: a single-center clinical experience, Clin. Transplant. 31 (9) (2017) e13042.

CHAPTER

12

Nutritional implications for the pathophysiology and treatment of autoimmune disorders

Catherine J. Andersen[a,b,*] *and Julia M. Greco*[a]

[a]Department of Biology, Fairfield University, Fairfield, CT, United States [b]Department of Nutritional Sciences, University of Connecticut, Storrs, CT, United States

*Corresponding author

Abstract

Autoimmune diseases are complex conditions that are increasing in incidence worldwide. Autoimmune disorders are often associated clinical challenges in regards to clear diagnoses, comorbidities, and effective disease management and treatment strategies. Importantly, research suggests that an individual's nutritional status and metabolic health, such as the presence of obesity or metabolic syndrome, may play a role in the risk, pathophysiology, and management of autoimmune diseases. Further, adherence to Western or Mediterranean-style dietary patterns, as well as intake of specific macronutrients (e.g., carbohydrates, protein, fatty acids), micronutrients (e.g., vitamin D, selenium, sodium) and non-nutrient dietary factors (e.g., food contaminants, gut microbiome profiles), may modulate autoimmune disease development and complications. Thus, nutritional interventions may represent an effective approach to mitigate risk and support the management of autoimmune disorders.

Keywords

Overweight and obesity, Metabolic syndrome, Western diet, Mediterranean diet, Macronutrients, Omega-3 fatty acids, Vitamin D, Selenium, Sodium, Non-nutrient dietary factors

1 Introduction

Autoimmune diseases affect approximately 8% of the US population (78% of whom are women), with numbers steadily increasing worldwide in recent years [1, 2]. Given the complex nature of diagnosing and managing autoimmune disorders, the comorbidities associated with them, and the adverse immunosuppressive side effects of some treatments, effective strategies to reduce risk and optimize treatment are essential [3]. While the etiology of autoimmune disorders is largely unknown, research suggests that an individual's nutritional status and metabolic health may play a role in the risk, pathophysiology, and management of autoimmune diseases, including rheumatoid arthritis (RA), systemic lupus erythematous (SLE), multiple sclerosis (MS), psoriasis, type 1 diabetes mellitus (T1DM), thyroid autoimmunity, and inflammatory bowel diseases (IBD) [4, 5]. Furthermore, studies have shown that adherence to certain dietary patterns, as well as intake of specific nutrients and non-nutrient dietary factors, may modulate autoimmune disease development and complications [6–11]. Thus, this chapter presents an overview of the nutritional implications for the pathophysiology and treatment of autoimmune disorders, with a specific emphasis on evidence derived from human studies.

2 Body composition and metabolic health

It has been well established that body mass index (BMI) is associated with immune profiles and inflammatory status. For example, obesity is associated with a chronic state of low-grade inflammation, increased white blood cell counts, and proinflammatory leukocyte profiles, in addition to increased risk of chronic inflammatory conditions, complications related to viral and bacterial infections, and reduced efficacy of vaccines [12–14]. Immune dysfunction may further be exasperated by the presence of metabolic syndrome—a constellation of risk factors that include elevated blood pressure, increased waist circumference, high levels of fasting blood glucose and triglycerides, and low HDL-cholesterol—or nutritional deficiencies, which can be observed in individuals with both low and elevated BMIs [15–17]. Accordingly, body composition, metabolic health, and nutritional status have similarly been associated with autoimmune complications, as discussed below [4, 5, 18].

2.1 Overweight and obesity

Risk and incidence of a wide range of autoimmune disorders has been shown to be increased in individuals with elevated BMI. Metabolic complications in obesity have been shown to impair mechanisms regulating self-tolerance, in addition to promoting proinflammatory T helper 1 (Th1) and T helper 17 (Th17) cell activity, while downregulating antiinflammatory B regulatory (Breg) and T regulatory (Treg) cells [19]. Accordingly, obesity is associated with increased levels of autoantibodies in humans and animal models [20–23]. In a systematic literature review of 329 articles, Versini et al. [4] reported strong evidence for positive associations between obesity and risk of RA, MS, and psoriasis or psoriatic arthritis (PsA). Furthermore, the disease progression, management, and responsiveness to treatment have been reported to be further impaired by obesity in RA, psoriasis or PsA, and IBD. In a prospective cohort study analysis of 238,130 US women in the Nurses' Health Studies (NHS), obesity was associated with an 85% increased risk of SLE in the NHSII 1989–2013 cohort, but no associations between obesity and SLE were observed in the NHS 1976–2012 cohort, which may be explained by the NHS 1976–2012 cohort having a lower average BMI and incidence of obesity—particularly during reproductive age, when incidence of SLE in women is more prevalent [24]. In a study analyzing data from 75,008 women from the Danish National Birth Cohort, risk of developing any autoimmune diseases (out of 43 included in the analysis) was increased in women with obesity as compared to women with a BMI in the normal range (18.5 to <25 kg/m^2), with autoimmune disease risk increasing by 2% for every unit increase in BMI [25]. Elevated BMI has further been shown to be a predictor of autoantibodies against pancreatic islets in adolescents and children older than 9 years of age prior to clinical manifestation of T1DM [26], whereas islet autoantibodies are additionally observed in overweight and obese adults with type 2 diabetes mellitus (T2DM) [27]. Interestingly, there may be sex-dependent differences in the relationship between obesity and specific autoimmune diseases. Zynat et al. [28] found that waist circumference—a measure of abdominal obesity—was associated with greater risk of thyroid autoantibodies in men, whereas no associations between obesity measures and thyroid autoimmunity were observed in women.

Many dietary interventions and functional foods have been shown to improve markers of inflammation and immune dysfunction associated with obesity, including some of the dietary patterns and nutrients described below [29, 30]. Weight loss following bariatric surgery has additionally been shown to reduce autoantibodies against A disintegrin and metalloproteinase with a thrombospondin type 1 motif, member 13 (ADAMTS13), which is associated with increased risk of thrombosis [31]. Weight loss has additionally been shown to improve inflammation, quality of life, and responsiveness to treatment in autoimmune conditions such as RA and psoriasis or PsA [32, 33]. Thus, dietary intervention and weight loss may be an important strategy to improve autoimmune disease severity and complications in patients with obesity.

2.2 Metabolic syndrome

Metabolic syndrome (MetS) is a collection of three or more cardiovascular pathologies including abdominal obesity, decreased HDL levels, elevated blood pressure, increased fasting blood glucose levels, and elevated triglycerides. MetS increases the risk of developing T2DM, cardiovascular disease (CVD), and stroke [34]. MetS is additionally associated with chronic low-grade inflammation, characterized by elevated levels of inflammatory markers including C-reactive protein (CRP), IL-18, tumor necrosis factor-α (TNF-α), IL-6, type I interferons, and self-nucleic acid-driven Toll-like receptor (TLR) activation in plasmacytoid dendritic cells (pDCs) [35–38]. Furthermore, research suggests that MetS may increase the risk of developing autoimmune disorders, whereas the presence of autoimmunity may additionally increase the risk of MetS. For instance, individuals with T1DM, psoriasis, SLE, RA, antiphospholipid syndrome, Behçet's disease, lichen planus, Sjögren syndrome, chronic urticaria, vasculitis, ankylosing spondylitis, and vasculitis have a higher incidence of MetS [5, 38–42]. Despite this evidence, the association between MetS and autoimmunity has been debated [43–45].

In order to mitigate the progression or development of symptoms associated with MetS-associated inflammation, which may lead to autoimmune complications, a wide range of dietary patterns, functional foods, and dietary bioactives has been analyzed. For example, fruits serve as a rich source of vitamins, antioxidant phytochemicals, and antiinflammatory compounds. Many fruits demonstrate beneficial effects in MetS, including black raspberries, blueberries, bilberries, grapes, açaí and agraz, as well as red-fleshed sweet orange and pomegranate juice [46–52]. Moreover, Pu'er tea extract has been observed to improve several MetS parameters [53]. Some animal products, including eggs and nonfat fortified yogurt, have been shown to reduce levels of inflammation and oxidative stress in MetS [54–60]. Nuts, including walnuts, almonds, hazelnuts, and pistachios have positively impacted CVD markers [61, 62], whereas seasonings such as cinnamon, raw crushed garlic, saffron, and curcumin may improve MetS progression [63–66]. As a whole, the Nordic diet and Mediterranean diet, which includes the frequent intake of fruits, berries, vegetables, potatoes, nuts, and whole grains, has been shown to decrease MetS lipid levels and adipose tissue inflammatory gene expression [29, 67–70]. With increasing research on the link between MetS and the prevalence of autoimmune disorders, additional research is warranted to elucidate whether these dietary strategies further improve disease outcomes in patients with autoimmunity.

3 Dietary patterns

Dietary patterns are defined as the overall combination of foods and beverages consumed within an individual's habitual diet, taking into account the frequency, quantity, and variety in which they are consumed [71, 72]. A number of dietary patterns have been investigated to determine their role in the risk and treatment of autoimmune disorders [6, 7]. In the following section, we specifically review evidence to support the role of Western and Mediterranean dietary patterns, as they have been most extensively investigated within the context of autoimmunity.

3.1 Western diet

Western dietary patterns are characterized by greater intake of highly-processed or "fast" foods, total and saturated fat, cholesterol, animal-based protein, refined grains, sugar, and sodium, in addition to a reduced intake of fruits, vegetables, and whole grains [6, 73]. While Western-style dietary patterns have long been associated with increased risk of obesity, cardiovascular disease, and type 2 diabetes, more recent evidence suggests that Western diets may play an important role in the pathophysiology and management of autoimmune disorders, including RA, IBD, and psoriasis [6, 74, 75]. Western diets have been shown to promote proinflammatory and Th17-based immune responses, in addition to altered B cell activity and the development of autoantibodies, which may be attributable to altered cellular cholesterol loading and metabolism within leukocytes [59, 76, 77].

In a case–control study by Nezamoleslami et al. [78] conducted with 297 adults in Iran, Western dietary patterns were associated with greater risk of RA. Positive associations between Western diet patterns and Psoriasis Area and Severity Index (PASI) score have similarly been observed [79]. However, results are not consistent across autoimmune disorders. For example, risk and severity of MS has been linked to individual food components that are associated with Western diet patterns, such as meat and dairy [6, 80, 81]. Conversely, in a case–control study utilizing data from the 2003–2006 Ausimmune Study, Black et al. [82] reported that Western dietary patterns (defined as high in meat and full-fat dairy products, and low in low-fat dairy, fresh fruit, whole grains, and nuts) as a whole were not associated with risk of a first clinical diagnosis of central nervous system demyelination, which is a commonly observed precursor to MS. The role of specific nutrients associated with Western diet patterns in autoimmune diseases are described in greater detail in the sections below.

3.2 Mediterranean diet

Broadly, the Mediterranean diet is considered to be a high-quality comprehensive diet that positively impacts human health and longevity. This is because the diet involves the regular intake of foods abundant in antioxidants and antiinflammatory properties [83]. The Mediterranean diet typically consists of an increased consumption of fresh vegetables, fruits, legumes, nuts, wheat, and olive oil; a moderate intake of fish and wine during meals; and a low consumption of certain low-fat dairy products and meat—with an emphasis on the avoidance of red meats [83, 84]. In countries where the Mediterranean diet is common, the total lipid intake comprises about 30%–40% of daily calories, with the ratio of monounsaturated to saturated fats being the greatest in these regions across the globe [83, 85]. The Mediterranean diet has been observed to reduce the risk of cardiovascular disease, cancer, morbidity, as well as decrease mortality by 17% [86, 87]. Furthermore, the essential nutrients contained in the Mediterranean diet not only lower the risk of atherosclerosis, but an abundance of research has provided evidence for its ability to modulate markers of inflammation [70, 88]. Thus, the Mediterranean diet may potentially serve as a method to mitigate the development or symptoms of autoimmune disorders, as well as their associated comorbidities, including increased risk of cardiovascular disease and low levels of HDL [89, 90].

Accordingly, several researchers have examined the effects of the Mediterranean diet in individuals with autoimmune disorders, with a large number of studies conducted with RA patients. RA is characterized by the reduction in the lining of the synovial joints and can lead to functional impairments and premature death [91]. A randomized parallel study showed that individuals following a Mediterranean diet had improved RA as compared to the Western diet group, which reported no detected changes. For instance, the Mediterranean diet group had a decrease in their disease activity index and disease symptom compared with 1 year earlier, and an increase in vitality [92]. In patients with Crohn's disease, greater adherence to the Mediterranean diet has been associated with a reduction in inflammatory markers and lower risk of later-onset disease. Comparatively, lower Mediterranean diet adherence had a 12% greater risk for development of later-onset of Crohn's disease [93, 94]. In addition to RA and Crohn's disease, the Mediterranean diet has been associated with improved anthropometric measures, decreased cardiovascular risk, and lower disease activity in SLE patients [7].

In addition to evaluating the effects of Mediterranean dietary patterns on autoimmune symptoms as a whole, scientists have evaluated how the presence or absence of certain foods with in the Mediterranean diet may attenuate autoimmune symptoms [92]. Fish supplementation in the Mediterranean diet has been largely analyzed. In a cross-sectional study with RA patients ($n = 176$), participants that consumed fish more than two times per week had a lower Disease Activity Score-28 for RA with CRP (DAS28-CRP) as compared to those who ate fish

0 to <1 time per month, with DAS28-CRP decreasing by 0.18 with each additional serving of fish consumed per week [95]. In adolescents, consumption of fish within Mediterranean dietary patterns has been associated with a reduction in CRP blood concentrations and improved airway inflammation for pediatric asthma cases [96, 97]. Thus, a moderate fish intake may provide nutritional benefits to those suffering from various autoimmune disorders.

In addition to fish, other nutritional factors in the Mediterranean diet have been investigated. For instance, plasma levels of vitamin C, retinol (vitamin A), and uric acid following the consumption of a Mediterranean diet showed an inverse association to RA disease activity [98]. Further, although Mediterranean diets are frequently associated with weight loss, improvements in RA metrics have been demonstrated that are independent of weight loss [99]. Additionally, consumption of highly processed foods and added sugars are avoided in the Mediterranean diet, which can further impact disease outcomes. In individuals with ulcerative colitis (UC) or Crohn's disease, higher intake of "high sugar and soft drinks" with a low vegetable intake had a positive association with UC risk [100]. It is important to note that some foods associated with Mediterranean-style dietary patterns can promote autoimmune symptoms.

In a study focusing on the relationship between dietary components and palindromic rheumatism (PR) severity, foods that are low-to-moderately consumed in the Mediterranean diet, such as fish, eggs, canned vegetables, and processed cheese were shown to trigger PR attacks, while their cessation eliminated PR symptoms [101]. Thus, although these foods tend to be consumed in low to moderate amounts as part of Mediterranean diets [84], it is important to determine whether incorporation of these foods attenuates vs. exacerbates autoimmune symptoms across individuals.

In addition to considering the total amount of specific foods within Mediterranean-style diet patterns, the type or preparation of foods should also be considered within the context of autoimmune disease management. After the adjustment for lifestyle and dietary variables, increased adherence to the Mediterranean diet did not impact risk developing of RA in 174,638 women from the NHS 1980–2008 and NHS II 1991–2009 cohorts [102]. However, the researchers noted several possibilities for their null result. However, information on food type and preparation was limited in these databases. For example, the researchers were unable to control for vegetable form, whereas a previous report found that cooked as opposed to raw vegetables were associated with a reduced RA risk [102, 103]. Further, the researchers were unable to distinguish between types of fish. In a study conducted by Pedersen et al., fatty fish ($\geq$ 8 g fat/100 g fish) was found to reduce risk of RA by 49%, whereas medium fat fish (3–7 g fat/100 g fish) significantly increased the risk of developing RA [102, 104]. In this cohort, a majority of the source of monounsaturated fats was derived from meats, including beef, instead of olive oil, which is often the most common source of monounsaturated fats in the Mediterranean diet, as it can be used as a cooking substitute and as a dressing [84, 102].

Olive oil, more specifically extra virgin olive oil (EVOO), is extracted using methods that do not alter its natural composition, and has a high percentage of monounsaturated fatty acids, such as oleic acid and oleocanthal [105–107]. Increased consumption of olive oil has been shown to decrease inflammation in individuals with Hashimoto's thyroiditis (HT) and SLE [107, 108]. In SLE patients, EVOO reduced the secretion of IFN-γ, TNF-α, IL-6, IL-1β, and IL-10, the frequency of CD69$^+$ cells, extracellular signal regulated kinase phosphorylation of peripheral blood mononuclear cells, and increased expression of I-kappa-B-α nuclear factor

[108]. Additionally, olive oil capsules (6.8 g oleic acid) consistently reduced the number of swollen joints throughout the entirety of the study in RA participants [109].

Overall, a decrease in autoimmune symptoms may be a combination of various nutritional factors, as opposed to a specific, single nutritional factor [83]. Transcriptomic analysis has shown multiple small, beneficial synergistic changes in gene expression after the consumption of a Mediterranean diet in Crohn's disease patients [93]. Additionally, the "Mediterranean life-style" includes both a healthy diet and also a proponent of physical exercise, which has shown to decrease inflammatory symptoms [110–112]. Thus, greater insight into long-term effects of the Mediterranean diet for preventative and progression of autoimmune diseases is essential.

4 Macronutrients

In addition to being contributors to the immunomodulatory effects of dietary patterns, individual macronutrients have been shown to impact the health outcomes of various autoimmune disorders. In the following section, the role of carbohydrates, proteins, and fatty acids—specifically omega-3 polyunsaturated fatty acids (PUFA)—in the pathophysiology and treatment of autoimmune disorders is described.

4.1 Carbohydrates

Carbohydrates are composed of digestible sugars and indigestible fibers that may modulate autoimmunity. The effects of low carbohydrate diets (LCD) on autoimmune disorders have been investigated, with much of the research focused on T1DM. LCD have been shown to decrease high blood glucose and the need for medication and insulin doses in individuals with T1DM [113, 114]. Consistent and moderated 70–90 g carbohydrate diets have been shown to improve glycemic control and may serve as feasible long-term treatment alternatives for some patients [115, 116]. Furthermore, in case study of a 19-year old T1DM patient, adherence to a low carbohydrate, high protein paleolithic diet for two months increased C-peptide levels, indicating the decline in and retrogression of autoimmune pancreatic beta-cell destruction, and the patient was able to discontinue insulin treatments [117]. It is also well recognized that foods of similar macronutrient composition can impact glycemic responses in T1DM patients differently. Consumption of white rice increased postprandial glucose levels as compared to high and regular pasta [118]. However, in T1DM patients, Rabasa-Lhoret et al. found that glycemic control is not affected by increased carbohydrate consumption with appropriate premeal insulin adjustments, that basal premeal insulin requirements do not change as a result of high or low carbohydrate meals, and that the glycemic index and overall lipid and caloric content of meals does not change insulin requirements [119].

Aside from T1DM, LCDs have been reported to reduce body weight, fat mass, and sentinel autoantibodies in Hashimoto's thyroiditis [120]. In humans and mouse models, improvements in MS resulted from a paleolithic diet in addition to a fasting and ketogenic diets [121, 122]. These diets have been shown to decrease symptoms of fatigue [122], reduce disease severity, regulate immunity, and increase remyelination [121].

Fiber has additionally been shown to mitigate effects of autoimmune disease. For instance, long-term dietary fiber intake from fruit has been associated with reduced risk of Crohn's disease [123] and an early consumption of non-fermentable fibers prevents the development of spontaneous autoimmune encephalomyelitis in a mouse model of MS [124]. Non-fermentable fibers are suggested to change the gut microbiota composition and increase the amount of long-chain fatty acids which promote Th2 immune responses that mitigate autoimmune dysfunction [124]. In individuals with T1DM, high-fiber diet variations improve glycemic control, and reduce hypoglycemia [125, 126], insulin requirements, total cholesterol, and increases peripheral glucose disposal [127]. The presence of fiber in the diet may further mitigate the impact of consuming high- vs. low-glycemic foods on T1DM outcomes [128]. Taken together, these findings support the significance of carbohydrate intake in a range of autoimmune diseases.

4.2 Protein

A growing body of research has investigated the effects of protein in autoimmunity, with evidence suggesting that animal vs. plant-derived proteins may differentially impact symptoms and progression of autoimmune disorders. Vegetarian and vegan diets have been shown to lessen or mitigate inflammatory, autoimmune symptoms in various disorders [129–134]. These studies have shown an improvement in fatigue [129], lower risk of disease development [132], association with reduced levels of serum high-sensitivity C-reactive protein (hs-CRP) [133], and decreased immunoglobulin G antibodies levels against gliadin and beta-lactoglobulin—markers of immunoreactivity to gluten and cow's milk, respectively [134]. The beneficial impact of a vegetarian diet has been reported to last 1 year post-intervention in individuals with RA [131]. In a prospective study of 131,342 individuals in the NHS and Health Professionals Follow-up Study, increased intake of plant-derived protein was found to be inversely associated with all-cause and cardiovascular mortality, whereas diets high in animal protein positively correlated with cardiovascular mortality [135]. Greater consumption of whole grain bread has been associated with reduced inflammatory marker levels of gamma-glutamyl transferase (GGT), alanine transaminase (ALT), and hs-CRP whereas the converse is true for high red meat intake [136]. Thus, adopting a plant-based diet has suggests a greater likelihood to decrease inflammation and promote health and in general and autoimmune populations.

Accordingly, plant-based diets have been shown to be beneficial in a range of autoimmune diseases. In laboratory rats, a diet high in animal protein aggravates dextran sulfate sodium (DSS)-induced colitis resulting in monocyte pro-inflammatory activity whereas a plant protein-rich diet does not [137]. Furthermore, the elimination of all animal foods has been associated with reduced incidence of hypothyroidism, whereas intermediate protection may be provided by lacto-ovo and pesco-vegetarian diets [138]. In RA patients, a raw, uncooked vegan diet rich in lactobacilli was found to improve subjective symptoms and measures of disease activity, whereas a switch to an omnivorous diet aggravated RA symptoms [139]. Vegetarian diets have also been indirectly linked to T1DM incidence, whereas animal foods—including dairy and meat—have been directly associated with T1DM prevalence. This may be due to the presence of protein, nitrosamines, nitrates, and nitrites present in meat. Additionally, meat may negatively interact with microbiota causing a gut epithelium inflammatory response [140]. Additionally, the consumption of cow's milk, particularly one containing A1 beta-casein and consumed prematurely, may increase risk of islet autoimmunity and T1DM development [140–142]. In obese patients, vegan, vegetarian, and pesco-vegetarian diets resulted in significant short-term inflammatory improvements [143]. Furthermore, standard and low-carbohydrate vegan diets with protein sources from gluten, soy, nuts, and vegetable oils have led to weight loss and decreased lipid levels, which may further support a reduction in autoimmune risk and complications [143–145].

As a common component of plant-based diets, soybeans may improve autoinflammatory symptoms. In laboratory pigs with IBD, soy peptide supplementation suppressed innate Th1 and Th17 proinflammatory pathways in the colon and ileum. In addition, upregulation of the ileal FOXP3$^+$ regulatory T cells was also observed [146]. Similar results were found when analyzing the effects of anthocyanin—a flavonoid extracted from a black soybean seed coat—in mice and human peripheral blood mononuclear cells with RA. A decrease in the presence of Th17 cells, proinflammatory cytokines, nuclear factor κ B (NF-κB) signaling, osteoclastogenesis, and oxidative stress was observed [147]. Additionally, the soybean-derived serine protease Bowman-Birk inhibitor (BBI) may provide a new treatment for MS as it has shown to decrease Th17 cells, IFN-γ, IL-17, and increase IL-10 production (mainly from CD4$^+$ T cells) as well as Foxp3 expression in laboratory rats [148]. However, it has also been shown that a soy diet as compared to a casein diet promoted the progression of SLE in laboratory mice [149].

Certain amino acids may also influence autoimmune diseases. For example, elevated branched-chain amino acids have been reported to be present before the occurrence of autoinflammation and insulinogenic activity may further increase the risk [140]. However, in patients with MS, a daily dose of threonine has shown to improve spasticity and a whey–protein mixture containing tryptophan was reported to improve memory process [150, 151]. Further, amino acid polymorphisms such as CD24Ala/Val has been reported to increase susceptibility to SLE and MS [152, 153] Thus, dietary protein and protein metabolism may have a significant impact on a range of autoimmune disorders.

4.3 Omega-3 polyunsaturated fatty acids

The effects of saturated and monounsaturated fatty acids on autoimmunity have often been studied within the context of Western and Mediterranean diet patterns, as described above. Thus, this section will focus on evidence to support the role of omega-3 PUFA in the risk and management of autoimmune disorders.

The role of omega-3 PUFAs in inflammatory diseases is well documented [154–156]. Dietary sources of omega-3 PUFAs include fatty fish (e.g., mackerel and salmon) and fish oil, seafood, flaxseeds and flax oil, as well as walnuts, greens, and soybean oil [157]. By serving as precursors to eicosanoid mediators, omega-3 PUFAs—specifically the very long-chain omega-3 PUFAs, eicosapentaenoic acid (EPA) and docosapentaenoic acid (DHA)—exhibit antiinflammatory and pro-resolving activity, as compared to omega-6 PUFA-derived eicosanoids that are known to promote proinflammatory pathways [157, 158]. Accordingly, omega-3 PUFA-rich diets have been shown to reduce risk and lower inflammation in a number of different autoimmune conditions, including SLE, RA, MS, and psoriasis [159–162]. However, it is important to note that evidence for the protective and therapeutic potentials of omega-3

PUFAs in autoimmune disease is often stronger in animal studies, whereas clinical trials have yielded conflicting results, which may be related to the study population/disease being studied, and the use of supplements rather than whole foods [160, 161].

DHA supplementation has been shown to protect against inflammatory lupus flaring in a crystalline silica-induced NZBWF1 mouse model of lupus [163]. Greater overall Omega-3 Index scores were additionally associated with reduced inflammation, leukocyte infiltration into lung tissue, glomerulonephritis, and autoantibody production [164]. In a randomized placebo-controlled clinical trial, Arriens et al. [165] observed that 6 months of fish oil supplementation improved Physical Global Assessment scores and reduced erythrocyte sedimentation rate (ESR) in SLE patients; however, no significant changes were observed in SLE Disease Activity Index (SLEDAI) or Fatigue Severity Scale (FSS) scores. A similar study found that supplementation with 3 g EPA with or without 3 mg copper for up to 6 months reduced revised Systemic Lupus Activity Measure (SLAM-R) scores in SLE patients as compared to taking placebos [162].

Omega-3 PUFA supplementation has additionally been shown to confer benefits in RA [166, 167]. In RA patients, daily supplementation with EPA (1.8 g) and DHA (2.1 g) for 3 months was similarly shown to improve clinical indicators of disease severity, including degree of morning stiffness, number of tender and swollen joints, and ESR level, while additionally reducing use of analgesic medications [168]. Observational studies have additionally reported reduced risk of MS in individuals with greater intake of omega-3 fatty acids [169, 170]. However, a number of clinical trials have demonstrated a lack of improvement in clinical outcomes of MS following omega-3 PUFA supplementation as compared to the intake of omega-6 PUFAs [171–173], while others have reported benefits when patients supplemented with fish oil while following a low-fat (15% of energy) diet [174]. Thus, further research into the autoimmune disease-specific effects of omega-3 PUFAs in humans is warranted—particularly studies that evaluate mechanistic pathways of action and the role of whole foods and dietary patterns in influencing omega-3 PUFA effects.

5 Micronutrients

A variety of micronutrients, or vitamins and minerals, have further been shown to play a significance role in the pathophysiology and treatment of autoimmune disorders [175]. Vitamin A-related pathways are protective against Th17-mediated autoimmunity in animal models [176], whereas antioxidant vitamin E has been shown to have therapeutic effects in animal studies and clinical trials targeting RA, SLE, inflammatory bowel diseases, and systemic sclerosis [177]. Deficiency and reduced serum levels of minerals such as zinc have additionally been implicated in autoimmune disease risk of incidence [178, 179]. In this section, we specifically highlight the roles of vitamin D, as well as selenium and sodium.

5.1 Vitamin D

Many autoimmune diseases are associated with levels of vitamin D below the homeostatic range. With this in mind, several studies have investigated the effects of low serum vitamin

D and vitamin D supplementation on the progression and treatment of autoimmune pathologies [180, 181]. Ascherio et al. [182] observed that higher 25-hydroxy vitamin D_3 (25(OH)D_3) serum levels were correlated with reduced disease activity, disability, and progression in MS patients. In particular, increases in serum 25(OH)D_3 levels were associated with a decrease in rates of new lesions and lesion volume, relapse rate, and a reduction in yearly brain volume loss, suggesting the potential beneficial impacts of vitamin D supplements in MS [182]. Correale et al. [183] found decreased levels of vitamin D in periods of MS relapse vs remission, as well as lower levels of 25(OH)D_3 and 1,25-dihydroxy vitamin D_3 (1,25(OH)$_2D_3$) in relapsed MS patients vs healthy controls. Furthermore, the researchers proposed $CD4^+$ and myelin basic protein (MBP)-specific T cell proliferation inhibition by 1,25(OH)$_2D_3$ as a potential mechanism responsible for reducing the risk of MS development. Additionally, T cells presented the ability to convert vitamin D into its active form. Active vitamin D was found to decrease IL-6 and IL-17 secreting cells, while increasing the maturation of IL-10 producing cells and the production of $CD4^+CD25^+$ Treg cells [183]. However, it is important to note that high-dose vitamin D has been shown to exacerbate MS markers in murine models and ex vivo murine and human T cells [184].

In addition to MS, vitamin D insufficiencies have been linked to other autoimmune disorders. In patients with T1DM, studies administering vitamin D supplements have shown both beneficial and null effects on inflammation. Cholecalciferol, or vitamin D_3 supplementation increased Treg cells' suppressive activities and frequency [185, 186]. Cholecalciferol supplements have also shown to improve painful diabetic neuropathy [187]. In addition to its inflammatory modulating properties, when paired with insulin for adjunctive therapy, cholecalciferol reduces β-cell function decline in patients with new-onset T1DM and may provide greater significant glycemic control [188, 189]. Similarly, when alphacalcidol—an active vitamin D3 analog—was added to insulin therapy, β-cell protection was increased in individuals with adult-onset latent autoimmune diabetes [190]. Alphacalcidol was observed to beneficially impact immunity by reducing the Th1- and Th17-related cytokine levels, restoring the natural Treg cells (nTreg cells) as well as the nTreg/Th7 balance [191]. Beneficial effects of vitamin D and alphacalcidol supplementation have been observed to decrease the incidence of T1DM in infants as well as preserve β-cell function [192, 193]. However, despite these positive effects of vitamin D on T1DM, several researchers have found null or weak effects of vitamin D [194–197]. Thus, this calls for additional research to further solidify the use of vitamin D supplements to support the management of autoimmune disorders.

5.2 Selenium

In patients with autoimmune disorders, selenium (Se) levels tend to be below the normal physiological range. Clinical trials have investigated the effects Se supplementation on treating and preventing inflammatory diseases; however, the effects of Se supplementation on autoimmune disorders remains unresolved, despite its known antioxidant effects [198].

Se supplements are typically administered through the naturally occurring amino acid, selenomethionine (SeMet). In subclinical and overt autoimmune thyroiditis (AIT), Se supplementation significantly decreased thyroid peroxidase antibodies (TPOAb) as well as its IgG1 and G3 subclasses [199–203]. During pregnancy and postpartum, L-Se-Met supplementation has shown beneficial modulation on autoantibodies in women with AIT [204]. Early Se supplementation by using SeMet gel capsules has even shown to slow down and delay the progression of Grave's disease [205, 206]. Furthermore, Se supplementation when paired with methimazole or L-thyroxine as adjuvant therapy has shown inflammatory improvements [206–209]. Se, when paired with antioxidants (β-carotene, vitamin C and E), has also shown effective results [210, 211]. Pork may additionally act as an important source of Se in the diet [212, 213].

However, the effects of Se supplementation in autoimmunity remains controversial, as several studies have demonstrated the lack of effectiveness of Se treatments [214–216]. In children with AIT, there was a reduction in thyroid volume by greater than or equal to 30% in 35% of the subjects, but TPOAb and thyroglobulin antibody (TgAb) did not have improvements in thyroid echogenicity [217]. Furthermore, Se supplements did not show improvement in TPOAb, cytokine production, and peripheral T lymphocyte activity in other studies [218–220]. Additionally, short-term control of hyperthyroidism was unaffected by Se adjuvant therapy [221]. Thus, research on the impact of Se supplementation on autoimmune diseases is encouraged.

5.3 Sodium

As a common component of Western dietary patterns, sodium has additionally been implicated in the pathophysiology of autoimmune diseases. Sodium chloride promotes polarization of macrophages to proinflammatory phenotypes, while also promoting proinflammatory Th17-mediated immune responses [222, 223]. Higher skeletal muscle tissue levels of sodium in SLE patients have additionally been reported, which was associated with greater disease activity as assessed by SLEDAI scores. Accordingly, increased intake of sodium has been associated with a greater risk of developing new lesions in MS patients, with risk increasing from 2.8-fold to 3.4-fold with intakes over 2.0 g/day and 4.8 g/day, respectively [75, 224]. Greater sodium intake was additionally found to be associated with self-reported diagnosis of RA [225]. Thus, sodium restriction may be an effective strategy to reduce risk and support the management of autoimmune disorders.

6 Additional non-nutrient dietary factors

It is important to note that non-nutrient dietary factors additionally play a role in autoimmunity. For example, a variety of antioxidant phytochemicals have been suggested to have protective and antiinflammatory properties within the context of autoimmunity [10, 226]. Conversely, conflicting studies have shown that alcohol consumption may promote or reduce the risk and inflammatory complications associated with a variety of different autoimmune disorders [11, 227–231]. Dietary contaminants, such as bisphenol A (BPA) and tetramethylpentadecane (TMPD), have additionally been implicated as inducers of autoimmunity [232, 233]. Furthermore, increasing evidence suggests that the microbiome plays a significant role in autoimmune disease pathophysiology [234]. Distinct microbiome profiles have been observed between MS patients with high- vs low-disease activity, with greater disease activity further associated with increased frequency of Th17 cells within the small intestine tissue samples [235]. Emerging data from human and animal studies further suggests that fecal microbiome transplantation supports improved clinical autoimmune outcomes in chronic inflammatory bowel disease and MS [236–238]. Given the potential significance of non-nutrient factors in autoimmune pathology, future studies should consider the contribution or confounding effects of these compounds when investigating the relationship between diet, nutritional status, and autoimmunity.

7 Conclusion

It is clear that a wide range of nutritional factors play important roles in the pathophysiology and treatment of autoimmune disorders. As described above, an individual's body composition and metabolic status, in addition to their adherence to Western- vs Mediterranean-style dietary patterns and intake of specific nutrient and non-nutrient dietary compounds may impact their risk of incidence and management of autoimmune complications (Fig. 1). Continuing studies are warranted to elucidate disease- and patient-specific effects of nutritional interventions in order to mitigate risk and optimize complementary therapies of autoimmune disorders through personalized nutrition.

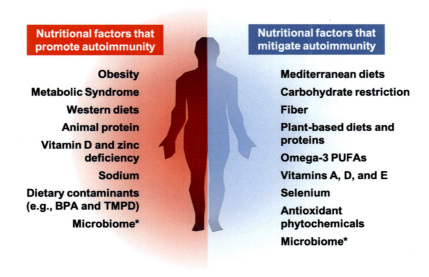

FIG. 1 Overview of nutritional factors that promote vs mitigate autoimmune disease. A variety of nutritional factors, including individual's body composition and metabolic status, in addition to their adherence to dietary patterns and intake of specific nutrient and non-nutrient dietary compounds, may impact their risk and management autoimmune complications.

References

[1] A. Lerner, P. Jeremias, T. Matthias, The world incidence and prevalence of autoimmune diseases is increasing, Int. J. Celiac Dis. 3 (4) (2015) 151–155.

[2] G.E. Dinse, T.A. Jusko, I.Z. Whitt, C.A. Co, C.G. Parks, M. Satoh, E.K. Chan, K.M. Rose, N.J. Walker, L.S. Birnbaum, D.C. Zeldin, C.R. Weinberg, F.W. Miller, Associations between selected xenobiotics and antinuclear antibodies in the national health and nutrition examination survey, 1999–2004, Environ. Health Perspect. 124 (4) (2016) 426–436.

[3] S. Chandrashekara, The treatment strategies of autoimmune disease may need a different approach from conventional protocol: a review, Indian J. Pharm. 44 (6) (2012) 665–671.

[4] M. Versini, P.Y. Jeandel, E. Rosenthal, Y. Shoenfeld, Obesity in autoimmune diseases: not a passive bystander, Autoimmun. Rev. 13 (9) (2014) 981–1000.

[5] G. Medina, O. Vera-Lastra, A.L. Peralta-Amaro, M.P. Jimenez-Arellano, M.A. Saavedra, M.P. Cruz-Dominguez, L.J. Jara, Metabolic syndrome, autoimmunity and rheumatic diseases, Pharmacol. Res. 133 (2018) 277–288.

[6] A. Manzel, D.N. Muller, D.A. Hafler, S.E. Erdman, R.A. Linker, M. Kleinewietfeld, Role of "Western diet" in inflammatory autoimmune diseases, Curr. Allergy Asthma Rep. 14 (1) (2014) 404.

[7] G. Pocovi-Gerardino, M. Correa-Rodriguez, J.L. Callejas-Rubio, R. Rios-Fernandez, M. Martin-Amada, M.G. Cruz-Caparros, B. Rueda-Medina, N. Ortego-Centeno, Beneficial effect of Mediterranean diet on disease activity and cardiovascular risk in systemic lupus erythematosus patients: a cross-sectional study, Rheumatology (Oxford) 60 (1) (2021) 160–169.

[8] X. Li, X. Bi, S. Wang, Z. Zhang, F. Li, A.Z. Zhao, Therapeutic potential of omega-3 polyunsaturated fatty acids in human autoimmune diseases, Front. Immunol. 10 (2019) 2241.

[9] C.Y. Yang, P.S. Leung, I.E. Adamopoulos, M.E. Gershwin, The implication of vitamin D and autoimmunity: a comprehensive review, Clin Rev Allergy Immunol 45 (2) (2013) 217–226.

[10] S. Hushmendy, L. Jayakumar, A.B. Hahn, D. Bhoiwala, D.L. Bhoiwala, D.R. Crawford, Select phytochemicals suppress human T-lymphocytes and mouse splenocytes suggesting their use in autoimmunity and transplantation, Nutr. Res. 29 (8) (2009) 568–578.

[11] V. Azizov, K. Dietel, F. Steffen, K. Durholz, J. Meidenbauer, S. Lucas, M. Frech, Y. Omata, N. Tajik, L. Knipfer, A. Kolenbrander, S. Seubert, D. Lapuente, M.V. Sokolova, J. Hofmann, M. Tenbusch, A. Ramming, U. Steffen, F. Nimmerjahn, R. Linker, S. Wirtz, M. Herrmann, V. Temchura, K. Sarter, G. Schett, M.M. Zaiss, Ethanol consumption inhibits TFH cell responses and the development of autoimmune arthritis, Nat. Commun. 11 (1) (2020) 1998.

[12] C.J. Andersen, K.E. Murphy, M.L. Fernandez, Impact of obesity and metabolic syndrome on immunity, Adv. Nutr. 7 (1) (2016) 66–75.

[13] J.B. Dixon, P.E. O'Brien, Obesity and the white blood cell count: changes with sustained weight loss, Obes. Surg. 16 (3) (2006) 251–257.

[14] V. Catalan, J. Gomez-Ambrosi, A. Rodriguez, B. Ramirez, V. Valenti, R. Moncada, C. Silva, J. Salvador, G. Fruhbeck, Peripheral mononuclear blood cells contribute to the obesity-associated inflammatory state independently of glycemic status: involvement of the novel proinflammatory adipokines chemerin, chitinase-3-like protein 1, lipocalin-2 and osteopontin, Genes Nutr. 10 (3) (2015) 460.

[15] P.L. Huang, A comprehensive definition for metabolic syndrome, Dis. Model. Mech. 2 (5–6) (2009) 231–237.

[16] A. Astrup, S. Bugel, Overfed but undernourished: recognizing nutritional inadequacies/deficiencies in patients with overweight or obesity, Int. J. Obes. (Lond) 43 (2) (2019) 219–232.

[17] M. Via, The malnutrition of obesity: micronutrient deficiencies that promote diabetes, ISRN Endocrinol. 2012 (2012) 103472.

[18] Y. Alwarawrah, K. Kiernan, N.J. MacIver, Changes in nutritional status impact immune cell metabolism and function, Front. Immunol. 9 (2018) 1055.

[19] C. Tsigalou, N. Vallianou, M. Dalamaga, Autoantibody production in obesity: is there evidence for a link between obesity and autoimmunity? Curr. Obes. Rep. 9 (3) (2020) 245–254.

[20] D. Frasca, A. Diaz, M. Romero, S. Thaller, B.B. Blomberg, Secretion of autoimmune antibodies in the human subcutaneous adipose tissue, PLoS One 13 (5) (2018), e0197472.

[21] S. Arai, N. Maehara, Y. Iwamura, S. Honda, K. Nakashima, T. Kai, M. Ogishi, K. Morita, J. Kurokawa, M. Mori, Y. Motoi, K. Miyake, N. Matsuhashi, K. Yamamura, O. Ohara, A. Shibuya, E.K. Wakeland, Q.Z. Li, T. Miyazaki, Obesity-associated autoantibody production requires AIM to retain the immunoglobulin M immune complex on follicular dendritic cells, Cell Rep. 3 (4) (2013) 1187–1198.

[22] D. Frasca, A. Diaz, M. Romero, D. Garcia, D. Jayram, S. Thaller, M. Del Carmen Piqueras, S. Bhattacharya, B.B. Blomberg, Identification and characterization of adipose tissue-derived human antibodies with "anti-self" specificity, Front. Immunol. 11 (2020) 392.

[23] I. Blanco, M. Labitigan, M.K. Abramowitz, The association between anti-nuclear antibodies and obesity is likely mediated by abdominal adiposity and systemic inflammation, J. Clin. Cell Immun. 8 (2017).

[24] S.K. Tedeschi, M. Barbhaiya, S. Malspeis, B. Lu, J.A. Sparks, E.W. Karlson, W. Willett, K.H. Costenbader, Obesity and the risk of systemic lupus erythematosus among women in the Nurses' health studies, Semin. Arthritis Rheum. 47 (3) (2017) 376–383.

[25] M.C. Harpsoe, S. Basit, M. Andersson, N.M. Nielsen, M. Frisch, J. Wohlfahrt, E.A. Nohr, A. Linneberg, T. Jess, Body mass index and risk of autoimmune diseases: a study within the Danish National Birth Cohort, Int. J. Epidemiol. 43 (3) (2014) 843–855.

[26] C. Ferrara-Cook, S.M. Geyer, C. Evans-Molina, I.M. Libman, D.J. Becker, S.E. Gitelman, M.J. Redondo, Type 1 Diabetes TrialNet Study Group, Excess BMI accelerates islet autoimmunity in older children and adolescents, Diabetes Care 43 (3) (2020) 580–587.

[27] S.J. Pilla, A. Balasubramanyam, W.C. Knowler, M. Lazo, D.M. Nathan, X. Pi-Sunyer, J.M. Clark, N.M. Maruthur, A.R.G. Look, Islet autoantibody positivity in overweight and obese adults with type 2 diabetes, Autoimmunity 51 (8) (2018) 408–416.

[28] J. Zynat, S. Li, Y. Ma, L. Han, F. Ma, Y. Zhang, B. Xing, X. Wang, Y. Guo, Impact of abdominal obesity on thyroid auto-antibody positivity: abdominal obesity can enhance the risk of thyroid autoimmunity in men, Int. J. Endocrinol. 2020 (2020) 6816198.

[29] C.J. Andersen, M.L. Fernandez, Dietary strategies to reduce metabolic syndrome, Rev. Endocr. Metab. Disord. 14 (3) (2013) 241–254.

[30] H. Lee, I.S. Lee, R. Choue, Obesity, inflammation and diet, Pediatr. Gastroenterol. Hepatol. Nutr. 16 (3) (2013) 143–152.

[31] V. Zanato, A.M. Lombardi, L. Busetto, C.D. Pra, M. Foletto, L. Prevedello, G.B. De Marinis, F. Fabris, R. Vettor, R. Fabris, Weight loss reduces anti-ADAMTS13 autoantibodies and improves inflammatory and coagulative parameters in obese patients, Endocrine 56 (3) (2017) 521–527.

[32] E. Gremese, B. Tolusso, M.R. Gigante, G. Ferraccioli, Obesity as a risk and severity factor in rheumatic diseases (autoimmune chronic inflammatory diseases), Front. Immunol. 5 (2014) 576.

[33] M.N. Di Minno, R. Peluso, S. Iervolino, A. Russolillo, R. Lupoli, R. Scarpa, R.S.G. Ca, Weight loss and achievement of minimal disease activity in patients with psoriatic arthritis starting treatment with tumour necrosis factor alpha blockers, Ann. Rheum. Dis. 73 (6) (2014) 1157–1162.

[34] Y. Rochlani, N.V. Pothineni, S. Kovelamudi, J.L. Mehta, Metabolic syndrome: pathophysiology, management, and modulation by natural compounds, Ther. Adv. Cardiovasc. Dis. 11 (8) (2017) 215–225.

[35] P.M. Ridker, J.E. Buring, N.R. Cook, N. Rifai, C-reactive protein, the metabolic syndrome, and risk of incident cardiovascular events: an 8-year follow-up of 14 719 initially healthy American women, Circulation 107 (3) (2003) 391–397.

[36] R. Ahmad, R. Thomas, S. Kochumon, S. Sindhu, Increased adipose tissue expression of IL-18R and its ligand IL-18 associates with inflammation and insulin resistance in obesity, Immun. Inflamm. Dis. 5 (3) (2017) 318–335.

[37] D. Ganguly, Do type I interferons link systemic autoimmunities and metabolic syndrome in a pathogenetic continuum? Trends Immunol. 39 (1) (2018) 28–43.

[38] B. Unlu, U. Tursen, Autoimmune skin diseases and the metabolic syndrome, Clin. Dermatol. 36 (1) (2018) 67–71.

[39] V. Gingras, C. Leroux, A. Fortin, L. Legault, R. Rabasa-Lhoret, Predictors of cardiovascular risk among patients with type 1 diabetes: a critical analysis of the metabolic syndrome and its components, Diabetes Metab. 43 (3) (2017) 217–222.

[40] P. Gisondi, G. Tessari, A. Conti, S. Piaserico, S. Schianchi, A. Peserico, A. Giannetti, G. Girolomoni, Prevalence of metabolic syndrome in patients with psoriasis: a hospital-based case-control study, Br. J. Dermatol. 157 (1) (2007) 68–73.

[41] S.K. Raychaudhuri, S. Chatterjee, C. Nguyen, M. Kaur, I. Jialal, S.P. Raychaudhuri, Increased prevalence of the metabolic syndrome in patients with psoriatic arthritis, Metab. Syndr. Relat. Disord. 8 (4) (2010) 331–334.

[42] M. Vadacca, D. Margiotta, A. Rigon, F. Cacciapaglia, G. Coppolino, A. Amoroso, A. Afeltra, Adipokines and systemic lupus erythematosus: relationship with metabolic syndrome and cardiovascular disease risk factors, J. Rheumatol. 36 (2) (2009) 295–297.

[43] M.I. Hawa, C. Thivolet, D. Mauricio, I. Alemanno, E. Cipponeri, D. Collier, S. Hunter, R. Buzzetti, A. de Leiva, P. Pozzilli, R.D. Leslie, L.G. Action, Metabolic syndrome and autoimmune diabetes: action LADA 3, Diabetes Care 32 (1) (2009) 160–164.

[44] B. Pan, Q. Zhang, H. Zhou, Z.F. Ma, Prevalence of components of metabolic syndrome among adults with the presence of autoimmune thyroid condition in an iodine-sufficient region, Biol. Trace Elem. Res. 199 (8) (2020) 2837–2843.

[45] L. Mehran, A. Amouzegar, F. Azizi, Thyroid disease and the metabolic syndrome, Curr. Opin. Endocrinol. Diabetes Obes. 26 (5) (2019) 256–265.

[46] H.S. Jeong, S.J. Hong, T.B. Lee, J.W. Kwon, J.T. Jeong, H.J. Joo, J.H. Park, C.M. Ahn, C.W. Yu, D.S. Lim, Effects of black raspberry on lipid profiles and vascular endothelial function in patients with metabolic syndrome, Phytother. Res. 28 (10) (2014) 1492–1498.

[47] A.R. Nair, N. Mariappan, A.J. Stull, J. Francis, Blueberry supplementation attenuates oxidative stress within monocytes and modulates immune cell levels in adults with metabolic syndrome: a randomized, double-blind, placebo-controlled trial, Food Funct. 8 (11) (2017) 4118–4128.

[48] M. Kolehmainen, O. Mykkanen, P.V. Kirjavainen, T. Leppanen, E. Moilanen, M. Adriaens, D.E. Laaksonen, M. Hallikainen, R. Puupponen-Pimia, L. Pulkkinen, H. Mykkanen, H. Gylling, K. Poutanen, R. Torronen, Bilberries reduce low-grade inflammation in individuals with features of metabolic syndrome, Mol. Nutr. Food Res. 56 (10) (2012) 1501–1510.

[49] H. Kim, S.Y. Simbo, C. Fang, L. McAlister, A. Roque, N. Banerjee, S.T. Talcott, H. Zhao, R.B. Kreider, S.U. Mertens-Talcott, Acai (Euterpe oleracea Mart.) beverage consumption improves biomarkers for inflammation but not glucose- or lipid-metabolism in individuals with metabolic syndrome in a randomized, double-blinded, placebo-controlled clinical trial, Food Funct. 9 (6) (2018) 3097–3103.

[50] J. Espinosa-Moncada, C. Marin-Echeverri, Y. Galvis-Perez, G. Ciro-Gomez, J.C. Aristizabal, C.N. Blesso, M.L. Fernandez, J. Barona-Acevedo, Evaluation of Agraz consumption on adipocytokines, inflammation, and oxidative stress markers in women with metabolic syndrome, Nutrients 10 (11) (2018).

[51] J.Q. Silveira, G.K. Dourado, T.B. Cesar, Red-fleshed sweet orange juice improves the risk factors for metabolic syndrome, Int. J. Food Sci. Nutr. 66 (7) (2015) 830–836.

[52] M.I. Kojadinovic, A.C. Arsic, J.D. Debeljak-Martacic, A.I. Konic-Ristic, N.D. Kardum, T.B. Popovic, M.D. Glibetic, Consumption of pomegranate juice decreases blood lipid peroxidation and levels of arachidonic acid in women with metabolic syndrome, J. Sci. Food Agric. 97 (6) (2017) 1798–1804.

[53] S.L. Chu, H. Fu, J.X. Yang, G.X. Liu, P. Dou, L. Zhang, P.F. Tu, X.M. Wang, A randomized double-blind placebo-controlled study of Pu'er tea extract on the regulation of metabolic syndrome, Chin. J. Integr. Med. 17 (7) (2011) 492–498.

[54] C.E. Dugan, D. Aguilar, Y.K. Park, J.Y. Lee, M.L. Fernandez, Dairy consumption lowers systemic inflammation and liver enzymes in typically low-dairy consumers with clinical characteristics of metabolic syndrome, J. Am. Coll. Nutr. 35 (3) (2016) 255–261.

[55] R.A. Stancliffe, T. Thorpe, M.B. Zemel, Dairy attentuates oxidative and inflammatory stress in metabolic syndrome, Am. J. Clin. Nutr. 94 (2) (2011) 422–430.

[56] M. Mohammadi-Sartang, N. Bellissimo, J.O. Totosy de Zepetnek, N.R. Brett, S.M. Mazloomi, M. Fararouie, A. Bedeltavana, M. Famouri, Z. Mazloom, The effect of daily fortified yogurt consumption on weight loss in adults with metabolic syndrome: a 10-week randomized controlled trial, Nutr. Metab. Cardiovasc. Dis. 28 (6) (2018) 565–574.

[57] C.J. Andersen, Bioactive egg components and inflammation, Nutrients 7 (9) (2015) 7889–7913.

[58] C.J. Andersen, J.Y. Lee, C.N. Blesso, T.P. Carr, M.L. Fernandez, Egg intake during carbohydrate restriction alters peripheral blood mononuclear cell inflammation and cholesterol homeostasis in metabolic syndrome, Nutrients 6 (7) (2014) 2650–2667.

[59] C.J. Andersen, Impact of dietary cholesterol on the pathophysiology of infectious and autoimmune disease, Nutrients 10 (6) (2018).

[60] C.N. Blesso, C.J. Andersen, J. Barona, B. Volk, J.S. Volek, M.L. Fernandez, Effects of carbohydrate restriction and dietary cholesterol provided by eggs on clinical risk factors in metabolic syndrome, J. Clin. Lipidol. 7 (5) (2013) 463–471.

[61] P. Casas-Agustench, P. Lopez-Uriarte, M. Bullo, E. Ros, J.J. Cabre-Vila, J. Salas-Salvado, Effects of one serving of mixed nuts on serum lipids, insulin resistance and inflammatory markers in patients with the metabolic syndrome, Nutr. Metab. Cardiovasc. Dis. 21 (2) (2011) 126–135.

[62] S. Gulati, A. Misra, R.M. Pandey, S.P. Bhatt, S. Saluja, Effects of pistachio nuts on body composition, metabolic, inflammatory and oxidative stress parameters in Asian Indians with metabolic syndrome: a 24-wk, randomized control trial, Nutrition 30 (2) (2014) 192–197.

[63] S. Gupta Jain, S. Puri, A. Misra, S. Gulati, K. Mani, Effect of oral cinnamon intervention on metabolic profile and body composition of Asian Indians with metabolic syndrome: a randomized double -blind control trial, Lipids Health Dis. 16 (1) (2017) 113.

[64] P.R. Choudhary, R.D. Jani, M.S. Sharma, Effect of raw crushed garlic (*Allium sativum* L.) on components of metabolic syndrome, J. Diet Suppl. 15 (4) (2018) 499–506.

[65] M. Shemshian, S.H. Mousavi, A. Norouzy, T. Kermani, T. Moghiman, A. Sadeghi, M. Ghayour-Mobarhan, G.A. Ferns, Saffron in metabolic syndrome: its effects on antibody titers to heat-shock proteins 27, 60, 65 and 70, J. Complement. Integr. Med. 11 (1) (2014) 43–49.

[66] Y. Panahi, M.S. Hosseini, N. Khalili, E. Naimi, L.E. Simental-Mendia, M. Majeed, A. Sahebkar, Effects of curcumin on serum cytokine concentrations in subjects with metabolic syndrome: a post-hoc analysis of a randomized controlled trial, Biomed. Pharmacother. 82 (2016) 578–582.

[67] M. Uusitupa, K. Hermansen, M.J. Savolainen, U. Schwab, M. Kolehmainen, L. Brader, L.S. Mortensen, L. Cloetens, A. Johansson-Persson, G. Onning, M. Landin-Olsson, K.H. Herzig, J. Hukkanen, F. Rosqvist, D. Iggman, J. Paananen, K.J. Pulkki, M. Siloaho, L. Dragsted, T. Barri, K. Overvad, K.E.B. Knudsen, M.S. Hedemann, P. Arner, I. Dahlman, G.I. Borge, P. Baardseth, S.M. Ulven, I. Gunnarsdottir, S. Jonsdottir, I. Thorsdottir, M. Oresic, K.S. Poutanen, U. Riserus, B. Akesson, Effects of an isocaloric healthy Nordic diet on insulin sensitivity, lipid profile and inflammation markers in metabolic syndrome—a randomized study (SYSDIET), J. Intern. Med. 274 (1) (2013) 52–66.

[68] M. Kolehmainen, S.M. Ulven, J. Paananen, V. de Mello, U. Schwab, C. Carlberg, M. Myhrstad, J. Pihlajamaki, E. Dungner, E. Sjolin, I. Gunnarsdottir, L. Cloetens, M. Landin-Olsson, B. Akesson, F. Rosqvist, J. Hukkanen, K.H. Herzig, L.O. Dragsted, M.J. Savolainen, L. Brader, K. Hermansen, U. Riserus, I. Thorsdottir, K.S. Poutanen, M. Uusitupa, P. Arner, I. Dahlman, Healthy Nordic diet downregulates the expression of genes involved in inflammation in subcutaneous adipose tissue in individuals with features of the metabolic syndrome, Am. J. Clin. Nutr. 101 (1) (2015) 228–239.

[69] S.M. Ulven, K.B. Holven, A. Rundblad, M.C.W. Myhrstad, L. Leder, I. Dahlman, V.D. Mello, U. Schwab, C. Carlberg, J. Pihlajamaki, K. Hermansen, L.O. Dragsted, I. Gunnarsdottir, L. Cloetens, B. Akesson, F. Rosqvist, J. Hukkanen, K.H. Herzig, M.J. Savolainen, U. Riserus, I. Thorsdottir, K.S. Poutanen, P. Arner, M. Uusitupa, M. Kolehmainen, An isocaloric nordic diet modulates RELA and TNFRSF1A gene expression in peripheral blood mononuclear cells in individuals with metabolic syndrome—a SYSDIET sub-study, Nutrients 11 (12) (2019).

[70] J.L. Jones, D. Ackermann, J. Barona, M. Calle, C. Andersen, J.E. Kim, J.S. Volek, M. McIntosh, W. Najm, R.H. Lerman, M.L. Fernandez, A Mediterranean low-glycemic-load diet alone or in combination with a medical food improves insulin sensitivity and reduces inflammation in women with metabolic syndrome, Br. J. Med. Med. Res. 1 (4) (2011) 356–370.

[71] A. Sánchez-Villegas, E.H. Martínez-Lapiscina, Chapter 11—a healthy diet for your heart and your brain, in: A. Sánchez-Villegas, A. Sánchez-Tainta (Eds.), The Prevention of Cardiovascular Disease Through the Mediterranean Diet, Academic Press, 2018, pp. 169–197.

[72] M.C. Calle, C.J. Andersen, Assessment of dietary patterns represents a potential, yet variable, measure of inflammatory status: a review and update, Dis. Markers 2019 (2019) 3102870.

[73] D. Statovci, M. Aguilera, J. MacSharry, S. Melgar, The impact of Western diet and nutrients on the microbiota and immune response at mucosal interfaces, Front. Immunol. 8 (2017) 838.

[74] Z. Shi, X. Wu, S. Yu, M. Huynh, P.K. Jena, M. Nguyen, Y.Y. Wan, S.T. Hwang, Short-term exposure to a Western diet induces Psoriasiform dermatitis by promoting accumulation of IL-17A-producing gammadelta T cells, J. Invest. Dermatol. 140 (9) (2020) 1815–1823.

[75] O. Matveeva, J.F.J. Bogie, J.J.A. Hendriks, R.A. Linker, A. Haghikia, M. Kleinewietfeld, Western lifestyle and immunopathology of multiple sclerosis, Ann. N. Y. Acad. Sci. 1417 (1) (2018) 71–86.

[76] A. Ito, C. Hong, K. Oka, J.V. Salazar, C. Diehl, J.L. Witztum, M. Diaz, A. Castrillo, S.J. Bensinger, L. Chan, P. Tontonoz, Cholesterol accumulation in CD11c(+) immune cells is a causal and targetable factor in autoimmune disease, Immunity 45 (6) (2016) 1311–1326.

[77] P.K. Jena, L. Sheng, K. McNeil, T.Q. Chau, S. Yu, M. Kiuru, M.A. Fung, S.T. Hwang, Y.Y. Wan, Long-term Western diet intake leads to dysregulated bile acid signaling and dermatitis with Th2 and Th17 pathway features in mice, J. Dermatol. Sci. 95 (1) (2019) 13–20.

12. Nutritional implications for autoimmunity

[78] S. Nezamoleslami, R. Ghiasvand, A. Feizi, M. Salesi, M. Pourmasoumi, The relationship between dietary patterns and rheumatoid arthritis: a case-control study, Nutr. Metab. (Lond.) 17 (2020) 75.

[79] L. Barrea, P.E. Macchia, G. Tarantino, C. Di Somma, E. Pane, N. Balato, M. Napolitano, A. Colao, S. Savastano, Nutrition: a key environmental dietary factor in clinical severity and cardio-metabolic risk in psoriatic male patients evaluated by 7-day food-frequency questionnaire, J. Transl. Med. 13 (2015) 303.

[80] K. Lauer, The risk of multiple sclerosis in the U.S.A. in relation to sociogeographic features: a factor-analytic study, J. Clin. Epidemiol. 47 (1) (1994) 43–48.

[81] M.L. Esparza, S. Sasaki, H. Kesteloot, Nutrition, latitude, and multiple sclerosis mortality: an ecologic study, Am. J. Epidemiol. 142 (7) (1995) 733–737.

[82] L.J. Black, C. Rowley, J. Sherriff, G. Pereira, A.L. Ponsonby, R.M. Lucas, A healthy dietary pattern associates with a lower risk of a first clinical diagnosis of central nervous system demyelination, Mult. Scler. 25 (11) (2019) 1514–1525.

[83] M.A. Martinez-Gonzalez, N. Martin-Calvo, Mediterranean diet and life expectancy; beyond olive oil, fruits, and vegetables, Curr. Opin. Clin. Nutr. Metab. Care 19 (6) (2016) 401–407.

[84] A. Bach-Faig, E.M. Berry, D. Lairon, J. Reguant, A. Trichopoulou, S. Dernini, F.X. Medina, M. Battino, R. Belahsen, G. Miranda, L. Serra-Majem, Mediterranean Diet Foundation Expert Group, Mediterranean diet pyramid today. Science and cultural updates, Public Health Nutr. 14 (12A) (2011) 2274–2284.

[85] A. Trichopoulou, Mediterranean diet: the past and the present, Nutr. Metab. Cardiovasc. Dis. 11 (4 Suppl) (2001) 1–4.

[86] A. Trichopoulou, T. Costacou, C. Bamia, D. Trichopoulos, Adherence to a Mediterranean diet and survival in a Greek population, N. Engl. J. Med. 348 (26) (2003) 2599–2608.

[87] A. Trichopoulou, A. Kouris-Blazos, M.L. Wahlqvist, C. Gnardellis, P. Lagiou, E. Polychronopoulos, T. Vassilakou, L. Lipworth, D. Trichopoulos, Diet and overall survival in elderly people, BMJ 311 (7018) (1995) 1457–1460.

[88] J.L. Jones, M. Comperatore, J. Barona, M.C. Calle, C. Andersen, M. McIntosh, W. Najm, R.H. Lerman, M.L. Fernandez, A Mediterranean-style, low-glycemic-load diet decreases atherogenic lipoproteins and reduces lipoprotein (a) and oxidized low-density lipoprotein in women with metabolic syndrome, Metabolism 61 (3) (2012) 366–372.

[89] C.M. Madsen, A. Varbo, B.G. Nordestgaard, Low HDL cholesterol and high risk of autoimmune disease: two population-based cohort studies including 117341 individuals, Clin. Chem. 65 (5) (2019) 644–652.

[90] J. Frostegard, Atherosclerosis in patients with autoimmune disorders, Arterioscler. Thromb. Vasc. Biol. 25 (9) (2005) 1776–1785.

[91] Q. Guo, Y. Wang, D. Xu, J. Nossent, N.J. Pavlos, J. Xu, Rheumatoid arthritis: pathological mechanisms and modern pharmacologic therapies, Bone Res. 6 (2018) 15.

[92] L. Skoldstam, L. Hagfors, G. Johansson, An experimental study of a Mediterranean diet intervention for patients with rheumatoid arthritis, Ann. Rheum. Dis. 62 (3) (2003) 208–214.

[93] G. Marlow, S. Ellett, I.R. Ferguson, S. Zhu, N. Karunasinghe, A.C. Jesuthasan, D.Y. Han, A.G. Fraser, L.R. Ferguson, Transcriptomics to study the effect of a Mediterranean-inspired diet on inflammation in Crohn's disease patients, Hum. Genomics 7 (2013) 24.

[94] H. Khalili, N. Hakansson, S.S. Chan, Y. Chen, P. Lochhead, J.F. Ludvigsson, A.T. Chan, A.R. Hart, O. Olen, A. Wolk, Adherence to a Mediterranean diet is associated with a lower risk of later-onset Crohn's disease: results from two large prospective cohort studies, Gut 69 (9) (2020) 1637–1644.

[95] S.K. Tedeschi, J.M. Bathon, J.T. Giles, T.C. Lin, K. Yoshida, D.H. Solomon, Relationship between fish consumption and disease activity in rheumatoid arthritis, Arthritis Care Res. (Hoboken) 70 (3) (2018) 327–332.

[96] A.B. Arouca, A. Meirhaeghe, J. Dallongeville, L.A. Moreno, G.J. Lourenco, A. Marcos, I. Huybrechts, Y. Manios, C.P. Lambrinou, F. Gottrand, A. Kafatos, M. Kersting, M. Sjostrom, K. Widhalm, M. Ferrari, D. Molnar, M. Gonzalez-Gross, M. Forsner, S. De Henauw, N. Michels, H.S. Group, Interplay between the Mediterranean diet and C-reactive protein genetic polymorphisms towards inflammation in adolescents, Clin. Nutr. 39 (6) (2020) 1919–1926.

[97] M.M. Papamichael, C. Katsardis, K. Lambert, D. Tsoukalas, M. Koutsilieris, B. Erbas, C. Itsiopoulos, Efficacy of a Mediterranean diet supplemented with fatty fish in ameliorating inflammation in paediatric asthma: a randomised controlled trial, J. Hum. Nutr. Diet. 32 (2) (2019) 185–197.

[98] L. Hagfors, P. Leanderson, L. Skoldstam, J. Andersson, G. Johansson, Antioxidant intake, plasma antioxidants and oxidative stress in a randomized, controlled, parallel, Mediterranean dietary intervention study on patients with rheumatoid arthritis, Nutr. J. 2 (2003) 5.

[99] L. Skoldstam, L. Brudin, L. Hagfors, G. Johansson, Weight reduction is not a major reason for improvement in rheumatoid arthritis from lacto-vegetarian, vegan or Mediterranean diets, Nutr. J. 4 (2005) 15.

[100] A. Racine, F. Carbonnel, S.S. Chan, A.R. Hart, H.B. Bueno-de-Mesquita, B. Oldenburg, F.D. van Schaik, A. Tjonneland, A. Olsen, C.C. Dahm, T. Key, R. Luben, K.T. Khaw, E. Riboli, O. Grip, S. Lindgren, G. Hallmans, P. Karling, F. Clavel-Chapelon, M.M. Bergman, H. Boeing, R. Kaaks, V.A. Katzke, D. Palli, G. Masala, P. Jantchou, M.C. Boutron-Ruault, Dietary patterns and risk of inflammatory bowel disease in Europe: results from the EPIC study, Inflamm. Bowel Dis. 22 (2) (2016) 345–354.

[101] G. Nesher, M. Mates, Palindromic rheumatism: effect of dietary manipulation, Clin. Exp. Rheumatol. 18 (3) (2000) 375–378.

[102] Y. Hu, K.H. Costenbader, X. Gao, F.B. Hu, E.W. Karlson, B. Lu, Mediterranean diet and incidence of rheumatoid arthritis in women, Arthritis Care Res. (Hoboken) 67 (5) (2015) 597–606.

[103] A. Linos, V.G. Kaklamani, E. Kaklamani, Y. Koumantaki, E. Giziaki, S. Papazoglou, C.S. Mantzoros, Dietary factors in relation to rheumatoid arthritis: a role for olive oil and cooked vegetables? Am. J. Clin. Nutr. 70 (6) (1999) 1077–1082.

[104] M. Pedersen, C. Stripp, M. Klarlund, S.F. Olsen, A.M. Tjonneland, M. Frisch, Diet and risk of rheumatoid arthritis in a prospective cohort, J. Rheumatol. 32 (7) (2005) 1249–1252.

[105] M. Aparicio-Soto, M. Sanchez-Hidalgo, M.A. Rosillo, M.L. Castejon, C. Alarcon-de-la-Lastra, Extra virgin olive oil: a key functional food for prevention of immune-inflammatory diseases, Food Funct. 7 (11) (2016) 4492–4505.

[106] C. Santangelo, R. Vari, B. Scazzocchio, P. De Sanctis, C. Giovannini, M. D'Archivio, R. Masella, Anti-inflammatory activity of extra virgin olive oil polyphenols: which role in the prevention and treatment of immune-mediated inflammatory diseases? Endocr. Metab. Immune Disord. Drug Targets 18 (1) (2018) 36–50.

[107] D. Kalicanin, L. Brcic, K. Ljubetic, A. Baric, S. Gracan, M. Brekalo, V. Torlak Lovric, I. Kolcic, O. Polasek, T. Zemunik, A. Punda, V. Boraska Perica, Differences in food consumption between patients with Hashimoto's thyroiditis and healthy individuals, Sci. Rep. 10 (1) (2020) 10670.

[108] M. Aparicio-Soto, M. Sanchez-Hidalgo, A. Cardeno, J.M. Lucena, F. Gonzalez-Escribano, M.J. Castillo, C. Alarcon-de-la-Lastra, The phenolic fraction of extra virgin olive oil modulates the activation and the inflammatory response of T cells from patients with systemic lupus erythematosus and healthy donors, Mol. Nutr. Food Res. 61 (8) (2017).

[109] J.M. Kremer, D.A. Lawrence, W. Jubiz, R. DiGiacomo, R. Rynes, L.E. Bartholomew, M. Sherman, Dietary fish oil and olive oil supplementation in patients with rheumatoid arthritis. Clinical and immunologic effects, Arthritis Rheum. 33 (6) (1990) 810–820.

[110] D.B. Bartlett, L.H. Willis, C.A. Slentz, A. Hoselton, L. Kelly, J.L. Huebner, V.B. Kraus, J. Moss, M.J. Muehlbauer, G. Spielmann, W.E. Kraus, J.M. Lord, K.M. Huffman, Ten weeks of high-intensity interval walk training is associated with reduced disease activity and improved innate immune function in older adults with rheumatoid arthritis: a pilot study, Arthritis Res. Ther. 20 (1) (2018) 127.

[111] P. Katz, M. Margaretten, S. Gregorich, L. Trupin, Physical activity to reduce fatigue in rheumatoid arthritis: a randomized controlled trial, Arthritis Care Res. (Hoboken) 70 (1) (2018) 1–10.

[112] E. Grazioli, E. Tranchita, G. Borriello, C. Cerulli, C. Minganti, A. Parisi, The effects of concurrent resistance and aerobic exercise training on functional status in patients with multiple sclerosis, Curr. Sports Med. Rep. 18 (12) (2019) 452–457.

[113] R.D. Feinman, W.K. Pogozelski, A. Astrup, R.K. Bernstein, E.J. Fine, E.C. Westman, A. Accurso, L. Frassetto, B.A. Gower, S.I. McFarlane, J.V. Nielsen, T. Krarup, L. Saslow, K.S. Roth, M.C. Vernon, J.S. Volek, G.B. Wilshire, A. Dahlqvist, R. Sundberg, A. Childers, K. Morrison, A.H. Manninen, H.M. Dashti, R.J. Wood, J. Wortman, N. Worm, Dietary carbohydrate restriction as the first approach in diabetes management: critical review and evidence base, Nutrition 31 (1) (2015) 1–13.

[114] J.D. Krebs, A. Parry Strong, P. Cresswell, A.N. Reynolds, A. Hanna, S. Haeusler, A randomised trial of the feasibility of a low carbohydrate diet vs standard carbohydrate counting in adults with type 1 diabetes taking body weight into account, Asia Pac. J. Clin. Nutr. 25 (1) (2016) 78–84.

[115] T.M. Wolever, S. Hamad, J.L. Chiasson, R.G. Josse, L.A. Leiter, N.W. Rodger, S.A. Ross, E.A. Ryan, Day-to-day consistency in amount and source of carbohydrate intake associated with improved blood glucose control in type 1 diabetes, J. Am. Coll. Nutr. 18 (3) (1999) 242–247.

[116] J.V. Nielsen, E. Jonsson, A. Ivarsson, A low carbohydrate diet in type 1 diabetes: clinical experience—a brief report, Ups. J. Med. Sci. 110 (3) (2005) 267–273.

12. Nutritional implications for autoimmunity

[117] C. Tóth, Z. Clemens, Type 1 diabetes mellitus successfully managed with the paleolithic ketogenic diet, Int. J. Case Rep. Images 5 (2014).

[118] S. Zavitsanou, J. Massa, S. Deshpande, J.E. Pinsker, M.M. Church, C. Andre, F.J. Doyle Iii, A. Michelson, J. Creason, E. Dassau, D.M. Eisenberg, The effect of two types of pasta versus White Rice on postprandial blood glucose levels in adults with type 1 diabetes: a randomized crossover trial, Diabetes Technol. Ther. 21 (9) (2019) 485–492.

[119] R. Rabasa-Lhoret, J. Garon, H. Langelier, D. Poisson, J.L. Chiasson, Effects of meal carbohydrate content on insulin requirements in type 1 diabetic patients treated intensively with the basal-bolus (ultralente-regular) insulin regimen, Diabetes Care 22 (5) (1999) 667–673.

[120] T. Esposito, J.M. Lobaccaro, M.G. Esposito, V. Monda, A. Messina, G. Paolisso, B. Varriale, M. Monda, G. Messina, Effects of low-carbohydrate diet therapy in overweight subjects with autoimmune thyroiditis: possible synergism with ChREBP, Drug Des. Devel. Ther. 10 (2016) 2939–2946.

[121] L.S. Bahr, M. Bock, D. Liebscher, J. Bellmann-Strobl, L. Franz, A. Pruss, D. Schumann, S.K. Piper, C.S. Kessler, N. Steckhan, A. Michalsen, F. Paul, A. Mahler, Ketogenic diet and fasting diet as nutritional approaches in multiple sclerosis (NAMS): protocol of a randomized controlled study, Trials 21 (1) (2020) 3.

[122] B. Bisht, W.G. Darling, R.E. Grossmann, E.T. Shivapour, S.K. Lutgendorf, L.G. Snetselaar, M.J. Hall, M.B. Zimmerman, T.L. Wahls, A multimodal intervention for patients with secondary progressive multiple sclerosis: feasibility and effect on fatigue, J. Altern. Complement. Med. 20 (5) (2014) 347–355.

[123] A.N. Ananthakrishnan, H. Khalili, G.G. Konijeti, L.M. Higuchi, P. de Silva, J.R. Korzenik, C.S. Fuchs, W.C. Willett, J.M. Richter, A.T. Chan, A prospective study of long-term intake of dietary fiber and risk of Crohn's disease and ulcerative colitis, Gastroenterology 145 (5) (2013) 970–977.

[124] K. Berer, I. Martinez, A. Walker, B. Kunkel, P. Schmitt-Kopplin, J. Walter, G. Krishnamoorthy, Dietary non-fermentable fiber prevents autoimmune neurological disease by changing gut metabolic and immune status, Sci. Rep. 8 (1) (2018) 10431.

[125] R. Giacco, M. Parillo, A.A. Rivellese, G. Lasorella, A. Giacco, L. D'Episcopo, G. Riccardi, Long-term dietary treatment with increased amounts of fiber-rich low-glycemic index natural foods improves blood glucose control and reduces the number of hypoglycemic events in type 1 diabetic patients, Diabetes Care 23 (10) (2000) 1461–1466.

[126] L. Lafrance, R. Rabasa-Lhoret, D. Poisson, F. Ducros, J.L. Chiasson, Effects of different glycaemic index foods and dietary fibre intake on glycaemic control in type 1 diabetic patients on intensive insulin therapy, Diabet. Med. 15 (11) (1998) 972–978.

[127] J.W. Anderson, J.A. Zeigler, D.A. Deakins, T.L. Floore, D.W. Dillon, C.L. Wood, P.R. Oeltgen, R.J. Whitley, Metabolic effects of high-carbohydrate, high-fiber diets for insulin-dependent diabetic individuals, Am. J. Clin. Nutr. 54 (5) (1991) 936–943.

[128] A.M. Fontvieille, S.W. Rizkalla, A. Penfornis, M. Acosta, F.R. Bornet, G. Slama, The use of low glycaemic index foods improves metabolic control of diabetic patients over five weeks, Diabet. Med. 9 (5) (1992) 444–450.

[129] V. Yadav, G. Marracci, E. Kim, R. Spain, M. Cameron, S. Overs, A. Riddehough, D.K. Li, J. McDougall, J. Lovera, C. Murchison, D. Bourdette, Low-fat, plant-based diet in multiple sclerosis: a randomized controlled trial, Mult. Scler. Relat. Disord. 9 (2016) 80–90.

[130] L. Skoldstam, Fasting and vegan diet in rheumatoid arthritis, Scand. J. Rheumatol. 15 (2) (1986) 219–221.

[131] J. Kjeldsen-Kragh, M. Haugen, C.F. Borchgrevink, E. Laerum, M. Eek, P. Mowinkel, K. Hovi, O. Forre, Controlled trial of fasting and one-year vegetarian diet in rheumatoid arthritis, Lancet 338 (8772) (1991) 899–902.

[132] S. Tonstad, E. Nathan, K. Oda, G. Fraser, Vegan diets and hypothyroidism, Nutrients 5 (11) (2013) 4642–4652.

[133] F. Haghighatdoost, N. Bellissimo, J.O. Totosy de Zepetnek, M.H. Rouhani, Association of vegetarian diet with inflammatory biomarkers: a systematic review and meta-analysis of observational studies, Public Health Nutr. 20 (15) (2017) 2713–2721.

[134] I. Hafstrom, B. Ringertz, A. Spangberg, L. von Zweigbergk, S. Brannemark, I. Nylander, J. Ronnelid, L. Laasonen, L. Klareskog, A vegan diet free of gluten improves the signs and symptoms of rheumatoid arthritis: the effects on arthritis correlate with a reduction in antibodies to food antigens, Rheumatology (Oxford) 40 (10) (2001) 1175–1179.

[135] M. Song, T.T. Fung, F.B. Hu, W.C. Willett, V.D. Longo, A.T. Chan, E.L. Giovannucci, Association of animal and plant protein intake with all-cause and cause-specific mortality, JAMA Intern. Med. 176 (10) (2016) 1453–1463.

[136] J. Montonen, H. Boeing, A. Fritsche, E. Schleicher, H.G. Joost, M.B. Schulze, A. Steffen, T. Pischon, Consumption of red meat and whole-grain bread in relation to biomarkers of obesity, inflammation, glucose metabolism and oxidative stress, Eur. J. Nutr. 52 (1) (2013) 337–345.

[137] K. Kostovcikova, S. Coufal, N. Galanova, A. Fajstova, T. Hudcovic, M. Kostovcik, P. Prochazkova, Z. Jiraskova Zakostelska, M. Cermakova, B. Sediva, M. Kuzma, H. Tlaskalova-Hogenova, M. Kverka, Diet rich in animal protein promotes pro-inflammatory macrophage response and exacerbates colitis in mice, Front. Immunol. 10 (2019) 919.

[138] S. Tonstad, E. Nathan, K. Oda, G.E. Fraser, Prevalence of hyperthyroidism according to type of vegetarian diet, Public Health Nutr. 18 (8) (2015) 1482–1487.

[139] M.T. Nenonen, T.A. Helve, A.L. Rauma, O.O. Hanninen, Uncooked, lactobacilli-rich, vegan food and rheumatoid arthritis, Br. J. Rheumatol. 37 (3) (1998) 274–281.

[140] E.J. Feskens, D. Sluik, G.J. van Woudenbergh, Meat consumption, diabetes, and its complications, Curr. Diab. Rep. 13 (2) (2013) 298–306.

[141] M.M. Lamb, M. Miller, J.A. Seifert, B. Frederiksen, M. Kroehl, M. Rewers, J.M. Norris, The effect of childhood cow's milk intake and HLA-DR genotype on risk of islet autoimmunity and type 1 diabetes: the diabetes autoimmunity study in the Young, Pediatr. Diabetes 16 (1) (2015) 31–38.

[142] J.S.J. Chia, J.L. McRae, A.K. Enjapoori, C.M. Lefevre, S. Kukuljan, K.M. Dwyer, Dietary Cows' Milk protein A1 Beta-casein increases the incidence of T1D in NOD mice, Nutrients 10 (9) (2018).

[143] G.M. Turner-McGrievy, M.D. Wirth, N. Shivappa, E.E. Wingard, R. Fayad, S. Wilcox, E.A. Frongillo, J.R. Hebert, Randomization to plant-based dietary approaches leads to larger short-term improvements in dietary inflammatory index scores and macronutrient intake compared with diets that contain meat, Nutr. Res. 35 (2) (2015) 97–106.

[144] G.M. Turner-McGrievy, C.R. Davidson, E.E. Wingard, S. Wilcox, E.A. Frongillo, Comparative effectiveness of plant-based diets for weight loss: a randomized controlled trial of five different diets, Nutrition 31 (2) (2015) 350–358.

[145] D.J. Jenkins, J.M. Wong, C.W. Kendall, A. Esfahani, V.W. Ng, T.C. Leong, D.A. Faulkner, E. Vidgen, G. Paul, R. Mukherjea, E.S. Krul, W. Singer, Effect of a 6-month vegan low-carbohydrate ('Eco-Atkins') diet on cardiovascular risk factors and body weight in hyperlipidaemic adults: a randomised controlled trial, BMJ Open 4 (2) (2014), e003505.

[146] D. Young, M. Ibuki, T. Nakamori, M. Fan, Y. Mine, Soy-derived di- and tripeptides alleviate colon and ileum inflammation in pigs with dextran sodium sulfate-induced colitis, J. Nutr. 142 (2) (2012) 363–368.

[147] H.K. Min, S.M. Kim, S.Y. Baek, J.W. Woo, J.S. Park, M.L. Cho, J. Lee, S.K. Kwok, S.W. Kim, S.H. Park, Anthocyanin extracted from black soybean seed coats prevents autoimmune arthritis by suppressing the development of Th17 cells and synthesis of proinflammatory cytokines by such cells, via Inhibition of NF-kappaB, PLoS One 10 (11) (2015), e0138201.

[148] H. Dai, B. Ciric, G.X. Zhang, A. Rostami, Interleukin-10 plays a crucial role in suppression of experimental autoimmune encephalomyelitis by Bowman-Birk inhibitor, J. Neuroimmunol. 245 (1–2) (2012) 1–7.

[149] J.H. Zhao, S.J. Sun, H. Horiguchi, Y. Arao, N. Kanamori, A. Kikuchi, E. Oguma, F. Kayama, A soy diet accelerates renal damage in autoimmune MRL/Mp-lpr/lpr mice, Int. Immunopharmacol. 5 (11) (2005) 1601–1610.

[150] S.L. Hauser, T.H. Doolittle, M. Lopez-Bresnahan, B. Shahani, D. Schoenfeld, V.E. Shih, J. Growdon, J.R. Lehrich, An antispasticity effect of threonine in multiple sclerosis, Arch. Neurol. 49 (9) (1992) 923–926.

[151] C.K. Lieben, A. Blokland, N.E. Deutz, W. Jansen, G. Han, R.M. Hupperts, Intake of tryptophan-enriched whey protein acutely enhances recall of positive loaded words in patients with multiple sclerosis, Clin. Nutr. 37 (1) (2018) 321–328.

[152] P. Piotrowski, M. Lianeri, M. Wudarski, J.K. Lacki, P.P. Jagodzinski, CD24 Ala57Val gene polymorphism and the risk of systemic lupus erythematosus, Tissue Antigens 75 (6) (2010) 696–700.

[153] W. Yang, W. Zhou, B.K. Zhang, L.S. Kong, X.X. Zhu, R.X. Wang, Y. Yang, Y.F. Chen, L.R. Chen, Association between CD24 Ala/Val polymorphism and multiple sclerosis risk: a meta analysis, Medicine (Baltimore) 99 (15) (2020), e19530.

[154] U. Akbar, M. Yang, D. Kurian, C. Mohan, Omega-3 fatty acids in rheumatic diseases: a critical review, J. Clin. Rheumatol. 23 (6) (2017) 330–339.

[155] P.C. Calder, n-3 polyunsaturated fatty acids, inflammation, and inflammatory diseases, Am. J. Clin. Nutr. 83 (6 Suppl) (2006) 1505S–1519S.

12. Nutritional implications for autoimmunity

[156] M. Simonetto, M. Infante, R.L. Sacco, T. Rundek, D. Della-Morte, A novel anti-inflammatory role of Omega-3 PUFAs in prevention and treatment of atherosclerosis and vascular cognitive impairment and dementia, Nutrients 11 (10) (2019).

[157] P.C. Calder, Mechanisms of action of (n-3) fatty acids, J. Nutr. 142 (3) (2012) 592S–599S.

[158] P.C. Calder, The relationship between the fatty acid composition of immune cells and their function, Prostaglandins Leukot. Essent. Fatty Acids 79 (3–5) (2008) 101–108.

[159] G.M. Balbas, M.S. Regana, P.U. Millet, Study on the use of omega-3 fatty acids as a therapeutic supplement in treatment of psoriasis, Clin. Cosmet. Investig. Dermatol. 4 (2011) 73–77.

[160] I. Kostoglou-Athanassiou, L. Athanassiou, P. Athanassiou, The effect of Omega-3 fatty acids on rheumatoid arthritis, Mediterr. J. Rheumatol. 31 (2) (2020) 190–194.

[161] I. Katz Sand, The role of diet in multiple sclerosis: mechanistic connections and current evidence, Curr. Nutr. Rep. 7 (3) (2018) 150–160.

[162] E.M. Duffy, G.K. Meenagh, S.A. McMillan, J.J. Strain, B.M. Hannigan, A.L. Bell, The clinical effect of dietary supplementation with omega-3 fish oils and/or copper in systemic lupus erythematosus, J. Rheumatol. 31 (8) (2004) 1551–1556.

[163] K.N. Gilley, K.A. Wierenga, P.S. Chauhuan, J.G. Wagner, R.P. Lewandowski, E.A. Ross, A.L. Lock, J.R. Harkema, A.D. Benninghoff, J.J. Pestka, Influence of total western diet on docosahexaenoic acid suppression of silica-triggered lupus flaring in NZBWF1 mice, PLoS One 15 (5) (2020), e0233183.

[164] K.A. Wierenga, R.S. Strakovsky, A.D. Benninghoff, L.D. Rajasinghe, A.L. Lock, J.R. Harkema, J.J. Pestka, Requisite Omega-3 HUFA biomarker thresholds for preventing murine lupus flaring, Front. Immunol. 11 (2020) 1796.

[165] C. Arriens, L.S. Hynan, R.H. Lerman, D.R. Karp, C. Mohan, Placebo-controlled randomized clinical trial of fish oil's impact on fatigue, quality of life, and disease activity in systemic lupus erythematosus, Nutr. J. 14 (2015) 82.

[166] P. Geusens, C. Wouters, J. Nijs, Y. Jiang, J. Dequeker, Long-term effect of omega-3 fatty acid supplementation in active rheumatoid arthritis. A 12-month, double-blind, controlled study, Arthritis Rheum. 37 (6) (1994) 824–829.

[167] B. Bahadori, E. Uitz, R. Thonhofer, M. Trummer, I. Pestemer-Lach, M. McCarty, G.J. Krejs, omega-3 fatty acids infusions as adjuvant therapy in rheumatoid arthritis, J. Parenter. Enteral. Nutr. 34 (2) (2010) 151–155.

[168] E. Rajaei, K. Mowla, A. Ghorbani, S. Bahadoram, M. Bahadoram, M. Dargahi-Malamir, The effect of Omega-3 fatty acids in patients with active rheumatoid arthritis receiving DMARDs therapy: double-blind randomized controlled trial, Global J. Health Sci. 8 (7) (2015) 18–25.

[169] M. Baarnhielm, T. Olsson, L. Alfredsson, Fatty fish intake is associated with decreased occurrence of multiple sclerosis, Mult. Scler. 20 (6) (2014) 726–732.

[170] S. Hoare, F. Lithander, I. van der Mei, A.L. Ponsonby, R. Lucas, G. Ausimmune Investigator, Higher intake of omega-3 polyunsaturated fatty acids is associated with a decreased risk of a first clinical diagnosis of central nervous system demyelination: results from the Ausimmune study, Mult. Scler. 22 (7) (2016) 884–892.

[171] D. Bates, N.E. Cartlidge, J.M. French, M.J. Jackson, S. Nightingale, D.A. Shaw, S. Smith, E. Woo, S.A. Hawkins, J.H. Millar, et al., A double-blind controlled trial of long chain n-3 polyunsaturated fatty acids in the treatment of multiple sclerosis, J. Neurol. Neurosurg. Psychiatry 52 (1) (1989) 18–22.

[172] D. Bates, P.R. Fawcett, D.A. Shaw, D. Weightman, Polyunsaturated fatty acids in treatment of acute remitting multiple sclerosis, Br. Med. J. 2 (6149) (1978) 1390–1391.

[173] O. Torkildsen, S. Wergeland, S. Bakke, A.G. Beiske, K.S. Bjerve, H. Hovdal, R. Midgard, F. Lilleas, T. Pedersen, B. Bjornara, F. Dalene, G. Kleveland, J. Schepel, I.C. Olsen, K.M. Myhr, omega-3 fatty acid treatment in multiple sclerosis (OFAMS Study): a randomized, double-blind, placebo-controlled trial, Arch. Neurol. 69 (8) (2012) 1044–1051.

[174] B. Weinstock-Guttman, M. Baier, Y. Park, J. Feichter, P. Lee-Kwen, E. Gallagher, J. Venkatraman, K. Meksawan, S. Deinehert, D. Pendergast, A.B. Awad, M. Ramanathan, F. Munschauer, R. Rudick, Low fat dietary intervention with omega-3 fatty acid supplementation in multiple sclerosis patients, Prostaglandins Leukot. Essent. Fatty Acids 73 (5) (2005) 397–404.

[175] I. Wessels, L. Rink, Micronutrients in autoimmune diseases: possible therapeutic benefits of zinc and vitamin D, J. Nutr. Biochem. 77 (2020) 108240.

[176] S. Manicassamy, R. Ravindran, J. Deng, H. Oluoch, T.L. Denning, S.P. Kasturi, K.M. Rosenthal, B.D. Evavold, B. Pulendran, Toll-like receptor 2-dependent induction of vitamin A-metabolizing enzymes in dendritic cells promotes T regulatory responses and inhibits autoimmunity, Nat. Med. 15 (4) (2009) 401–409.

[177] Z. Rezaieyazdi, M. Sahebari, N. Saadati, M. Khodashahi, Vitamin E and autoimmune diseases: a narrative review, Rev. Clin. Med. 5 (2) (2018) 42–48.

[178] M. Bredholt, J.L. Frederiksen, Zinc in multiple sclerosis: a systematic review and meta-analysis, ASN Neuro 8 (3) (2016).

[179] A. Sanna, D. Firinu, P. Zavattari, P. Valera, Zinc status and autoimmunity: a systematic review and meta-analysis, Nutrients 10 (1) (2018).

[180] S.M. Attar, A.M. Siddiqui, Vitamin d deficiency in patients with systemic lupus erythematosus, Oman Med. J. 28 (1) (2013) 42–47.

[181] Y. Zhang, G. Liu, X. Han, H. Dong, J. Geng, The association of serum 25-hydroxyvitamin D levels with multiple sclerosis severity and progression in a case-control study from China, J. Neuroimmunol. 297 (2016) 127–131.

[182] A. Ascherio, K.L. Munger, R. White, K. Kochert, K.C. Simon, C.H. Polman, M.S. Freedman, H.P. Hartung, D.H. Miller, X. Montalban, G. Edan, F. Barkhof, D. Pleimes, E.W. Radu, R. Sandbrink, L. Kappos, C. Pohl, Vitamin D as an early predictor of multiple sclerosis activity and progression, JAMA Neurol. 71 (3) (2014) 306–314.

[183] J. Correale, M.C. Ysrraelit, M.I. Gaitan, Immunomodulatory effects of vitamin D in multiple sclerosis, Brain 132 (Pt 5) (2009) 1146–1160.

[184] D. Hausler, S. Torke, E. Peelen, T. Bertsch, M. Djukic, R. Nau, C. Larochelle, S.S. Zamvil, W. Bruck, M.S. Weber, High dose vitamin D exacerbates central nervous system autoimmunity by raising T-cell excitatory calcium, Brain 142 (9) (2019) 2737–2755.

[185] G. Treiber, B. Prietl, E. Frohlich-Reiterer, E. Lechner, A. Ribitsch, M. Fritsch, B. Rami-Merhar, C. Steigleder-Schweiger, W. Graninger, M. Borkenstein, T.R. Pieber, Cholecalciferol supplementation improves suppressive capacity of regulatory T-cells in young patients with new-onset type 1 diabetes mellitus—a randomized clinical trial, Clin. Immunol. 161 (2) (2015) 217–224.

[186] G. Bock, B. Prietl, J.K. Mader, E. Holler, M. Wolf, S. Pilz, W.B. Graninger, B.M. Obermayer-Pietsch, T.R. Pieber, The effect of vitamin D supplementation on peripheral regulatory T cells and beta cell function in healthy humans: a randomized controlled trial, Diabetes Metab. Res. Rev. 27 (8) (2011) 942–945.

[187] U. Alam, A. Fawwad, F. Shaheen, B. Tahir, A. Basit, R.A. Malik, Improvement in neuropathy specific quality of life in patients with diabetes after vitamin D supplementation, J. Diabetes Res. 2017 (2017) 7928083.

[188] M.A. Gabbay, M.N. Sato, C. Finazzo, A.J. Duarte, S.A. Dib, Effect of cholecalciferol as adjunctive therapy with insulin on protective immunologic profile and decline of residual beta-cell function in new-onset type 1 diabetes mellitus, Arch. Pediatr. Adolesc. Med. 166 (7) (2012) 601–607.

[189] K.S. Aljabri, S.A. Bokhari, M.J. Khan, Glycemic changes after vitamin D supplementation in patients with type 1 diabetes mellitus and vitamin D deficiency, Ann. Saudi Med. 30 (6) (2010) 454–458.

[190] X. Li, L. Liao, X. Yan, G. Huang, J. Lin, M. Lei, X. Wang, Z. Zhou, Protective effects of 1-alpha-hydroxyvitamin D3 on residual beta-cell function in patients with adult-onset latent autoimmune diabetes (LADA), Diabetes Metab. Res. Rev. 25 (5) (2009) 411–416.

[191] E. Zold, P. Szodoray, B. Nakken, S. Barath, J. Kappelmayer, L. Csathy, A. Hajas, S. Sipka, E. Gyimesi, J. Gaal, Z. Barta, J. Hallay, G. Szegedi, E. Bodolay, Alfacalcidol treatment restores derailed immune-regulation in patients with undifferentiated connective tissue disease, Autoimmun. Rev. 10 (3) (2011) 155–162.

[192] E. Hypponen, E. Laara, A. Reunanen, M.R. Jarvelin, S.M. Virtanen, Intake of vitamin D and risk of type 1 diabetes: a birth-cohort study, Lancet 358 (9292) (2001) 1500–1503.

[193] A. Ataie-Jafari, S.C. Loke, A.B. Rahmat, B. Larijani, F. Abbasi, M.K. Leow, Z. Yassin, A randomized placebo-controlled trial of alphacalcidol on the preservation of beta cell function in children with recent onset type 1 diabetes, Clin. Nutr. 32 (6) (2013) 911–917.

[194] M. Walter, T. Kaupper, K. Adler, J. Foersch, E. Bonifacio, A.G. Ziegler, No effect of the 1alpha,25-dihydroxyvitamin D3 on beta-cell residual function and insulin requirement in adults with new-onset type 1 diabetes, Diabetes Care 33 (7) (2010) 1443–1448.

[195] D. Pitocco, A. Crino, E. Di Stasio, S. Manfrini, C. Guglielmi, S. Spera, G.B. Anguissola, N. Visalli, C. Suraci, M.C. Matteoli, I.P. Patera, M.G. Cavallo, C. Bizzarri, P. Pozzilli, I. Group, The effects of calcitriol and nicotinamide on residual pancreatic beta-cell function in patients with recent-onset type 1 diabetes (IMDIAB XI), Diabet. Med. 23 (8) (2006) 920–923.

[196] C. Bizzarri, D. Pitocco, N. Napoli, E. Di Stasio, D. Maggi, S. Manfrini, C. Suraci, M.G. Cavallo, M. Cappa, G. Ghirlanda, P. Pozzilli, I. Group, No protective effect of calcitriol on beta-cell function in recent-onset type 1 diabetes: the IMDIAB XIII trial, Diabetes Care 33 (9) (2010) 1962–1963.

12. Nutritional implications for autoimmunity

[197] E.M. Shih, S. Mittelman, P. Pitukcheewanont, C.G. Azen, R. Monzavi, Effects of vitamin D repletion on glycemic control and inflammatory cytokines in adolescents with type 1 diabetes, Pediatr. Diabetes 17 (1) (2016) 36–43.

[198] K.H. Winther, S.J. Bonnema, F. Cold, B. Debrabant, M. Nybo, S. Cold, L. Hegedus, Does selenium supplementation affect thyroid function? Results from a randomized, controlled, double-blinded trial in a Danish population, Eur. J. Endocrinol. 172 (6) (2015) 657–667.

[199] L. Zhu, X. Bai, W.P. Teng, Z.Y. Shan, W.W. Wang, C.L. Fan, H. Wang, H.M. Zhang, Effects of selenium supplementation on antibodies of autoimmune thyroiditis, Zhonghua Yi Xue Za Zhi 92 (32) (2012) 2256–2260.

[200] R. Gartner, B.C. Gasnier, Selenium in the treatment of autoimmune thyroiditis, Biofactors 19 (3–4) (2003) 165–170.

[201] R. Gartner, B.C. Gasnier, J.W. Dietrich, B. Krebs, M.W. Angstwurm, Selenium supplementation in patients with autoimmune thyroiditis decreases thyroid peroxidase antibodies concentrations, J. Clin. Endocrinol. Metab. 87 (4) (2002) 1687–1691.

[202] I. Pirola, E. Gandossi, B. Agosti, A. Delbarba, C. Cappelli, Selenium supplementation could restore euthyroidism in subclinical hypothyroid patients with autoimmune thyroiditis, Endokrynol. Pol. 67 (6) (2016) 567–571.

[203] O. Turker, K. Kumanlioglu, I. Karapolat, I. Dogan, Selenium treatment in autoimmune thyroiditis: 9-month follow-up with variable doses, J. Endocrinol. 190 (1) (2006) 151–156.

[204] G. Mantovani, A.M. Isidori, C. Moretti, C. Di Dato, E. Greco, P. Ciolli, M. Bonomi, L. Petrone, A. Fumarola, G. Campagna, G. Vannucchi, S. Di Sante, C. Pozza, A. Faggiano, A. Lenzi, E. Giannetta, Selenium supplementation in the management of thyroid autoimmunity during pregnancy: results of the "SERENA study", a randomized, double-blind, placebo-controlled trial, Endocrine 66 (3) (2019) 542–550.

[205] L.H. Duntas, A. Boutsiadis, A. Tsakris, Impaired metabolism of Selenomethionine in Graves' disease: a biokinetics study of soft gel capsule formulation, Horm. Metab. Res. 49 (8) (2017) 589–594.

[206] A. Peretz, J. Neve, J. Duchateau, J.P. Famaey, Adjuvant treatment of recent onset rheumatoid arthritis by selenium supplementation: preliminary observations, Br. J. Rheumatol. 31 (4) (1992) 281–282.

[207] K. Heinle, A. Adam, M. Gradl, M. Wiseman, O. Adam, Selenium concentration in erythrocytes of patients with rheumatoid arthritis. Clinical and laboratory chemistry infection markers during administration of selenium, Med. Klin. (Munich) 92 (Suppl 3) (1997) 29–31.

[208] B. Xu, D. Wu, H. Ying, Y. Zhang, A pilot study on the beneficial effects of additional selenium supplementation to methimazole for treating patients with Graves' disease, Turk. J. Med. Sci. 49 (3) (2019) 715–722.

[209] C. Balazs, The effect of selenium therapy on autoimmune thyroiditis, Orv. Hetil. 149 (26) (2008) 1227–1232.

[210] V.B. Vrca, F. Skreb, I. Cepelak, Z. Romic, L. Mayer, Supplementation with antioxidants in the treatment of Graves' disease; the effect on glutathione peroxidase activity and concentration of selenium, Clin. Chim. Acta 341 (1–2) (2004) 55–63.

[211] F. Karimi, G.R. Omrani, Effects of selenium and vitamin C on the serum level of antithyroid peroxidase antibody in patients with autoimmune thyroiditis, J. Endocrinol. Invest. 42 (4) (2019) 481–487.

[212] J. Mrazova, M. Gazarova, J. Kopcekova, A. Kolesarova, O. Bucko, B. Bobcek, The effect of consumption of pork enriched by organic selenium on selenium status and lipid profile in blood serum of consumers, J. Environ. Sci. Health B 55 (1) (2020) 69–74.

[213] Z. Fajt, J. Drabek, L. Steinhauser, Z. Svobodova, The significance of pork as a source of dietary selenium—an evaluation of the situation in the Czech Republic, Neuro Endocrinol. Lett. 30 (Suppl 1) (2009) 17–21.

[214] G.J. Kahaly, M. Riedl, J. Konig, T. Diana, L. Schomburg, Double-Blind, placebo-controlled, randomized trial of selenium in graves hyperthyroidism, J. Clin. Endocrinol. Metab. 102 (11) (2017) 4333–4341.

[215] U. Tarp, K. Overvad, E.B. Thorling, H. Graudal, J.C. Hansen, Selenium treatment in rheumatoid arthritis, Scand. J. Rheumatol. 14 (4) (1985) 364–368.

[216] A. Peretz, V. Siderova, J. Neve, Selenium supplementation in rheumatoid arthritis investigated in a double blind, placebo-controlled trial, Scand. J. Rheumatol. 30 (4) (2001) 208–212.

[217] H. Onal, G. Keskindemirci, E. Adal, A. Ersen, O. Korkmaz, Effects of selenium supplementation in the early stage of autoimmune thyroiditis in childhood: an open-label pilot study, J. Pediatr. Endocrinol. Metab. 25 (7–8) (2012) 639–644.

[218] W. Bonfig, R. Gartner, H. Schmidt, Selenium supplementation does not decrease thyroid peroxidase antibody concentration in children and adolescents with autoimmune thyroiditis, ScientificWorldJournal 10 (2010) 990–996.

[219] G. Karanikas, M. Schuetz, S. Kontur, H. Duan, S. Kommata, R. Schoen, A. Antoni, K. Kletter, R. Dudczak, M. Willheim, No immunological benefit of selenium in consecutive patients with autoimmune thyroiditis, Thyroid 18 (1) (2008) 7–12.

[220] S.A. Eskes, E. Endert, E. Fliers, E. Birnie, B. Hollenbach, L. Schomburg, J. Kohrle, W.M. Wiersinga, Selenite supplementation in euthyroid subjects with thyroid peroxidase antibodies, Clin. Endocrinol. (Oxf) 80 (3) (2014) 444–451.

[221] M. Leo, L. Bartalena, G. Rotondo Dottore, E. Piantanida, P. Premoli, I. Ionni, M. Di Cera, E. Masiello, L. Sassi, M.L. Tanda, F. Latrofa, P. Vitti, C. Marcocci, M. Marino, Effects of selenium on short-term control of hyperthyroidism due to Graves' disease treated with methimazole: results of a randomized clinical trial, J. Endocrinol. Invest. 40 (3) (2017) 281–287.

[222] S. Hucke, M. Eschborn, M. Liebmann, M. Herold, N. Freise, A. Engbers, P. Ehling, S.G. Meuth, J. Roth, T. Kuhlmann, H. Wiendl, L. Klotz, Sodium chloride promotes pro-inflammatory macrophage polarization thereby aggravating CNS autoimmunity, J. Autoimmun. 67 (2016) 90–101.

[223] M. Kleinewietfeld, A. Manzel, J. Titze, H. Kvakan, N. Yosef, R.A. Linker, D.N. Muller, D.A. Hafler, Sodium chloride drives autoimmune disease by the induction of pathogenic TH17 cells, Nature 496 (7446) (2013) 518–522.

[224] M.F. Farez, M.P. Fiol, M.I. Gaitan, F.J. Quintana, J. Correale, Sodium intake is associated with increased disease activity in multiple sclerosis, J. Neurol. Neurosurg. Psychiatry 86 (1) (2015) 26–31.

[225] E. Salgado, M. Bes-Rastrollo, J. de Irala, L. Carmona, J.J. Gomez-Reino, High sodium intake Is associated with self-reported rheumatoid arthritis: a cross sectional and case control analysis within the SUN cohort, Medicine (Baltimore) 94 (37) (2015), e0924.

[226] K.R.R. Rengasamy, H. Khan, S. Gowrishankar, R.J.L. Lagoa, F.M. Mahomoodally, Z. Khan, S. Suroowan, D. Tewari, G. Zengin, S.T.S. Hassan, S.K. Pandian, The role of flavonoids in autoimmune diseases: therapeutic updates, Pharmacol. Ther. 194 (2019) 107–131.

[227] B. Lu, D.H. Solomon, K.H. Costenbader, E.W. Karlson, Alcohol consumption and risk of incident rheumatoid arthritis in women: a prospective study, Arthritis Rheumatol. 66 (8) (2014) 1998–2005.

[228] M. Barbhaiya, B. Lu, J.A. Sparks, S. Malspeis, S.C. Chang, E.W. Karlson, K.H. Costenbader, Influence of alcohol consumption on the risk of systemic lupus erythematosus among women in the Nurses' health study cohorts, Arthritis Care Res. (Hoboken) 69 (3) (2017) 384–392.

[229] G. Effraimidis, J.G. Tijssen, W.M. Wiersinga, Alcohol consumption as a risk factor for autoimmune thyroid disease: a prospective study, Eur. Thyroid J. 1 (2) (2012) 99–104.

[230] L.G. Zhang, J. Chen, J.L. Meng, Y. Zhang, Y. Liu, C.S. Zhan, X.G. Chen, L. Zhang, C.Z. Liang, Effect of alcohol on chronic pelvic pain and prostatic inflammation in a mouse model of experimental autoimmune prostatitis, Prostate 79 (12) (2019) 1439–1449.

[231] K.J. Zhu, C.Y. Zhu, Y.M. Fan, Alcohol consumption and psoriatic risk: a meta-analysis of case-control studies, J. Dermatol. 39 (9) (2012) 770–773.

[232] G. Aljadeff, E. Longhi, Y. Shoenfeld, Bisphenol a: a notorious player in the mosaic of autoimmunity, Autoimmunity 51 (8) (2018) 370–377.

[233] K.M. Pollard, P. Hultman, D.H. Kono, Toxicology of autoimmune diseases, Chem. Res. Toxicol. 23 (3) (2010) 455–466.

[234] C. Dehner, R. Fine, M.A. Kriegel, The microbiome in systemic autoimmune disease: mechanistic insights from recent studies, Curr. Opin. Rheumatol. 31 (2) (2019) 201–207.

[235] I. Cosorich, G. Dalla-Costa, C. Sorini, R. Ferrarese, M.J. Messina, J. Dolpady, E. Radice, A. Mariani, P.A. Testoni, F. Canducci, G. Comi, V. Martinelli, M. Falcone, High frequency of intestinal TH17 cells correlates with microbiota alterations and disease activity in multiple sclerosis, Sci. Adv. 3 (7) (2017), e1700492.

[236] R. Mahajan, V. Midha, A. Singh, V. Mehta, Y. Gupta, K. Kaur, R. Sudhakar, A. Singh Pannu, D. Singh, A. Sood, Incidental benefits after fecal microbiota transplant for ulcerative colitis, Intest Res. 18 (3) (2020) 337–340.

[237] A.R. Weingarden, B.P. Vaughn, Intestinal microbiota, fecal microbiota transplantation, and inflammatory bowel disease, Gut Microbes 8 (3) (2017) 238–252.

[238] S. Makkawi, C. Camara-Lemarroy, L. Metz, Fecal microbiota transplantation associated with 10 years of stability in a patient with SPMS, Neurol. Neuroimmunol. Neuroinflamm. 5 (4) (2018), e459.

CHAPTER

13

Dysbiosis and probiotic applications in autoimmune diseases

Larissa Vedovato Vilela de Salis[a], Luísa Sales Martins[a], Guilherme Siqueira Pardo Rodrigues[b], and Gislane Lelis Vilela de Oliveira[a,c,]*

[a]Microbiology Program, Institute of Biosciences, Humanities and Exact Sciences (IBILCE), São Paulo State University (UNESP), São Paulo, Brazil [b]Department of Pediatrics, Hospital from School of Medicine from Botucatu (HCFMB), São Paulo State University (UNESP), Botucatu, Brazil [c]Department of Food Engineering and Technology, Institute of Biosciences, Humanities and Exact Sciences, São Paulo State University (UNESP), São Paulo, Brazil

*Corresponding author

Abstract

Several evidence in animal models and humans pointed to the involvement of oral and intestinal dysbiosis in the development of autoimmune diseases. Dysbiosis is associated with decreased bacterial function and diversity, as well as decreased beneficial microbes, increased pathobionts, impaired barrier function, bacterial translocation, systemic inflammation, and decreased immune regulatory mechanisms in the gut mucosa. The mechanisms proposed to link dysbiosis with autoimmune diseases include molecular mimicry, bystander T-cell activation, T helper cell skewing, epitope spreading, dual T-cell receptors, posttranslational modification of luminal proteins by dysbiotic microbiota, and amplification by inflammatory cytokines. Studies suggest that probiotics influence systemic immune responses, ensure the homeostasis of the healthy microbiota in the intestinal mucosa, and therefore, could be used as adjuvant therapy to treat immune-mediated diseases. The mechanisms to achieve these effects include mucus secretion, antimicrobial peptide production, cross-feeding other resident microbes, production of organic acids and enzymes, gastrointestinal epithelial barrier maintenance, decreasing oxidative stress, competition with pathogens, and finally, modulation of the host immunity. Here, we described several reports concerning dysbiosis and probiotic applications in animal models of autoimmune diseases, human studies, and clinical trials concerning the applicability of probiotics in autoimmune diabetes, autoimmune thyroid diseases, rheumatoid arthritis, systemic lupus erythematosus, and Sjögren syndrome.

Keywords

Microbiota, Dysbiosis, Inflammation, Autoimmunity, Probiotics

13. Dysbiosis and probiotic applications in autoimmune diseases

1 Introduction

Different surfaces of the human body, including the skin and all mucosal surfaces from the oral-gastrointestinal, respiratory, and urogenital tracts, are densely colonized by more than a trillion commensal and mutualistic microorganisms from all three domains of life (Archaea, Bacteria, and Eukarya) [1–3]. The gastrointestinal tract has the highest density and diversity of symbiotic microorganisms, which through millions of years of coevolution have become part of the human organism as a whole, playing essential role in immunity, metabolism, and behavior [4, 5].

The intestinal microbiota plays an essential role in the development and maturation of host immune system, and in turn, the mucosal immune system controls the microbiota through epithelial barrier maintenance and immune exclusion [1, 6, 7]. The interactions of intestinal microbiota and mucosal immune system are tightly regulated and homeostatic, contributing to eubiosis conditions in the gastrointestinal tract [1, 2, 8]. However, a combination of environmental and genetic factors can result in a tolerance breakdown and intestinal dysbiosis, with decrease in commensal bacteria groups, diversity, and function of this ecosystem, and increase in pathobionts [1, 9]. The outcomes of these deregulated interactions at the intestinal mucosa present systemic effects in host immunity and contribute to the development of chronic inflammatory and autoimmune diseases [7, 10] (Fig. 1).

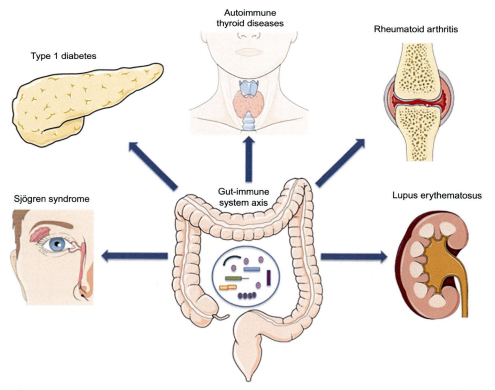

FIG. 1 The gut-immune system axis and the relationship with autoimmune diseases development, including autoimmune thyroid diseases, type 1 diabetes, rheumatoid arthritis, Sjögren syndrome, and lupus erythematosus.

In this chapter, several studies concerning dysbiosis and probiotic applications in autoimmune diseases, and data from ongoing clinical trials in autoimmune diabetes, autoimmune thyroid diseases, rheumatoid arthritis, systemic lupus erythematosus, and Sjögren's syndrome are discussed.

2 Dysbiosis in autoimmune diseases

Several studies performed in animal models pointed to the involvement of altered intestinal microbiota in the development of autoimmune diseases [11–22]. Dysbiosis observed in autoimmune diseases is associated with impaired epithelial barrier function, also known as the leaky gut, systemic inflammation, and decreased regulatory T cells (Tregs) in the gastrointestinal mucosa [23–26] (Fig. 2). The leaky gut can be triggered by an imbalance between microbes that potentiate the mucous barrier and mucolytic species, which leads not only to high exposure of antigens but also to local inflammation, prior to disease manifestation [27, 28]. The mechanisms to link dysbiosis with autoimmune diseases include molecular mimicry, bystander T-cell activation, T helper cell polarization, epitope spreading, dual T-cell receptors, posttranslational

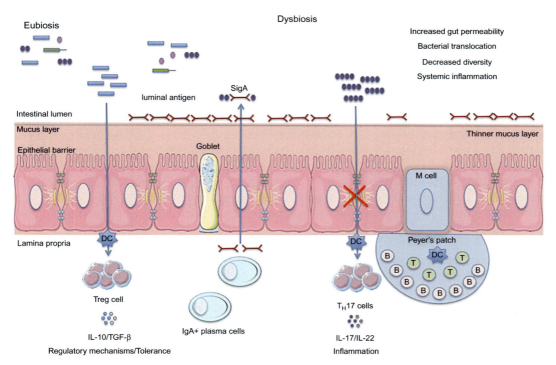

FIG. 2 Schematic representation of the interaction between the commensal microbiota and the mucosal immune system in the gastrointestinal tract. In eubiosis conditions, there is microbiota diversity and prevalence of beneficial microbes, favoring regulatory and tolerogenic mechanisms. In dysbiosis conditions, there is a decrease in the microbiota function and diversity, increase in pathobionts and barrier hyperpermeability, and deregulated interactions between immune cells and microbiota, resulting in local and further systemic inflammation.

modification of luminal proteins by microbiota, generating immunogenic neoepitopes, and amplification by inflammatory cytokines, which is elicited by a dysbiotic microbiota [25, 29].

3 Dysbiosis in autoimmune diabetes

Autoimmune diabetes or type 1 diabetes (T1D) is a chronic inflammatory disease characterized by immune reactions against pancreatic β-cells, resulting in hyperglycemia and insulin dependence to control the blood glucose [30, 31]. According to the International Diabetes Federation Atlas (2019), more than 132,600 individuals under 20 years of age are estimated to develop T1D every year. Multiple genetic and environmental factors seem to be involved in the T1D development, but the exact etiology remains unknown [31].

The role of intestinal dysbiosis in T1D etiology has been the target of research over the recent years to develop possible preventive approaches, including diet manipulation and probiotic administration [32, 33]. It was hypothesized that the immune tolerance breakdown in childhood, associated with intestinal dysbiosis, promotes autoreactive T-cell activation and autoantibody generation, thus increasing the chances of developing autoimmune diseases. Dysbiosis can also predispose children with genetic susceptibility and detectable autoantibodies to develop clinical manifestations of diseases [34].

In animal models, in germ-free nonobese diabetic (NOD) mice, significant alterations in the balance of T helper 1 (Th1), T helper 17 (Th17), and Tregs skewing in the gastrointestinal mucosa were detected, favoring the differentiation of inflammatory cells, insulitis, and pancreatitis [35]. Moreover, the intestinal microbiota modulates the mucosal immune system and induces diabetes in MyD88$^{-/-}$ NOD mouse model [36]. Interestingly, segmented filamentous bacteria (SFB), involved in Th17 induction in other autoimmune diseases, are involved in protection against diabetes in NOD mice [37]. In biobreeding diabetes-prone rats, prediabetic and diabetic patients, the predominance of gram-negative Bacteroidetes species induces an increase in intestinal permeability and precedes the clinical onset of diabetes [38, 39]. Finally, a study in germ-free NOD mice colonized with feces from T1D children with β-cell destruction showed a decrease in alpha diversity compared to human stool samples. The humanized recipient mice did not replicate the phenotype of the microbiota donor in relation to the progression toward T1D [20].

Previous studies have demonstrated that the intestinal microbiota from prediabetic children, with genetic predisposition and positive antibodies against β-cells, presents a dearth of *Bifidobacterium adolescentis* and *Bifidobacterium pseudocatenulatum*, increased abundance of *Bacteroides* species, and lower abundance of lactate and butyrate-producing bacteria [40]. Increased gram-negative bacteria *Bacteroides dorei* and *Bacteroides vulgatus* in seroconverted diabetes patients are detected 8 months prior to β-cell autoimmunity, indicating that early dysbiosis may predict T1D in genetically predisposal individuals [41]. Children with anti-β-cell autoantibodies exhibited decreased lactate and butyrate-producing bacteria [42], supporting the hypothesis that there is a gut microbiome signature associated with T1D development in seropositive children [43]. Additionally, there are decreased microbiota diversity and mucin-degrading microbes besides reduced Firmicutes/Bacteroidetes proportion, along with *Lactobacillus*, *Bifidobacterium*, and *Prevotela* species [44]. Decreased lactate-producing bacteria, such as *Bifidobacterium longum*, and increased *Clostridium*, *Bacteroides*, and *Veillonella* are equally observed [45].

Our research group evaluated the intestinal microbiota in 20 T1D patients and 28 healthy controls, and we detected dysbiosis and significant differences in β-diversity when compared with the control group. Moreover, gram-negative microbes including *Bacteroides vulgatus, Bacteroides rodentium, Prevotella copri,* and *Bacteroides xylanisolvens* dominated the gut microbiota in diabetes patients and were positively correlated with increased IL-6 plasma levels. Finally, we reported an association among T1D patients with poor glycemic control, with higher hemoglobin HbA1c levels and members of Bacteroidetes phylum and *Bacteroides dorei,* suggesting a possible role of gut microbiota in leaky gut, bacterial translocation, inflammation, and altered glycemia [46].

A study examining 53 T1D patients and 50 age and sex-matched controls reported significant alterations in oral and intestinal microbiota, according to β-diversity analysis. In fecal samples, *Christensenella* genus in T1D patients inversely correlated with fecal acetate, whereas *Subdoligranulum* genus correlated with LPS-binding protein (LBP) and C-reactive protein (CRP). Furthermore, HbA1c positively correlated with plasma LBP, and fecal IgA strongly correlated with fecal butyrate in T1D patients. Oral microbiota was dominated by species from Actinobacteria and Firmicutes phyla, including *Streptococcus, Actinomyces,* and *Rothia,* and were not correlated with glycemic and inflammatory markers or short-chain fatty acids [47]. In addition to oral and intestinal bacterial dysbiosis, researchers found fungal dysbiosis in children with β-cell autoantibodies, with predominance of fecal *Saccharomyces* and *Candida* species [48].

Finally, a study examined the inflammatory status and microbiota composition in duodenal mucosa biopsies from 19 T1D patients and 16 control subjects and found a T1D-specific inflammatory status compared with healthy control, especially characterized by increased monocyte/macrophage infiltration. The T1D duodenal microbiota showed an increase in Firmicutes and Firmicutes/Bacteroidetes ratio and a decrease in Proteobacteria and Bacteroidetes phyla [49].

The interaction between the intestinal microbiota and the mucosal immune system of the gastrointestinal tract plays a critical role in triggering diabetes. The cells of the immune system have receptors for the antigens and metabolites of the intestinal microbiota, and this bidirectional interaction can modulate the mucosal immune system, which may influence the protection or progression of the pathogenesis of diabetes [50].

Even though studies have shown that intestinal dysbiosis can affect gut permeability via bacterial metabolites and play a role in T1D development, the real role of intestinal microbiota in the development of autoimmunity against β-cells and in pancreas damage in humans remains controversial [51]. Additional studies are needed to find the specific microbial ligands that signal through immune cells in the gut mucosa and may be involved in the induction of autoreactivity against β-cells [52].

4 Dysbiosis in autoimmune thyroid diseases

Autoimmune thyroid diseases (AITD), including Hashimoto's thyroiditis (HT) and Graves' disease (GD), are the most common autoimmune disorders in humans and affect 10%–20% of all women, and approximately 5% of the general population [53]. Both diseases, GD and HT share some immune-mediated mechanisms including autoreactive B and T lymphocytes' infiltration, presence of thyroid autoantibodies, and thyroid hormone dysfunction, despite being clinically distinct [53, 54].

HT, also known as chronic lymphocytic thyroiditis, is characterized by chronic inflammation and increased circulating autoantibodies against thyroid peroxidase (TPO) and thyroglobulin (TG) and represents the main cause of hypothyroidism in the iodine-sufficient areas [55, 56]. GD affects the thyroid gland and represents the main cause of hyperthyroidism, with autoantibodies against the thyroid-stimulating hormone (TSH) receptor that act as agonists and induce excessive thyroid hormone secretion, compromising the control of the thyroid gland by the pituitary, and Graves' orbitopathy [57]. HT patients often require a lifelong hormone replacement therapy with levothyroxine while GD patients usually need thyreostatic drugs such as propylthiouracil and methimazole and often also radioiodine therapy or surgery to control the disease in long term [58, 59].

The etiology of the AITD might be a combination of genetic susceptibility and environmental factors that promote the immune tolerance breakdown and autoimmune attack to the thyroid gland and disease development [53]. Intestinal microbiota alterations are among the environmental factors involved in triggering autoimmune thyroid diseases [7, 55]. Moreover, some other related environmental risk factors of AITD are also known determinants of microbiota composition, such as diet, drugs, and infections [60].

The intestinal microbiota plays an important role in bile acid metabolism, carrying out the conversion of primary bile acids (BAs) to secondary BAs that are involved in lipid metabolism and stimulate type 2 iodothyronine deiodinase (D2) in brown adipose tissue, increasing local production of bioactive thyroid hormone T3 [61]. In addition, microbiota influences the absorption of minerals, including iodine, selenium, zinc, and iron, which are important to the thyroid function and homeostasis, including the enterohepatic cycle of thyroid hormones, iodothyronines metabolism, and oral thyroxine absorption [62, 63]. The intestinal bacteria that express β-glucuronidases and sulfatases are able to hydrolyze glucuronide and iodothyronine sulfate metabolites, which leads to the inactivation of thyroid hormones in the liver [64]. Thus, dysbiosis can be related to the prevalence of the disease, hormonal modulation, and therapeutic response.

There is increasing evidence for the presence of an important thyroid–gut axis and the intestinal dysbiosis appears to negatively influence the immune system and the regulation of inflammatory processes, and consequently, the thyroid function [27]. The role of the intestinal microbiota in autoimmune thyroid diseases was proposed after observing that the transfer of feces from conventional to specific pathogen-free rats increased the susceptibility to HT development [27]. In addition, some researchers have observed a cross-reaction between amino acid sequences from TPO/TG with *Lactobacillus* and *Bifidobacterium* species from the gut, which can induce an autoimmune reaction by autoantibodies [65]. In GD, intestinal dysbiosis plays an important role in susceptibility in different mice strains, in which some specific genera were significantly increased in C57BL/6J when compared to the less susceptible model, BALB/c strain [18]. Finally, alterations in composition and diversity of the gut microbiota seem to be a common feature shared by HT and GD [27].

Two recent studies, conducted in China, have demonstrated alterations of the gut microbiota in HT patients, one of them carried out in 2017, with 29 patients and 12 healthy individuals, showed an increase in the *Escherichia*, *Shigella*, and *Parasutterella* genera and a decrease in *Dialister* and *Prevotella* genera [66]. The other study, conducted in 2018, including 28 HT patients and 16 healthy controls reported an increase in *Blautia*, *Eubacterium*, *Fusicatenibacter*, and *Romboutsia* and a decrease in *Bacteroides*, *Fecalibacterium*, and *Prevotella* species [67].

It is necessary to note that some alterations detected in fecal microbiota can be explained by differences in thyroid function and treatments. However, independent of the thyroid status, studies identified a reduction in relative abundance of *Prevotella* species in HT [66, 67].

In a recent study, Cayres and colleagues evaluated the gut microbiota in 40 Hashimoto thyroiditis' Brazilian patients and 53 healthy controls and observed a significant increase in *Bacteroides* species and a decrease in *Bifidobacterium*. Besides that, *Lactobacillus* species were higher in patients without hormone replacement, compared with those that use oral levothyroxine. Researchers also found a negative correlation between animal-derived protein consumption and *Bacteroides* abundance, and increased zonulin concentrations in patients' serum, suggesting a barrier disruption in these patients [68].

Regarding GD, a Chinese study carried in 2018 with 27 patients and 11 healthy subjects evidenced significantly raised *Prevotella* and *Haemophilus* genera and significantly decreased *Alistipes* and *Faecalibacterium* genera [69]. Another study including 14 patients with hyperthyroidism and 7 healthy controls pointed to a decrease of *Bifidobacterium* and *Lactobacillus* and an increase of *Enterococcus* in the hyperthyroid group, suggesting an intestinal dysbiosis in these patients [70]. Besides, it was suggested that the gut microbiota could modulate the clinical presentation of Graves' orbitopathy (GO) in experimental models established in different environments [17]. Furthermore, a study with 33 patients with severe and active GO and 32 controls demonstrated that microbiota diversity was significantly lower and the proportion of Bacteroidetes increased in patients with GO. Therefore, intestinal dysbiosis can be related to extrathyroid manifestations of GD [71].

Although an exact composition of a healthy microbiota or a dysbiotic microbiota related to AITD is not yet clearly defined, alteration in the composition of intestinal bacteria, bacterial overgrowth, increased intestinal permeability, alteration of hormonal metabolism, and shift to proinflammatory immune cells are some of the factors of microbial impact on the thyroid gland [28].

5 Dysbiosis in rheumatoid arthritis

Rheumatoid arthritis (RA) is a systemic autoimmune disease characterized by chronic synovitis, bone erosion, and cartilage destruction [72]. The disease can affect internal organs including lungs, heart, and kidneys. The autoreactive immune cells induce autoantibodies, including anticyclic citrullinated peptide (anti-CCP) and rheumatoid factor (RF) [73]. According to World Health Organization, the worldwide prevalence of RA is 1%, and the disease affects mainly women between 50 and 60 years old. The triggers of RA incidence involve the interaction of HLA genes and environmental factors, such as smoking and infections [74]. Intestinal dysbiosis has been identified as a possible environmental factor that can trigger RA [75].

Dysbiosis might be involved in joint inflammation and the proposed mechanisms include dendritic cells activation, loss of tolerance to citrullinated antigens, molecular mimicry, leaky gut, and interference of microbiota with immunity, by triggering T-cell skewing and activation of Th17-mediated mucosal inflammation [76, 77].

Previous studies in animal models demonstrated that the antibiotic administration exacerbates the RA and induces an increase in IL-6, IFN-γ, and IL-17 inflammatory concentrations in collagen-induced arthritic mice [78]. Further investigations showed increased serum levels of IL-17 and CD4 Th17 cells in the spleen [79]. An increase in epithelial barrier permeability and a Th17 profile in RA susceptible mice were detected, indicating that genetic background potentially affects the microbiota profile [80]. Moreover, Th17 lymphocytes, induced by segmented filamentous bacteria in the intestinal lamina propria might stimulate the formation of autoantibodies involved in the initiation of RA in animal models [81]. The fecal transplantation from RA patients to germ-free arthritis-prone SKG mice induced an increase in Th17 cells in the gut mucosa and severe disease. Additionally, the SKG dendritic cells and *Prevotella copri* co-culture induce IL-17 secretion in response to autoantigens, indicating that intestinal microbiota could induce autoreactive T cells and joint inflammation [13].

Regarding oral dysbiosis, *Porphyromonas gingivalis*, a periodontitis-associated bacteria, has been implicated in triggering RA due to the peptidyl arginine deiminase expression, which induces autoantigen spreading that is a common finding in RA. Oral administration of *Porphyromonas gingivalis* promoted changes in the intestinal microbiota, increase in inflammatory markers, serum endotoxin, and impaired barrier function. The intestinal dysbiosis, induced by *Porphyromonas gingivalis* and *Prevotella intermedia*, is associated with collagen-induced arthritis in mice as well as increased bone loss and joint destruction, suggesting a connection between microbiota and bone metabolism [82, 83]. Antigens from the dysbiotic microbiota activate the immune system and can promote osteoclast differentiation and bone erosion by the secretion of TNF-α, IL-17, and RANK [83, 84]. Moreover, the *Porphyromonas gingivalis* administration in DBA/1J mice augments the disease severity, serum IL-17 concentration, and Th17 lymphocytes count in the mesenteric lymph nodes, suggesting a connection between periodontitis and RA that might affect the intestinal microbiota and consequently, the systemic immune responses [85].

In humans, researchers identified an intestinal microbiota signature and showed a decreased α-diversity (species richness), which positively correlated with higher RF and disease progression [11]. A study from Scher et al. in 2013 reported that the gram-negative *Prevotella* dominated the intestinal microbiota in newly diagnosed RA patients, mainly the *Prevotella copri* [86]. Regarding the microbiota from untreated newly diagnosed patients, *Lactobacillus salivarius*, *Lactobacillus iners*, and *Lactobacillus ruminis* were prevalent [87]. On the other hand, methotrexate-treated patients presented dominance of *Actinomyces*, *Collinsela*, *Eggerthella*, *Streptococcus*, and *Turibacter* species, with direct correlation with IL-17 inflammatory cytokine levels. Furthermore, CRP level, RF concentration, disease progression, and methotrexate administration are correlated with β-diversity in RA patients, suggesting that the gut microbiota modulation influences clinical parameters [11, 88].

Our research group investigated the presence of some specific microbes in the gut microbiota from 20 RA patients receiving disease-modifying anti-rheumatic drugs (DMARDs) and 30 healthy subjects. We observed an increase in *Bacteroides* and *Prevotella* species in samples from RA patients and a decrease in *Clostridium leptum* when compared to control group, suggesting that dysbiosis is not reestablished by DMARDs. Moreover, RF levels positively correlated with *Prevotella* abundance [89].

Increasing evidence indicate the crucial role of intestinal microbiota in RA development and the role of dysbiosis in disease progression and induction of inflammatory microenvironment, and led us to a greater understanding of RA etiopathogenesis [90]. Currently, the challenge is to explore the microbiota signatures as possible biomarkers of diseases' clinical activity and response to treatment, since the microbiota is able to interact with drugs and change the body's response to them [91]. Other questions to be answered are in relation to the participation of the virome and mycobiome, and the discovery of the cellular and molecular mechanisms involved in these interactions between the microbiota itself in its ecosystem [90]. In addition, a new interesting research field in relation to dysbiotic microbiota and RA involves osteomicrobiology, which analyzes the possible role of the microbiota and its metabolites in bone metabolism [83]. All of these studies will allow the development of therapies aimed at modulating the interactions of microbiota and the immune system, and complex metabolic pathways involved in these interactions [90].

6 Dysbiosis in systemic lupus erythematosus

Systemic lupus erythematosus (SLE) is a multisystem autoimmune disease characterized by damage to the skin, kidneys, lungs, joints, heart, and brain (94). The disease affects mainly women in a 9:1 ratio and presents a great clinical variability and significant morbidity and mortality [92, 93]. SLE pathogenesis may involve genetic and environmental factors, including viral infections, ultraviolet light exposure, abnormal apoptosis, and increased oxidative stress, resulting in tolerance breakdown and immune dysregulation, with autoantibodies production against nuclear and cytoplasmic antigens [94, 95]. Recent evidence pointed to an important role of intestinal dysbiosis in SLE development, and considering the reports that antibiotic use exacerbates SLE flares, suggest that microbiota plays an important role in the disease status [16, 96].

In animal models, in female lupus-prone mice, there is a decrease in *Lactobacillus* species while the early disease onset and severe symptoms correlated with increased *Lachnospiraceae* members [97]. In agreement with this study, Luo et al. in 2018 showed a decrease in *Lactobacillaceae* and an increase in *Lachnospiraceae* in lupus-prone strain, MRL/Mp-Faslpr (MRL/lpr), and mild disease phenotype was associated with recovered *Lactobacillus* species [16]. In SLE-prone mice, SWR x NZB (SNF1), higher abundance of *Rikenellaceae* family was found to be related to disease severity [98]. The leaky gut added up dysbiosis may explain the *Enterococcus gallinarum* translocation from the gut to the liver and the activation of the production of autoantibodies via TLR7/8 signaling in mice [99]. Interestingly, fecal samples from SLE mice induce the production of anti-dsDNA autoantibodies in germ-free mice, activate an inflammatory response, and alter the expression of SLE susceptibility genes [19]. In addition, depletion of the intestinal microbes exacerbates proteinuria and proinflammatory cytokines in SNF1 females, suggesting the essential role of the gut microbiota [84].

In humans, decreased Firmicutes/Bacteroidetes ratio in SLE patients was reported in some studies [100–102], even in the disease remission phase [103, 104]. The α-diversity and richness were decreased in SLE patients, along with a reduction in *Faecalibacterium prausnitzii* and *Roseburia*. *Ruminococcus gnavus* was increased in SLE and is associated with disease severity and lupus nephritis [105]. This species possibly share the epitope Ro60 with autoantigens, which is present in SLE patients [96, 106, 107]. Additionally, in silico analysis suggested that the dysbiosis observed in SLE patients could be linked to an increase in oxidative phosphorylation and glycan metabolism pathways induced by intestinal microbiota [100].

In treated patients, the gut microbiota from SLE patients undergoing glucocorticoid use was different when compared with nontreated patients and more similar to healthy controls, suggesting that glucocorticoid might downregulate inflammation via microbiota modulation [108].

Based on these reports showing dysbiosis in SLE patients, scientists evaluated the role of microbes from fecal samples by the in vitro differentiation of Th1, Th17, and Tregs. Patients' samples induced Th17 differentiation and the supplementation with Treg-inducing bacteria significantly decreased the inflammatory Th1/Th17 balance, supporting the use of specific strains as a promising therapeutic tool for SLE patients [100, 109].

The role of intestinal dysbiosis in the development of autoimmune diseases, including lupus, has already been recognized. The oral–intestinal microbiota axis represents an important link for human health and disease. However, some researchers did not recognize the relationship between oral microbes and SLE. Oral dysbiosis was detected in SLE patients, with decreased diversity, increased *Lactobacillaceae*, *Veillonellaceae*, and *Moraxellaceae* members, and no differences between newly diagnosed and treated patients [110]. Species frequently found in periodontitis were detected in higher amounts in SLE patients, including *Fretibacterium*, *Prevotella nigrescens*, and *Selenomonas*, as well as increased local inflammation, with increased IL-6, IL-17, and IL-33 concentrations in SLE patients with periodontal disease [111].

Studies performed in animal models and humans concerning intestinal microbiota provided new insights into the crucial role of dysbiosis in SLE. Intestinal pathobionts can translocate to systemic tissues and activate immune responses and anti-dsDNA autoantibodies production. Molecular mimicry is critical in autoimmunity induction by intestinal microorganisms. Proteins from intestinal microbiota have homologous epitopes with the Ro60 autoantigen found in SLE patients. These proteins bind to B and T lymphocytes to induce cellular and humoral autoreactive responses. Moreover, increased abundance of specific gut microbes is associated with disease activity and predicts lupus nephritis. Studies about intestinal microbiota have increased our understanding of the SLE pathogenesis, however, further studies are necessary to determine possible biomarkers of disease activity, predictors of lupus nephritis, and cardiovascular damage in lupus patients [96].

7 Dysbiosis in Sjögren's syndrome

Sjögren syndrome (SS) is a systemic autoimmune disease that essentially affects the exocrine glands, mainly the lacrimal and salivary glands, resulting in dry mucous surfaces, including eyes, mouth, nose, oropharynx, upper respiratory tract, and vagina [112]. SS predominantly affects middle-aged women in a 9:1 ratio, but can also be observed in children, men, and the elderly [113]. Despite being neglected, the disease is the second most prevalent systemic rheumatic autoimmune disease [113, 114]. The immune mechanism involved in the SS development includes epithelium destruction of the exocrine glands mediated by autoreactive B and T cells against autoantigens (Ro/SSA and La/SSB), lymphocytic infiltration, and immune complexes deposition [112, 115]. The clinical presentation of SS is heterogeneous and can vary from oral and ocular mucosal dryness (sicca symptoms) to systemic symptoms, including fatigue, musculoskeletal complaints, pulmonary complications, hepatic, renal and nervous system involvement [115].

In an experimental SS model, germ-free CD25KO mice presented epithelial barrier dysfunction, decreased number of goblet cells, higher lymphocytic infiltration and inflammatory cytokines, all reversed aspects after the fecal microbiota transplantation from conventional control mice [116].

Stool samples from SS patients presented higher relative abundances of *Blautia*, *Escherichia*, *Pseudobutyrivibrio*, *Shigella*, and *Streptococcus* genera, while *Bacteroides*, *Faecalibacterium*, *Parabacteroides*, and *Prevotella* genera were reduced compared to controls [12]. Moreover, while microbiota diversity decreases, the disease severity increases and overall intestinal dysbiosis was highly associated with ocular disease severity [117]. Mandl et al. examined the gut microbiota from 42 primary SS patients and 35 controls and detected a severe dysbiosis in SS patients that was associated with increased fecal calprotectin and the disease activity, as well as decreased relative abundances of *Bifidobacterium* and *Alistipes* genera [118].

Another recent work evaluated the intestinal microbiota in 13 SS patients, 8 subjects with features of SS, and 21 healthy controls and showed that all individuals with dry eyes presented depletion of Firmicutes and increased Proteobacteria, Actinobacteria, and Bacteroidetes phyla. There was a reduction in *Bacteroides*, *Faecalibacterium*, and *Veillonella* genera in SS patients compared to healthy controls. In addition, some bacterial families, including *Methanobacteriaceae*, *Bifidobacteriaceae*, *Flavobacteriaceae*, *Eubacteriaceae*, *Peptococcaceae*, and *Ruminococcaceae* correlated with symptoms (dry eye questionnaire and ocular surface disease index) and ocular surface inflammation, corneal staining, and tear production [119].

Oral dysbiosis was also detected in saliva from primary SS patients, with increase in *Candida* and *Streptococcus mutans*, and decreased *Fusobacterium nucleatum* [120]. Salivary microbiota from primary SS patients were found to be different from healthy individuals, with increased *Leucobacter*, *Delftia*, *Pseudochrobactrum*, *Ralstonia*, *Mitsuaria*, *Tannerella*, and *Treponema* genera, and *Streptococcus intermedius*, *Prevotella intermedia*, *Fusobacterium nucleatum* subspecie vincentii, *Porphyromonas endodontalis*, and *Prevotella nanceiensis* [121, 122]. Finally, Sembler-Møller et al. did not find significant differences between oral microbiota from primary SS and patients with non-Sjögren-related sicca symptoms [123].

Sjögren syndrome remains underdiagnosed and undertreated, and the latest breakthroughs in human microbiome studies revealed the connection with dysbiosis and helped us to understand the SS pathogenesis. However, further studies are needed to identify possible biomarkers for diagnosis, disease severity, and determination of the therapeutic response, in addition to identification of the molecular mechanisms involved in SS trigger by the gut microbes. The supplementation with prebiotics and probiotics offers a very promising future concerning SS therapies with diet interventions and may prove to be the ultimate immunomodulatory factor to suppress autoimmunity [113].

8 Probiotic applications in autoimmune diseases

According to the International Scientific Association for Probiotics and Prebiotics, the definition of probiotics is "live microorganisms that, when administered in adequate amounts, confer a health benefit on the host." Probiotics can be found in fermented foods and several supplements, but only well-defined strains, with scientifically demonstrated benefit should be used [124]. Most commonly used probiotic includes lactic acid-producing bacteria, such as *Lactobacillus*, *Bifidobacterium*, and *Streptococcus* species. Nonlactic, acid-producing bacteria, such as *Bacillus*, *Propionibacterium* species, and nonpathogenic yeasts, including *Saccharomyces boulfecesardii*, nonspore-forming and nonflagellated rod or coccobacilli, could have also been used as probiotics [125]. Other bacterial strains, including *Roseburia*, *Akkermansia*, *Propionibacterium*, and *Faecalibacterium* have shown to be promising for being used as probiotics [126]. Some of these strains were chosen based on origin, in vitro adherence to intestinal cells, and survival during passage through the gastrointestinal tract [127]. Despite the focus on probiotics, there are other modulators of the microbiota, including prebiotics, synbiotics, and postbiotics. Prebiotic is "a substrate that is selectively utilized by host microorganisms conferring a health benefit," i.e., the prebiotic dietary fiber needs to function as substrate for health-promoting microbes in the intestine [128]. Moreover, synbiotics are defined as "mixtures of probiotics and prebiotics that beneficially affect the host" [129]. Postbiotics include functional bioactive substances resulting from the microbial fermentation processes, including metabolites such as short-chain fatty acids and bacterial cell components, which confer beneficial impact on the host health [130, 131].

Studies suggest that probiotics influence systemic host immunity, ensure the eubiosis condition in the intestinal mucosa, and therefore, could be used as adjuvant therapy to treat immune-mediated diseases. The mechanisms proposed to achieve this notion include mucus secretion, antimicrobial peptide production, cross-feeding other resident microbes, production of organic acids and enzymes, the maintenance of the gastrointestinal-epithelial barrier, decreasing oxidative stress, competing with pathogens, and finally, modulation of the host immunity [126, 132]. The immunomodulatory effects of probiotics are associated with the release of antiinflammatory cytokines, proinflammatory cytokines, and chemokines from mucosal immune cells, including macrophages, neutrophils, mast cells, epithelial cells, dendritic cells, and lymphocytes, which further regulate the innate and adaptive immune responses [133].

In this section, we described several studies concerning probiotic applications in autoimmune diseases in animal models, in vitro experiments, and human studies. Table 1 summarizes the ongoing clinical trials using probiotics in autoimmune diabetes, autoimmune thyroid diseases, rheumatoid arthritis, systemic lupus erythematosus, and Sjögren syndrome.

9 Probiotics in autoimmune diabetes

Several studies are underway to verify whether the probiotic administration can improve the diabetes prognosis by modulating the intestinal microbiota [34, 50, 134, 135]. Probiotics influence innate and adaptive immune responses to environmental antigens, supporting the healthy intestinal microbiota, and thus, it was hypothesized that it could prevent the onset of T1D-associated islet autoimmunity and possibly treat the disease already established [6].

Early oral administration of *Lactobacillus* probiotics abrogated insulitis and β-cell destruction in NOD mice, and this protection was correlated with increased IL-10 secretion in Peyer's patches, spleen, and pancreas. This positive effect was transferable to irradiated mice, receiving diabetogenic cells and splenocytes from treated mice [136]. Likewise, the administration of *Lactobacillus*, alone or in combination with retinoic acid, protects NOD mice from diabetes by suppressing inflammasome formation, IL-1β, and by inducing indoleamine 2,3-dioxygenase and IL-33 secretion. In addition, treated NOD mice showed modulation of the intestinal immunity, by induction of CD103 dendritic cell differentiation along with the Th1 and Th17 suppression in the gut mucosa [137].

TABLE 1 Ongoing clinical trials testing the effectiveness of using probiotics in autoimmune diseases (ClinicalTrials.gov).

Registration	Country	Study design	Evaluations	Target subjects	Intervention	Administration route	Duration	Participants
NCT03880760	China	Randomized, double-blind clinical trial	Effect on serum cytokines and β-cell insulin secretion	T1D patients (+) autoantibodies (6 to 18 years)	*L. salivarius* AP-32 *L. johnsonii* MH-68 *B. lactis* CP-9	Orally (twice daily)	6 months	80
NCT03423589	United States of America	Nonrandomized, open label clinical trial	Effect on disease progression, endogenous innate inflammation	Full siblings of diagnosed T1D patients (5 to 17 years)	*B. longum*, *B. infantis*, *B. breve*, *L. acidophilus*, *L. casei*, *L. bulgaricus*, *L. plantarum* $(4.5 \times 10^{11}$ CFU)	Orally (twice daily)	6 weeks	30
NCT03032354	Poland	Randomized, double-blind, placebo-controlled clinical trial	Effect on β-cell function	T1D patients (+) autoantibodies fasting C-peptide ≥0.4 ng/mL (8 to 17 years)	*Lactobacillus rhamnosus* GG, *Bifidobacterium lactis* BB12	Orally (daily capsule)	6 months	96
NCT03556631	China	Randomized, single-blind, par-allel- controlled clinical trial	Effect on glycemic control and other T1D-related outcomes	T1D patients BMI ≤30Kg/m2, fasting blood glucose >7 mmol and <13 mmol HbA1c ≤10% (18 to 60 years)	*Bifidobacterium Lactobacillus* (strains not determined)	Orally (6 tablets/ twice daily)	3 months	30
NCT04141761	United States of America	Randomized, single-blind, placebo-controlled clinical trial	Effect on increased risk of developing T1D in those with genetic suscepti-bility	T1D patients (+) autoantibodies C-peptide AUC ≥0.2 nmol/L (5 to 17 years)	*L. paracasei*, *L. plantarum*, *L. acidophilus* *L. helveticus*, *B. lactis*, *B. breve* $(11 \times 10^{10}$ CFU)	Orally (powder form/ daily)	3 years	60
NCT03961347	United States of America	Randomized, double-blind, placebo-controlled clinical trial	Effect on β-cell function immunity and gut microbiota resto-ration	T1D patients (+) autoantibodies C-peptide ≥0.2 pmoL/mL (18 to 45 years)	*Lactobacillus johnsonii* N6.2 $(1.0 \times 10^9$ CFU)	Orally (daily capsule)	24 weeks	52

Continued

Registration	Country	Study design	Evaluations	Target subjects	Intervention	Administration route	Duration	Participants
NCT04335656	United States of America	Randomized, double-blind, placebo-controlled clinical trial	Effect on systemic inflammation and residual β-cell function	≤100 days diagnosed T1D (+) autoantibodies C-peptide ≥0.2 nmol/L (3 to 45 years)	*Lactobacillus plantarum* 299v	Orally (daily capsule)	6 months	60
NCT02605148	Sweden	Randomized, single-blind, controlled clinical trial	Effect of gluten-free diet on β-cell function and glucose metabolism	Prediabetes T1D patients (+) autoantibodies (2 to 49 years)	Vitamin D 800 U, Omega 3 fatty acids, Probiotics (not informed)	Orally (daily capsules)	18 months	240
NCT04014660	Sweden	Randomized, double-blind clinical trial	Effect on autoimmune process in the small intestine and permeability	T1D patients celiac disease thyroid disease (+) autoantibodies (10 to 18 years)	*L. plantarum* Heal 9 *L. paracasei* 8700:2 + corn starch	Orally (daily capsule)	12 months	200
NCT02373995	Italy	Randomized, single-blind clinical trial	Effect on gut microbiota and immune status	Untreated Graves' hyperthyroidism or 4 weeks of treatment, with orbitopathy (18 to 65 years)	*L. acidophilus*, CUL60 CUL21 *Bifidobacterium bifidum* CUL20 *B. animalis* subsp. *lactis* CUL34	Orally (2 capsules/ twice daily)	6 months	60
NCT00664820	England Canada	Randomized, double-blind clinical trial	Effect on symptom relief and patient activity	RA clinically diagnosed, at least four swollen and tender joints on a 64/66 scale (18 to 80 years)	*Lactobacillus rhamnosus* GR-1 *L. reuteri* RC-14	Orally (2 capsules/ daily)	3 months	50
NCT02941055	Sweden	Randomized, double-blind, cross-over clinical trial	Effect on disease activity and quality of life	Established RA, disease duration >2 years, disease activity DAS28 ≥2.6 (18 to 75 years)	Antiinflammatory diet, rich in fiber, fish and probiotics (not informed)	Orally (5 days/week)	10 weeks	56
NCT03840538	Egypt	Randomized, double-blind clinical trial	Effect on prophylaxis against oral candidiasis	Primary or secondary Sjögren syndrome (30 to 70 years)	*L. acidophilus*, *L. bulgaricus*, *Bifidobacterium bifidus*	Orally (twice daily)	5 weeks	32

The administration of probiotic *Clostridium butyricum* induces regulatory T cells in pancreas and consequently inhibits the onset of diabetes in NOD mice. The probiotic supplementation suppressed the insulitis, delayed the disease onset, and improved the glucose metabolism. These beneficial effects could involve the migration of intestinal Treg cells to the pancreatic lymph nodes, alterations in the Th1/Th2/Th17 balance, favoring an antiinflammatory milieu in the gut and pancreas. Additionally, probiotic supplementation increased the Firmicutes/Bacteroidetes ratio, *Clostridium* species, and butyrate-producing bacteria in the gut [138].

The *Akkermansia muciniphila*, a commensal microbe that resides in the mucous layer, is considered to be a promising candidate as probiotics [139]. The abundance of *Akkermansia muciniphila* is inversely correlated with the risk of developing antibodies against pancreatic beta cells. Thus, researchers transferred these bacteria to high diabetes incidence mice and reported an increased production of mucus and antimicrobial peptides, decreased serum endotoxin concentrations, and reduced Toll-like receptor expression in the pancreas, in addition to increased regulatory immune mechanisms and delayed disease onset [140].

In humans, a TEDDY study group evaluated the association between probiotic supplementation and islet autoimmunity in children with genetic risk for T1D, during their first year of life. The multicenter prospective cohort study investigated 7473 children ranging from 4 to 10 years old. The study indicated that early probiotic administration (0–27 days of life) was correlated with a decreased risk of islet autoimmunity when compared with control group [141].

In a recent double-blinded clinical trial, scientists examined the effect of *Lactobacillus sporogenes* GBI-30 plus fructooligosaccharide in 50 T1D patients for 8 weeks. They observed a significant reduction in HbA1c and CRP levels, as well as increased insulin levels [142].

The *Lactobacillus* and *Bifidobacterium* are the major bacteria genera that make up the colon microbiota in humans and help in the intestinal microbial homeostasis, inhibit the growth of pathobionts, improve the gut mucosal barrier, and modulate local and systemic immune responses [143]. Intestinal dysbiosis may influence the immune system by increasing gut permeability, intestinal inflammation, and impaired oral tolerance in T1D patients. Beneficial effect of *Lactobacillus rhamnosus* GG and *Bifidobacterium lactis* BB12 on β-cell function would create a rationale for its routine use in patients with newly diagnosed T1D [144]. Taken together, the studies imply that bacteriotherapy may potentially be used as a tool to modulate the immune system for preventing islet autoimmunity [143, 144].

10 Probiotics in autoimmune thyroid diseases

Studies have demonstrated the beneficial effect of probiotics in the modulation of gut microbiota, limiting the intestinal colonization from pathogenic bacteria, improving the physiological intestinal barrier function, and influencing the proinflammatory and antiinflammatory cytokines production [6, 145]. Besides that, in overt thyroid disorders, the microbiota can affect the uptake of levothyroxine (LT4) and influence the efficacy and toxicity of propylthiouracil (PTU), drugs used to treat hypothyroidism and hyperthyroidism, respectively. Therefore, probiotics, through the modulation of gut microbiota, may be effective in the maintenance of thyroid hormone homeostasis, contributing to the AITD management [27].

In animal models, *Lactobacillus reuteri* supplementation seems to benefit the thyroid function by increasing thyroid mass, free T4 levels, and by affecting the physiological parameters, such as more active behavior, slimness, and skin structure [146]. In murine experimental auto-immune thyroiditis (EAT), which mimics the cellular and pathological aspects of Hashimoto thyroiditis, the influence of oral supplementation of *Lactobacillus rhamnosus* HN001 and *Bifidobacterium lactis* HN019 in immune system, development, and disease progression were examined. Probiotic administration did not induce the entire EAT. In addition, no differences were observed in spleen weight, splenocytes proliferation in response to phorbol myristate acetate (PMA) when comparing probiotic-administrated group with control group [147].

In humans, a randomized, single-blinded, controlled clinical trial evaluated the effect of oral probiotic supplementation in LT4 metabolism in hypothyroid patients, for 2 months. The probiotic formulation includes *Bifidobacterium breve, B. longum, B. infantis, Lactobacillus aci-dophilus, L. plantarum, L. paracasei, L. bulgaricus,* and *Streptococcus thermophilus.* In this study, 39 patients took one capsule daily and 41 patients did not. There was no significant impact in thyroid function, just a decrease in LT4 levels in the probiotic group [148]. However, considering that the iodothyronines deconjugation can be mediated by bacterial sulfatases and β-glucuronidases, the microbiota modulation by probiotics could allow an increased LT4 bio-availability, and the thyroid hormones' gut reservoir could return to the blood circulation through enterohepatic recycling [148].

In GD, the metabolism of PTU is mediated by liver flavin-dependent monooxygenase (FMO3) enzyme. Meanwhile, some gut microbes have a similar enzyme, known as trimethyl-amine monooxygenase, which is able to metabolize PTU [27, 149]. Therefore, the intestinal microbiota can act on PTU stability and probiotics could interfere positively or negatively in the treatment of hyperthyroidism.

Current data do not support the hypothesis of the presence of a specific microbiota composition for thyroid diseases. However, since *Lactobacillaceae* and *Bifidobacteriaceae* members are often reduced in hypothyroidism and hyperthyroidism [69, 150, 151], studies suggest that bacteria from these families may have positive effects in suppressing inflammatory responses, through IL-10 secretion [152].

11 Probiotics in rheumatoid arthritis

Experiments in animal models suggest that the gut microbiota influences local and systemic immunity and might trigger joint inflammation [78]. A study investigating the role of *Bacillus coagulans* probiotic and inulin on the immune responses and RA progression in rat models showed that the spore-forming probiotic strain presents an antiinflammatory effect and significantly inhibits serum amyloid A and decreases TNF-α levels [153, 154].

Another study evaluated the effect of *Lactobacillus helveticus* SBT2171 on collagen-induced arthritis (CIA) in mice and on the antigen-specific antibody production. Probiotics induced a decrease in joint swelling and the serum level of bovine type II collagen-specific antibodies. In addition, the intraperitoneal route of *Lactobacillus helveticus* SBT2171 administration decreased the arthritis incidence, joint damage, and serum IL-6 concentration [155]. The *Lactobacillus helveticus* SBT2171 inhibits lymphocytes' proliferation through JNK signaling pathway suppression and exerts an immunosuppressive effect in vivo, supporting their beneficial effects in immune-mediated diseases [156].

Moreover, a study by Pan et al. (2019) evaluated the effect of *Lactobacillus casei* ATCC334 on arthritis, intestinal dysbiosis, and immune system in arthritis induced by adjuvant (AIA) rats. The results demonstrated a reduced joint swelling and bone destruction, in addition to decreased inflammatory cytokines, proposing that the beneficial effect of *L. casei* on AIA is associated with the suppressive effect on inflammatory pathways [157]. Similarly, Fan et al. examined the impact of *Bifidobacterium adolescentis* in CIA rats and reported that early supplementation reduces clinical symptoms, such as edema and pain, decreases inflammatory response, improves regulatory mechanisms, and restores eubiosis [158].

In clinical trials in RA patients, the oral administration of *Lactobacillus rhamnosus* and *Lactobacillus reuteri* for 3 months promoted an improvement in the Health Assessment Questionnaire Score and a functional improvement within the probiotic group, compared to the control group [159]. Another clinical trial showed improvement in disease activity score, increased levels of serum IL-10, and decreased levels of inflammatory mediators such as TNF-α, IL-6, and IL-12 cytokines in patients treated with oral *Lactobacillus casei* [160]. Likewise, oral administration of *Lactobacillus acidophilus*, *Lactobacillus casei*, and *Bifidobacterium bifidum*, for 8 weeks improved the Disease Activity Score of 28 joints (DAS-28). In addition, a significant decrease in serum insulin levels, homeostatic model assessment-B cell function (HOMA-B), and serum high-sensitivity C-reactive protein (hs-CRP) concentration in RA patients was reported [161, 162].

A systematic review and meta-analysis studies have been conducted in this area as well. It was demonstrated that probiotics, such as *Lactobacillus* and *Bifidobacterium* strains, used on average for 60 days, can improve the quality of life, reduce pain, decrease CRP and IL-6 inflammatory concentrations [163, 164]. The extrapolation of the results to clinical practice must be cautious due to the samples containing older patients, outside the therapeutic window of intervention. Small but statistically significant benefits require confirmation by randomized, double-blinded, placebo-controlled clinical studies as well as large cohort studies, considering confounding factors, in addition to differences in sex, age, and individuals' microbiota signature [164].

12 Probiotics in systemic lupus erythematous

Some *Lactobacillus* species have immunomodulatory activities in the gut mucosa and inhibit neutrophil extracellular traps (NETs) formation, improving antioxidant status and expression of adhesion molecules in the gut barrier [16, 165]. The administration of retinoic acid that potentially restored *Lactobacillus* species in lupus-like animal model and improved symptoms suggests the use of these species as a probiotic [97]. In addition, *Lactobacillus* spp. treatment of MRL/lpr mice ameliorated lupus nephritis and prolonged the survival [16, 166].

A study investigating the impact of *Lactobacillus paracasei* GMNL-32, *Lactobacillus reuteri* GMNL-89, and *Lactobacillus reuteri* GMNL-263 administration in NZB/WF1 mice reported a significant decrease in serum level of IL-6 and TNF-α and an increase in antioxidant activity in serum and liver. Additionally, the probiotic supplementation induced CD4$^+$CD25$^+$FoxP3$^+$ cell differentiation, suggesting that these strains could be used as adjuvant treatment for SLE patients due to their immunoregulatory activity [167]. Another investigation demonstrated that supplementation with these three probiotic strains improved hepatic apoptosis, matrix metalloproteinase-9 activity, inflammatory CRP, and inducible nitric oxide synthase. In addition, this supplementation reduced the hepatic IL-1β, IL-6, and TNF-α protein expression, by suppressing the mitogen-activated protein kinase and NF-κB signaling pathways [168].

An imbalance in Tregs involved in SLE pathogenesis and tolerogenic probiotics has shown beneficial impact in autoimmunity regulation. Therefore, researchers examined the prophylactic and therapeutic impact of *Lactobacillus delbrueckii* and *Lactobacillus rhamnosus* in pristane-induced lupus mice model. Probiotics promote a decrease in antinuclear antibodies (ANA), antidouble-stranded DNA (anti-dsDNA), and IL-6 and develop an increase in Tregs and *Foxp3* gene expression [169].

A recent study examined the effect of *Lactobacillus fermentum* CECT5716 in protecting the kidney function in a female NZBWF1 lupus mouse model. The probiotic administration decreased the plasma levels of anti-dsDNA, LPS, creatinine, urea excretion, and kidney injury. Moreover, the immune complex depositions and inflammatory infiltration were also reduced, as well as inflammatory cytokines (TNF-α, IFN-γ, and IL-17), Th1/Th17 infiltration, and NADPH oxidase activity [170]. Moreover, it was demonstrated that *Lactobacillus fermentum* promotes a reduction in disease activity, blood pressure, cardiac and renal hypertrophy, and splenomegaly, and an increase in *Bifidobacterium* abundance in the intestinal microbiota and Tregs in mesenteric lymph nodes, as well as an improvement of the vascular damage in female NZBWF1. These data open new possibilities for the prevention of renal and vascular complications related to high blood pressure observed in lupus [171].

The risk of atherosclerosis and cardiovascular diseases (CVD) represents the main cause of morbidity and mortality in SLE patients. Therefore, researchers evaluated the effects of heat-killed *Lactobacillus reuteri* GMNL-263 on the cardiac tissue in NZB/WF1 mice. Probiotics suppressed the enlargement of interstitial spaces, averted the abnormal myocardial structures in the heart of treated mice, decreased fibrosis, and restricted cardiac apoptotic signaling pathways, which all these observations suggest the potential *Lactobacillus reuteri* probiotic application in the treatment of SLE-related cardiovascular diseases [172].

Although several studies in SLE animal models showed promising data regarding the application of probiotic supplements, currently there is no published or ongoing clinical trial investigating the role of probiotics as an adjuvant therapy in the treatment of SLE patients.

13 Probiotics in Sjögren's syndrome

Several studies have shown that there is a connection between alterations in the intestinal microbiota and the SS manifestation, disease severity, and response to therapy. Dysbiosis, defined as decreased microbiota diversity and function, increases the disease severity in SS animal models and humans [114]. Interventions aimed at restoring eubiosis conditions and intestinal homeostasis, including modulation of the intestinal microbiota through diet, prebiotics, probiotics, synbiotics, and postbiotics, are considered modern strategies and are being studied in experimental models, in vitro studies, and clinical trials [113].

Patients with SS are at high risk for oral candidiasis development when compared to the general population. Due to the side effects of antifungals, treatment approaches such as probiotic supplementation can be very promising to solve this problem. Therefore, a recent randomized, double-blinded, placebo-controlled clinical trial evaluated the effect of *Lactobacillus acidophilus*, *Lactobacillus bulgaricus*, *Bifdobacterium bifdum*, and *Streptococcus thermophiles* administration in 32 SS patients, for 5 weeks. The probiotic administration promoted a decrease in the fungal load and may be effective to reduce colonization and prevent oral candidiasis in SS patients [173].

14 Conclusion

Several studies have presumed an association between dysbiosis and autoimmune diseases pathogenesis and highlighted the importance of maintenance of a healthy microbiota. The gastrointestinal mucosa could represent a predisposed site for the initiation of autoimmunity, by neoantigen generation under dysbiotic conditions. Ongoing studies are discovering specific microbes that could function as biomarkers in disease prediction, severity, and progression, as well as in optimizing or predicting the therapeutic response. Moreover, emerging findings point to the use of probiotics as an adjuvant treatment of autoimmune diseases, and researchers are looking for new probiotic strains, capable of modulating the immune system in specific diseases. However, further randomized, double-blinded, placebo-controlled clinical trials and larger cohorts are mandatory to evaluate the safety and efficacy of the probiotic supplementation in patients with autoimmune diseases.

References

[1] G.P. Donaldson, S.M. Lee, S.K. Mazmanian, Gut biogeography of the bacterial microbiota, Nat. Rev. Microbiol. 14 (1) (2016) 20–32.

[2] N.W. Palm, M.R. Zoete, R.A. Flavell, Immune-microbiota interactions in health and disease, Clin. Immunol. 159 (2) (2015) 122–127.

[3] F. De Luca, Y. Shoenfeld, The microbiome in autoimmune diseases, Clin. Exp. Immunol. 195 (1) (2019) 74–85.

[4] H. Anwar, S. Irfan, G. Hussain, M.N. Faisal, H. Muzaffar, et al., Gut microbiome: a new organ system in body, in: G.A.B. Pacheco, A.A. Kamboh (Eds.), Parasitology and Microbiology Research, first ed., IntechOpen, London, 2019, pp. 1–23.

[5] A.N. Skelly, Y. Sato, S. Kearney, K. Honda, Mining the microbiota for microbial and metabolite-based immunotherapies, Nat. Rev. Microbiol. 19 (5) (2019) 305–323.

[6] G.L.V. de Oliveira, A.Z. Leite, B.S. Higuchi, M.I. Gonzaga, V.S. Mariano, Intestinal dysbiosis and probiotic applications in autoimmune diseases, Immunology 152 (1) (2017) 1–12.

[7] E.M. Brown, D.J. Kenny, R.J. Xavier, Gut microbiota regulation of T cells during inflammation and autoimmunity, Annu. Rev. Immunol. 37 (2019) 599–624.

[8] G.L.V. de Oliveira, The gut microbiome in autoimmune diseases, in: J. Faintuch, S. Faintuch (Eds.), Microbiome and Metabolome in Diagnosis, Therapy, and Other Strategic Applications, first ed., Elsevier, Amsterdam, 2019, pp. 325–332.

[9] Y. Jiao, L. Wu, N.D. Huntington, X. Zhang, Crosstalk between gut microbiota and innate immunity and its implication in autoimmune diseases, Front. Immunol. 11 (2020) 282.

[10] M. Levy, A.A. Kolodziejczyk, C.A. Thaiss, E. Elinav, Dysbiosis and the immune system, Nat. Rev. Microbiol. 17 (4) (2017) 219–232.

[11] J. Chen, K. Wright, J.M. Davis, P. Jeraldo, E.V. Marietta, J. Murray, et al., An expansion of rare lineage intestinal microbes characterizes rheumatoid arthritis, Genome Med. 8 (1) (2016) 43.

[12] C.S. de Paiva, D.B. Jones, M.E. Stern, F. Bian, Q.L. Moore, S. Corbiere, et al., Altered mucosal microbiome diversity and disease severity in Sjögren's syndrome, Sci. Rep. 6 (2016) 23561.

[13] Y. Maeda, T. Kurakawa, E. Umemoto, D. Motooka, Y. Ito, K. Gotoh, et al., Dysbiosis contributes to arthritis development via activation of autoreactive T cells in the intestine, Arthritis Rheumatol. 68 (11) (2016) 2646–2661.

13. Dysbiosis and probiotic applications in autoimmune diseases

[14] Y. Hu, J. Peng, F. Li, F.S. Wong, L. Wen, Evaluation of different mucosal microbiota leads to gut microbiota-based prediction of type 1 diabetes in NOD mice, Sci. Rep. 8 (1) (2018) 15451.

[15] W.K. Jubair, J.D. Hendrickson, E.L. Severs, H.M. Schulz, S. Adhikari, et al., Modulation of inflammatory arthritis in mice by gut microbiota through mucosal inflammation and autoantibody generation, Arthritis Rheumatol. 70 (8) (2018) 1220–1233.

[16] X.M. Luo, M.R. Edwards, Q. Mu, Y. Yu, M.D. Vieson, C.M. Reilly, et al., Gut microbiota in human systemic lupus erythematosus and a mouse model of lupus, Appl. Environ. Microbiol. 84 (4) (2018). e02288–17.

[17] G. Masetti, S. Moshkelgosha, H.-L. Köhling, D. Covelli, J.P. Banga, et al., Gut microbiota in experimental murine model of graves' orbitopathy established in different environments may modulate clinical presentation of disease, Microbiome 6 (1) (2018) 97.

[18] S. Moshkelgosha, G. Masetti, U. Berchner-Pfannschmidt, H.L. Verhasselt, et al., Gut microbiome in BALB/c and C57BL/6J mice undergoing experimental thyroid autoimmunity associate with differences in immunological responses and thyroid function, Horm. Metab. Res. 50 (12) (2018) 932–941.

[19] Y. Ma, X. Xu, M. Li, J. Cai, Q. Wei, H. Niu, Gut microbiota promote the inflammatory response in the pathogenesis of systemic lupus erythematosus, Mol. Med. 25 (1) (2019) 35.

[20] V. Neuman, O. Cinek, D.P. Funda, T. Hudcovic, J. Golias, et al., Human gut microbiota transferred to germ-free NOD mice modulate the progression towards type 1 diabetes regardless of the pace of beta cell function loss in the donor, Diabetologia 62 (7) (2019) 1291–1296.

[21] B.M. Johnson, M.-C. Gaudreau, R. Gudi, R. Brown, G. Gilkeson, C. Vasu, Gut microbiota differently contributes to intestinal immune phenotype and systemic autoimmune progression in female and male lupus-prone mice, J. Autoimmun. 108 (2020) 102420.

[22] M.-C. Simon, A.L. Reinbeck, C. Wessel, J. Heindirk, T. Jelenik, K. Kaul, et al., Distinct alterations of gut morphology and microbiota characterize accelerated diabetes onset in nonobese diabetic mice, J. Biol. Chem. 295 (4) (2020) 969–980.

[23] H.-J. Wu, E. Wu, The role of gut microbiota in immune homeostasis and autoimmunity, Gut Microbes 3 (1) (2012) 4–14.

[24] E.C. Rosser, C. Mauri, A clinical update on the significance of the gut microbiota in systemic autoimmunity, J. Autoimmun. 74 (2016) 85–93.

[25] W.E. Ruff, T.M. Greiling, M.A. Kriegel, Host-microbiota interactions in immune-mediated diseases, Nat. Rev. Microbiol. 18 (9) (2020) 521–538.

[26] Q. Mu, J. Kirby, C.M. Reilly, X.M. Luo, Leaky gut as a danger signal for autoimmune diseases, Front. Immunol. 8 (2017) 598.

[27] E. Fröhlich, R. Wahl, Microbiota and thyroid interaction in health and disease, Trends Endocrinol. Metab. 30 (8) (2019) 479–490.

[28] A.C. Fenneman, E. Rampanelli, Y.S. Yin, J. Ames, M.J. Blaser, et al., Gut microbiota and metabolites in the pathogenesis of endocrine disease, Biochem. Soc. Trans. 48 (3) (2020) 915–931.

[29] A. Lerner, R. Aminov, T. Matthias, Dysbiosis may trigger autoimmune diseases via inappropriate post-translational modification of host proteins, Front. Microbiol. 7 (2016) 84.

[30] L.A. DiMeglio, C. Evans-Molina, R.A. Oram, Type 1 diabetes, Lancet 391 (10138) (2018) 2449–2462.

[31] J. Ilonen, J. Lempainen, R. Veijola, The heterogeneous pathogenesis of type 1 diabetes mellitus, Nat. Rev. Microbiol. 15 (11) (2019) 635–650.

[32] M.A. Atkinson, A. Chervonsky, Does the gut microbiota have a role in type 1 diabetes? Early evidence from humans and animal models of the disease, Diabetologia 55 (11) (2012) 2868–2877.

[33] O. Vaarala, Human intestinal microbiota and type 1 diabetes, Curr. Diab. Rep. 13 (5) (2013) 601–607.

[34] M. Knip, J. Honkanen, Modulation of type 1 diabetes risk by the intestinal microbiome, Curr. Diab. Rep. 17 (11) (2017) 105.

[35] C. Alam, E. Bittoun, D. Bhagwat, S. Valkonen, A. Saari, et al., Effects of a germ-free environment on gut immune regulation and diabetes progression in non-obese diabetic (NOD) mice, Diabetologia 54 (6) (2011) 1398–1406.

[36] L. Wen, R.E. Ley, P.Y. Volchkov, P.B. Stranges, L. Avanesyan, et al., Innate immunity and intestinal microbiota in the development of type 1 diabetes, Nature 455 (7216) (2008) 1109–1113.

[37] M.A. Kriegel, E. Sefik, J.A. Hill, H.-J. Wu, C. Benoist, D. Mathis, Naturally transmitted segmented filamentous bacteria segregate with diabetes protection in nonobese diabetic mice, Proc. Natl. Acad. Sci. U. S. A. 108 (28) (2011) 11548–11553.

[38] E. Bosi, L. Molteni, M.G. Radaelli, L. Folini, I. Fermo, E. Bazzigaluppi, et al., Increased intestinal permeability precedes clinical onset of type 1 diabetes, Diabetologia 49 (12) (2006) 2824–2827.

[39] L.F.W. Roesch, G.L. Lorca, G. Casella, A. Giongo, A. Naranjo, et al., Culture-independent identification of gut bacteria correlated with the onset of diabetes in a rat model, ISME J. 3 (5) (2009) 536–548.

[40] M.C. de Goffau, K. Luopajärvi, M. Knip, J. Ilonen, T. Ruohtula, et al., Fecal microbiota composition differs between children with β-cell autoimmunity and those without, Diabetes 62 (4) (2013) 1238–1244.

[41] A.G. Davis-Richardson, A.N. Ardissone, R. Dias, V. Simell, M.T. Leonard, et al., *Bacteroides dorei* dominates gut microbiome prior to autoimmunity in Finnish children at high risk for type 1 diabetes, Front. Microbiol. 5 (2014) 678.

[42] X. Li, M.A. Atkinson, The role for gut permeability in the pathogenesis of type 1 diabetes- -a solid or leaky concept? Pediatr. Diabetes 16 (7) (2015) 485–492.

[43] M.E. Mejía-León, J.F. Petrosino, N.J. Ajami, M.G. Domínguez-Bello, A.M.C. Barca, Fecal microbiota imbalance in Mexican children with type 1 diabetes, Sci. Rep. 4 (2014) 3814.

[44] A. Giongo, K.A. Gano, D.B. Crabb, N. Mukherjee, L.L. Novelo, et al., Toward defining the autoimmune microbiome for type 1 diabetes, ISME J. 5 (1) (2011) 82–91.

[45] M. Murri, I. Leiva, J.M. Gomez-Zumaquero, F.J. Tinahones, F. Cardona, et al., Gut microbiota in children with type 1 diabetes differs from that in healthy children: a case-control study, BMC Med. 11 (2013) 46.

[46] B.S. Higuchi, N. Rodrigues, M.I. Gonzaga, J.C.C. Paiolo, N. Stefanutto, et al., Intestinal Dysbiosis in autoimmune diabetes is correlated with poor glycemic control and increased Interleukin-6: a pilot study, Front. Immunol. 9 (2018) 1689.

[47] P.F. de Groot, C. Belzer, Ö. Aydin, E. Levin, J.H. Levels, S. Aalvink, et al., Distinct fecal and oral microbiota composition in human type 1 diabetes, an observational study, PLoS One 12 (12) (2017), e0188475.

[48] J. Honkanen, A. Vuorela, D. Muthas, L. Orivuori, K. Luopajärvi, et al., Fungal Dysbiosis and intestinal inflammation in children with Beta-cell autoimmunity, Front. Immunol. 11 (2020) 468.

[49] S. Pellegrini, V. Sordi, A.M. Bolla, D. Saita, R. Ferrarese, et al., Duodenal mucosa of patients with type 1 diabetes shows distinctive inflammatory profile and microbiota, J. Clin. Endocrinol. Metab. 102 (5) (2017) 1468–1477.

[50] S.P. Mishra, S. Wang, R. Nagpal, B. Miller, R. Singh, et al., Probiotics and prebiotics for the amelioration of type 1 diabetes: present and future perspectives, Microorganisms 7 (3) (2019) 67.

[51] H. Zhou, L. Sun, S. Zhang, X. Zhao, X. Gang, G. Wang, Evaluating the causal role of gut microbiota in type 1 diabetes and its possible pathogenic mechanisms, Front. Endocrinol. 11 (2020) 125.

[52] A. Paun, C. Yau, J.S. Danska, The influence of the microbiome on type 1 diabetes, J. Immunol. 198 (2) (2017) 590–595.

[53] H.J. Lee, C.W. Li, S.S. Hammerstad, M. Stefan, Y. Tomer, Immunogenetics of autoimmune thyroid diseases: a comprehensive review, J. Autoimmun. 64 (2015) 82–90.

[54] J.P. Banga, M. Schott, Autoimmune thyroid diseases, Horm. Metab. Res. 50 (12) (2018) 837–839.

[55] E. Fröhlich, R. Wahl, Thyroid autoimmunity: role of anti-thyroid antibodies in thyroid and extra-thyroidal diseases, Front. Immunol. 8 (2017) 521.

[56] F. Ragusa, P. Fallahi, G. Elia, D. Gonnella, S.R. Paparo, et al., Hashimotos' thyroiditis: epidemiology, pathogenesis, clinic and therapy, Best Pract. Res. Clin. Endocrinol. Metab. 33 (6) (2019) 101367.

[57] T.F. Davies, S. Andersen, R. Latif, Y. Nagayama, G. Barbesino, et al., Graves' disease, Nat. Rev. Dis. Primers. 6 (1) (2020) 52.

[58] I. Subekti, L.A. Pramono, Current diagnosis and Management of Graves' disease, Acta Med. Indones. 50 (2) (2018) 177–182.

[59] P. Caturegli, A. De Remigis, N.R. Rose, Hashimoto thyroiditis: clinical and diagnostic criteria, Autoimmun. Rev. 13 (4–5) (2014) 391–397.

[60] S.M. Ferrari, P. Fallahi, A. Antonelli, S. Benvenga, Environmental issues in thyroid diseases, Front. Endocrinol. 8 (2017) 50.

[61] R. Mullur, Y.Y. Liu, G.A. Brent, Thyroid hormone regulation of metabolism, Physiol. Rev. 94 (2) (2014) 355–382.

[62] C. Virili, M. Centanni, "With a little help from my friends" - the role of microbiota in thyroid hormone metabolism and enterohepatic recycling, Mol. Cell. Endocrinol. 458 (2017) 39–43.

[63] J. Knezevic, C. Starchl, A. Tmava Berisha, K. Amrein, Thyroid-gut-Axis: how does the microbiota influence thyroid function? Nutrients 12 (6) (2020) 1769.

[64] M. Kunc, A. Gabrych, J.M. Witkowski, Microbiome impact on metabolism and function of sex, thyroid, growth and parathyroid hormones, Acta Biochim. Pol. 63 (2) (2016) 189–201.

13. Dysbiosis and probiotic applications in autoimmune diseases

[65] E.P. Kiseleva, K.I. Mikhailopulo, O.V. Sviridov, G.I. Novik, Y.A. Knirel, E. Szwajcer Dey, The role of components of Bifidobacterium and Lactobacillus in pathogenesis and serologic diagnosis of autoimmune thyroid diseases, Benefic. Microbes 2 (2) (2011) 139–154.

[66] H.M. Ishaq, I.S. Mohammad, H. Guo, M. Shahzad, Y.J. Hou, et al., Molecular estimation of alteration in intestinal microbial composition in Hashimoto's thyroiditis patients, Biomed. Pharmacother. 95 (2017) 865–874.

[67] F. Zhao, J. Feng, J. Li, L. Zhao, Y. Liu, et al., Alterations of the gut microbiota in hashimoto's thyroiditis patients, Thyroid 28 (2) (2018) 175–186.

[68] L.C.F. Cayres, L.V.V. de Salis, G.S.P. Rodrigues, A.H. Lengert, et al., Detection of alterations in the gut microbiota and intestinal permeability in Hashimoto thyroiditis patients, Front. Immunol. 12 (2021) 579140.

[69] H.M. Ishaq, I.S. Mohammad, M. Shahzad, C. Ma, M.A. Raza, et al., Molecular alteration analysis of human gut microbial composition in graves' disease patients, Int. J. Biol. Sci. 14 (11) (2018) 1558–1570.

[70] L. Zhou, X. Li, A. Ahmed, Gut microbe analysis between hyperthyroid and healthy individuals, Curr. Microbiol. 69 (2014) 675–680.

[71] T.T. Shi, Z. Xin, L. Hua, R.X. Zhao, Y.L. Yang, H. Wang, et al., Alterations in the intestinal microbiota of patients with severe and active graves' orbitopathy: a cross-sectional study, J. Endocrinol. Investig. 42 (8) (2019) 967–978.

[72] J.A. Sparks, Rheumatoid arthritis, Ann. Intern. Med. 170 (1) (2019) ITC1–16.

[73] J.S. Smolen, D. Aletaha, A. Barton, G.R. Burmester, P. Emery, et al., Rheumatoid arthritis, Nat. Rev. Dis. Primers. 4 (2018) 18001.

[74] C. Croia, R. Bursi, D. Sutera, F. Petrelli, A. Alunno, I. Puxeddu, One year in review 2019: pathogenesis of rheumatoid arthritis, Clin. Exp. Rheumatol. 37 (3) (2019) 347–357.

[75] A.-S. Bergot, R. Giri, R. Thomas, The microbiome and rheumatoid arthritis, Best Pract. Res. Clin. Rheumatol. 33 (6) (2019) 101497.

[76] S.B. Brusca, S.B. Abramson, J.U. Scher, Microbiome and mucosal inflammation as extra-articular triggers for rheumatoid arthritis and autoimmunity, Curr. Opin. Rheumatol. 26 (1) (2014) 101–107.

[77] G. Horta-Baas, M.D.S. Romero-Figueroa, A.J. Montiel-Jarquín, et al., Intestinal Dysbiosis and rheumatoid arthritis: a link between gut microbiota and the pathogenesis of rheumatoid arthritis, J Immunol Res 2017 (2017) 4835189.

[78] I. Dorożyńska, M. Majewska-Szczepanik, K. Marcińska, M. Szczepanik, Partial depletion of natural gut flora by antibiotic aggravates collagen induced arthritis (CIA) in mice, Pharmacol. Rep. 66 (2) (2014) 250–255.

[79] X. Liu, B. Zeng, J. Zhang, W. Li, F. Mou, et al., Role of the gut microbiome in modulating arthritis progression in mice, Sci. Rep. 6 (2016) 30594.

[80] A. Gomez, D. Luckey, C.J. Yeoman, E.V. Marietta, M.E. Berg Miller, et al., Loss of sex and age driven differences in the gut microbiome characterize arthritis-susceptible 0401 mice but not arthritis-resistant 0402 mice, PLoS One 7 (4) (2012), e36095.

[81] H.-J. Wu, I.I. Ivanov, J. Darce, K. Hattori, T. Shima, et al., Gut-residing segmented filamentous bacteria drive autoimmune arthritis via T helper 17 cells, Immunity 32 (6) (2010) 815–827.

[82] S.H. Jeong, Y. Nam, H. Jung, J. Kim, Y.A. Rim, et al., Interrupting oral infection of *Porphyromonas gingivalis* with anti-FimA antibody attenuates bacterial dissemination to the arthritic joint and improves experimental arthritis, Exp. Mol. Med. 50 (3) (2018), e460.

[83] R.M. Jones, J.G. Mulle, R. Pacifici, Osteomicrobiology: the influence of gut microbiota on bone in health and disease, Bone 115 (2018) 59–67.

[84] C.M. Novince, C.R. Whittow, J.D. Aartun, J.D. Hathaway, N. Poulides, et al., Commensal gut microbiota immunomodulatory actions in bone marrow and liver have catabolic effects on skeletal homeostasis in health, Sci. Rep. 7 (1) (2017) 5747.

[85] K. Sato, N. Takahashi, T. Kato, Y. Matsuda, M. Yokoji, et al., Aggravation of collagen-induced arthritis by orally administered *Porphyromonas gingivalis* through modulation of the gut microbiota and gut immune system, Sci. Rep. 7 (1) (2017) 6955.

[86] J.U. Scher, A. Sczesnak, R.S. Longman, N. Segata, C. Ubeda, et al., Expansion of intestinal *Prevotella copri* correlates with enhanced susceptibility to arthritis, elife 2 (2013), e01202.

[87] X. Liu, Q. Zou, B. Zeng, Y. Fang, H. Wei, Analysis of fecal Lactobacillus community structure in patients with early rheumatoid arthritis, Curr. Microbiol. 67 (2) (2013) 170–176.

[88] M. Di Paola, D. Cavalieri, D. Albanese, M. Sordo, M. Pindo, et al., Alteration of Fecal microbiota profiles in Juvenile Idiopathic Arthritis. Associations with HLA-B27 allele and disease status, Front. Microbiol. 7 (2016) 1703.

[89] G.S.P. Rodrigues, L.C.F. Cayres, F.P. Gonçalves, N.N.C. Takaoka, et al., Detection of increased relative expression units of Bacteroides and Prevotella, and decreased *Clostridium leptum* in stool samples from Brazilian rheumatoid arthritis patients: a pilot study, Microorganisms 7 (10) (2019) 413.

[90] Z. Reyes-Castillo, E. Valdés-Miramontes, M. Llamas-Covarrubias, J.F. Muñoz-Valle, Troublesome friends within us: the role of gut microbiota on rheumatoid arthritis etiopathogenesis and its clinical and therapeutic relevance, Clin. Exp. Med. 21 (1) (2021) 1–13.

[91] J.U. Scher, R.R. Nayak, C. Ubeda, P.J. Turnbaugh, S.B. Abramson, Pharmacomicrobiomics in inflammatory arthritis: gut microbiome as modulator of therapeutic response, Nat. Rev. Rheumatol. 16 (5) (2020) 282–292.

[92] T. Dörner, R. Furie, Novel paradigms in systemic lupus erythematosus, Lancet 393 (10188) (2019) 2344–2358.

[93] J. Narváez, Systemic lupus erythematosus 2020, Med. Clin. (Barc.) 155 (11) (2020) 494–501.

[94] A. Kaul, C. Gordon, M.K. Crow, Z. Touma, M.B. Urowitz, et al., Systemic lupus erythematosus, Nat. Rev. Dis. Primers. 2 (2016) 16039.

[95] R. Illescas-Montes, C.C. Corona-Castro, L. Melguizo-Rodríguez, C. Ruiz, V.J. Costela-Ruiz, Infectious processes and systemic lupus erythematosus, Immunology 158 (3) (2019) 153–160.

[96] J.-W. Kim, S.-K. Kwok, J.-Y. Choe, S.-H. Park, Recent advances in our understanding of the link between the intestinal microbiota and systemic lupus erythematosus, Int. J. Mol. Sci. 20 (19) (2019) 4871.

[97] H. Zhang, X. Liao, J.B. Sparks, X.M. Luo, Dynamics of gut microbiota in autoimmune lupus, Appl. Environ. Microbiol. 80 (24) (2014) 7551–7560.

[98] B.M. Johnson, M.-C. Gaudreau, M.M. Al-Gadban, R. Gudi, C. Vasu, Impact of dietary deviation on disease progression and gut microbiome composition in lupus-prone SNF1 mice, Clin. Exp. Immunol. 181 (2) (2015) 323–337.

[99] S. Manfredo Vieira, M. Hiltensperger, V. Kumar, D. Zegarra-Ruiz, C. Dehner, et al., Translocation of a gut pathobiont drives autoimmunity in mice and humans, Science 359 (6380) (2018) 1156–1161.

[100] A. Hevia, C. Milani, P. López, A. Cuervo, S. Arboleya, et al., Intestinal dysbiosis associated with systemic lupus erythematosus, mBio 5 (5) (2014). e01548–01514.

[101] T.M. Greiling, C. Dehner, X. Chen, K. Hughes, A.J. Iñiguez, et al., Commensal orthologs of the human autoantigen Ro60 as triggers of autoimmunity in lupus, Sci. Transl. Med. 10 (434) (2018) eaan2306.

[102] Z. He, T. Shao, H. Li, Z. Xie, C. Wen, Alterations of the gut microbiome in Chinese patients with systemic lupus erythematosus, Gut Pathog. 8 (2016) 64.

[103] N. Katz-Agranov, G. Zandman-Goddard, The microbiome and systemic lupus erythematosus, Immunol. Res. 65 (2) (2017) 432–437.

[104] Y. Li, H.-F. Wang, X. Li, H.-X. Li, Q. Zhang, et al., Disordered intestinal microbes are associated with the activity of systemic lupus erythematosus, Clin. Sci. (Lond). 133 (7) (2019) 821–838.

[105] D. Azzouz, A. Omarbekova, A. Heguy, D. Schwudke, et al., Lupus nephritis is linked to disease-activity associated expansions and immunity to a gut commensal, Ann. Rheum. Dis. 78 (7) (2019) 947–956.

[106] I. Peene, D. Elewaut, Changing the wolf from outside: how microbiota trigger systemic lupus erythematosus, Ann. Rheum. Dis. 78 (7) (2019) 867–869.

[107] G.J. Silverman, D.F. Azzouz, A.V. Alekseyenko, Systemic lupus erythematosus and dysbiosis in the microbiome: cause or effect or both? Curr. Opin. Immunol. 61 (2019) 80–85.

[108] M. Guo, H. Wang, S. Xu, Y. Zhuang, J. An, et al., Alteration in gut microbiota is associated with dysregulation of cytokines and glucocorticoid therapy in systemic lupus erythematosus, Gut Microbes 11 (6) (2020) 1758–1773.

[109] P. López, B. de Paz, J. Rodríguez-Carrio, A. Hevia, B. Sánchez, et al., Th17 responses and natural IgM antibodies are related to gut microbiota composition in systemic lupus erythematosus patients, Sci. Rep. 6 (2016) 24072.

[110] B.-Z. Li, H.-Y. Zhou, B. Guo, W.-J. Chen, J.-H. Tao, et al., Dysbiosis of oral microbiota is associated with systemic lupus erythematosus, Arch. Oral Biol. 113 (2020) 104708.

[111] J.D. Corrêa, D.C. Calderaro, G.A. Ferreira, S.M.S. Mendonça, G.R. Fernandes, et al., Subgingival microbiota dysbiosis in systemic lupus erythematosus: association with periodontal status, Microbiome 5 (1) (2017) 34.

[112] P. Brito-Zerón, C. Baldini, H. Bootsma, S.J. Bowman, R. Jonsson, et al., Sjögren's syndrome, Nat. Rev. Dis. Primers. 2 (2016) 16047.

[113] C. Tsigalou, E. Stavropoulou, E. Bezirtzoglou, Current insights in microbiome shifts in Sjogren's syndrome and possible therapeutic interventions, Front. Immunol. 9 (2018) 1106.

[114] T.A. van der Meulen, A. Vissink, H. Bootsma, F.K.L. Spijkervet, F.G.M. Kroese, Microbiome in Sjögren's syndrome: here we are, Ann. Rheum. Dis. (2020) (annrheumdis-2020-218213).

13. Dysbiosis and probiotic applications in autoimmune diseases

[115] C.P. Mavragani, H.M. Moutsopoulos, Sjögren's syndrome: old and new therapeutic targets, J. Autoimmun. 110 (2020) 102364.

[116] M. Zaheer, C. Wang, F. Bian, Z. Yu, H. Hernandez, et al., Protective role of commensal bacteria in Sjögren's syndrome, J. Autoimmun. 93 (2018) 45–56.

[117] J. Moon, S.H. Choi, C.H. Yoon, M.K. Kim, Gut dysbiosis is prevailing in Sjögren's syndrome and is related to dry eye severity, PLoS One 15 (2) (2020), e0229029.

[118] T. Mandl, J. Marsal, P. Olsson, B. Ohlsson, K. Andréasson, Severe intestinal dysbiosis is prevalent in primary Sjögren's syndrome and is associated with systemic disease activity, Arthritis Res. Ther. 19 (1) (2017) 237.

[119] R. Mendez, A. Watane, M. Farhangi, K.M. Cavuoto, T. Leith, et al., Gut microbial dysbiosis in individuals with Sjögren's syndrome, Microb. Cell Factories 19 (1) (2020) 90.

[120] A. Almståhl, M. Wikström, I. Stenberg, A. Jakobsson, B. Fagerberg-Mohlin, Oral microbiota associated with hyposalivation of different origins, Oral Microbiol. Immunol. 18 (1) (2003) 1–8.

[121] M. Li, Y. Zou, Q. Jiang, L. Jiang, Q. Yu, et al., A preliminary study of the oral microbiota in Chinese patients with Sjögren's syndrome, Arch. Oral Biol. 70 (2016) 143–148.

[122] S. Rusthen, A.K. Kristoffersen, A. Young, H.K. Galtung, B.É. Petrovski, et al., Dysbiotic salivary microbiota in dry mouth and primary Sjögren's syndrome patients, PLoS One 14 (6) (2019), e0218319.

[123] M.L. Sembler-Møller, D. Belstrøm, H. Locht, C. Enevold, A.M.L. Pedersen, Next-generation sequencing of whole saliva from patients with primary Sjögren's syndrome and non-Sjögren's sicca reveals comparable salivary microbiota, J. Oral Microbiol. 11 (1) (2019) 1660566.

[124] C. Hill, F. Guarner, G. Reid, G.R. Gibson, D.J. Merenstein, et al., Expert consensus document. The International Scientific Association for Probiotics and Prebiotics consensus statement on the scope and appropriate use of the term probiotic, Nat. Rev. Gastroenterol. Hepatol. 11 (8) (2014) 506–514.

[125] M. Bermudez-Brito, J. Plaza-Díaz, S. Muñoz-Quezada, C. Gómez-Llorente, A. Gil, Probiotic mechanisms of action, Ann. Nutr. Metab. 61 (2) (2012) 160–174.

[126] M.E. Sanders, D.J. Merenstein, G. Reid, G.R. Gibson, R.A. Rastall, Probiotics and prebiotics in intestinal health and disease: from biology to the clinic, Nat. Rev. Gastroenterol. Hepatol. 16 (10) (2019) 605–616.

[127] G.L.V. de Oliveira, Probiotic applications in autoimmune diseases, in: S. Enany (Ed.), Probiotics—Current Knowledge and Future Prospects, first ed., IntechOpen, London, 2018, pp. 1–23.

[128] G.R. Gibson, R. Hutkins, M.E. Sanders, S.L. Prescott, R.A. Reimer, et al., Expert consensus document: the international scientific Association for Probiotics and Prebiotics (ISAPP) consensus statement on the definition and scope of prebiotics, Nat. Rev. Gastroenterol. Hepatol. 14 (8) (2017) 491–502.

[129] K.S. Swanson, G.R. Gibson, R. Hutkins, R.A. Reimer, G. Reid, et al., The international scientific Association for Probiotics and Prebiotics (ISAPP) consensus statement on the definition and scope of synbiotics, Nat. Rev. Gastroenterol. Hepatol. 17 (11) (2020) 687–701.

[130] J. Żółkiewicz, A. Marzec, M. Ruszczyński, W. Feleszko, Postbiotics-a step beyond pre- and probiotics, Nutrients 12 (8) (2020) 2189.

[131] C.A.M. Wegh, S.Y. Geerlings, J. Knol, G. Roeselers, C. Belzer, Postbiotics and their potential applications in early life nutrition and beyond, Int. J. Mol. Sci. 20 (19) (2019) 4673.

[132] P.A. Bron, M. Kleerebezem, R.-J. Brummer, P.D. Cani, A. Mercenier, et al., Can probiotics modulate human disease by impacting intestinal barrier function? Br. J. Nutr. 117 (1) (2017) 93–107.

[133] M.A.K. Azad, M. Sarker, D. Wan, Immunomodulatory effects of probiotics on cytokine profiles, Biomed. Res. Int. 2018 (2018) 8063647.

[134] C. He, Y. Shan, W. Song, Targeting gut microbiota as a possible therapy for diabetes, Nutr. Res. 35 (5) (2015) 361–367.

[135] R. Insel, M. Knip, Prospects for primary prevention of type 1 diabetes by restoring a disappearing microbe, Pediatr. Diabetes 19 (8) (2018) 1400–1406.

[136] F. Calcinaro, S. Dionisi, M. Marinaro, P. Candeloro, V. Bonato, et al., Oral probiotic administration induces interleukin-10 production and prevents spontaneous autoimmune diabetes in the non-obese diabetic mouse, Diabetologia 48 (8) (2005) 1565–1575.

[137] J. Dolpady, C. Sorini, C. Di Pietro, I. Cosorich, R. Ferrarese, et al., Oral probiotic VSL#3 prevents autoimmune diabetes by modulating microbiota and promoting Indoleamine 2,3-dioxygenase-enriched Tolerogenic intestinal environment, J. Diabetes Res. 2016 (2016) 7569431.

[138] L. Jia, K. Shan, L.-L. Pan, N. Feng, Z. Lv, et al., *Clostridium butyricum* CGMCC0313.1 protects against autoimmune diabetes by modulating intestinal immune homeostasis and inducing pancreatic regulatory T cells, Front. Immunol. 8 (2017) 1345.

[139] T. Zhang, Q. Li, L. Cheng, H. Buch, F. Zhang, *Akkermansia muciniphila* is a promising probiotic, Microb. Biotechnol. 12 (6) (2019) 1109–1125.

[140] A. Hänninen, R. Toivonen, S. Pöysti, C. Belzer, H. Plovier, et al., *Akkermansia muciniphila* induces gut microbiota remodelling and controls islet autoimmunity in NOD mice, Gut 67 (8) (2018) 1445–1453.

[141] U. Uusitalo, X. Liu, J. Yang, C.A. Aronsson, S. Hummel, et al., Association of Early Exposure of probiotics and islet autoimmunity in the TEDDY study, JAMA Pediatr. 170 (1) (2016) 20–28.

[142] A. Zare Javid, M. Aminzadeh, M.H. Haghighi-Zadeh, M. Jamalvandi, The effects of synbiotic supplementation on glycemic status, lipid profile, and biomarkers of oxidative stress in type 1 diabetic patients. A placebo-controlled, double-blind, randomized clinical trial, Diabetes Metab. Syndr. Obes. 13 (2020) 607–617.

[143] M. Papizadeh, M. Rohani, H. Nahrevanian, A. Javadi, M.R. Pourshafie, Probiotic characters of Bifidobacterium and Lactobacillus are a result of the ongoing gene acquisition and genome minimization evolutionary trends, Microb. Pathog. 111 (2017) 118–131.

[144] L. Groele, H. Szajewska, A. Szypowska, Effects of *Lactobacillus rhamnosus* GG and *Bifidobacterium lactis* Bb12 on beta-cell function in children with newly diagnosed type 1 diabetes: protocol of a randomised controlled trial, BMJ Open 7 (10) (2017), e017178.

[145] V.B.M. Peters, E. van de Steeg, J. van Bilsen, M. Meijerink, Mechanisms and immunomodulatory properties of pre- and probiotics, Benefic. Microbes 10 (3) (2019) 225–236.

[146] B.J. Varian, T. Poutahidis, T. Levkovich, Y.M. Ibrahim, J.R. Lakritz, et al., Beneficial Bacteria stimulate youthful thyroid gland activity, J. Obes. Weight Loss Ther. 4 (2014) 220.

[147] J.S. Zhou, H.S. Gill, Immunostimulatory probiotic *Lactobacillus rhamnosus* HN001 and *Bifidobacterium lactis* HN019 do not induce pathological inflammation in mouse model of experimental autoimmune thyroiditis, Int. J. Food Microbiol. 103 (1) (2005) 97–104.

[148] G. Spaggiari, G. Brigante, S. Vincentis, U. Cattini, L. Roli, et al., Probiotics ingestion does not directly affect thyroid hormonal parameters in hypothyroid patients on levothyroxine treatment, Front. Endocrinol. 8 (2017) 1–9.

[149] K.A. Romano, E.I. Vivas, D. Amador-Noguez, F.E. Rey, Intestinal microbiota composition modulates choline bioavailability from diet and accumulation of the proatherogenic metabolite trimethylamine-N-oxide, mBio 6 (2) (2015) 1–8.

[150] J. Knezevic, C. Starchl, A.T. Berisha, K. Amrein, Thyroid-gut-axis: how does the microbiota influence thyroid function? Nutrients 12 (6) (2020) 1–16.

[151] N.R. Shin, S. Bose, J.-H. Wang, Y.-D. Nam, E.-J. Song, et al., Chemically or surgically induced thyroid dysfunction altered gut microbiota in rat models, FASEB J. 34 (6) (2020) 8686–8701.

[152] H. Liang, Z. Luo, Z. Miao, X. Shen, M. Li, X. Zhang, et al., Lactobacilli and bifidobacteria derived from infant intestines may activate macrophages and lead to different IL-10 secretion, Biosci. Biotechnol. Biochem. 84 (12) (2020) 2558–2568.

[153] D.R. Mandel, K. Eichas, J. Holmes, *Bacillus coagulans*: a viable adjunct therapy for relieving symptoms of rheumatoid arthritis according to a randomized, controlled trial, BMC Complement. Altern. Med. 10 (2010) 1.

[154] K. Abhari, S.S. Shekarforoush, S. Hosseinzadeh, S. Nazifi, J. Sajedianfard, M.H. Eskandari, The effects of orally administered *Bacillus coagulans* and inulin on prevention and progression of rheumatoid arthritis in rats, Food Nutr. Res. 60 (2016) 30876.

[155] M. Yamashita, K. Matsumoto, T. Endo, K. Ukibe, T. Hosoya, et al., Preventive effect of *Lactobacillus helveticus* SBT2171 on collagen-induced arthritis in mice, Front. Microbiol. 8 (2017) 1159.

[156] T. Hosoya, F. Sakai, M. Yamashita, T. Shiozaki, T. Endo, et al., *Lactobacillus helveticus* SBT2171 inhibits lymphocyte proliferation by regulation of the JNK signaling pathway, PLoS One 9 (9) (2014), e108360.

[157] H. Pan, R. Guo, Y. Ju, Q. Wang, J. Zhu, et al., A single bacterium restores the microbiome dysbiosis to protect bones from destruction in a rat model of rheumatoid arthritis, Microbiome 7 (1) (2019) 107.

[158] Z. Fan, B. Yang, R.P. Ross, C. Stanton, G. Shi, et al., Protective effects of *Bifidobacterium adolescentis* on collagen-induced arthritis in rats depend on timing of administration, Food Funct. 11 (5) (2020) 4499–4511.

[159] M.L.A. Pineda, S.F. Thompson, K. Summers, F. Leon, J. Pope, G. Reid, A randomized, double-blinded, placebo-controlled pilot study of probiotics in active rheumatoid arthritis, Med. Sci. Monit. 17 (6) (2011) CR347–354.

[160] E. Vaghef-Mehrabany, B. Alipour, A. Homayouni-Rad, S.-K. Sharif, M. Asghari-Jafarabadi, S. Zavvari, Probiotic supplementation improves inflammatory status in patients with rheumatoid arthritis, Nutrition 30 (4) (2014) 430–435.

[161] B. Zamani, H.R. Golkar, S. Farshbaf, M. Emadi-Baygi, M. Tajabadi-Ebrahimi, et al., Clinical and metabolic response to probiotic supplementation in patients with rheumatoid arthritis: a randomized, double-blind, placebo-controlled trial, Int. J. Rheum. Dis. 19 (9) (2016) 869–879.

[162] B. Zamani, S. Farshbaf, H.R. Golkar, F. Bahmani, Z. Asemi, Synbiotic supplementation and the effects on clinical and metabolic responses in patients with rheumatoid arthritis: a randomised, double-blind, placebo-controlled trial, Br. J. Nutr. 117 (8) (2017) 1095–1102.

[163] A.T. Mohammed, M. Khattab, A.M. Ahmed, T. Turk, N. Sakr, et al., The therapeutic effect of probiotics on rheumatoid arthritis: a systematic review and meta-analysis of randomized control trials, Clin. Rheumatol. 36 (12) (2017) 2697–2707.

[164] J.R. Lowe, A.M. Briggs, S. Whittle, M.D. Stephenson, A systematic review of the effects of probiotic administration in inflammatory arthritis, Complement. Ther. Clin. Pract. 40 (2020) 101207.

[165] L. Vong, R.J. Lorentz, A. Assa, M. Glogauer, P.M. Sherman, Probiotic *Lactobacillus rhamnosus* inhibits the formation of neutrophil extracellular traps, J. Immunol. 192 (4) (2014) 1870–1877.

[166] Q. Mu, H. Zhang, X. Liao, K. Lin, H. Liu, et al., Control of lupus nephritis by changes of gut microbiota, Microbiome 5 (1) (2017) 73.

[167] B.-S. Tzang, C.-H. Liu, K.-C. Hsu, Y.-H. Chen, C.-Y. Huang, T.-C. Hsu, Effects of oral Lactobacillus administration on antioxidant activities and CD4+CD25+forkhead box P3 (FoxP3)+ T cells in NZB/W F1 mice, Br. J. Nutr. 118 (5) (2017) 333–342.

[168] T.-C. Hsu, C.-Y. Huang, C.-H. Liu, K.-C. Hsu, Y.-H. Chen, B.-S. Tzang, *Lactobacillus paracasei* GMNL-32, *Lactobacillus reuteri* GMNL-89 and *L. reuteri* GMNL-263 ameliorate hepatic injuries in lupus-prone mice, Br. J. Nutr. 117 (8) (2017) 1066–1074.

[169] S. Khorasani, M. Mahmoudi, M.R. Kalantari, F.L. Arab, S.-A. Esmaeili, et al., Amelioration of regulatory T cells by *Lactobacillus delbrueckii* and *Lactobacillus rhamnosus* in pristane-induced lupus mice model, J. Cell. Physiol. 234 (6) (2019) 9778–9786.

[170] N. de la Visitación, I. Robles-Vera, M. Toral, F. O'Valle, J. Moleon, et al., *Lactobacillus fermentum* CECT5716 prevents renal damage in the NZBWF1 mouse model of systemic lupus erythematosus, Food Funct. 11 (6) (2020) 5266–5274.

[171] M. Toral, I. Robles-Vera, M. Romero, N. de la Visitación, M. Sánchez, et al., *Lactobacillus fermentum* CECT5716: a novel alternative for the prevention of vascular disorders in a mouse model of systemic lupus erythematosus, FASEB J. 33 (9) (2019) 10005–10018.

[172] Y.-L. Yeh, M.-C. Lu, B.C.-K. Tsai, B.-S. Tzang, S.-M. Cheng, et al., Heat-killed *Lactobacillus reuteri* GMNL-263 inhibits systemic lupus erythematosus-induced cardiomyopathy in NZB/W F1 mice, Probiotics Antimicrob. Proteins 13 (1) (2021) 51–59.

[173] Y. Kamal, M. Kandil, M. Eissa, R. Yousef, B. Elsaadany, Probiotics as a prophylaxis to prevent oral candidiasis in patients with Sjogren's syndrome: a double-blinded, placebo-controlled, randomized trial, Rheumatol. Int. 40 (6) (2020) 873–879.

CHAPTER
14

Precision medicine to manage chronic immune-related conditions

David S. Gibson*, Phil Egan, Guangran Guo, Catriona Kelly, Paula McClean, Victoria McGilligan, Roisin McAllister, Kyle B. Matchett, Chloe A. Martin, Elaine K. Murray, Coral R. Lapsley, Taranjit Singh Rai, and Anthony J. Bjourson

Northern Ireland Centre for Stratified Medicine, Ulster University, Londonderry, United Kingdom
*Corresponding author

Abstract

The dysregulated immune system represents a major target for improving health outcomes in a range of chronic conditions. This chapter describes key changes in the immune system as we age and showcases its dysregulation across five chronic conditions including diabetes, cardiovascular disease, and cancer, highlighting dysregulated key immune system pathways and resultant inflammatory sequelae. Precision medicine aims to subdivide patients into different groups who will respond to specific treatments and could offer a novel way of addressing the complexity of immune system involvement in these conditions. The potential for precision medicine-led therapeutic strategies is discussed for each condition and considered in the context of multimorbidity.

Keywords

Immunosenescence, Diabetes mellitus, Cardiovascular disease, Rheumatoid arthritis, Depression, Cancer, Precision medicine, Genomics, Multimorbidity

1 Introduction

Immune system dysfunction is a central feature of many chronic health conditions including allergy, asthma, autoimmune diseases like rheumatoid arthritis (RA) or type I diabetes (T1D), autoinflammatory diseases such as Crohn's disease, and immunological deficiency syndromes. Decades of research have pinpointed molecular and cellular mechanisms within specific immune system pathways, which has greatly improved our understanding of the etiology, pathology, diagnosis, and therapeutic targeting of these classical immunological conditions. However, it has also emerged that the immune system is involved in the development and persistence of several chronic diseases that may not be considered immunological in origin, and therefore, these may benefit from similar therapeutic targeting strategies. These conditions with a strong immunopathological component and inflammatory backdrop include cardiovascular disease, mental health disorders, and cancers.

Advances in genomic, proteomic, and imaging technologies, and bioinformatic analyses to explore clinical phenotype associations are now leading the development of precision medicine strategies. Precision medicine aims to optimize the selection and allocation of treatment that is most likely to benefit particular subgroups of patients. A central premise of precision medicine is that heterogenous patient populations with the same index disease can be subdivided or stratified into clinically meaningful groups by combined dataset analyses. Though precision medicine approaches have predominated in cancer care, where genomic characterization of tumors can assist in the treatment triage, there is a great promise for it to assist in the management of the collective groups of chronic conditions with an immune system component.

This chapter describes immune system involvement in five key disease areas, highlighting dysregulated key immune system pathways and resultant inflammatory sequelae, and indicating potential areas for precision medicine-led diagnostics and therapies. The chapter begins by discussing these topics in the context of age-related changes in the immune system, also known as immunosenescence.

2 Immunosenescence

Immune function declines as we age [1]. One cellular process potentially involved in this functional decline is cellular senescence. Senescence is a state of stable cell cycle arrest when cells encounter unscheduled stress [2, 3]. Cells of the immune system such as T cells and B cells also encounter stresses and enter a similar state called immunosenescence [4]. Several factors such as aging, tumor-associated stresses, DNA damage, telomere attrition, regulatory T cells, and infections with pathogens such as cytomegalovirus (CMV) [5] can cause cells to enter into an immunosenescent state [6–9] (Fig. 1). Senescent cells are metabolically active and secrete numerous inflammatory factors, cytokines, immune modulators, and growth factors that are collectively termed as senescence-associated secretory phenotype (SASP) [10]. SASP is conserved among species [11] and plays a key role in immune regulation [12], inflammation [13], and senescence in neighboring cells [14].

Senescent cells are resistant to apoptotic pathways through regulation of antiapoptotic genes such as *BCL2* [15] and *MCL1* [16]. By secreting SASP, senescent cells attract immune cells and act as targets for immune clearance [17]. When the immune system is young and fully functional, this results in efficient clearance of senescent cells from the body. However, functional decline of the immune system with age (immunosenescence) results in impaired senescent cell clearance, which in turn causes an accumulation of various types of senescent cells [18]. In addition, immunosenescence increases susceptibility to infections and decreases immune responses such as those to vaccination in older individuals [19]. Understanding immunosenescence mechanistically may help in finding useful interventions to restore the immune system in old age and treat the related diseases that are discussed in subsequent sections (Fig. 1).

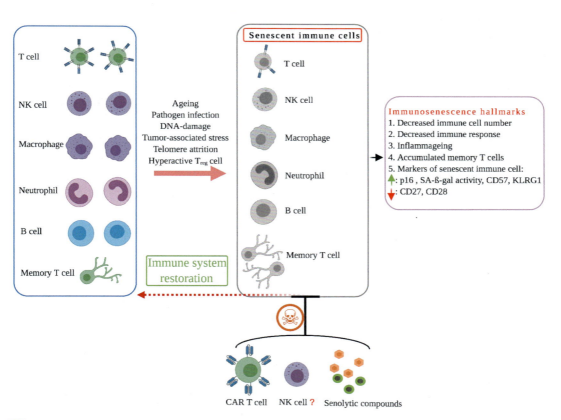

FIG. 1 Immune cells that encounter aging, pathogen infection, DNA damage, tumor-associated stress, telomere attrition, and hyperactive Treg cells develop immunosenescence. An immunosenescent state is defined by decreased cell numbers, weaker antigen responses, increased memory T lymphocytes, inflammaging, and many other senescence markers. Targeting immunosenescent cells through senolytic compounds, chimeric antigen receptor (CAR) T cells, and normal immune cells may help restore the immune system.

2.1 Hallmarks of immunosenescence and inflammatory pathways

Hallmarks of immunosenescence consist of decreased immune cell numbers and diminished antigen responses, accumulation of memory T lymphocytes, and "inflammaging," which is a chronic low-grade inflammation that contributes to the development of age-related diseases [20, 21]. In response to various stresses, immunosenescence can also occur in natural killer (NK) cells, T lymphocytes, B cells, macrophages, and neutrophils [22, 23]. Senescent immune cells exhibit increased p16 [24], senescence-associated β-galactosidase (SA-β-gal) activity [24], CD57 [25], and killer cell lectin-like receptor 1 (KLRG1) expression [26]; and decreased expression of immune cell costimulatory molecules such as CD27 [27] and CD28 [9]. Immunosenescence may contribute to aging of immune cells. Aged individuals show fewer naïve CD4$^+$ and CD8$^+$ T cells and higher levels of differentiation, increasing the risk of infections with viruses such as cytomegalovirus [28]. Senescent NK cells also show a decrease in cell numbers, altered secretion of chemokines [29], and reduced cytotoxicity, which could expose older individuals to bacterial, viral, and fungal infections [30]. Neutrophils can also enter senescence in response to microbial infections [31], which results in increased heterogeneity and impaired formation of neutrophil extracellular traps (NETs) required for restricting the pathogens. Eliminating senescent neutrophils led to improvement in sickle cell disease and septic shock cases, suggesting that targeting immunosenescence may have therapeutic potential [31].

Signal pathways involved in immunosenescence still remain largely unknown. MAPK, AMPK, p38, mTOR, and JAK/STAT pathways are involved in establishment of immunosenescence [32]. For example, senescent T cells activate AMPK and p38 pathways, downregulate the T-cell receptor (TCR) complex, and inhibit T-cell proliferation [33]. mTOR pathway plays a key role in T-cell proliferation and maturation. It has been reported that treatment of mice with mTOR inhibitor, rapamycin, decreased immunosenescence hallmarks that in turn improved health span and life span [34]. By targeting immunosenescence, potential treatments may be developed to recover the immune system and optimize immune responses to pathogens and vaccines.

2.2 Senolytic therapies

Eliminating senescent cells have been shown to alleviate symptoms of many age-associated diseases such as osteoarthritis and Alzheimer's disease [35, 36]), extend life span [37], and restore hemostasis among tissues [38]. Compounds that preferentially target senescent cells are known as senolytics [39]. Combination of dasatinib & quercetin (D&Q) [40], ABT-263 (also known as Navitoclax) [41], ABT-737 [42], fisetin [43], FOXO4-DRI peptide [38], cardiac glycosides [44, 45], and many others were recently reported as effective senolytic compounds. Various senolytics and their combinations are now undergoing clinical trials. D&Q is being evaluated in alleviating symptoms of Alzheimer's disease (NCT04063124) and chronic kidney disease (NCT02848131), fisetin in alleviating articular cartilage degeneration caused by osteoarthritis (NCT04210986), and combination of D&Q and fisetin for attenuating skeletal dysfunctions (NCT04313634).

Immune cells carry out natural senolytic activities, for instance, T cells cooperate with macrophages to preferentially eliminate senescent hepatocytes [46]. DNA damage-induced senescent hepatic stellate cells activate the immune system and increase immune modulators. Senescent hepatic stellate cells are cleared by NK cells that clear the fibrosis caused by dysfunctional cells

[47]. Moreover, NK cells recruit macrophages and neutrophils for immune clearance in murine liver [48]. Immune cells can be engineered to target senescent cells in vivo. Elevated cell surface expression of urokinase-type plasminogen activator receptor (uPAR) was found exclusively in senescent cells [49], while uPAR-targeting chimeric antigen receptor (CAR) T cells efficiently and selectively cleared senescent cells. In addition, liver fibrosis was reduced after the engineered CAR T-cell therapy, indicating that this therapeutic method has the potential to treat related diseases [49]. Thus, targeting senescence could improve immune cell functionality and extend human health and life span. Senescence of specific immune cell subtypes and pathways can evidently be a major contributor to the development of several aging-associated chronic conditions. As an example, elevated levels of CD57[+] and CD28[null] senescent T cells have been implicated in diabetes and cardiovascular conditions [50]. Exemplar diseases associated with immune dysregulation are discussed in the next sections.

3 Diabetes mellitus

Diabetes mellitus encompasses a group of metabolic disorders driven by insufficient production or action of the glucose-lowering hormone, insulin. Uncontrolled hyperglycemia presents as polyuria, polydipsia, and polyphagia, and requires treatment to prevent the onset of diabetes-associated complications including cardiovascular disease, neuropathies, nephropathies, and ocular disturbances.

Type 1 and type 2 diabetes (T1D and T2D, respectively) are the predominant forms of the disease. However, diabetes is also observed during pregnancy, in individuals with cystic fibrosis, and as a monogenic disease. There is clear evidence for genetic involvement in the pathogenesis of both primary forms. Genome-wide association studies (GWAS) have identified over 50 risk loci for T1D [51] and in the region of 100 loci for T2D [52]. Many genes that predispose development of hyperglycemia have immune regulatory capacity and, together with environmental factors such as obesity in the case of T2D, contribute to immune-mediated reductions in insulin production and uptake.

3.1 Immune system and inflammatory factors in diabetes

Immune involvement in T1D is well defined and leads to autoimmune destruction of the insulin-producing pancreatic beta cells resulting in an absolute insulin requirement that is most commonly treated with daily administration of exogenous insulin. Several autoantigens are associated with beta-cell demise in T1D including islet cell antibodies (ICA), antibodies to glutamic acid decarboxylase (GAD-65), insulin autoantibodies (IAA), and zinc transporter 8 autoantibodies (ZnT8A), which are released during the spontaneous turnover of beta cells [53]. Presentation of these antibodies to CD4[+] T cells lead to the production of proinflammatory cytokines including tumor necrosis factor alpha (TNF-α), TNF-β, interleukin (IL)-2, and interferon (IFN)γ. IFN-γ causes macrophages to become cytotoxic and release substantial quantities of cytokines (including IFN-γ, TNF-α, and IL-1β) leading to beta-cell apoptosis [53].

T2D is characterized by insulin resistance or insensitivity that is overcome by hypersecretion of insulin from beta cells in the early stages of disease. However, this compensatory mechanism fails over time, and insulin secretion becomes insufficient to meet metabolic demands [54]. Insulin resistance is driven by obesity and central adiposity. Indeed, fat deposition in the liver is associated with reduced hepatic insulin sensitivity [55]. Obesity, even in the absence of T2D, is considered an inflammatory condition and results in a heightened profile of inflammatory cytokines. Studies have shown that elevated IL-6 is predictive of insulin resistance and the development of T2D [56]. Both the c-Jun N-terminal kinase (JNK) and nuclear factor kappa B (NF-κB) pathways underlie chronic inflammation in obesity [57–60]. Indeed, insulin-resistant individuals have increased basal NF-κB activity in muscle [61].

3.2 Immunomodulatory therapies for diabetes

In recent years, a range of immunomodulatory therapies have been trialed for the treatment of T1D and T2D and are reviewed in detail by Tsalamandris et al. [54] and Cabello-Olmo et al. [62]. Since risk loci associated with T1D account for around 80% of the heritability of disease, early trials aimed at preventing the onset of T1D focused on the administration of insulin to relatives of those with a confirmed diagnosis [63, 64]. Insulin signaling has recently been shown to modulate the immune system through amplification of T-cell responses during inflammation and infection [65]. However, the Diabetes Prevention Trial-Type1 (DPT-1) found little effect of exogenous insulin administration on the incidence of T1D, with the exception of a small subset of participants who had higher autoantibody counts at baseline [63, 64]. Subsequent trials on immunomodulatory therapies in T1D have had some success in preserving beta-cell mass. Promisingly, treatment with two humanized anti-CD3 monoclonal antibodies (mAb), teplizumab and otelixizumab, was associated with enhanced beta-cell function [66]. The anti-TNF-α therapy, etanercept, improved insulin secretion and metabolic control in children with newly diagnosed T1D [67]. Vitamin D supplementation has been associated with some preservation of beta-cell function in cases of new onset T1D, but the observed effects were modest [68]. Although several studies of immunomodulatory therapies in T1D have reached their target of improved or preserved beta-cell function, these studies have been unable to reverse the initial beta-cell loss precipitating T1D onset, and islet transplantation remains the only route to reach long-term insulin independence.

Many drugs used for routine treatment of T2D have multiple effects on the immune system, for example, statins, metformin, and exogenous insulin. However, the complex etiology of T2D has resulted in limited clear-cut data in relation to the use of immunomodulatory drugs. For example, a systematic review suggests that people with RA who are receiving methotrexate are less likely to develop T2D [69]. However, in a large-scale clinical trial, the antiinflammatory benefit of methotrexate was not observed in those with cardiovascular disease with comorbid T2D [70]. Biological agents such as anakinra and gevokizumab (IL-1R antagonists) have been associated with improved beta-cell function and reduced inflammatory profiles [71, 72], while treatment with the TNF-α antagonist, infliximab, was found to improve insulin sensitivity and reduce the incidence of diabetes [73]. The following section discusses the cardiovascular disease, which is frequently comorbid in diabetes patients.

4 Atherosclerotic cardiovascular disease

Cardiovascular disease (CVD) is the leading cause of mortality and morbidity worldwide and represents a major healthcare burden. It accounts for up to 30% of worldwide deaths [74] and its incidence increases with age [75]. CVD pathogenesis is driven by atherosclerosis (Fig. 2) and risk factors including hyperlipidemia, obesity, smoking, and hypertension, in

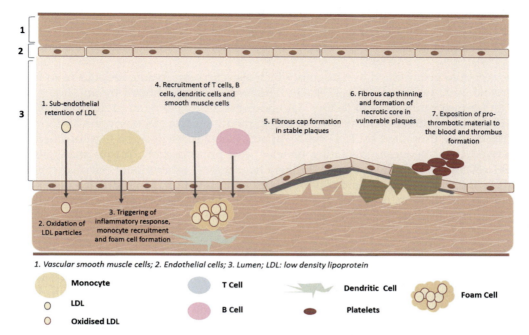

FIG. 2   Atherosclerotic plaque formation and progression. (1) Atherosclerosis starts with an endothelial injury/subendothelial retention of low-density lipoprotein (LDL) particles in the arterial wall. (2) LDL particles undergo oxidation which (3) triggers an inflammatory response with the recruitment of monocytes and foam cell formation. (4) This is followed by the recruitment of T cells, B cells, dendritic cells, and smooth muscle cells. (5) This results in the formation of a fibrous cap in stable plaques. (6) Vulnerable plaques may undergo thinning and the subsequent formation of a necrotic core. This leads to the exposition of thrombotic material to the blood circulation and the formation of thrombus.

addition to previously mentioned factors, aging and diabetes. These drivers can initiate endothelial dysfunction and atherosclerotic plaque formation. An unresolved cycle of chronic inflammation within the arterial intima results in plaque progression that is accompanied by varying degrees of fibrosis and calcification. The disease trajectory terminates in plaque destabilization, erosion, rupture, and occlusive thrombosis. An acute coronary syndrome (ACS) event may result and present along a severity spectrum: from STEMI (ST wave-elevated myocardial infarction) to NSTEMI (non-ST wave-elevated myocardial infarction) to UA (unstable angina).

4.1 Immune system involvement in cardiovascular pathology

Endothelial damage, induced by lipoproteins (especially low-density lipoprotein (LDL)), hypertension-induced shear stress, protein glycation, and toxins, promotes lipoprotein uptake into the intima, where it is chemically modified (e.g., by oxidation to ox-LDL). Modified lipoprotein antigens serve as pathogen-associated molecular patterns (PAMPs) or damage-associated molecular patterns (DAMPs) to induce a low-grade inflammatory response characterized by vascular cell activation, innate and subsequently adaptive immune cell recruitment. "Foam cells," resulting from macrophage uptake of ox-LDL, accumulate to form a lipid core. They upregulate scavenger receptor (e.g., CD36) and Toll-like-receptor (e.g., TLR4) expression and secrete proinflammatory cytokines to orchestrate inflammatory processes [76].

The response is amplified by Th1 cells which also can react to autoantigens from the apolipoprotein B100 protein of LDL [77]. The Th1 response is countered by antiinflammatory IL-10 and transforming growth factor (TGF)-βexpressing Treg and, more controversially, Th2 cells. Partial resolution is achieved by vascular smooth muscle cell migration and formation of a fibrotic cap, promoted by Th17 cells [78] and vascular calcification that together form a protective barrier between circulating platelets and prothrombotic plaque materials. Most plaques remain stabilized. However, "vulnerable plaques" exhibit foam cell death and accumulation of proinflammatory and prothrombotic stimuli within the lipid-laden necrotic core, the hallmark of such plaques. Eventually, the chronic inflammatory processes can propagate plaque rupture, leading to thrombotic coronary occlusion.

4.2 Inflammatory pathways in cardiovascular disease

The nucleotide-binding and oligomerization domain-like receptor, leucine-rich repeat and pyrin domain-containing 3 (NRLP3) inflammasome, is a master inflammatory mediator that proteolytically processes IL-1β (and IL-18) within activated foam cells and endothelial cells. Initial priming is TLR, TNFα, and IL-1 dependent; endocytosed cholesterol crystals and ox-LDL provide the activation signals. In addition to inducing the production of IL-1β and IL-18, the activation of the NLRP3 inflammasome boosts the migratory capacity of macrophages and augments lipid deposition in macrophage lysosomes. These events facilitate entry of macrophages into the arterial wall, stimulate foam cell formation, and ultimately promote atherosclerosis [79]. The self-perpetuating inflammatory cycle continues to induce other proinflammatory cytokines, including TNF-α, IL-6, and C-reactive protein (CRP), within the vasculature. These proteins and other TNF-pathway members (e.g., TNF receptor (TNFR)1/2 and the membrane-associated protease, tumor necrosis factor alpha converting enzyme (TACE)) have all been implicated in plaque progression and rupture [80, 81].

CVD has a genetic and environmental etiology, with a heritability rate of 40%–60% [82, 83]. GWASs have identified hundreds of CVD-associated variants, with many modulating proinflammatory protein expression to aggravate coexisting classic risk factors [84]. In situ DNA damage in vascular cells results from oxidative damage inflicted by ox-LDL and other reactive oxygen species. The resultant genomic instability and cell cycle deregulation underpin the age-dependent vasculature dysfunction and "inflammaging" increasingly seen in aging populations [85–87].

The gut microbiome produces metabolic products that modulate lipid metabolism and the immune response in many chronic diseases, including CVD. Trimethylamine N-oxide (TMAO) induces endothelial cell dysfunction and platelet hyperactivity [88]. Several studies have also reported bacterial organisms in arterial plaques [89]. Emerging research reports bacterial DNA in the blood associated with a personal microbiotic fingerprint as a predictor of cardiovascular events and stool microbiome as a signature of cardiovascular disease [90–92].

4.3 Potentials for novel therapies and diagnostics

Cholesterol-lowering statins are the mainstay of CVD treatment, but the residual risk is still very important. Statins can reduce cardiovascular events by no more than 40% [93]. The seminal CANTOS trial demonstrated that therapeutic targeting of IL-1β in atherosclerosis using the mAb, canakinumab, could reduce recurrent cardiovascular events by up to 15%, independent of their lipid-lowering effect [94]. Other preclinical studies have shown that direct NLRP3 inflammasome inhibition has efficacy in targeting plaque progression [95] with potentially less systemic immunosuppression and susceptibility to infection [96, 97].

CVD risk assessment and prognosis are made by empirical consideration of risk factors or the use of formal risk algorithms (e.g., SCORE, GRACE, and TIMI). However, not all patients at risk of a primary or recurrent CVD event are identified [98]. Several studies have investigated the diagnostic potential of various biomarkers such as high-sensitivity C-reactive protein (hs-CRP) but many have nonspecific prognostic value [99]. However, multimarker predictive panels are gaining traction [100]. Additionally, ACS diagnosis has traditionally relied upon the 12-lead ECG in combination with ischemic symptoms and elevation in serum troponin. However, ECG changes are often absent [101, 102]. New diagnostic tools are certainly required and in response to this, machine learning approaches to identify panels or "biosignatures" of immune responses and plaque progression plasma proteomic biomarkers capable of being predictive of CVD event occurrence/reoccurrence are being explored. Adoption of such biomarkers into patients' decision pathways offers the potential for referral streamlining and management standardization.

Other chronic inflammatory conditions, especially musculoskeletal diseases which are discussed next, can increase CVD morbidity and mortality by up to 50%. In these patients, increased proinflammatory cytokines, autoantibodies (e.g., anticyclic citrullinated peptide (anti-CCP) antibody), and various T-cell subpopulations promote plaque progression [103, 104].

5 Musculoskeletal conditions and arthritis

The term arthritis is used to describe a range of inflammatory or immune-related disorders affecting the musculoskeletal system. Musculoskeletal conditions are leading causes of morbidity and disability, which carry serious societal and personal impacts including growing healthcare costs and high risk of loss of work [105]. Osteoarthritis (OA), the most common form of arthritis, involves degeneration of articular cartilages in high usage joints including knees, hips, fingers, and lower spine. Worldwide estimates are that 9.6% of men and 18.0% of women aged over 60 years have symptomatic OA. RA is a chronic systemic disease associated with joint pain, swelling, and deformity of musculoskeletal tissue and is associated with cardiovascular, diabetic, and mental health comorbidities. RA is more common in women, has a prevalence between 0.3% and 1% and an onset between the ages 20–40 years, and as many as half of individuals are unable to work 10 years after diagnosis. There are many other arthritic disorders such as psoriatic arthritis (PsA), systemic lupus erythematosus (SLE), and ankylosing spondylitis (AS) that affect tissues beyond the musculoskeletal system.

Early diagnosis and treatment are key to effective management of arthritic disorders to prevent permanent damage. Precision medicine, driven by advances in omics analyses, promises to improve patient care with phenotypic and molecular markers to guide diagnostic and therapeutic decisions. There are major efforts to identify clinically actionable biomarkers and define pathobiological endotypes to aid risk stratification, drug selection, and treatment response prediction [106, 107]. Here, we overview immune system involvement in arthritic disorders, describe how these pathways contribute to pathology, act as therapeutic targets, and briefly mention efforts to stratify patients.

5.1 Immune system involvement in arthritis

Using RA as an initial exemplar arthritic disorder, though its etiology is still not fully understood, it is an inflammatory, autoimmune disease that is associated with autoantibodies that target various molecules including modified self-epitopes. Several risk factors predispose the development of RA including female sex, smoking, and silica exposure, and genetic variants involved in immune and inflammatory pathways [108]. For instance, specific class II human leukocyte antigen (HLA) loci especially HLA-DRB1*01 and HLA-DRB1*04 are significantly associated with the risk of developing RA [109]. Differential methylation patterns in the HLA region may also add to the development risk [110].

RA pathogenesis is broadly considered as a continuum, whereby loss of self-tolerant helper T-cell responses drive the production of specific autoantibodies by B cells for years in advance of symptom onset [111, 112] (Fig. 3). Early-stage RA (postdiagnosis) is characterized by inflammation of the fine synovial tissue that encapsulates joints. The synovial membrane

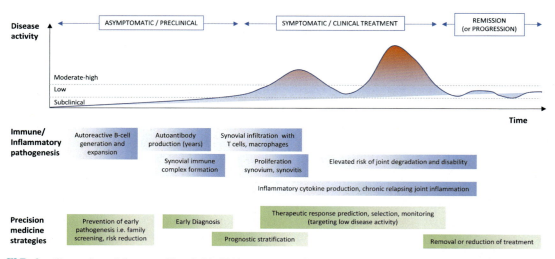

FIG. 3 Illustration of rheumatoid arthritis (RA) progression from asymptomatic stage through the disease's process to diagnosis and treatment, with the goal of targeting low disease activity and remission. The evolving immune system role in pathogenesis and opportunities for precision medicine strategies are signposted along a timeline representing an exemplar RA patient. In this idealized scenario, the patient responds to the first-line treatment, though later becomes refractory to treatment. With precision medicine-guided drug selection, such a patient could achieve remission and reduced long-term risk of joint damage.

(also known as the synovium) becomes infiltrated by mononuclear cells, primarily CD4+ T cells and macrophages, along with stromal cell activation [113]. Autoantibody complexes detected in the synovium, including rheumatoid factor which targets IgG and anti-CCP antibodies, may act as an inflammatory trigger. Macrophage-like synoviocytes produce a variety of proinflammatory cytokines and if left untreated, proliferate over time invading and proliferate over time invading and degrading bone and cartilage in adjacent articular structures, causing permanent joint damage and increasing disability [108].

5.2 Potential for precision medicine in arthritis

Discrete innate and adaptive immunopathogenic mechanisms operate across the RA pathological continuum, creating opportunities for stage-specific and personalized interventions that could suppress disease activity. Understanding the mixed innate and adaptive immune system backdrop may also be a key to preventing the chronic relapsing nature of RA and arthritic disorders with an immune system component. Immunophenotyping presents opportunities for molecular stratification of clinically relevant subgroups and targeted treatment in OA, SLE, and PsA [114–116].

Targeting specific pathological endotypes through novel biomarker tests could offer new ways to improve outcomes and health economics in both OA and RA. Albeit recent RA discovery studies are modest and may use lower throughput or newer, unvalidated analytical technologies, they advance the laudable goals of endotype-tailored drug development, therapeutic precision [117], and disease prediction and prevention [118]. Synovial biopsy to determine treatment selection or modification is one such novel approach being trialed in RA [119, 120].

In OA, differences in complement and innate immune response can differentiate subgroups of knee pathology [121]. Other OA early-stage patient subgroups have been suggested based on pain or tenderness and functional scoring along with knee radiographs of joint erosion and narrowing [122]. Though the majority of OA cases progress slowly, rapidly progressing OA likely has different pathogenic pathways that may help stratify this subgroup for precision medicine approaches [123]. Mobasheri et al. have proposed four potential molecular OA endotypes including inflammatory (including IL-1, IL-6, IL-17, and TNF-α), bone remodeling, metabolic syndrome, and senescent age-related [124]. Activated neutrophil and macrophage biomarkers are elevated in a knee with OA inflammatory endotype patient group at higher risk of radiographic progression [125]. However, treatment options are currently much more limited for OA with poor results from trials of potential disease-modifying osteoarthritis drugs (DMOADs).

It has been postulated that cytokine perturbations in early RA, due to dysregulation in the evolving immune system, could prime synovial stromal cells to propagate a persistent proinflammatory phenotype, which in turn could partially explain the failure of RA to spontaneously resolve [126]. Specific cytokine families are engaged via innate and adaptive immune responses and drive disease manifestations and persistence. A cytokine hierarchy, whereby factors such as IL-6 and TNF-α elicit potent proinflammatory responses, has helped to prioritize therapeutic targets [127]. Recombinant receptor or chimeric antibody-based (biologic) therapies, such as etanercept or adalimumab that target TNFα, can be extremely effective in RA patients refractive to conventional disease-modifying antirheumatic drugs (cDMARDs) such as methotrexate. In the absence of effective treatment, persistent secretion of proinflammatory cytokines contributes to the systemic nature of RA, with an increased risk of cardiovascular complications and depression, the latter of which is described in the following section.

6 Mental health conditions

Depression is a highly prevalent and complex mental health disorder, affecting around 264 million people worldwide [128]. Depression has a wide range of debilitating symptoms which can affect daily life, making it the leading cause of global disability. The most common symptoms include low mood, lack of motivation or interest (anhedonia), and lack of self-esteem.

Epidemiological research indicates that people with chronic inflammatory conditions are often comorbid with depression, up to 70% of individuals with RA and 20% of CVD patients will experience depression [129, 130]. Similarly, depression is associated with an increased prevalence of a wide range of physical health conditions, many with an inflammatory phenotype, suggesting an overlap in the underlying pathophysiology. Depression also manifests in many otherwise medically healthy individuals, without the presence of inflammatory illness, but in both cases the immune system and inflammatory cytokines are considered to play a prominent role in the pathology of depression [129].

6.1 Inflammation as a cardinal feature in depression

Stress, a major psychosocial risk factor in the development of depression can activate inflammatory response in both the peripheral and central nervous system (CNS) through the hypothalamic pituitary adrenal (HPA) axis, the primary stress response mechanism. Chronic stress disrupts negative feedback in the HPA axis by desensitizing glucocorticoid receptors, resulting in abnormally high cortisol levels and ultimately production of proinflammatory cytokines, chemokines, and acute-phase proteins from macrophages through the activation of NF-kB. These molecules enter the blood perivascular space from the blood vessels and, once inside the brain, inflammatory signals are detected by microglia and astroglia, which then initiate the production of CNS cytokines including TNF-α and IL-6 that induce the breakdown of tryptophan, a precursor of serotonin [131]). This decrease in serotonin is thought to contribute to the low mood and subsequent behavioral changes associated with depression (Fig. 4).

Peripheral levels of proinflammatory cytokines and associated innate immune system proteins have been studied in connection with depression and response to antidepressant treatments. Activation of the innate immune system and associated increase in proinflammatory cytokines including CRP, IL-6, IL-1β, and TNF-α have been consistently reported in individuals with depression [132–134]. In particular, patients with comorbid chronic inflammatory conditions, treatment-resistant patients, and those who have experienced childhood adversities show elevated levels of inflammasome-related cytokines.

Elevated proinflammatory cytokine levels are associated with treatment resistance whereas successful antidepressant treatment is associated with a decrease in proinflammatory cytokine levels. Meta-analyses of proinflammatory cytokine levels and response to antidepressant

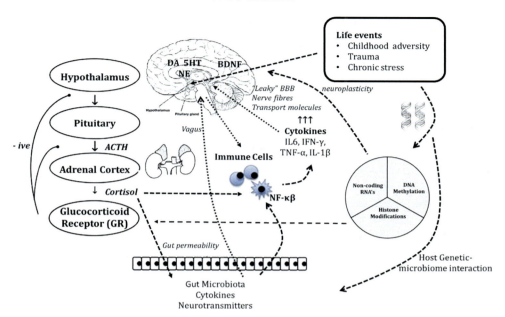

FIG. 4 Key neurotransmitter, endocrine, microbial and inflammatory systems interact in the complex pathology of depression.

treatment have demonstrated that IL-6 is reduced following the antidepressant treatment, regardless of treatment outcome, whereas a decrease in TNF-α levels is predictive of the response [135, 136]. An elevated inflammatory state, using a composite measure of IL-6, TNF-α, and CRP levels, was also useful in predicting treatment outcomes [135].

In addition to circulating cytokine levels, measuring gene expression of immune-related genes in whole blood is potentially useful in predicting response to antidepressant treatment. Expression of a 13-gene panel predicts response to treatment with citalopram with approximately 80% accuracy, and analysis of the functionality of these genes indicated a role in immune activation and elevated inflammation [137, 138]. Higher levels of proinflammatory gene mRNA expression have been found in blood cells of untreated and treatment-resistant individuals with depression, compared to those in remission. Furthermore, expression of a panel of six genes linked to inflammasome activation and glucocorticoid insensitivity (P2RX7, IL-1-β, IL-6, TNF-α, CXCL12, and GR) was sufficient to separate responders and nonresponders to antidepressant treatment [139].

6.2 Antiinflammatory treatments to target depression

Given the accumulating evidence for a proinflammatory phenotype in depression, particularly in association with antidepressant treatment resistance, antiinflammatory medications are being investigated as an alternative or to augment antidepressant treatment. Nonsteroidal antiinflammatory drugs (NSAIDs) and cytokine-inhibitors have been the most widely studied to date [140], and early indications are that there may be therapeutic benefits [141]. For example, adjunctive treatment with the COX-2 inhibitor NSAID, celecoxib, was associated with 6.6 times higher rates of remission than placebo in a meta-analysis of four randomized controlled trials [142]. Targeting specific immune pathways using mAb against proinflammatory cytokines is also a promising approach. In a randomized, placebo-controlled trial of infliximab, an anti-TNF-α mAb treatment, resistant depression patients with high levels of CRP showed a significant improvement compared to placebo treatment [143]. In addition, a recent mega-analysis of depressive symptoms in clinical trials on patients with inflammatory disorders indicates that novel immunomodulatory drugs have antidepressant effects [144].

Although these approaches are intriguing and hold great promise in a move toward more targeted treatment for depression, more research is required in larger and more representative patient populations. Future studies will continue to investigate the clinical utility of screening patients for their inflammatory status at baseline to identify those who may not respond to traditional antidepressant therapy and those who are most likely to benefit from adjunct antiinflammatory treatment. Indeed, it is postulated that the efficacy of novel immunotherapies used to treat cancers, such as programmed cell death protein 1 (PD1) checkpoint inhibitors described in the next section, may be improved by simultaneous inhibition of the kynurenine catabolic pathway [145]. Inhibitors of the immunosuppressant indoleamine dioxygenase (IDO1) can restore diversion of tryptophan metabolism to serotonin production.

7 Cancer

Cancer is the second leading cause of death globally with an estimated 18.1 million new cases and 9.6 million deaths in 2018 [128]. Although it is known as an extremely complex and diverse disease, it can be characterized by an accumulation of mutated cells that proliferate without regulation. Tumors can be graded on their histology, physical size, and stage of disease progression and, in some cases, classified by their molecular landscape [146–148]. The complexity and variability of the disease make it difficult to treat patients often receiving the same standard chemotherapy regimens despite presenting with different cancer subtypes [149].

7.1 Immune system involvement and inflammatory pathways in cancer

The first link between the immune system and cancer was made over 150 years ago by Rudolph Virchow [150]. Immunosurveillance, originally proposed by Burnet and Thomas in the 1950s, details the ability of the immune system to recognize not only foreign pathogens but also those belonging to the host that has undergone transformation. This allows the immune system to protect the body against the development of cancers originating from genetic changes in normal cells [151, 152]. In recent years, the role of the immune system in cancer pathogenesis can be viewed as a double-edged sword as it has both the ability to protect against cancer but also to promote its progression. This delicate balance is often referred to as immunoediting and is made up of three major phases known as elimination, equilibrium, and escape (Fig. 5) [151, 153, 154].

The capability of the immune system to eliminate cancer cells relies not only on the complex genetic and cellular changes with which cancer is characterized but also on the associated

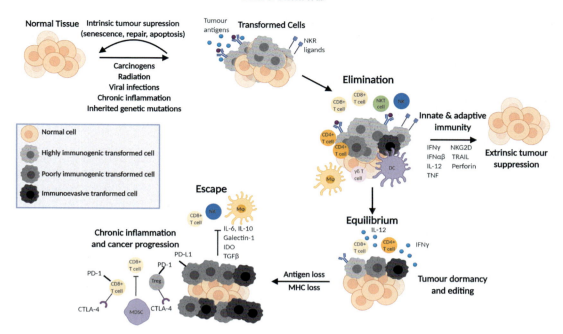

FIG. 5 The cancer immunoediting process showing the three phases. Elimination through innate and adaptive immune responses inducing cancer cell death; equilibrium between cancer and the immune system; and escape as cancer cells evade immune system checkpoints leading to expansion of neoplastic cells, disease progression, and metastasis. *Adapted from M.D. Vesely, M.H. Kershaw, R.D. Schreiber, M.J. Smyth, Natural innate and adaptive immunity to cancer, Annu. Rev. Immunol. 29 (2011) 235–271.*

inflammation, a hallmark of the disease [153, 155]. Inflammatory markers such as IL-1 and TNF-α are expressed in at least 25% of patients [156]. This, coupled with the expression of tumor-associated antigens (TAA), or neoantigens, summons cells of the innate immune system, including NK, NKT, and γδ T cells and macrophages [154, 157]. Mechanisms by which cancer cell lysis occurs are via secretion of perforin from cytolytic immune cells (NK cells, NKT cells, γδ T cells, and CD8$^+$ T cells), antibody-dependent cellular cytotoxicity (ADCC), and complement-dependent cytotoxicity (CDC) [151].

The ability of cancer cells to evade modulated control checkpoints and breach the host's immune system leads to the escape phase which is mediated through several immunosuppressive mechanisms, such as downregulation of MHC Class I expression [151, 154, 158]. Multiple mechanisms including defective antigen presentation, suppression of TAA expression, and induction of antiapoptotic pathways aid in the escape of cancer cells from the elimination and equilibrium phases [154, 157].

7.2 Potential for precision medicine in cancer diagnostics and novel therapies

The use of diagnostic inflammatory markers CRP, erythrocyte sedimentation rate (ESR), and plasma viscosity (PV) along with levels of circulating blood cells including neutrophils, lymphocytes, and platelets have the potential to provide earlier diagnosis and generate valuable information for improved patient risk stratification and more targeted cancer care [156, 159, 160].

Efforts to treat cancer using a more precise and personalized approach have highlighted the potential of molecular markers and mechanisms of the innate and adaptive immune system as targets for oncology therapy [152, 161]. Immunotherapies can act passively (mAb, cytokines, and adoptive cell transfer of ex vivo immune cells) or actively (anticancer vaccines and immune checkpoint inhibitors), with many of these therapies already approved by the Food and Drug Administration (FDA) [162].

To date, mAb have become the largest class of immunotherapies approved in the last decade and their promise lies in their high specificity, low cytotoxicity, and scalability [162–164]. Currently, 30 mAb-based drugs for oncology have been approved by the FDA including trastuzumab (Herceptin), which targets HER2 positive breast cancer, and rituximab (Rituxan) for non-Hodgkins lymphoma which targets CD20 [165].

Recently, immune checkpoint inhibitors have become one of the most promising types of immunotherapy with specific attention on cytotoxic T-lymphocyte antigen-4 (CTLA-4) and PD-1. Both checkpoint molecules function as negative regulators of T-cell activation [166]. In 2011, the first antibody-based immune checkpoint blockade (ICB) treatment, ipilimumab (a CTLA-4 inhibitor), was approved. This was followed by mAb targeting PD-1, nivolumab and pembrolizumab, and mAb targeting PD-L1, atezolizumab and durvalumab [149, 162, 166, 167].

Currently, there is only one FDA-approved cancer vaccine, sipuleucel-T (Provenge), a personalized vaccine encompassing a patient's ex vivo dendritic cells that have been treated with prostatic acid phosphatase (PAP), enhancing antigen presentation. The re-administered dendritic cells enable the patient's T cells to target PAP-expressing tumor cells [168].

CAR T-cell therapies exemplify a personalized approach to oncology therapy as they directly prime a patient's cells to more effectively combat the existing malignancy [162, 169]. There are currently two approved CAR T-cell therapies, tisagenlecleucel (Kymriah) and axicabtagene ciloleucel (Yescarta). Both therapies are genetically modified autologous T cells expressing CD19-specific CAR, targeting and lysing CD19 positive cancer cells [169, 170].

Although some immune-oncology pathways require biological targeting, there are those that can be most effectively or solely targeted by small-molecule medicines [171]. Small molecules require much less time and money to develop and are also easily delivered compared to large, high molecular weight biologics. Success has already been achieved in targeting vascular endothelial growth factor (VEGF), expression of which promotes cancer cell growth and metastasis [172]. A collection of small-molecule VEGF inhibitors, including sunitinib, sorafenib, axitinib, lenvatinib, and pazopanib, has been identified and approved for the treatment of various cancers [173].

8 Conclusion

There is ample evidence implicating inflammation and aberrant immune responses in multiple, ostensibly unrelated conditions as per exemplars described in the preceding sections. However, many of these conditions do not exist in isolation and multimorbid disease associations continue to present major clinical challenges. Multimorbidity has been defined as "the co-occurrence of multiple chronic or acute diseases and medical conditions within one person" [174]. Multimorbidity becomes progressively more common with age. In a 2012 UK-based epidemiology study, by the age of 65 years, 66% of people had two or more coexisting long-term conditions [175]. As multimorbidity has become the norm, optimizing multiple simultaneous treatments and making healthcare system changes to move away from a single-disease framework are increasingly important [176]. A UK Biobank study reveals patterns or clusters of multimorbid conditions. Diabetes, for example, is commonly associated with 14 chronic cardiovascular, musculoskeletal, respiratory, and neurodegenerative conditions [177].

Progress in identifying molecular proinflammatory subclasses or endotypes is also challenging, largely because of the current clinical research paradigm. Research naturally uses a single index, disease-specific approach, based on clinical symptoms and geared largely toward symptomatic or late stages of disease. There is thus a recognized need to identify genetic and environmental drivers that are shared between complex multimorbid diseases but are currently studied via assigned classical diagnostic labels. Consequently, the early, presymptomatic causes and disease mechanisms may be missed and the role of inflammation and immune regulation in multimorbid disease mechanisms need to be carefully dissected out from underlying causal pathways.

Personalized, stratified, or precision medicine approaches assisted by advanced bioinformatic analyses are needed to analyze large complex multimorbid datasets composed of genomic, proteomic, prescribed medication, imaging, clinical, and lifestyle data. A central premise of precision medicine is that heterogeneous patient populations with the same index disease can be subdivided, or stratified, into clinically meaningful groups by combined dataset analyses [178]. The approach aims to more precisely subclassify diseases and optimize the selection and allocation of treatment that is most likely to benefit particular patient subgroups or endotypes [179]. Specific multimorbid disease subclasses may actually represent a syndrome (analogous to a rare disease) encompassing several disease endotypes and there may be merit in regarding multimorbidity as a collection of multiple rare diseases. Future research will need to focus on the identification of multimorbid disease endotypes, along with new targeted approaches and modified clinical care pathways for better management of multimorbid disease endotypes.

Acknowledgments

The *NI Centre for Stratified Medicine* has been funded by a grant to AB under the EU Regional Development Fund and EU Sustainable Competitiveness Programme for NI & the NI Public Health Agency. The authors also wish to acknowledge the award of Ph.D. fellowships from the Department for Economy and support from Northern Ireland Rheumatism Trust, Versus Arthritis, Invest Northern Ireland, Little Princess Trust, Cystic Fibrosis Trust, Western Health & Social Care Trust, and the Research and Development Office of the Public Health Authority.

References

[1] C.B. Vaughn, D. Jakimovski, K.S. Kavak, et al., Epidemiology and treatment of multiple sclerosis in elderly populations, Nat. Rev. Neurol. 15 (6) (2019) 329–342.

[2] J.M. van Deursen, The role of senescent cells in ageing, Nature 509 (7501) (2014) 439–446.

14. Precision medicine to manage chronic immune-related conditions

[3] N. Herranz, J. Gil, Mechanisms and functions of cellular senescence, J. Clin. Invest. 128 (4) (2018) 1238–1246.

[4] D. Weiskopf, B. Weinberger, B. Grubeck-Loebenstein, The aging of the immune system, Transpl. Int. 22 (11) (2009) 1041–1050.

[5] P. Sansoni, R. Vescovini, F.F. Fagnoni, et al., New advances in CMV and immunosenescence, Exp. Gerontol. 55 (2014) 54–62.

[6] J. Campisi, Senescent cells, tumor suppression, and organismal aging: good citizens, bad neighbors, Cell 120 (4) (2005) 513–522.

[7] M.E.C. Waaijer, D. Goldeck, D.A. Gunn, et al., Are skin senescence and immunosenescence linked within individuals? Aging Cell 18 (4) (2019), e12956.

[8] O.O. Onyema, L. Decoster, R. Njemini, et al., Chemotherapy-induced changes and immunosenescence of CD8+ T-cells in patients with breast cancer, Anticancer Res. 35 (3) (2015) 1481–1489.

[9] W.X. Huff, J.H. Kwon, M. Henriquez, K. Fetcko, M. Dey, The evolving role of CD8(+)CD28(−) immunosenescent T cells in cancer immunology, Int. J. Mol. Sci. 20 (11) (2019) 2810.

[10] J.P. Coppe, C.K. Patil, F. Rodier, et al., Senescence-associated secretory phenotypes reveal cell-nonautonomous functions of oncogenic RAS and the p53 tumor suppressor, PLoS Biol. 6 (12) (2008) 2853–2868.

[11] J.P. Coppe, C.K. Patil, F. Rodier, et al., A human-like senescence-associated secretory phenotype is conserved in mouse cells dependent on physiological oxygen, PLoS One 5 (2) (2010), e9188.

[12] M. Ruscetti, J. Leibold, M.J. Bott, et al., NK cell-mediated cytotoxicity contributes to tumor control by a cytostatic drug combination, Science 362 (6421) (2018) 1416–1422.

[13] C. Kang, Q. Xu, T.D. Martin, et al., The DNA damage response induces inflammation and senescence by inhibiting autophagy of GATA4, Science 349 (6255) (2015) aaa5612.

[14] L. Prata, I.G. Ovsyannikova, T. Tchkonia, J.L. Kirkland, Senescent cell clearance by the immune system: emerging therapeutic opportunities, Semin. Immunol. 40 (2018) 101275.

[15] E. Wang, Senescent human fibroblasts resist programmed cell death, and failure to suppress bcl2 is involved, Cancer Res. 55 (11) (1995) 2284–2292.

[16] D. Dikovskaya, J.J. Cole, S.M. Mason, et al., Mitotic stress is an integral part of the oncogene-induced senescence program that promotes multinucleation and cell cycle arrest, Cell Rep. 12 (9) (2015) 1483–1496.

[17] A. Kale, A. Sharma, A. Stolzing, P.Y. Desprez, J. Campisi, Role of immune cells in the removal of deleterious senescent cells, Immun. Ageing 17 (2020) 16.

[18] D. Ray, R. Yung, Immune senescence, epigenetics and autoimmunity, Clin. Immunol. 196 (2018) 59–63.

[19] A. Pera, C. Campos, N. Lopez, et al., Immunosenescence: implications for response to infection and vaccination in older people, Maturitas 82 (1) (2015) 50–55.

[20] A. Aiello, F. Farzaneh, G. Candore, et al., Immunosenescence and its hallmarks: how to oppose aging strategically? A review of potential options for therapeutic intervention, Front. Immunol. 10 (2019) 2247.

[21] C. Franceschi, P. Garagnani, P. Parini, C. Giuliani, A. Santoro, Inflammaging: a new immune-metabolic viewpoint for age-related diseases, Nat. Rev. Endocrinol. 14 (10) (2018) 576–590.

[22] C.M. Weyand, J.J. Goronzy, Aging of the immune system. mechanisms and therapeutic targets, Ann. Am. Thorac. Soc. 13 (Suppl. 5) (2016) S422–S428.

[23] P. Song, Q. Zhao, M.H. Zou, Targeting senescent cells to attenuate cardiovascular disease progression, Ageing Res. Rev. 60 (2020) 101072.

[24] B.M. Hall, V. Balan, A.S. Gleiberman, et al., Aging of mice is associated with p16(Ink4a)- and beta-galactosidase-positive macrophage accumulation that can be induced in young mice by senescent cells, Aging (Albany NY) 8 (7) (2016) 1294–1315.

[25] J.M. Brenchley, N.J. Karandikar, M.R. Betts, et al., Expression of CD57 defines replicative senescence and antigen-induced apoptotic death of CD8+ T cells, Blood 101 (7) (2003) 2711–2720.

[26] Q. Ouyang, W.M. Wagner, D. Voehringer, et al., Age-associated accumulation of CMV-specific CD8+ T cells expressing the inhibitory killer cell lectin-like receptor G1 (KLRG1), Exp. Gerontol. 38 (8) (2003) 911–920.

[27] W. Xu, A. Larbi, Markers of T cell senescence in humans, Int. J. Mol. Sci. 18 (8) (2017) 1742.

[28] K. Wistuba-Hamprecht, D. Frasca, B. Blomberg, G. Pawelec, E. Derhovanessian, Age-associated alterations in gammadelta T-cells are present predominantly in individuals infected with cytomegalovirus, Immun. Ageing 10 (1) (2013) 26.

[29] E. Mariani, A. Meneghetti, S. Neri, et al., Chemokine production by natural killer cells from nonagenarians, Eur. J. Immunol. 32 (6) (2002) 1524–1529.

[30] J. Hazeldine, J.M. Lord, The impact of ageing on natural killer cell function and potential consequences for health in older adults, Ageing Res. Rev. 12 (4) (2013) 1069–1078.

[31] D. Zhang, G. Chen, D. Manwani, et al., Neutrophil ageing is regulated by the microbiome, Nature 525 (7570) (2015) 528–532.

[32] T. Fulop, J.M. Witkowski, A. Le Page, C. Fortin, G. Pawelec, A. Larbi, Intracellular signalling pathways: targets to reverse immunosenescence, Clin. Exp. Immunol. 187 (1) (2017) 35–43.

[33] A. Lanna, S.M. Henson, D. Escors, A.N. Akbar, The kinase p38 activated by the metabolic regulator AMPK and scaffold TAB1 drives the senescence of human T cells, Nat. Immunol. 15 (10) (2014) 965–972.

[34] H.E. Walters, L.S. Cox, mTORC inhibitors as broad-spectrum therapeutics for age-related diseases, Int. J. Mol. Sci. 19 (8) (2018) 2325.

[35] O.H. Jeon, C. Kim, R.M. Laberge, et al., Local clearance of senescent cells attenuates the development of post-traumatic osteoarthritis and creates a pro-regenerative environment, Nat. Med. 23 (6) (2017) 775–781.

[36] T.J. Bussian, A. Aziz, C.F. Meyer, B.L. Swenson, J.M. van Deursen, D.J. Baker, Clearance of senescent glial cells prevents tau-dependent pathology and cognitive decline, Nature 562 (7728) (2018) 578–582.

[37] D.J. Baker, T. Wijshake, T. Tchkonia, et al., Clearance of p16Ink4a-positive senescent cells delays ageing-associated disorders, Nature 479 (7372) (2011) 232–236.

[38] M.P. Baar, R.M.C. Brandt, D.A. Putavet, et al., Targeted apoptosis of senescent cells restores tissue homeostasis in response to chemotoxicity and aging, Cell 169 (1) (2017) 132–147. e116.

[39] B.G. Childs, M. Durik, D.J. Baker, J.M. van Deursen, Cellular senescence in aging and age-related disease: from mechanisms to therapy, Nat. Med. 21 (12) (2015) 1424–1435.

[40] Y. Zhu, T. Tchkonia, T. Pirtskhalava, et al., The Achilles' heel of senescent cells: from transcriptome to senolytic drugs, Aging Cell 14 (4) (2015) 644–658.

[41] Y. Zhu, T. Tchkonia, H. Fuhrmann-Stroissnigg, et al., Identification of a novel senolytic agent, navitoclax, targeting the Bcl-2 family of anti-apoptotic factors, Aging Cell 15 (3) (2016) 428–435.

[42] R. Yosef, N. Pilpel, R. Tokarsky-Amiel, et al., Directed elimination of senescent cells by inhibition of BCL-W and BCL-XL, Nat. Commun. 7 (2016) 11190.

[43] M.J. Yousefzadeh, Y. Zhu, S.J. McGowan, et al., Fisetin is a senotherapeutic that extends health and lifespan, EBioMedicine 36 (2018) 18–28.

[44] A. Guerrero, N. Herranz, B. Sun, et al., Cardiac glycosides are broad-spectrum senolytics, Nat. Metab. 1 (11) (2019) 1074–1088.

[45] F. Triana-Martinez, P. Picallos-Rabina, S. Da Silva-Alvarez, et al., Identification and characterization of cardiac glycosides as senolytic compounds, Nat. Commun. 10 (1) (2019) 4731.

[46] T.W. Kang, T. Yevsa, N. Woller, et al., Senescence surveillance of pre- malignant hepatocytes limits liver cancer development, Nature 479 (7374) (2011) 547–551.

[47] V. Krizhanovsky, M. Yon, R.A. Dickins, et al., Senescence of activated stellate cells limits liver fibrosis, Cell 134 (4) (2008) 657–667.

[48] W. Xue, L. Zender, C. Miething, et al., Senescence and tumour clearance is triggered by p53 restoration in murine liver carcinomas, Nature 445 (7128) (2007) 656–660.

[49] C. Amor, J. Feucht, J. Leibold, et al., Senolytic CAR T cells reverse senescence-associated pathologies, Nature 583 (7814) (2020) 127–132.

[50] Y.H. Lee, S.R. Kim, D.H. Han, et al., Senescent T cells predict the development of hyperglycemia in humans, Diabetes 68 (1) (2019) 156–162.

[51] I. Santin, D.L. Eizirik, Candidate genes for type 1 diabetes modulate pancreatic islet inflammation and beta-cell apoptosis, Diabetes Obes. Metab. 15 (Suppl. 3) (2013) 71–81.

[52] J. Fernandez-Tajes, K.J. Gaulton, M. van de Bunt, et al., Developing a network view of type 2 diabetes risk pathways through integration of genetic, genomic and functional data, Genome Med. 11 (1) (2019) 19.

[53] L. Sun, S. Xi, G. He, et al., Two to tango: dialogue between adaptive and innate immunity in type 1 diabetes, J. Diabetes Res. 2020 (2020) 4106518.

[54] S. Tsalamandris, A.S. Antonopoulos, E. Oikonomou, et al., The role of inflammation in diabetes: current concepts and future perspectives, Eur. Cardiol. 14 (1) (2019) 50–59.

[55] A.L. Birkenfeld, G.I. Shulman, Nonalcoholic fatty liver disease, hepatic insulin resistance, and type 2 diabetes, Hepatology 59 (2) (2014) 713–723.

[56] M. Akbari, V. Hassan-Zadeh, IL-6 signalling pathways and the development of type 2 diabetes, Inflammopharmacology 26 (3) (2018) 685–698.

[57] G.S. Hotamisligil, Inflammation and metabolic disorders, Nature 444 (7121) (2006) 860–867.

[58] S. Nishimura, I. Manabe, M. Nagasaki, et al., CD8+ effector T cells contribute to macrophage recruitment and adipose tissue inflammation in obesity, Nat. Med. 15 (8) (2009) 914–920.

[59] J.M. Olefsky, C.K. Glass, Macrophages, inflammation, and insulin resistance, Annu. Rev. Physiol. 72 (2010) 219–246.

[60] A.S. Andreasen, M. Kelly, R.M. Berg, K. Moller, B.K. Pedersen, Type 2 diabetes is associated with altered NF-kappaB DNA binding activity, JNK phosphorylation, and AMPK phosphorylation in skeletal muscle after LPS, PLoS One 6 (9) (2011), e23999.

[61] P. Tantiwong, K. Shanmugasundaram, A. Monroy, et al., NF-kappaB activity in muscle from obese and type 2 diabetic subjects under basal and exercise-stimulated conditions, Am. J. Physiol. Endocrinol. Metab. 299 (5) (2010) E794–E801.

[62] M. Cabello-Olmo, M. Arana, I. Radichev, P. Smith, E. Huarte, M. Barajas, New insights into immunotherapy strategies for treating autoimmune diabetes, Int. J. Mol. Sci. 20 (19) (2019) 4789.

[63] Diabetes Prevention Trial—Type 1 Diabetes Study G, Effects of insulin in relatives of patients with type 1 diabetes mellitus, N. Engl. J. Med. 346 (22) (2002) 1685–1691.

[64] J.S. Skyler, J.P. Krischer, J. Wolfsdorf, et al., Effects of oral insulin in relatives of patients with type 1 diabetes: the Diabetes Prevention Trial—Type 1, Diabetes Care 28 (5) (2005) 1068–1076.

[65] S. Tsai, X. Clemente-Casares, A.C. Zhou, et al., Insulin receptor-mediated stimulation boosts T cell immunity during inflammation and infection, Cell Metab. 28 (6) (2018) 922–934. e924.

[66] A.G. Daifotis, S. Koenig, L. Chatenoud, K.C. Herold, Anti-CD3 clinical trials in type 1 diabetes mellitus, Clin. Immunol. 149 (3) (2013) 268–278.

[67] L. Mastrandrea, J. Yu, T. Behrens, et al., Etanercept treatment in children with new-onset type 1 diabetes: pilot randomized, placebo-controlled, double-blind study, Diabetes Care 32 (7) (2009) 1244–1249.

[68] A. Ataie-Jafari, S.C. Loke, A.B. Rahmat, et al., A randomized placebo-controlled trial of alphacalcidol on the preservation of beta cell function in children with recent onset type 1 diabetes, Clin. Nutr. 32 (6) (2013) 911–917.

[69] L.R. Baghdadi, Effect of methotrexate use on the development of type 2 diabetes in rheumatoid arthritis patients: a systematic review and meta-analysis, PLoS One 15 (7) (2020), e0235637.

[70] P.M. Ridker, B.M. Everett, A. Pradhan, et al., Low-dose methotrexate for the prevention of atherosclerotic events, N. Engl. J. Med. 380 (8) (2019) 752–762.

[71] M. Boni-Schnetzler, J. Thorne, G. Parnaud, et al., Increased interleukin (IL)-1beta messenger ribonucleic acid expression in beta-cells of individuals with type 2 diabetes and regulation of IL-1beta in human islets by glucose and autostimulation, J. Clin. Endocrinol. Metab. 93 (10) (2008) 4065–4074.

[72] C. Cavelti-Weder, A. Babians-Brunner, C. Keller, et al., Effects of gevokizumab on glycemia and inflammatory markers in type 2 diabetes, Diabetes Care 35 (8) (2012) 1654–1662.

[73] B. Yazdani-Biuki, H. Stelzl, H.P. Brezinschek, et al., Improvement of insulin sensitivity in insulin resistant subjects during prolonged treatment with the anti-TNF-alpha antibody infliximab, Eur. J. Clin. Investig. 34 (9) (2004) 641–642.

[74] E.J. Benjamin, S.S. Virani, C.W. Callaway, et al., Heart disease and stroke statistics-2018 update: a report from the American Heart Association, Circulation 137 (12) (2018) e67–e492.

[75] C. Andersson, A.D. Johnson, E.J. Benjamin, D. Levy, R.S. Vasan, 70-year legacy of the Framingham Heart Study, Nat. Rev. Cardiol. 16 (11) (2019) 687–698.

[76] L. Chavez-Sanchez, M.G. Garza-Reyes, J.E. Espinosa-Luna, K. Chavez-Rueda, M.V. Legorreta-Haquet, F. Blanco-Favela, The role of TLR2, TLR4 and CD36 in macrophage activation and foam cell formation in response to oxLDL in humans, Hum. Immunol. 75 (4) (2014) 322–329.

[77] A. Gistera, G.K. Hansson, The immunology of atherosclerosis, Nat. Rev. Nephrol. 13 (6) (2017) 368–380.

[78] D. Wolf, K. Ley, Immunity and inflammation in atherosclerosis, Circ. Res. 124 (2) (2019) 315–327.

[79] Y. Jin, J. Fu, Novel insights into the NLRP 3 inflammasome in atherosclerosis, J. Am. Heart Assoc. 8 (12) (2019) e012219.

[80] J.W. Williams, L.H. Huang, G.J. Randolph, Cytokine circuits in cardiovascular disease, Immunity 50 (4) (2019) 941–954.

[81] M. Chemaly, V. McGilligan, M. Gibson, et al., Role of tumour necrosis factor alpha converting enzyme (TACE/ADAM17) and associated proteins in coronary artery disease and cardiac events, Arch. Cardiovasc. Dis. 110 (12) (2017) 700–711.

[82] M. Fischer, U. Broeckel, S. Holmer, et al., Distinct heritable patterns of angiographic coronary artery disease in families with myocardial infarction, Circulation 111 (7) (2005) 855–862.

[83] B. Mayer, J. Erdmann, H. Schunkert, Genetics and heritability of coronary artery disease and myocardial infarction, Clin. Res. Cardiol. 96 (1) (2007) 1–7.

[84] H. Schunkert, Genetics of CVD in 2017: expanding the spectrum of CVD genetics, Nat. Rev. Cardiol. 15 (2) (2018) 77–78.

[85] A.P. Patel, P. Natarajan, Completing the genetic spectrum influencing coronary artery disease: from germline to somatic variation, Cardiovasc. Res. 115 (5) (2019) 830–843.

[86] Z. Ungvari, S. Tarantini, A.J. Donato, V. Galvan, A. Csiszar, Mechanisms of vascular aging, Circ. Res. 123 (7) (2018) 849–867.

[87] I.M. Rea, D.S. Gibson, V. McGilligan, S.E. McNerlan, H.D. Alexander, O.A. Ross, Age and age-related diseases: role of inflammation triggers and cytokines, Front. Immunol. 9 (2018) 586.

[88] N. Kazemian, M. Mahmoudi, F. Halperin, J.C. Wu, S. Pakpour, Gut microbiota and cardiovascular disease: opportunities and challenges, Microbiome 8 (1) (2020) 36.

[89] L.L. Håheim, The infection hypothesis revisited: oral infection and cardiovascular disease, Epidemiol. Res. Int. 735378 (2014) 1–9, https://www.hindawi.com/journals/eri/2014/735378/.

[90] J. Renko, K.A. Koskela, P.W. Lepp, et al., Bacterial DNA signatures in carotid atherosclerosis represent both commensals and pathogens of skin origin, Eur. J. Dermatol. 23 (1) (2013) 53–58.

[91] J. Amar, C. Lange, G. Payros, et al., Blood microbiota dysbiosis is associated with the onset of cardiovascular events in a large general population: the D.E.S.I.R. study, PLoS One 8 (1) (2013) e54461.

[92] Z. Jie, H. Xia, S.L. Zhong, et al., The gut microbiome in atherosclerotic cardiovascular disease, Nat. Commun. 8 (1) (2017) 845.

[93] M.J. Chapman, J.S. Redfern, M.E. McGovern, P. Giral, Niacin and fibrates in atherogenic dyslipidemia: pharmacotherapy to reduce cardiovascular risk, Pharmacol. Ther. 126 (3) (2010) 314–345.

[94] P.M. Ridker, B.M. Everett, T. Thuren, et al., Antiinflammatory therapy with canakinumab for atherosclerotic disease, N. Engl. J. Med. 377 (12) (2017) 1119–1131.

[95] S. Donnelly, R. McAllister, M. Chemaly, A.J. Bjourson, A. Peace, V. McGilligan, The NLRP3 inflammasome as a promising target for coronary artery disease: current and pipeline NLRP3 inhibitors, Online J. Cardiovasc. Res. 3 (2) (2019) 1–7, https://irispublishers.com/ojcr/fulltext/the-nlrp3-inflammasome-as-a-promising-target-for-coronary-artery-disease-current-and-pipeline.ID.000556.php.

[96] E. Ozaki, M. Campbell, S.L. Doyle, Targeting the NLRP3 inflammasome in chronic inflammatory diseases: current perspectives, J. Inflamm. Res. 8 (2015) 15–27.

[97] A. Grebe, F. Hoss, E. Latz, NLRP3 inflammasome and the IL-1 pathway in atherosclerosis, Circ. Res. 122 (12) (2018) 1722–1740.

[98] D.M. Lloyd-Jones, L.T. Braun, C.E. Ndumele, et al., Use of risk assessment tools to guide decision-making in the primary prevention of atherosclerotic cardiovascular disease: a special report from the American Heart Association and American College of Cardiology, Circulation 139 (25) (2019) e1162–e1177.

[99] P.M. Ridker, J.G. MacFadyen, B.M. Everett, et al., Relationship of C-reactive protein reduction to cardiovascular event reduction following treatment with canakinumab: a secondary analysis from the CANTOS randomised controlled trial, Lancet 391 (10118) (2018) 319–328.

[100] C.P. McCarthy, R.R.J. van Kimmenade, H.K. Gaggin, et al., Usefulness of multiple biomarkers for predicting incident major adverse cardiac events in patients who underwent diagnostic coronary angiography (from the Catheter Sampled Blood Archive in Cardiovascular Diseases [CASABLANCA] study), Am. J. Cardiol. 120 (1) (2017) 25–32.

[101] V. McGilligan, S. Watterson, K. Rjoob, et al., An exploratory analysis investigating blood protein biomarkers to augment ECG diagnosis of ACS, J. Electrocardiol. 57S (2019) S92–S97.

[102] G.W. Rouan, T.H. Lee, E.F. Cook, D.A. Brand, M.C. Weisberg, L. Goldman, Clinical characteristics and outcome of acute myocardial infarction in patients with initially normal or nonspecific electrocardiograms (a report from the Multicenter Chest Pain Study), Am. J. Cardiol. 64 (18) (1989) 1087–1092.

[103] D.J. DeMizio, L.B. Geraldino-Pardilla, Autoimmunity and inflammation link to cardiovascular disease risk in rheumatoid arthritis, Rheumatol. Ther. 7 (1) (2020) 19–33.

[104] F.J. Lopez-Longo, D. Oliver-Minarro, I. de la Torre, et al., Association between anti-cyclic citrullinated peptide antibodies and ischemic heart disease in patients with rheumatoid arthritis, Arthritis Rheum. 61 (4) (2009) 419–424.

[105] World Health Organisation, Musculoskeletal conditions (2021). Available from: from https://www.who.int/news-room/fact-sheets/detail/musculoskeletal-conditions.

[106] J.R. Tarn, D.W. Lendrem, J.D. Isaacs, In search of pathobiological endotypes: a systems approach to early rheumatoid arthritis, Expert. Rev. Clin. Immunol. 16 (6) (2020) 621–630.

[107] R. Castillo, J.U. Scher, Not your average joint: towards precision medicine in psoriatic arthritis, Clin. Immunol. 217 (2020) 108470.

[108] J.S. Smolen, D. Aletaha, A. Barton, et al., Rheumatoid arthritis, Nat. Rev. Dis. Primers 4 (2018) 18001.

[109] P.K. Gregersen, J. Silver, R.J. Winchester, The shared epitope hypothesis. An approach to understanding the molecular genetics of susceptibility to rheumatoid arthritis, Arthritis Rheum. 30 (11) (1987) 1205–1213.

[110] Y. Liu, M.J. Aryee, L. Padyukov, et al., Epigenome-wide association data implicate DNA methylation as an intermediary of genetic risk in rheumatoid arthritis, Nat. Biotechnol. 31 (2) (2013) 142–147.

[111] D. McGonagle, A. Watad, S. Savic, Mechanistic immunological based classification of rheumatoid arthritis, Autoimmun. Rev. 17 (11) (2018) 1115–1123.

[112] L.B. Kelmenson, B.D. Wagner, B.K. McNair, et al., Timing of elevations of autoantibody isotypes prior to diagnosis of rheumatoid arthritis, Arthritis Rheumatol. 72 (2) (2020) 251–261.

[113] G.S. Firestein, I.B. McInnes, Immunopathogenesis of rheumatoid arthritis, Immunity 46 (2) (2017) 183–196.

[114] S. Slight-Webb, M. Smith, A. Bylinska, et al., Autoantibody-positive healthy individuals with lower lupus risk display a unique immune endotype, J. Allergy Clin. Immunol. 146 (6) (2020) 1419–1433.

[115] I. Miyagawa, Y. Tanaka, The approach to precision medicine for the treatment of psoriatic arthritis, Immunol. Med. 43 (3) (2020) 98–102.

[116] Y. Tanaka, S. Kubo, I. Miyagawa, S. Iwata, S. Nakayamada, Lymphocyte phenotype and its application to precision medicine in systemic autoimmune diseases, Semin. Arthritis Rheum. 48 (6) (2019) 1146–1150.

[117] D. Aletaha, Precision medicine and management of rheumatoid arthritis, J. Autoimmun. 110 (2020) 102405.

[118] M. Mahler, L. Martinez-Prat, J.A. Sparks, K.D. Deane, Precision medicine in the care of rheumatoid arthritis: focus on prediction and prevention of future clinically-apparent disease, Autoimmun. Rev. 19 (5) (2020) 102506.

[119] A. Barton, C. Pitzalis, Stratified medicine in rheumatoid arthritis-the MATURA programme, Rheumatology (Oxford) 56 (8) (2017) 1247–1250.

[120] A. Small, M.D. Wechalekar, Synovial biopsies in inflammatory arthritis: precision medicine in rheumatoid arthritis, Expert. Rev. Mol. Diagn. 20 (3) (2020) 315–325.

[121] J. Soul, S.L. Dunn, S. Anand, et al., Stratification of knee osteoarthritis: two major patient subgroups identified by genome-wide expression analysis of articular cartilage, Ann. Rheum. Dis. 77 (3) (2018) 423.

[122] F.P. Luyten, S. Bierma-Zeinstra, F. Dell'Accio, et al., Toward classification criteria for early osteoarthritis of the knee, Semin. Arthritis Rheum. 47 (4) (2018) 457–463.

[123] A. Mobasheri, S. Saarakkala, M. Finnila, M.A. Karsdal, A.C. Bay-Jensen, W.E. van Spil, Recent advances in understanding the phenotypes of osteoarthritis, F1000Res 8 (2019).

[124] A. Mobasheri, W.E. van Spil, E. Budd, et al., Molecular taxonomy of osteoarthritis for patient stratification, disease management and drug development: biochemical markers associated with emerging clinical phenotypes and molecular endotypes, Curr. Opin. Rheumatol. 31 (1) (2019) 80–89.

[125] C.A. Haraden, J.L. Huebner, M.F. Hsueh, Y.J. Li, V.B. Kraus, Synovial fluid biomarkers associated with osteoarthritis severity reflect macrophage and neutrophil related inflammation, Arthritis Res. Ther. 21 (1) (2019) 146.

[126] L.A. Ridgley, A.E. Anderson, A.G. Pratt, What are the dominant cytokines in early rheumatoid arthritis? Curr. Opin. Rheumatol. 30 (2) (2018) 207–214.

[127] I.B. McInnes, C.D. Buckley, J.D. Isaacs, Cytokines in rheumatoid arthritis – shaping the immunological landscape, Nat. Rev. Rheumatol. 12 (1) (2016) 63–68.

[128] World Health Organisation, Cancer (2021). Available from https://www.who.int/news-room/fact-sheets/detail/cancer (Accessed 21 September 2021).

[129] M. Almond, Depression and inflammation: examining the link, Curr. Psychiatr. Ther. 12 (2013) 24–32.

[130] D.S. Gibson, S. Drain, C. Kelly, et al., Coincidence versus consequence: opportunities in multi-morbidity research and inflammation as a pervasive feature, Expert Rev. Precis. Med. Drug Dev. 2 (3) (2017) 147–156.

[131] A.H. Miller, V. Maletic, C.L. Raison, Inflammation and its discontents: the role of cytokines in the pathophysiology of major depression, Biol. Psychiatry 65 (9) (2009) 732–741.

[132] R. Dantzer, J.C. O'Connor, G.G. Freund, R.W. Johnson, K.W. Kelley, From inflammation to sickness and depression: when the immune system subjugates the brain, Nat. Rev. Neurosci. 9 (1) (2008) 46–56.

[133] Y. Dowlati, N. Herrmann, W. Swardfager, et al., A meta-analysis of cytokines in major depression, Biol. Psychiatry 67 (5) (2010) 446–457.

[134] C.A. Kohler, T.H. Freitas, M. Maes, et al., Peripheral cytokine and chemokine alterations in depression: a meta-analysis of 82 studies, Acta Psychiatr. Scand. 135 (5) (2017) 373–387.

[135] R. Strawbridge, D. Arnone, A. Danese, A. Papadopoulos, A. Herane Vives, A.J. Cleare, Inflammation and clinical response to treatment in depression: a meta-analysis, Eur. Neuropsychopharmacol. 25 (10) (2015) 1532–1543.

[136] J.J. Liu, Y.B. Wei, R. Strawbridge, et al., Peripheral cytokine levels and response to antidepressant treatment in depression: a systematic review and meta-analysis, Mol. Psychiatry 25 (2) (2020) 339–350.

[137] F. Mamdani, M.T. Berlim, M.M. Beaulieu, A. Labbe, C. Merette, G. Turecki, Gene expression biomarkers of response to citalopram treatment in major depressive disorder, Transl. Psychiatry 1 (2011), e13.

[138] J.P. Guilloux, S. Bassi, Y. Ding, et al., Testing the predictive value of peripheral gene expression for non-remission following citalopram treatment for major depression, Neuropsychopharmacology 40 (3) (2015) 701–710.

[139] A. Cattaneo, C. Ferrari, L. Turner, et al., Whole-blood expression of inflammasome- and glucocorticoid-related mRNAs correctly separates treatment-resistant depressed patients from drug-free and responsive patients in the BIODEP study, Transl. Psychiatry 10 (1) (2020) 232.

[140] O. Kohler, M.E. Benros, M. Nordentoft, et al., Effect of anti-inflammatory treatment on depression, depressive symptoms, and adverse effects: a systematic review and meta-analysis of randomized clinical trials, JAMA Psychiatry 71 (12) (2014) 1381–1391.

[141] M.K. Jha, Anti-inflammatory treatments for major depressive disorder: what's on the horizon? J. Clin. Psychiatry 80 (6) (2019).

[142] F. Faridhosseini, R. Sadeghi, L. Farid, M. Pourgholami, Celecoxib: a new augmentation strategy for depressive mood episodes. A systematic review and meta-analysis of randomized placebo-controlled trials, Hum. Psychopharmacol. 29 (3) (2014) 216–223.

[143] C.L. Raison, R.E. Rutherford, B.J. Woolwine, et al., A randomized controlled trial of the tumor necrosis factor antagonist infliximab for treatment-resistant depression: the role of baseline inflammatory biomarkers, JAMA Psychiatry 70 (1) (2013) 31–41.

[144] G.M. Wittenberg, A. Stylianou, Y. Zhang, et al., Effects of immunomodulatory drugs on depressive symptoms: a mega-analysis of randomized, placebo-controlled clinical trials in inflammatory disorders, Mol. Psychiatry 25 (6) (2020) 1275–1285.

[145] I. Cervenka, L.Z. Agudelo, J.L. Ruas, Kynurenines: tryptophan's metabolites in exercise, inflammation, and mental health, Science 357 (6349) (2017).

[146] H.A. Loomans-Kropp, A. Umar, Cancer prevention and screening: the next step in the era of precision medicine, NPJ Precis. Oncol. 3 (2019) 3.

[147] J. Guinney, R. Dienstmann, X. Wang, et al., The consensus molecular subtypes of colorectal cancer, Nat. Med. 21 (11) (2015) 1350–1356.

[148] S.M. Fragomeni, A. Sciallis, J.S. Jeruss, Molecular subtypes and local-regional control of breast cancer, Surg. Oncol. Clin. N. Am. 27 (1) (2018) 95–120.

[149] P. Krzyszczyk, A. Acevedo, E.J. Davidoff, et al., The growing role of precision and personalized medicine for cancer treatment, Technology (Singap. World Sci.) 6 (3–4) (2018) 79–100.

[150] F. Balkwill, A. Mantovani, Inflammation and cancer: back to Virchow? Lancet 357 (9255) (2001) 539–545.

[151] P.H. Pandya, M.E. Murray, K.E. Pollok, J.L. Renbarger, The immune system in cancer pathogenesis: potential therapeutic approaches, J. Immunol. Res. 2016 (2016) 4273943.

[152] G.P. Dunn, C.M. Koebel, R.D. Schreiber, Interferons, immunity and cancer immunoediting, Nat. Rev. Immunol. 6 (11) (2006) 836–848.

[153] D.S. Chen, I. Mellman, Oncology meets immunology: the cancer-immunity cycle, Immunity 39 (1) (2013) 1–10.

[154] M.J. Smyth, G.P. Dunn, R.D. Schreiber, Cancer immunosurveillance and immunoediting: the roles of immunity in suppressing tumor development and shaping tumor immunogenicity, Adv. Immunol. 90 (2006) 1–50.

[155] J.N. Kather, N. Halama, Harnessing the innate immune system and local immunological microenvironment to treat colorectal cancer, Br. J. Cancer 120 (9) (2019) 871–882.

[156] H. Gonzalez, C. Hagerling, Z. Werb, Roles of the immune system in cancer: from tumor initiation to metastatic progression, Genes Dev. 32 (19–20) (2018) 1267–1284.

[157] A. Rotte, M. Bhandaru, Mechanisms of immune evasion by cancer, Immunother. Melanoma (2016) 199–232.

[158] D. Mittal, M.M. Gubin, R.D. Schreiber, M.J. Smyth, New insights into cancer immunoediting and its three component phases—elimination, equilibrium and escape, Curr. Opin. Immunol. 27 (2014) 16–25.

[159] J.L. Sylman, A. Mitrugno, M. Atallah, et al., The predictive value of inflammation-related peripheral blood measurements in cancer staging and prognosis, Front. Oncol. 8 (2018) 78.

[160] R. Pio, L. Corrales, J.D. Lambris, The role of complement in tumor growth, Adv. Exp. Med. Biol. 772 (2014) 229–262.

[161] A.P. Sokolenko, E.N. Imyanitov, Molecular diagnostics in clinical oncology, Front. Mol. Biosci. 5 (2018) 76.

[162] N.E. Papaioannou, O.V. Beniata, P. Vitsos, O. Tsitsilonis, P. Samara, Harnessing the immune system to improve cancer therapy, Ann. Transl. Med. 4 (14) (2016) 261.

[163] E.V. Jensen, Estrogen receptors in hormone-dependent breast cancers, Cancer Res. 35 (11 Pt 2) (1975) 3362–3364.

[164] L.M. Weiner, M.V. Dhodapkar, S. Ferrone, Monoclonal antibodies for cancer immunotherapy, Lancet 373 (9668) (2009) 1033–1040.

[165] R.M. Lu, Y.C. Hwang, I.J. Liu, et al., Development of therapeutic antibodies for the treatment of diseases, J. Biomed. Sci. 27 (1) (2020) 1.

[166] E.S. Webb, P. Liu, R. Baleeiro, N.R. Lemoine, M. Yuan, Y.H. Wang, Immune checkpoint inhibitors in cancer therapy, J. Biomed. Res. 32 (5) (2018) 317–326.

[167] C. Robert, A decade of immune-checkpoint inhibitors in cancer therapy, Nat. Commun. 11 (1) (2020) 3801.

[168] E. Anassi, U.A. Ndefo, Sipuleucel-T (provenge) injection: the first immunotherapy agent (vaccine) for hormone-refractory prostate cancer, Pharm. Ther. 36 (4) (2011) 197–202.

[169] G. Dotti, S. Gottschalk, B. Savoldo, M.K. Brenner, Design and development of therapies using chimeric antigen receptor-expressing T cells, Immunol. Rev. 257 (1) (2014) 107–126.

[170] P.P. Zheng, J.M. Kros, J. Li, Approved CAR T cell therapies: ice bucket challenges on glaring safety risks and long-term impacts, Drug Discov. Today 23 (6) (2018) 1175–1182.

[171] J.L. Adams, J. Smothers, R. Srinivasan, A. Hoos, Big opportunities for small molecules in immuno-oncology, Nat. Rev. Drug Discov. 14 (9) (2015) 603–622.

[172] A. Calvo, R. Catena, M.S. Noble, et al., Identification of VEGF-regulated genes associated with increased lung metastatic potential: functional involvement of tenascin-C in tumor growth and lung metastasis, Oncogene 27 (40) (2008) 5373–5384.

[173] B.R. Huck, L. Kotzner, K. Urbahns, Small molecules drive big improvements in Immuno-oncology therapies, Angew. Chem. Int. Ed. Engl. 57 (16) (2018) 4412–4428.

[174] M. van den Akker, F. Buntinx, S. Roos, J.A. Knottnerus, Problems in determining occurrence rates of multimorbidity, J. Clin. Epidemiol. 54 (7) (2001) 675–679.

[175] K. Barnett, S.W. Mercer, M. Norbury, G. Watt, S. Wyke, B. Guthrie, Epidemiology of multimorbidity and implications for health care, research, and medical education: a cross-sectional study, Lancet 380 (9836) (2012) 37–43.

[176] J. Heaton, N. Britten, J. Krska, J. Reeve, Person-centred medicines optimisation policy in England: an agenda for research on polypharmacy, Prim. Health Care Res. Dev. 18 (1) (2017) 24–34.

[177] D.T. Zemedikun, L.J. Gray, K. Khunti, M.J. Davies, N.N. Dhalwani, Patterns of multimorbidity in middle-aged and older adults: an analysis of the UK biobank data, Mayo Clin. Proc. 93 (7) (2018) 857–866.

[178] A.S. Bierman, M.E. Tinetti, Precision medicine to precision care: managing multimorbidity, Lancet 388 (10061) (2016) 2721–2723.

[179] J.F. Schlender, V. Vozmediano, A.G. Golden, et al., Current strategies to streamline pharmacotherapy for older adults, Eur. J. Pharm. Sci. 111 (2018) 432–442.

CHAPTER
15

New advanced therapy medicinal products in treatment of autoimmune diseases

Shahrbanoo Jahangir[a,b,†], Sareh Zeydabadinejad[c,†], Zhila Izadi[d,†], Mahdi Habibi-Anbouhi[e], and Ensiyeh Hajizadeh-Saffar[b,f,g,]*

[a]Department of Stem Cells and Developmental Biology, Cell Science Research Center, Royan Institute for Stem Cell Biology and Technology, Tehran, Iran [b]Advanced Therapy Medicinal Product Technology Development Center (ATMP-TDC), Cell Science Research Center, Royan Institute for Stem Cell Biology and Technology, Tehran, Iran [c]Cellular and Molecular Endocrine Research Center, Research Institute for Endocrine Sciences, Shahid Beheshti University of Medical Sciences, Tehran, Iran [d]Pharmaceutical Sciences Research Center, Health Institute, Kermanshah University of Medical Sciences, Kermanshah, Iran [e]National Cell Bank of Iran, Pasteur Institute of Iran, Tehran, Iran [f]Department of Regenerative Medicine, Cell Science Research Center, Royan Institute for Stem Cell Biology and Technology, Tehran, Iran [g]Department of Diabetes, Obesity, and Metabolism, Cell Science Research Center, Royan Institute for Stem Cell Biology and Technology, Tehran, Iran
*Corresponding author

Abstract

Autoimmune diseases are the third common group of diseases in the industrialized world after cardiovascular diseases and cancers and their care are challenging with routine medical treatments. Meanwhile, advanced therapy medicinal products (ATMPs) have been very attractive in recent years, as a new candidate for the treatment of autoimmune diseases. Along with the scope of this book, this chapter is devoted to the description of different ATMPs, which have been used for the treatment of autoimmune diseases. Although a lot of

[†] These authors contributed equally in this chapter.

different experiments have been done on animal models of autoimmune diseases, some of them could reach the clinical phases. Here, we describe the ATMPs which have been used in different clinical settings for the treatment of autoimmune diseases such as type I diabetes, rheumatoid arteritis, multiple sclerosis, vitiligo, scleroderma, pemphigus, psoriasis, celiac disease, inflammatory bowel diseases, systemic lupus erythematosus, and autoimmune vasculitis.

Keywords

ATMP, Cell therapy, Gene therapy, Tissue engineering, Autoimmune diseases, Diabetes, Rheumatoid arteritis

1 Introduction

Cell-based therapies have attracted remarkable attention from not only researchers and clinicians, but also from industry, especially for incurable diseases such as inherited genetic diseases, blood-related disorders, malignancies, neurodegenerative diseases, and conditions which required tissue regeneration. Advanced therapy medicinal products (ATMPs) are classified into four types of products: gene therapy medicinal products (GTMPs), somatic cell therapy medicinal products (SCTMPs), tissue-engineered products (TEPs), and the combined ATMPs (cATMPs). As a scientific definition, GTMPs are products with therapeutic, prophylactic, or diagnostic effects with the use of a recombinant nucleic acid sequence. SCTMPs are defined as products that contain substantially manipulated cells or tissues, with nonhomologous function which means the cells or tissues are not intended to be used for the same essential function(s) in the recipient and the donor body. TEPs are described as engineered cells or tissues that have the properties to regenerate, repair, or replace human destructed tissue, and finally cATMPs is a subcategory of ATMPs that contains one or several medical devices as an integral part of the medicine [1–4]. These advanced therapies are regulated as biologic products, in different regulatory authorities of different countries. The regulatory guidelines to describe the details of submission and product approval procedures until getting marketing authorization have been described in related authorities [1, 5–7]. A significant growth in the commercialization speed of ATMPs has occurred in the recent two decades. In this regard, based on the results of different clinical trials databases, more than 900 clinical trials of ATMPs have been conducted from 1999 to 2015 [2]. This would also show a remarkable industrial investment by big pharma sponsors for this type of product [8].

The biologic origin of ATMPs is an important issue in their development phase to be considered, since the use of autologous, allogeneic, or xenogeneic cell sources would have a substantial effect on the product's regulatory concerns and financial policies of the producer companies. The allogeneic products have an extra advantage for their capability to be manufactured in large scale and consequent large market, which has been created by export strategies. Nevertheless, most CTMPs and GTMPs have an autologous source, because of the medicinal limitations raised from immune rejection concerns and the massive required tests for proving the safety of allogeneic products. Notably, the TEPs with almost local clinical indications have the same number of allogeneic and autologous products [9].

However, many challenges still remain in regard to the development of ATMPs including the necessity of high-technology equipment for large-scale cell production strategies, complicated manufacturing processes, need for the specialized technical staff, need of cold chain transfer, requirement of validated quality control assays to prove cell identity and functionality, concern of long-term adverse events, regulatory limitations such as lack of certain guidelines and prolonged approval pathways, small target populations for some of the rare diseases, and financial issues [10–14]. However, since ATMPs show to be a promising solution for treatment of incurable diseases, this field has the potential to overcome these mentioned challenges in the near future. Here in this chapter, the ATMPs that have published their results in different clinical settings for the treatment of autoimmune diseases are described and the ongoing clinical trials in each field are reviewed in the related table (Fig. 1).

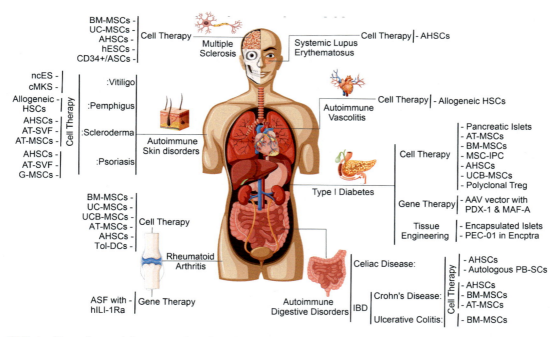

FIG. 1 New advanced therapy medicinal products in treatment of autoimmune diseases. The ATMPs which have been used for treatment of different autoimmune diseases have been mentioned in this figure. The autoimmune diseases including type I diabetes, rheumatoid arteritis, multiple sclerosis, vitiligo, scleroderma, pemphigus, psoriasis, celiac disease, inflammatory bowel diseases (IBD), systemic lupus erythematosus, and autoimmune vasculitis. *ASF*, autologous synovial fibroblast; *IL-1Ra*, interleukin-1 receptor antagonist; *Tol-DC*, tolerogenic dendritic cells; *CD34+/ASC*, CD34+ selected autologous stem cell; *hESCs*, human embryonic stem cells; *AT-SVF*, adipose tissue stromal vascular fraction; *AHSCs*, autologous hematopoietic stem cells; *AT-MSCs*, adipose tissue-derived mesenchymal stem cells; *BM-MSCs*, bone marrow-derived mesenchymal stem cells; *G-MSCs*, gingival mesenchymal stem cells; *UC-MSCs*, umbilical cord-derived mesenchymal stem cells; *UCB-MSCs*, umbilical cord blood derived mesenchymal stem cells; *cMKS*, cultured melanocyte-keratinocyte suspensions; *ncES*, noncultured epidermal suspensions; *PB-SC*, peripheral blood stem cells; *MSC-IPC*, mesenchymal stem cell-derived insulin producing cells; *AAV*, adeno-associated virus.

15. New advanced therapy medicinal products

2 Autoimmune disorders

2.1 Type 1 diabetes

Type 1 diabetes is an autoimmune metabolic disorder, in which insulin-producing beta cells in pancreatic islets of Langerhans are destroyed by the immune system. Insulin replacement therapy has been recognized as the sole treatment for diabetes, which is not an ideal treatment. Therefore, researchers have focused on new treatments based on regenerative medicine approaches including replacement of the destroyed beta cells, application of tissue engineering and biomaterials to prevent rejection of transplanted cells by the host immune system, and gene therapy strategies. Ultimately, it seems that the real treatment for type 1 diabetes will be a combination of these approaches in the future.

2.1.1 Cell therapy

After two decades of research on animal models, a process of clinical islet transplantation was carried out at the University of Alberta in Canada in 1989 on two patients. However, it failed to achieve an insulin independence status [15]. The first semisuccessful islet transplant, which was associated with insulin independence for 12 days in the patient, was reported by the Lacy group at the University of Washington in 1990. A patient with diabetes received transplantation of approximately 800,000 islet equivalents via injection into the portal vein, through which they were formerly receiving immunosuppressive drugs [16].

Islet transplantation was continued by various groups in Europe, the United States, and Canada in later years. Nevertheless, the results were not promising and only 10% of 270 patients receiving islet transplant until 1999 remained insulin-independent for 1 year.

Shapiro et al. in 2000 have published the results of their study on seven patients with brittle diabetes aged 29–54 years who underwent islet transplantation through the portal vein injection, that in the end, seven patients achieved insulin independence after the second or third transplant for 1 year. The success of this group depended on three major changes in the study compared to previous studies; first, immunosuppressive drugs applied in the research included sirolimus, tacrolimus, and daclizumab, and also corticosteroids were omitted from the drug regimen. Second, the duration between islet preparation and transplantation decreased, and third, more islets were transplanted in each patient (from two to three donors) [17]. This method, known as the Edmonton protocol [18], became a turning point for clinical islet transplantation and was used by other groups after that. In another report by the same group, the profit-loss ratio in this type of transplantation was in favor of its performance, since 11 out of 12 patients achieved insulin independence [19]. In their 5-year report in 2005, they reported the presence of C-peptide in the blood of 80% of the patients. Nevertheless, only 10% of the participants remained insulin-independent [20].

The national institute of health performed the Edmonton Protocol on six patients in 2003. Half of the patients remained insulin-independent after 1 year, and all of them experienced lower levels of hypoglycemia. Nonetheless, the problems pointed out by the group included complications caused by islet injection into the portal vein and increased portal blood pressure and complications caused by immunosuppressive drugs [21]. Hering et al. published an article in 2005, in which eight patients with diabetes received islet transplantation after experiencing multiple periods of loss of consciousness due to hypoglycemia. In total, 7000 islets (only from one pancreas) per kg of body weight were injected into each patient, and immunosuppression was induced by applying antithymocyte globulin (ATG), daclizumab, and etanercept. In the end, eight patients achieved insulin independence and did not experience another period of loss of consciousness due to hypoglycemia. In addition, 1-year follow-up showed insulin independence in five patients [22].

In an international study in nine centers, 36 patients were enrolled and 44% and 28% of the subjects achieved completely and partially insulin independence after 1 year, respectively. Among those who were completely insulin independent by the end of the first year, 31% remained the same by the end of the second year. The transplanted tissue function prevented a severe drop in the blood glucose level and improved A1c hemoglobin (HbA1c) level, even with the need to use insulin [18].

The Collaborative Islet Transplant Registry (CITR), which included 19 islet transplantation centers in North America, Europe, and Australia, announced the transplant outcomes of 138 patients in 2007. Insulin independence was achieved in 67% and 58% of the patients after 6 months and 1 year, respectively. While 82% of all transplant recipients experienced one to several times of severe hypoglycemia 1 year before the transplantation, this number decreased to 2% of patients within 1 year after the transplantation, which was indicative of the outstanding effect of islet transplantation on the life-threatening complications of the disease [23]. In 2007, the GRAGIL group, which is a combination of several islet transplantation centers in Europe, published their results on six patients that they achieved insulin independence within 6 months of transplantation and also had successful metabolic control [24]. In diabetics, blood sugar thresholds were reduced, at which counterregulatory hormones, including growth hormones, glucagon, and epinephrine are secreted to increase the blood glucose; therefore, these patients are at a high risk of severe hypoglycemia, which can threaten their life. Rickels et al. showed that islet transplantation can improve this threshold and prevent a severe drop in blood glucose level [25, 26]. Another research group invented an immunosuppression protocol in 2008 known as UIC (University of Illinois) protocol. In this method, they used etanercept and exenatide in addition to the drugs used in the Edmonton Protocol. In total, two to three transplantations were required in the Edmonton Protocol group in order to achieve insulin independence in patients, but only one transplantation was enough in the UIC protocol. As a result, four out of six patients in the UIC group, and all six patients in the Edmonton group remained insulin-independent. In addition, HbA1c reached a normal level in both groups and there was no severe drop in blood glucose level of patients [27].

In the latest CITR report in 2012, 677 patients receiving islet transplantation with or without kidney transplantation during 1999–2010 were assessed. This report shows improvement in efficacy parameters following islet transplantation in the patients who received transplants in 2007–2010 compared with the older cases, with fewer adverse events. Today, islet transplantation has reached phase 3 of clinical trial [28].

An important issue regarding the use of islet transplantation for diabetic patients is proving its effectiveness, compared to insulin treatment. In this regard, the University of British Columbia in Canada monitored patients treated with traditional insulin treatment and islet transplantation for 3 years. According to the report of this group, islet transplantation significantly reduced the percentage of HbA1c and also the progression of diabetic retinopathy, compared to insulin treatment [29]. In addition, the group of the University of Miami evaluated 40 patients receiving islet transplantation, reporting a significant improvement in the quality of life of the patients within 40 months of the transplantation [30]. In a recent clinical trial initiated by Dr. Peter Stock under the supervision of UCFL University of California in 2019, pancreatic islets were transplanted simultaneously with allogeneic parathyroid gland to a diabetic patient at the intramuscular site. The results will continue to be obtained for 2 years [31].

One of the most important issues in islet engraftment is the chronic exhaustion of these cells and autoimmune responses, which reduces the survival and function of transplanted islets and ultimately leads to impaired blood sugar control in patients [32, 33]. Therefore, simultaneous transplantation of cells that can increase the survival of transplanted islets would be a good strategy to increase the effectiveness of this treatment [22, 34].

Recently, mesenchymal stem cells (MSCs) have attracted much attention as a cell population with the immunomodulatory and regeneration properties [35–37]. Mesples et al. in a study [17] treated the patients with autologous bone marrow stem cell stimulated (BM-MSCs) with filgrastim and transplanted through liver puncture. Their results demonstrated that BM-MSCs could reverse the production and action of antipancreatic islet antibodies and significantly increase blood C-peptide concentration [38]. In another study by Thakker et al., human adipose-derived MSCs were injected into the portal/thyroid circulation of patient that showed a significant reduction in plasma glucose and HbA1c levels, along with increase of C-peptide levels, and decreased exogenous insulin requirement following the administration of the cells [39]. Similar to this methodology, Dave et al. showed significant improvement in diabetes clinical indices after co-infusion of MSC-derived insulin-producing cells and autologous hematopoietic stem cells (HSC) into the portal circulation in 10 patients, after 27 months of follow-up [40]. On the other hand, a study in which BM-MSCs were transferred to T1DM patients showed only a transient improvement in insulin secretion and no significant long-term improvement was observed [41].

One of the methods used to reprogram the immune system in type 1 diabetic patients is the transplantation of autologous hematopoietic stem cells of the patient after treatment with high doses of immunosuppressive drugs. This method was first used in a clinical trial performed by Voltarelli et al. in 2007. In total, 15 recently diagnosed patients with type 1 diabetes were enrolled in this study, and their hematopoietic stem cells were isolated and stored after injecting granulocyte colony-stimulating factor and cyclophosphamide to transfer these cells from the bone marrow to the peripheral blood. Afterward, the patients were injected with immunosuppressive drugs, antithymocyte globulin and cyclophosphamide, and stem cells were returned to the patients' blood to reconstitute the immune system's active cells [42]. After the treatment, patients achieved insulin independence for various periods, and the process was recognized as a promising treatment for type 1 diabetes. Other groups yielded similar results [43] and confirmed this method could be one of the promising treatments for the disease in the future.

Regulatory T cells play a considerable role in the homeostasis of immune cells and induction of tolerance to native antigens [44]. A clinical trial is currently being performed to evaluate the effect of using self-regulatory T cells that have increased in culture medium in newly diagnosed type 1 diabetic patients.

Recently, a group at UIC University of the United States demonstrated that the treatment of lymphocytes with umbilical cord blood stem cells leads to inhibitory properties and increases the percentage of regulatory T cells in their blood [45]. The results were indicative of a lower need for exogenous insulin in patients, decreased blood level of HbA1C, and improved blood level of C-peptide. In addition, the percentage of regulatory T cells increased in treated patients, which can justify the adaptive immune system reaction [46].

In previous studies, a research group in Poland has demonstrated that the administration of autologous T regulatory (Treg) cells improves the functioning of β-cells and prolongs remission in recently diagnosed type 1 diabetes in children [47]. In 2015, Bluestone et al. reported the successful results of polyclonal Tregs transfer in type 1 diabetic patients. They showed the long-lived and long-term phenotype of ex vivo–expanded polyclonal Tregs after transfer in adult patients with recent-onset type I diabetes and entered the phase II clinical trial [48].

Previous data show that diabetic patients have a higher proportion of T cells compared to healthy controls that can produce interferon (IFN)-γ in response to peptides from the autoantigens. Petrich de Marquesini et al. have demonstrated for the first time in humans that first-degree relatives (FDRs) of new onset type 1 diabetes patients have a higher interleukin (IL)-10-producing to IFN-γ-producing T-cell ratio as compared to the diabetic patients. They suggested that a moderate regulatory response may be sufficient to prevent the development of clinical type 1 diabetes in genetically predisposed individuals [49].

2.1.2 *Tissue engineering*

One of the biggest challenges in transplanting insulin-secreting cells is the use of immunosuppressive drugs to prevent rejection by the host. Immunosuppressive drugs have severe complications such as damage to the implanted organs and weakening the body against pathogens and carcinogenesis [50]. Researchers have paid special attention to the use of biomaterials in order to encapsulate insulin-secreting cells with structures that can protect them from the intrusion of immune system active cells and molecules, to prevent transplant rejection without the use of immunosuppressive drugs. There are currently more than 10 clinical trials around the world using this approach, and the initial results have been very promising. In this approach, islets are encapsulated inside biomaterials, with proper biocompatibility and biodegradability characteristics, that prevent the passage of cells into the host immune system antibodies, while allowing the infiltration and exchange of nutrients, oxygen, glucose, and insulin. This is possible by controlling the size of nanopores of the enclosing material of islets, since the size of the immune system molecules (150–180 kDa) and cells are much larger than the nutrients, oxygen, glucose, and insulin.

In 1994, the world's first clinical trial using encapsulated human islets was conducted on a patient with type 1 diabetes, who remained insulin-independent and had a controlled level of blood glucose within 9 months of allogeneic transplantation of islets enclosed in alginate microparticles [51]. Many clinical trials have been performed using microencapsulation following the initial success of transplantation of enclosed islets [52]. Since islets are placed in a single device in the approach of macrocapsulation, the transplant can be easily retrieved from the host body, as a valuable advantage, which is contrary to the microencapsulation approach. In the first-generation microcapsule tools, the amount of oxygen supply is low due to the high volume of the enclosing material. Therefore, most encapsulated cells experience hypoxia. In general, several clinical studies have been performed on the encapsulation of insulin-secreting cells, including pancreatic islets, and cells derived from the source of pluripotent stem cells.

The first attempt to develop stem cells in the clinical trial was started in ViaCyte Company for the evaluation of PEC-01 combined with Encaptra device (a drug delivery system) in type 1 diabetes patients [53]. In 2017, PEC-Direct product was allowed by the FDA to test in the clinic and two other clinical trials were examined the efficacy of PEC-Encaptra device [54]. Similar clinical trials in Japan were also conducted using auto-hiPSC, which is not associated with a safe outcome so far [55]. Indeed, further investigations are needed to evaluate the efficacy of pluripotent stem cell therapy of diabetes. Inadequate oxygenation, the formation of fibrous tissue around the graft, and the infiltration of host cytokines into the enclosing structure are some of the challenges of this method [52].

2.1.3 *Gene therapy*

Major problems of islet transplantation are insufficient blood and oxygen perfusion, poor implantation and the immunological disposal of the transplanted islets. Therefore, various groups have conducted extensive research in the field of gene therapy to assess pancreatic islets or helper cells in the islets. Despite the successes of gene therapy in improving the islet transplantation results in animal models [56–58], there are still barriers to the use of this technique in humans in terms of safety.

Dr. George Gittes and his colleagues at UPMC Children's Hospital of Pittsburgh used an endoscope and an adeno-associated virus (AAV) vector to deliver Pdx1 and MafA genes to the patient's pancreas. The proteins which have been expressed by these genes, transform alpha cells in the pancreas into functional insulin-producing beta-like cells, but are distinct enough from native beta cells to evade from the body's immune system undesirable reactions [58]. Following preclinical studies, Dr. Gittes and his team achieve license agreement for potentially curative gene therapy candidate for diabetes and they plan to begin a phase I clinical trial in diabetic patients, which could be the first ever gene therapy tested in humans for diabetes.

However, this method can significantly contribute to the improvement of human islet transplantation results in the future with the advancement of methods in the field of gene therapy (Table 1).

2.2 Rheumatoid arthritis

Rheumatoid arthritis (RA) is a chronic inflammatory arthropathy characterized by synovial inflammation and hyperplasia that lead to extracellular matrix degradation and joint functional impairment [59–61]. The etiology of the disease is unclear and several cells involve in the disease progression, such as T cells and fibroblast-like synovial cells, so the treatment options remain limited [62]. Current therapies are based on inhibiting the symptoms of the disease by prescribing analgesics and antiinflammatory drugs such as steroids, but this treatment strategy does not regenerate damaged cartilage tissue. Cell-based therapeutic strategies using autologous chondrocytes have also been reported to be ineffective in RA because the local inflammatory conditions prevent cartilage formation and destroy newly formed cartilage [63].

2.2.1 *Cell therapy*

Since that MSCs have antiinflammatory, immunomodulatory, and regeneration properties, injection of these cells may lead to a reduction in inflammation and the new cartilage

TABLE 1 Ongoing clinical trials of type 1 diabetes with ATMP products.

| Type of ATMP | Cell type/intervention | Source | Administration route | | Start date | Study phase | Trial status | Trial number |
			Systemic	Local				
Cell therapy	Mesenchymal stromal cells	Umbilical cord	√			1/2	Recruiting	NCT03406585
	Beta cell	Pancreas		√	2000	1/2	Completed	NCT00623610
	Human pancreatic islets	Pancreas		√	2000	2	Ongoing	NCT00306098
	Human pancreatic islets and stem cells	Pancreas and bone marrow		√	2000	2	Completed	NCT00021801
	Human pancreatic islets	Pancreas		√	2000	2	Completed	NCT00021788
	Human pancreatic islets	Pancreas		√	2000	2	Completed	NCT00315588
	Human pancreatic islets	Pancreas		√	2000	2	Completed	NCT00006505
	Human pancreatic islets	Pancreas		√	2001	2	Completed	NCT00014911
	Human pancreatic islets	Pancreas		√	2002	1	Ongoing	NCT00706420
	Human pancreatic islets	Pancreas		√	2002	2	Completed	NCT00133809
	Hematopoietic stem cell	Peripheral blood		√	2003	1/2	Completed	NCT00315133
	Human pancreatic islets	Pancreas	√		2003	1/2	Ongoing	NCT00160732
	Human pancreatic islets	Pancreas		√	2004	1/2	Ongoing	NCT00566813

Continued

Type of ATMP	Cell type/ intervention	Source	Administration route		Start date	Study phase	Trial status	Trial number
			Systemic	Local				
	Human pancreatic islets	Pancreas		√	2005	1	Completed	NCT00214786
	Human pancreatic islets	Pancreas		√	2005	2	Completed	NCT00315627
	Hematopoietic stem cell	Peripheral blood	√		2006	2	Completed	NCT01341899
	Autologous dendritic cell	Peripheral blood		√	2007	1	Completed	NCT00445913
	Human pancreatic islets	Pancreas		√	2007	3	Completed	NCT00468117
	Adult CD34$^+$ stem cell subset	Peripheral blood	√		2008	1	Completed	NCT00788827
	Human pancreatic islets	Pancreas		√	2008	1	Completed	NCT00530686
	Human pancreatic islets	Pancreas		√	2008	Unknown	Completed	NCT00590876
	Mesenchymal stem cells	Peripheral blood	√		2008	2	Completed	NCT00690066
	Human pancreatic islets	Pancreas		√	2009	1/2	Completed	NCT00888628
	Multipotent stem cells	Umbilical cord blood		√	2010	2	Recruiting	NCT01350219
	Autologous hematopoietic stem cell	Peripheral blood	√		2010	2	Completed	NCT01121029
	Polyclonal regulatory T cells	Peripheral blood	√		2010	1	Completed	NCT01210664

Human pancreatic islets	Pancreas		√	2010	2	Recruiting	NCT01241864
Human pancreatic islets	Pancreas		√	2012	2	Completed	NCT01736228
Human pancreatic islets	Pancreas		√	2012	1/2	Recruiting	NCT01630850
Human pancreatic islets	Pancreas		√	2012	3	Ongoing	NCT01897688
Multipotent stem cells	Cord blood		√	2013	1/2	Recruiting	NCT01996228
Human pancreatic islets	Pancreas	√		2013	2	Recruiting	NCT01909245
Pancreatic islet	Porcine pancreas		√	2013	Not applicable	Completed	NCT03162237
Human pancreatic islets	Pancreas		√	2013	2	Recruiting	NCT01974674
Mesenchymal stem cells	Cord blood		√	2014	1/2	Completed	NCT02644759
Human pancreatic islets	Pancreas		√	2014	1/2	Recruiting	NCT02213003
Allogenic mesenchymal stem cells	Adipose tissue		√	2015	1	Ongoing	NCT03920397
Mesenchymal stem cells	Bone marrow	√		2015	1/2	Ongoing	NCT04078308
Mesenchymal stem cells	Umbilical cord		√	2015	1	Recruiting	NCT02745808
Human pancreatic islets	Pancreas		√	2016	1/2	Completed	NCT02821026

Continued

Type of ATMP	Cell type/ intervention	Source	Administration route		Start date	Study phase	Trial status	Trial number
			Systemic	Local				
	Polyclonal regulatory T cell	Peripheral blood	√		2016	1	Ongoing	NCT02772679
	"Educated" lymphocytes	Peripheral blood	√		2017	1	Recruiting	NCT02624804
	Mesenchymal cells and mononuclear cells	Adipose and bone marrow	√		2017	1	Recruiting	NCT02940418
	Hematopoietic stem cell	Peripheral-blood	√		2017	1/2	Recruiting	NCT03182426
	Regulatory T cells	Umbilical cord blood	√		2017	1/2	Recruiting	NCT03011021
	Human pancreatic islets	Pancreas		√	2017	1	Ongoing	NCT03073577
	Polyclonal regulatory T cell	Peripheral blood	√		2018	1	Recruiting	NCT03444064
	Mesenchymal stromal cells	Umbilical cord	√		2019	1/2	Recruiting	NCT03973827
	Stem cells	Exfoliated teeth	√		2019	1	Recruiting	NCT03912480
	Human pancreatic islets	Pancreas		√	2019	1/2	Recruiting	NCT03698396
	Stem cells and pancreatic islet	Umbilical cord and pancreas		√	2019	Not applicable	Recruiting	NCT03835312
	Mesenchymal stem/ stromal cells	Adipose tissue	√		2019	1	Recruiting	NCT03840343

	Human pancreatic islets and parathyroid gland	Pancreas		√	2019	1/2	Recruiting	NCT03977662
	Mesenchymal stem cells	Umbilical cord	√		2020	1	Recruiting	NCT04061746
Tissue engineering	Human pancreatic islets (CIT-01)	Pancreas		√	2008	2	Completed	NCT00789308
	Human pancreatic islets	Pancreas		√	2008	1	Withdrawn	NCT00790257
	Progenitor cells (ViaCyte ncaptra)	Human embryonic stem cells		√	2014	1/2	Ongoing	NCT02239354
	Human pancreatic islets	Pancreas		√	2014	1/2	Ongoing	NCT02064309
	Human pancreatic islets (VC-02)	Pancreas		√	2017	1/2	Recruiting	NCT03163511
	Human pancreatic islets (APS APP)	Pancreas		√	2018	2/3	Completed	NCT03504046
	Pancreatic islets (Sernova's Cell Pouch)	Pancreas		√	2019	1/2	Recruiting	NCT03513939

formation in RA [63, 64]. Accordingly, some clinical trials have already started to investigate MSCs for treatment of RA. So that, Aghdami et al. have demonstrated that intraarticular knee implantation of bone marrow derived-MSCs seem to be safe and well tolerated, they also observed a trend toward clinical efficacy. MSC-treated patients showed improvements during the first month after the treatment that continued until the end of the study. However, the trend in the placebo-treated group was that patients did not experience continuous improvement throughout the experiment [65]. Similarly, Wang et al. have investigated the treatment of RA patients with umbilical cord-derived MSCs (UC-MSCs) for up to 8 months [66]. Moreover, in another 3-year cohort study they investigated the safety and efficacy of UC-MSCs and confirmed that UC-MSC treatment was safe and able to control RA symptoms in the long term, when combined with DMARDs, there are no abnormalities in liver and kidney function and immunoglobulin examination [67]. Overall, they have shown the stable clinical outcomes of UC-MSC that can be maintained for 3 years, with expressively improved quality of life [66, 67].

It should be noted that UC-MSCs differ from human umbilical cord blood-derived MSCs (hUCB-MSCs) in terms of source and preparation of the investigational product [66]. Park et al. investigated the detailed mechanism by which hUCB-MSC injection might improve inflammatory arthritis, they also investigated the safety and tolerability of a single intravenous injection of hUCB-MSCs in Korean patients with a phase 1a study, which extended their preclinical research [68].

Adipose tissue is one of the most important sources of mesenchymal stem cells that have demonstrated therapeutic effect in experimental arthritis, however, little is known about its effect on RA. Accordingly, Álvaro-Gracia et al. examined the safety of intravenous injection of expanded allogeneic adipose-derived mesenchymal stem cells (AD-MSCs) in refractory RA. They showed that the intravenous administration of Cx611 is generally tolerated, without dose-related toxicity at the dose range and duration of study. It opens the possibility to evaluate the duration of the therapeutic effects, the appropriate dose strategy, and the most appropriate patient characteristics for this treatment in the future [69].

Hematopoietic stem cell transplantation (HSCT) was introduced as method of transplanting a source of cells for treating RA patients with poor prognosis [70, 71]. Burt et al. evaluated the safety and efficacy of immunosuppression with autologous HSCT in severe RA. They showed that in this series of patients, autologous HSCT was safe and effective in creating a major clinical improvement and maintained significant benefit for two patients at 9 and 20 months, respectively. Despite the initial improvement, the response was not sustained for the other two patients [72].

The ideal treatment for RA is one that restores the immune system to its tolerable state, and stops autoimmune manifestations, without long-term treatment. Dendritic cells (DCs) organize immune responses, by swallowing and presenting antigens to T cells [73, 74]. DCs also activate and differentiate T cells that are involved in the autoimmune reaction. Intraarticular (IA) injection of autologous tolerogenic dendritic cells (tol-DC) seems safe, feasible, and suitable. Knee symptoms stabilized in two patients who received tol-DC, but no clinical effect or systemic immune modulation was detectable [75].

2.2.2 *Gene therapy*

Current treatment approaches do not assure an ideal treatment for RA patients. In addition, classical regimes based on immunosuppression are nontargeted and have significant side effects. However, biologic therapy has advanced significantly, while some concerns about its efficacy and specificity remained to be solved [76, 77].

The development of technologies in gene therapy area has the potential to create a new direction for the treatment of RA. However, the beneficial effect of gene therapy for RA is still unknown. Several gene therapy experiments in animal models have been moderately successful so far, but they have not provided enough evidence to prove the improvement of RA patients treated with these strategies. Both viral and nonviral delivery systems are used for RA gene therapy in animal models [77]. Evans et al., in the first human clinical trials of gene therapy in RA, evaluated the safety and feasibility of autologous synovial fibroblasts that were genetically modified with a recombinant retrovirus (MFGIRAP) carrying the human interleukin-1 receptor antagonist (IL-1Ra) cDNA that transferred to human rheumatoid joints. In a dose-increasing manner, genetically modified or control cells were injected into the metacarpophalangeal (MCP) joints of nine patients with RA. One week later, MCP joints underwent unilateral systolic implant arthroplasty. Synovia was recovered and examined to prove its persistence and gene expression. Accordingly, they showed that a potential gene therapy product can be safely transferred to human rheumatoid joints and the intraarticular transgenic expression successfully occurred [78]. This group has reported the results of another study that determined a clinical response to gene transfer, with persistence of the transgene for at least 1 month [76] (Table 2).

2.3 Multiple sclerosis

Multiple sclerosis (MS) is an autoimmune disease affecting the central nervous system; the main feature of MS is the destruction of the myelin sheath and impaired conduction of nerve messages, which leads to the loss of axons [79, 80]. In the early stages of the disease, recurrence and recovery are frequently reported, and after an acute attack of the disease and myelin damage, its complications subside and myelin repair occurs endogenously. The endogenous repair capacity of the brain gradually declines, the myelin-free plaques remain in the brain and gradually increase, after which the disease enters a secondary chronic progressive stage. In advanced cases of the disease, due to the emergence and spread of myelinated lesions, the conduction of nerve messages is impaired and leads to a variety of sensory, motor, and cognitive complications. Current therapies often target the autoimmune aspect of disease and aim to control the inflammation, but have not had significant success in repairing myelin or stopping the disease [81–83].

2.3.1 Cell therapy

It is suggested that mesenchymal stem cells may play a therapeutic role in diseases such as MS, through strategies other than tissue replacement [84, 85], with increased evidence of neuroprotection and improved function following injection of mesenchymal stem cells in animal models of recurrent chronic MS [86–88].

Three recent reports have also described the use of intrathecal delivery of autologous mesenchymal stem cells in MS, without side effects or significant changes in general clinical outcomes [89–91].

TABLE 2 Ongoing clinical trials of rheumatoid arthritis with ATMP products.

Type of ATMP	Cell type/ intervention	Source	Administration route		Start date	Study phase	Trial status	Trial number
			Systemic	Local				
Cell therapy	Hematopoietic stem cell	Peripheral blood	√		1997	1	Completed	NCT00278551
	Placenta-derived stem cells	Placenta	√		2010	2	Completed	NCT01261403
	Mesenchymal stem cells	Adipose tissue	√		2011	1, 2	Completed	NCT01663116
	Mesenchymal stem cells	Umbilical cord	√		2013	1, 2	Ongoing	NCT01985464
	Allogeneic mesenchymal precursor cells	–	√		2013	2	Completed	NCT01851070
	Autologous stromal vascular fraction cells	Adipose tissue	√		2013	1, 2	Withdrawn	NCT01885819
	Mesenchymal stem cells	Umbilical cord	√		2013	1, 2	Recruiting	NCT01547091
	Autologous mesenchymal stem cells	Bone marrow	√		2016	1	Completed	NCT03333681
	Mesenchymal stem cells	Bone marrow	√		2016	1	Ongoing	NCT03067870
	Tolerogenic dendritic cells	Blood		√	2016	1	Completed	NCT03337165

	Mesenchymal stem cells	Bone marrow	√		2017	1	Completed	NCT03186417
	Mesenchymal stem cells	Umbilical cord blood	√		2017	Not applicable	Recruiting	NCT03798028
	Mesenchymal stem cells	Adipose tissue	√		2018	1, 2	Ongoing	NCT03691909
	Mesenchymal stem cell	Umbilical cord	√		2020	1	Ongoing	NCT03828344
	Mesenchymal stem cells	Adipose tissue	√		2020	1, 2	Ongoing	NCT04170426
	Autologous apoptotic cells	–	√		2020	1, 2	Ongoing	NCT02903212
Gene therapy	tgAAC94	AAV containing TNFR:Fc		√	2004	1	Completed	NCT00617032
	tgAAC94	AAV containing TNFR:Fc		√	2005	2	Completed	NCT00126724
	ART-I02	AAV containing NF-kB and IFN-β		√	2017	1	Ongoing	NCT02727764
	ART-I02	AAV containing NF-kB and IFN-β		√	2018	1	Ongoing	NCT03445715

Connick et al. demonstrated the safety and efficacy of autologous mesenchymal stem cells as a potential neuroprotective treatment for secondary progressive MS. Evidence for structural, functional, and physiological improvement after treatment at some endpoints of vision suggested neuroprotection of MSCs [84].

In the other pilot study, which evaluated the potential therapeutic application of autologous MSC in improving clinical symptoms of MS patients, 10 cases were included. They founded that intrathecal injection of MSC was not associated with any serious complications, but in some patients some improvement was observed and in others the progression of the disease was stopped. In five patients, MSC treatment had no effect in the progression of the disease [91]. Yamout et al. have evaluated the safety and feasibility of intrathecal injection of autologous BM-MSCs injection in MS patients. They have shown that autologous BM-MSC transplantation in cerebrospinal fluid of MS patients through lumbar and cisternal openings is a safe procedure. Large numbers of cells may cause transient encephalopathy, which may be secondary to inflammation, caused by a reaction to the by-products of cell lysis. Early signs of clinical improvement are seen in most patients for up to 3 months and last for up to 1 year [89]. In another study, the safety, feasibility, and immunological effects of intrathecal and intravenous administration of autologous MSCs were shown in MS patients. MSCs could alleviate the disease severity and improve cognitive function and quality of life of MS patients through the neuroprotective and antiinflammatory properties [90].

Several clinical trials have shown that hematopoietic stem cells cause clinical improvement in patients with MS and significantly reduce the progression of MS [92, 93]. Some other studies have shown that Hematopoietic stem cell therapy in patients with advanced MS improves nerve function and prevents mortality [92, 94, 95]. Carreras et al. have evaluated feasibility and toxicity of $CD34^+$ selected autologous stem cell transplantation ($CD34^+$/ASCT) for MS patients. They demonstrated a reduction in the progression of the disease and improvement of the patients' quality of life, evidently [96].

There is a report of successful treatment with human umbilical cord-derived MSC (hUC-MSC) in a patient with refractory progressive MS, the course of the disease was stabilized with signs of improved sensory function [97]. In subsequent clinical trials, during a 1-year observation period, no significant side effects were found in the hUCMSC-treated group, indicating better immunoreactivity profile of these stem cells [98]. Administration of hUC-MSC in MS patients showed lower recurrence rates and EDSS (Extensive Disability Status Scale) scores.

Clinical reports of human embryonic stem cells transplantation in patients with MS have shown significant improvements in functional skills, overall endurance, cognitive abilities, and muscle strength [99] (Table 3).

2.4 Autoimmune skin disorders

There are different types of skin-related autoimmune disorders, such as vitiligo, scleroderma, pemphigus, and psoriasis, for which cell-based therapy approaches could offer a novel method for their treatment.

TABLE 3 Ongoing clinical trials of multiple sclerosis with ATMP products.

Type of ATMP	Cell type/intervention	Source	Administration route		Start date	Study phase	Trial status	Trial number
			Systemic	Local				
Cell therapy	Hematopoietic stem cell	Peripheral blood	√		2003	1, 2	Completed	NCT00278655
	Autologous mesenchymal stem cells	Bone marrow	√	√	2006	1, 2	Completed	NCT00781872
	Allogeneic hematopoetic stem cell	–	√		2007	1, 2	Ongoing	NCT00497952
	Autologous hematopoietic cell	Peripheral blood	√		2008	2	Recruiting	NCT00716066
	Mesenchymal stem cells	–	√		2010	2	Completed	NCT01228266
	Mesenchymal stem cell	Umbilical cord			2010	1, 2	Ongoing	NCT01364246
	Autologous mesenchymal stem cells	Adipose tissue	√		2010	1, 2	Completed	NCT01056471
	Mesenchymal stem cells	–	√		2011	1	Completed	NCT00813969
	Autologous mesenchymal stem cells	Bone marrow		√	2012	1, 2	Completed	NCT01895439
	Autologous mesenchymal stem cells	Bone marrow	√		2012	1	Completed	NCT03778333
	Mesenchymal stem cells	Bone marrow	√		2013	1, 2	Completed	NCT01606215
	Mesenchymal stem cells	Bone marrow	√		2013	1, 2	Completed	NCT02035514
	Mesenchymal stem cells	Bone marrow	√		2013	1, 2	Recruiting	NCT01745783

Continued

Type of ATMP	Cell type/intervention	Source	Administration route		Start date	Study phase	Trial status	Trial number
			Systemic	Local				
	Mono-nuclear stem cell (MNCs)	Bone marrow	√		2014	1, 2	Recruiting	NCT01883661
	Mesenchymal stem cells	Adipose tissue	√		2014	1	Completed	NCT02326935
	Mesenchymal stem cells	Bone marrow	√		2015	1, 2	Completed	NCT02403947
	Mesenchymal stem cells	Bone marrow	√	√	2015	2	Completed	NCT02166021
	Autologous hematopoietic stem cell	–			2015	1	Recruiting	NCT03113162
	Mesenchymal stem cells	–	√		2015	2	Completed	NCT02239393
	Mesenchymal stem cells	Umbilical cord	√		2015	1, 2	Ongoing	NCT02587715
	Mesenchymal stem cells	Bone marrow	√	√	2016	1	Recruiting	NCT03069170
	Mesenchymal stem cells	Bone marrow	√	√	2016	Not applicable	Recruiting	NCT02795052
	Allogenic neural stem cells	Brain specimen of fetal human donors		√	2017	1	Ongoing	NCT03282760
	Mesenchymal stem cells	Umbilical cord		√	2017	1, 2	Completed	NCT03326505
	Hematopoietic stem cell	Peripheral blood	√		2017	3	Completed	NCT03342638
	Mesenchymal stem cell-derived neural progenitors	Bone marrow		√	2018	2	Ongoing	NCT03355365
	Hematopoietic stem cell	Blood	√		2019	3	Recruiting	NCT04047628
Gene therapy	Autologous mesenchymal stem cells secreting neurotrophic factors	Bone marrow		√	2019	2	Recruiting	NCT03799718

2.4.1 *Vitiligo*

Vitiligo is the most common human pigmentation disease characterized by the gradual destruction of mature epidermal melanocytes. The accepted mechanism for vitiligo pathogenesis is that genetic and nongenetic factors affect the function and viability of melanocytes and ultimately lead to their immune-mediated degradation [100]. First-line treatment in vitiligo includes nonsurgical treatments such as psoralen plus ultraviolet A (PUVA), narrowband ultraviolet B (NB-UVB), excimer lasers, immunosuppressive drugs, topical agents, and calcipotriol, even though they are not always effective [101, 102]. Surgical therapies are applied to treat stable vitiliginous lesions that do not respond to aforementioned medical treatments (Table 4).

Cell therapy

Recent studies highlighted potential therapeutic uses of stem cells of different origins in the treatment of vitiligo, even if the underlying mechanisms remained elusive [103, 104]. Significant advances in cell-based therapy have introduced melanocyte transplantation as a promising substitute for damaged cells [102]. In this approach, cultured or noncultured melanocyte-keratinocyte suspensions derived from a normal pigmented donor skin are transplanted into depigmented areas [105, 106].

Noncultured epidermal suspension transplant encompasses a type of cellular grafts, which involves separation of different cellular components of a split-thickness skin graft. The cellular suspension that consists of a mixture of epidermal keratinocytes and melanocytes is then applied to a dermabraded recipient area [102, 105, 107, 108]. Several clinical trials have revealed the safety and efficacy of autologous noncultured epidermal cellular grafting technique in patients with different types of vitiligo. This procedure achieved a high percentage of repigmentation; however, a perfect color match was seldom obtained [109–112].

In cultured epidermal suspension transplant, after separation of epidermis, the melanocytes and keratinocytes are dissociated and then the melanocytes are seeded in a proper melanocyte medium containing certain growth factors. The melanocytes are thus cultured and then transplanted as free suspension or as epidermal sheets on to dermabraded recipient skin [106, 107, 113, 114]. Cultured melanocyte transplantation creates a large number of cells from a small area of donor epidermis and is a promising option for patients with large depigmented areas. However, the method that uses noncultured autologous epidermal suspension is simpler, less expensive, less time consuming, does not require highly trained personnel and well-equipped tissue laboratories, and does not pose safety concerns regarding specific growth factors and additives in the culture medium [105, 106].

2.4.2 *Scleroderma*

Scleroderma or systemic sclerosis (SSc) is a heterogeneous autoimmune disease that is characterized by chronic inflammation, small vessel vasculopathy, and excessive collagen deposition in the skin and internal organs, resulting in devastating impairments. Treatment strategies are directed at improving circulation with vasodilators and antiplatelet therapy, preventing synthesis and release of harmful cytokines with immunosuppressants, and reducing fibrosis with collagen synthesis inhibitors or collagenases. The clinical benefit of these drugs is, however, limited by moderate- or short-term efficacy, along with severe side effects, including systemic toxicity, chronic immune suppression, and bleeding [115–117] (Table 5).

TABLE 4 Ongoing clinical trials of vitiligo with ATMP products.

Type of ATMP	Cell type/intervention	Source	Administration route		Start date	Study phase	Trial status	Trial number
			Systemic	Local				
Cell therapy	Autologous epidermal cells	Skin		√	2008	Not applicable	Completed	NCT00615355
	Autologous melanocytes and keratinocytes	Skin		√	2009	3	Completed	NCT00830713
	Melanocytes and keratinocytes	Skin		√	2010	2, 3	Withdrawn	NCT01822379
	Melanocytes and keratinocytes	Skin		√	2010	1	Completed	NCT02510651
	Autologous epidermal cells	Skin		√	2011	1, 2	Completed	NCT01511965
	Autologous epidermal cells	Skin		√	2011	2, 3	Completed	NCT01629979
	Epidermal cell suspension (ReCell)	Skin		√	2012	4	Unknown	NCT01640678
	Epidermal cells suspension (ReCell)	Skin		√	2015	4	Completed	NCT02458417
	Autologous epidermal cell suspension (ReNovaCell)	Skin		√	2016	Not applicable	Terminated	NCT03022019
	Autologous noncultured epidermal and dermal cells	Skin		√	2016	Not applicable	Unknown	NCT03013049
	Melanocytes and keratinocytes	Skin		√	2017	Not applicable	Recruiting	NCT04374435
	Autologous noncultured epidermal cells	Skin		√	2017	Not applicable	Recruiting	NCT03717025
	Autologous melanocytes and uncultured keratinocytes	Skin		√	2018	Not applicable	Unknown	NCT03497208
	Autologous noncultured epidermal cells	Skin		√	2018	Not applicable	Unknown	NCT03668834

TABLE 5 Ongoing clinical trials of scleroderma with ATMP products.

Type of ATMP	Cell type/intervention	Source	Administration route		Start date	Study phase	Trial status	Trial number
			Systemic	Local				
Cell therapy	Autologous stem cells	Peripheral blood	√		1999	1	Completed	NCT00058578
	Autologous stem cells	Peripheral blood	√		2000	1	Completed	NCT00010335
	Autologous stem cells		√		2005	2, 3	Completed	NCT00860548
	Allogenic hematopoietic stem cells	Peripheral blood	√		2005	1	Terminated	NCT00282425
	Allogeneic mesenchymal stem cells	–	√		2009	1, 2	Unknown	NCT00962923
	Autologous stem cells	Peripheral blood	√		2011	2	Active, not recruiting	NCT01413100
	Autologous stem cells	–		–	2012	2	Recruiting	NCT01895244
	Allogeneic mesenchymal stem cell	–		–	2014	1, 2	Unknown	NCT02213705
	Autologous regenerative cells	Adipose tissue		√	2015	Not applicable	Completed	NCT02396238
	Autologous regenerative cells	Adipose tissue		√	2015	–	Withdrawn	NCT02328625
	Autologous stromal vascular fraction	Adipose tissue		√	2016	Not applicable	Completed	NCT02975960
	Autologous stromal vascular fraction	Adipose tissue		√	2016	1	Active, not recruiting	NCT03060551
	Allogeneic mesenchymal stromal cells	Bone marrow		√	2018	1, 2	Not yet recruiting	NCT03211793
	Autologous hematopoietic stem cells	Peripheral blood	–		2019	–	Recruiting	NCT03444805
	Allogeneic hematopoietic stem cells		√		2020	1	Recruiting	NCT04380831
	Mesenchymal stem cells	Umbilical cord	√		2020	1, 2	Not yet recruiting	NCT04356287
	Autologous hematopoietic stem cells	Peripheral blood	√		2020	3	Not yet recruiting	NCT04464434
	Allogeneic mesenchymal stem cells	Wharton's jelly	√		2020	–	Available	NCT04432545
	Stem cells	Adipose tissue		√	2020	2	Not yet recruiting	NCT04356755
	Autologous human fibroblasts genetically modified with matrix metalloproteinase 1 (MMP-1) (FCX-013)	Skin		√	2019	1, 2	Recruiting	NCT03740724

Cell therapy

Since routine medications do not have regenerative properties and have only the potential to halt disease progression, cellular therapy has recently emerged as a credible option. Hematopoietic stem-cell transplantation (HSCT) has been demonstrated to be an effective treatment to cure some patients with rapidly progressive SSc.

The first study of an autologous HSCT for SSc was reported in 1977 [118]. Shortly thereafter, dramatic improvement in dermal fibrosis after autologous HSCT in SSc was observed. By 2009, the number of reported patients with SSc treated with autologous HSCT had reached 224 individuals in Europe and 97 in North and South America. After encouraging pilot studies showing beneficial effects of HSCT on immunomodulation, fibrosis, and angiogenesis, controlled clinical trials definitively established HSCT as a true disease-modifying treatment of SSc [119–121]. American Scleroderma Stem Cell versus Immune Suppression Trial (ASSIST) compared patients who received autologous HSCT with patients given cyclophosphamide (CYC) once per month for 6 months. All patients who received HSCT improved during 12 months of follow-up, while none of the CYC-received patients improved during their 6 months of treatment. Some patients were given HSCT at 12 months (i.e., 6 months after their 6-month CYC therapy), the results were not definitive, but supported the use of HSCT. Adverse events were poorly documented. Another randomized multicenter trial, Autologous Stem Cell Transplantation International Scleroderma (ASTIS), evaluated patients who received autologous HSCT, or patients given CYC once per month for 12 months. Patients receiving HCST showed higher mortality in the first 12 months, but had better long-term survival than patients receiving CYC. Adverse events in the HSCT group included lymphoproliferative disease, Epstein-Barr virus, cytomegalovirus and herpes zoster infections. The Scleroderma Cyclophosphamide or Transplantation (SCOT) trial compared the result of patients receiving autologous HSCT with patients receiving CYC per month until 12 months, during 54-month follow-up. The data demonstrated the efficacy of HSCT over CYC at 54 months. Overall, similar to ASTIS, SCOT provided clear data supporting the effectiveness of HSCT over CYC as well [120, 122].

More recently, some patients affected by linear scleroderma and different types of morphea have been treated by means of autologous fat grafting (AFG). Adipose tissue harvested with liposuction is processed to yield adipocytes and stromal vascular fraction cells. The stromal vascular fraction is composed of a mixture of adipose stem cells, endothelial cells, vascular smooth muscle cells, and immune cells. It has been shown that fat grafting reduced inflammation and fibrosis by limiting extracellular matrix proteins and increasing collagenase activity, and provided structural support through stem-cell proliferation and differentiation. Indeed, the adipocytes provide bulk and improve contour irregularities, and the endothelial and vascular smooth muscle cells assist in blood vessel regeneration. Onesti et al. have investigated the compression between the effects of lipotransfer and enriched ADSCs in systemic sclerosis patients. In the enriched ADSCs group, lipoaspirate from the abdomen was harvested and then processed for ADSC isolation. The ADSCs were injected into patients 3 weeks before the harvesting procedure by means of hyaluronic acid gels. After 1-year follow-up, both approaches provided significant results but neither procedure provided superior results. They did not observe severe adverse reactions. Taken together, these results prove the efficacy and safety of a variety of AFG procedures in the treatment of scleroderma-related fibrotic skin lesions, without considering the type of fat preparation and/or purification [123–127].

2.4.3 *Pemphigus*

Pemphigus encompasses a heterogeneous group of autoimmune chronic mucocutaneous blistering diseases. Patients with pemphigus suffer from chronic inflammation as well as blistering and scarring of the skin and mucous membranes. The pathogenic relevance of autoantibodies targeting desmosomal glycoproteins (dsg1, dsg3) has been well-documented. The overall prognosis of pemphigus has greatly improved since the advent of glucocorticoids. However, mortality remains high because long-term use of high-dose corticosteroids and immunosuppressive drugs enhance the risk of serious side effects, such as susceptibility to infections. A recent study showed superior efficacy of rituximab, a chimeric anti-CD20 monoclonal antibody that induces B-cell depletion, compared to immunosuppressive therapies and revealed that rituximab reduced incidence of immunosuppressant-related serious adverse events and overall mortality, leading to its approval as a first line treatment in pemphigus. The therapeutic option for patients with severe or refractory pemphigus is the administration of intravenous immunoglobulin (IVIg) or immunoadsorption. Current treatment options rely on nonspecific treatment, which in many cases do not lead to remission of the disease [128–131] (Table 6).

Cell therapy

Stem cell therapy in pemphigus not only has shown promises in treatment, but also brings about a shift toward nonsteroidal approach in autoimmune diseases. Two retrospective single-center studies by Vanikar et al. evaluated the effects of allogeneic HSCT delivered into thymus, bone marrow, and the portal and peripheral circulations in pemphigus patients who were resistant to steroids. They found that the existing skin lesions started to regress within 24 h of stem cell therapy and new lesions stopped after 6 months, while no lesions occurred during a mean follow-up of 8 years [132, 133].

2.4.4 *Psoriasis*

Psoriasis is an immune-mediated chronic systemic inflammatory disease, which causes red itchy scaly patches on the skin. It mainly affects the scalp, knees, elbows, hands, nails, and feet. Psoriasis occurs with several other serious illnesses such as diabetes, cardiovascular disease, lymphoma, and depression. There is no permanent cure for psoriasis, though steroid creams, vitamin D3 cream, ultraviolet light, and immunosuppressive medications (e.g., methotrexate) have been widely used to help controlling the symptoms. Therapeutic approaches such as biologics and cell transplantation are currently being developed and explored in search of disease-modifying cures [134–136].

Cell therapy

Currently, clinical trials are being conducted into the use of stem cells in the treatment of psoriasis. This idea originated from observation of the remission of lesions in patients treated with mesenchymal or hematopoietic stem cells because of other diseases such as lymphoma, leukemia, and aplastic anemia. Kaffenberger et al. performed a comprehensive search to

TABLE 6 Ongoing clinical trials of pemphigus with ATMP products.

Type of ATMP	Cell type/intervention	Source	Administration route		Start date	Study phase	Trial status	Trial number
			Systemic	Local				
Cell therapy	Autologous hematopoietic stem cells	Peripheral blood	√		2002	1	Terminated	NCT00278642
	Autologous polyclonal regulatory T cells	Peripheral blood	√		2017	1	Active, not recruiting	NCT03239470
	Autologous resmoglein 3 chimeric autoantibody receptor T cells (DSG3-CAART)	Peripheral blood	√		2020	1	Recruiting	NCT04422912

identify all previously reported cases of psoriasis that resolved after HSCT. According to their survey, 19 patients had been reported to have psoriasis resolution after allogeneic or autologous HSCT. In allogeneic conditions, 10 of 13 patients had long-term improvement in their psoriasis with an average follow-up of 49 months. Six patients had undergone autologous transplantation. Of these, five of six had developed a recurrence of their psoriasis within 2 years. It was hypothesized that T-cell receptor diversity preserved after autologous transplantation limits the effect of this method. Based on a limited number of patients, Kaffenberger et al. proposed that psoriasis is likely to remit after allogeneic HSCT, but it is likely to recur after autologous HSCT [137, 138].

Jesus et al. evaluated autologous adipose-derived MSCs (AD-MSCs) transplantation in psoriasis vulgaris and psoriatic arthritis patients. No serious adverse events were observed for either patient as a result of MSC infusions. They reported the safety and potential clinical utility of AD-MSCs for the treatment of psoriasis and served as preliminary evidence to support large clinical studies to investigate the long-term safety and efficacy of this approach [139].

Wang et al., for the first time, investigated the safety and efficacy of repeated infusion of gingival MSCs in a patient with severe plaque psoriasis refractory to multiple topical and systemic therapies. Complete regression was obtained after five injections without any adverse reaction. The patient has been followed for 3 years and has remained disease-free [140] (Table 7).

2.5 Autoimmune digestive disorders

Autoimmune digestive disorders, such as celiac disease and inflammatory bowel disease, are conditions that occur when the body's immune system wrongly attacks part of the gastrointestinal tract. In these conditions, cell-based therapy approaches could offer an effective method for their treatment.

2.5.1 *Celiac disease*

Celiac disease (CeD) occurs when a person becomes intolerant to gluten, a protein found in wheat, rye, and barley products. Therefore, the ingestion of gluten causes the immune system to attack the small intestine villi. CD has a wide spectrum of clinical manifestations that vary from asymptomatic to classic symptomatic form of the disease. Over time, damage to the small intestine can increase the risk of intestinal lymphoma. CeD treatment is mainly based on a gluten-free diet (GFD), which is troublesome for affected patients because of the lifelong interventional regimen. However, in a small percentage (2%–5%) of adult patients with CeD, a refractory state develops despite strict adherence to a GFD. Other therapies such as zonolin antagonists, immunosuppressive therapies, and glutenases have entered phase II/III clinical studies. Furthermore, stem cell transplantation is starting to be examined as a potential therapy for CeD [141–143].

Cell therapy

Several studies have reported the feasibility and effectiveness of allogenic HSCT in patients with refractory CD. One patient with CeD and acute myelogenous leukemia, one with severe aplastic anemia and CeD, and two patients affected by CeD and major β-thalassemia,

TABLE 7 Ongoing clinical trials of psoriasis with ATMP products.

Type of ATMP	Cell type/intervention	Source	Administration route		Start date	Study phase	Trial status	Trial number
			Systemic	Local				
Cell therapy	Allogeneic mesenchymal stem cells	Adipose tissue	√		2017	1, 2	Active, not recruiting	NCT03265613
	Mesenchymal stem cells	Umbilical cord	√		2018	1	Unknown	NCT03424629
	Allogeneic mesenchymal stem cells	Umbilical cord	√		2018	1	Recruiting	NCT02918123
	Mesenchymal stem cells	Umbilical cord	√		2018	1, 2	Recruiting	NCT03745417
	Mesenchymal stem cells	Umbilical cord	√		2019	1	Recruiting	NCT03765957
	Mesenchymal stem cells	Adipose tissue	√		2019	1, 2	Recruiting	NCT03392311
	Mesenchymal stem cells	Adipose tissue	√		2020	Not applicable	Recruiting	NCT04275024

who underwent allogeneic HSCT, achieved correction of CeD despite the initiation of a gluten-containing diet. Autologous peripheral blood stem cell (PB-SC) transplant has been tried in patients with refractory CeD as well. Al-Toma et al. subjected patients with refractory CeD type-II to autologous PB-SC transplant, it was found that not only the transplantation was well tolerated but also it led to rapid clinical response, which lasted for at least 2 years. Similar results were obtained by Tack et al. in refractory type-II CD patients that showed an impressive clinical improvement after autologous HSCT [143–145].

2.5.2 *Inflammatory bowel disease*

Inflammatory bowel disease (IBD) is a group of chronic inflammatory disorders characterized by gastrointestinal (GI) mucosal ulceration, rectal bleeding, diarrhea, and abdominal pain. Crohn's disease (CD) and ulcerative colitis (UC) are the two major diseases in this category. CD occurs when the immune system attacks parts of the digestive tract, from the mouth to the anus. UC happens when the immune system attacks the lining of the rectum and colon, causing ulcers that may bleed and produce pus. People with UC may also experience anemia, rectal bleeding, and fatigue. The differentiation between CD and UC is difficult in some cases due to some common manifestations [146, 147].

Treatments include antiinflammatory drugs, immune-suppressant drugs, and steroids. Patients who become refractory to medical management eventually require surgery; as up to 60% of patients with CD will require a surgical intervention during their disease course, and 15% of UC patients will need colectomy. There is growing evidence that cell-based therapy can be an alternative method to treat IBD patients through alteration of the mucosal immune response [148, 149] (Tables 8 and 9).

Cell therapy for CD

Cell therapy was initially applied for treating this disease in CD patients who developed lymphoma and leukemia. After transplantation, an improvement was also detected in their CD clinical symptoms. Since then, several case series and randomized studies have been published reporting transplantation of hematopoietic stem cells or mesenchymal stem cells to treat the disease itself [150].

Autologous HSCT in patients with severe CD unresponsive to treatment resulted in clinical relapse-free survival of 91% at 1 year and 19% at 5 years, with a rapid and sustained improvement in CD. One randomized trial of autologous HSCT for CD did not result in a statistically significant improvement in sustained disease remission at the end of 1 year, and concluded that the use of HSCT is not an acceptable treatment option for patients with refractory CD compared to conventional therapy. However, another multicenter retrospective study supported the safety and efficacy of autologous HSCT in patients with severe CD [151–154].

Moreover, bone marrow-derived MSC transplantation was associated with significantly lower clinical CD activity. Extended ex vivo autologous BM-MSC has been shown to be a safe and feasible method for intrafistular injection in patients with CD. Additionally, Local administration of ex vivo expanded adipose-derived MSC with a fibrin glue caused fistula healing in ~70% of treated patients when compared to those treated with fibrin glue alone as a control. Locally injected Alofisel, allogeneic adipose tissue derived mesenchymal stem cells, in perianal fistulas in patients with CD induced beneficial effects. This drug has been approved in Europe [155, 156]. On the contrary, systemic infusion of autologous BM-MSC

TABLE 8 Ongoing clinical trials of Crohn's disease with ATMP products.

Type of ATMP	Cell type/intervention	Source	Administration route		Start date	Study phase	Trial status	Trial number
			Systemic	Local				
Cell therapy	Mesenchymal stem cells	–	√		2007	3	Completed	NCT00482092
	Mesenchymal stem cells	–	√		2010	2	Completed	NCT01090817 NCT01233960
	Human placenta-derived cells	Placenta	√		2010	2	Completed	NCT01155362
	Allogenic mesenchymal stem cells	–	√		2012	1, 2	Unknown	NCT01540292
	Autologous stem cells	Peripheral blood	√		2012	1, 2	Recruiting	NCT00692939
	Mesenchymal stem cells	Umbilical cord	√		2012	1, 2	Completed	NCT02445547
	Human placenta-derived cells	Placenta	√		2013	1	Completed	NCT01769755
	Autologous antigen-specific regulatory T lymphocyte (Ovasave)	Peripheral blood	√		2014	2	Terminated	NCT02327221
	Stem cells	Umbilical cord blood	√		2014	1, 2	Unknown	NCT02000362
	Stromal vascular fraction	Adipose tissue		√	2015	1, 2	Completed	NCT02520843
	Autologous centrifuged adipose tissue	Adipose tissue		√	2016	Not applicable	Completed	NCT04326907
	Autologous regenerative cells	Adipose tissue		√	2018	Not applicable	Active, not recruiting	NCT03466515
	Autologous regulatory T cells	Peripheral blood	√		2018	1, 2	Not yet recruiting	NCT03185000
	Autologous hematopoietic stem cells	Peripheral blood	√		2019	2	Withdrawn	NCT04154735
	Allogenic mesenchymal stem cells	Bone marrow		√	2020	1, 2	Not yet recruiting	NCT04519697 NCT04519671

TABLE 9 Ongoing clinical trials of ulcerative colitis with ATMP products.

Type of ATMP	Cell type/intervention	Source	Administration route		Start date	Study phase	Trial status	Trial number
			Systemic	Local				
Cell therapy	Mesenchymal stem cells	Umbilical cord	√		2010	1, 2	Unknown	NCT01221428
	Allogenic mesenchymal stem cells	Adipose tissue		√	2013	1, 2	Unknown	NCT01914887
	Mesenchymal stem cells	Umbilical cord	√		2015	1, 2	Unknown	NCT02442037
	Allogenic mesenchymal stem cells	Adipose tissue		√	2018	1, 2	Recruiting	NCT03609905
	Allogenic mesenchymal stem cells	Bone marrow		√	2020	1, 2	Not yet recruiting	NCT04543994
	Autologous mesenchymal stem cells	Adipose tissue	√		2020	1	Not yet recruiting	NCT04312113

did not lead to disease remission, despite this, autologous MSC from all patients suppressed T-cell proliferation in vitro, indicating that differences in patient outcomes were not caused by defects in the MSC immunomodulatory capabilities but are potentially due to differences in the route of administration [157, 158].

Cell therapy for UC

Until now, four single-arm clinical trials evaluated MSC transplantation in patients with UC, in which the healing rate of MSC therapy was higher than that of the 5-aminosalicylic acids (5-ASA) and azathioprine therapies. Clinical trials with the control group showed that BM-MSCs were significantly associated with improved healing rate as compared with 5-ASA. Furthermore, in a phase I clinical trial of seven patients with IBD (four patients with CD and three with UC) were treated with intravenous allogeneic MSCs, while continuing their treatment regimens with steroids and/or immunosuppressive agents. After 3 months, a significant reduction in CD activity index (CDAI) and UC clinical activity index (CAI) scores were observed in all patients, as remission was achieved in five out of the seven patients (two patients with CD and three patients with UC). In addition, endoscopic improvement was observed. Due to the lack of data homogeneity compared with biological agents, more studies are needed to provide sufficient evidence [150, 159, 160].

2.6 Systemic lupus erythematosus

Systemic lupus erythematosus (SLE) is a systemic autoimmune disease characterized by aberrant activation of lymphocytes and generation of autoantibodies against a variety of autoantigens including DNA, RNA, ribonuclear proteins, phospholipids, and histones, which can lead to multiorgan dysfunction. There is a wide spectrum of symptoms attributed to SLE, however, manifested symptoms in each patient depend on what part of the body is being attacked [161, 162]. SLE treatment depends on the severity of the symptoms and the severity of organs' involvement. Conventional immunosuppressive therapies include cyclophosphamide (CYC) and mycophenolate mofetil (MMF). Several new strategies have been developed to target specific activation pathways relevant to SLE pathogenesis such as B cell-depleting therapies using the monoclonal antibodies, rituximab and belimumab. Patients are rarely cured using these treatments and lifelong treatment is often required [161–163] (Table 10).

2.6.1 *Cell therapy*

SLE has been treated with MSCs for over 10 years. Several single/multicenter clinical studies have been conducted on the safety and efficacy of MSC therapy for SLE. It has been shown that MSCs could improve the disease activity, proteinuria, and hypocomplementemia (markers of disease activity) in these patients. However, there existed some relapsed cases during long-term follow-up. Additionally, it has been revealed that although allogeneic MSCs are promising candidates for treating SLE, autologous MSCs may not be eligible to treat SLE patients because of their defective immunomodulatory function and poor regenerative characteristics. Moreover, HSCT has been reported to improve disease condition in refractory SLE, though relapse of the original disease increased with longer follow-up. As promising as the results of these studies sound, large-scale and high-quality randomized controlled trials are required to validate the efficacy of MSC treatment in SLE patients [164–167].

TABLE 10 Ongoing clinical trials of systemic lupus erythematosus with ATMP products.

Type of ATMP	Cell type/intervention	Source	Administration route		Start date	Study phase	Trial status	Trial number
			Systemic	Local				
Cell therapy	Allogenic hematopoietic stem cells	Peripheral blood	√		2004	1	Unknown	NCT00325741
	Hematopoietic stem cells	Peripheral blood			2005	2	Withdrawn	NCT00230035
	Autologous hematopoietic stem cells	Peripheral blood	√		2008	2	Unknown	NCT00750971
	Autologous regulatory T cells	Peripheral blood	√		2015	1	Terminated	NCT02428309
	Autologous EBV-specific cytotoxic T cells	Peripheral blood	√		2016	1, 2	Active, not recruiting	NCT02677688
	Mesenchymal stem cells	Umbilical cord	√		2017	1	Unknown	NCT03219801
	Allogenic mesenchymal stem cells	Bone marrow	√		2017	1	Recruiting	NCT03174587
	Allogeneic mesenchymal stem cells	Umbilical cord	√		2017	1	Completed	NCT03171194
	Mesenchymal stem cells	Umbilical cord	√		2018	1, 2	Not yet recruiting	NCT03562065
	Mesenchymal stem cells	Umbilical cord	√		2018	2	Recruiting	NCT02633163
	Mesenchymal stem cells	Umbilical cord	√		2019	2	Recruiting	NCT03917797
	Allogenic mesenchymal stem cells	Olfactory mucosa	√		2019	1, 2	Recruiting	NCT04184258

2.7 Autoimmune vasculitis

Vasculitis is a common autoimmune disease characterized by inflammation of the blood vessels. The inflamed blood vessel can be narrowed down obstructing the flow of blood to major body organs. In severe vasculitis, the blood vessel can become weak or stretched until it causes an aneurysm. The systemic signs of the disease are fever, headache, loss of appetite, fatigue, pain and aching of the body, night sweats, rash, nervous problems, and loss of pulse in the limb. Treatment of vasculitis depends on the cause and symptoms of the underlying disease and the specific organs of the body that are affected. Conventional drugs include prednisone, cyclophosphamide, methylprednisolone, and pentoxifylline. Refractory vasculitis has been treated through cell-based therapies [168, 169] (Table 11).

TABLE 11 Ongoing clinical trials of autoimmune vasculitis with ATMP products.

| Type of ATMP | Cell type/ intervention | Source | Administration route | | Start date | Study phase | Trial status | Trial number |
			Systemic	Local				
Cell therapy	Autologous hematopoietic stem cells	Peripheral blood	√		2003	1	Terminated	NCT00278512

2.7.1 *Cell therapy*

As published in European league against rheumatism (EULAR) and European bone marrow transplantation (EBMT) databases, autologous as well as allogeneic HSCT has resulted in long-lasting partial remission or even complete remission in refractory cases of systemic vasculitis. However, relapses occur in both treatments. Since the clinical data are sparse due to the limited number of patients, further studies and long-term documentation of the cases are necessary to assess the value and potentials of this treatment option in the future [169, 170].

3 Conclusion

Cell-based treatments have attracted tremendous attention from different researchers and clinicians, specifically for incurable diseases such as autoimmune disorders, inherited genetic diseases, blood related disorders, malignancies, neurodegenerative diseases, and conditions which required tissue regeneration.

Overall, with a note to antiinflammatory and regenerative characteristics of different cell-based products, the criteria regarding the efficacy of each ATMPs show optimistic results. Also, the total numbers of adverse events are not very high, so these products which have been approved by different regulatory agencies are considered as safe products.

Cellular therapy is expected to be a promising area used for the treatment of a noticeable quantity of incurable disorders, catching a special place in the future of medicine. However, limiting factors regarding the use of ATMPs should be still overcome, including the demand for high-technology systems for cell manufacturing and delivery, establishment of validated assays to check products potency, the high costs of these products, and their difficulties in the fund reimbursement. In this regard, since advanced therapy medicinal products strategies might become a solution for treatment of still incurable diseases and due to massive industrial investments in this field, it could be claimed that this field has the potential to overcome many of the mentioned limitations in a near future to reach a revolutionary phase in the pharma industry and the clinics.

References

[1] G. Detela, A. Lodge, EU regulatory pathways for ATMPs: standard, accelerated and adaptive pathways to marketing authorisation, Mol. Ther. Methods Clin. Dev. 13 (2019) 205–232.

[2] E. Hanna, et al., Advanced therapy medicinal products: current and future perspectives, J. Market Access Health Policy 4 (2016).

[3] C. Iglesias-Lopez, et al., Regulatory framework for advanced therapy medicinal products in Europe and United States, Front. Pharmacol. 10 (2019) 921.

[4] Cellular & Gene Therapy Products, FDA [Internet], [cited 2020 May 11], Available from: https://www.fda.gov/vaccines-blood-biologics/cellular-gene-therapy-products.

[5] M. Choi, et al., Regulatory oversight of gene therapy and cell therapy products in Korea, Adv. Exp. Med. Biol. 871 (2015) 163–179.

[6] Internet, P.O.o.t.E, Study on the Regulation of Advanced Therapies in Selected Jurisdictions, 2020, Available from: https://op.europa.eu/en/publication-detail/-/publication/78af6082-bc4a-11e6-a237-01aa75ed71a1.

[7] X.R. Luria Beate Schmidt, et al., BIOREG (SOE3/P1/E750)-Co-financed by the INTERREG IVB SUDOE Program with ERDF Funds Handbook about Regulatory Guidelines and Procedures for the Preclinical and Clinical Stages of Advanced Therapy Medicinal Products (ATMPs) Reviewers: Editor [Internet], 2020.

[8] E. Hanna, et al., Risk of discontinuation of advanced therapy medicinal products clinical trials, J. Mark. Access Health Policy 4 (2016).

[9] Y.S. Kim, et al., An overview of the tissue engineering market in the United States from 2011 to 2018, Tissue Eng. Part A 25 (1–2) (2019) 1–8.

[10] R.M.T. Ten Ham, et al., Challenges in advanced therapy medicinal product development: a survey among companies in Europe, Mol. Ther. Methods Clin. Dev. 11 (2018) 121–130.

[11] L. Buckler, 9 Challenges Keeping Cell and Gene Therapy Executives Up at Night [Internet], RepliCel Life Sciences Inc, 2018.

[12] N.M. Mount, et al., Cell-based therapy technology classifications and translational challenges, Philos. Trans. R. Soc. Lond. Ser. B Biol. Sci. 370 (1680) (2015) 20150017.

[13] A. Elsanhoury, et al., Accelerating patients' access to advanced therapies in the EU, Mol. Ther. Methods Clin. Dev. 7 (2017) 15–19.

[14] M. Vigano, et al., Tips and tricks for validation of quality control analytical methods in good manufacturing practice mesenchymal stromal cell production, Stem Cells Int. 2018 (2018) 3038565.

[15] G. Warnock, et al., Continued function of pancreatic islets after transplantation in type I diabetes, Lancet (London, England) 2 (8662) (1989) 570–572.

[16] D.W. Scharp, et al., Insulin independence after islet transplantation into type I diabetic patient, Diabetes 39 (4) (1990) 515–518.

[17] A.J. Shapiro, et al., Islet transplantation in seven patients with type 1 diabetes mellitus using a glucocorticoid-free immunosuppressive regimen, N. Engl. J. Med. 343 (4) (2000) 230–238.

[18] A.J. Shapiro, et al., International trial of the Edmonton protocol for islet transplantation, N. Engl. J. Med. 355 (13) (2006) 1318–1330.

[19] E.A. Ryan, et al., Clinical outcomes and insulin secretion after islet transplantation with the Edmonton protocol, Diabetes 50 (4) (2001) 710–719.

[20] E.A. Ryan, et al., Five-year follow-up after clinical islet transplantation, Diabetes 54 (7) (2005) 2060–2069.

[21] B. Hirshberg, et al., Benefits and risks of solitary islet transplantation for type 1 diabetes using steroid-sparing immunosuppression: the National Institutes of Health experience, Diabetes Care 26 (12) (2003) 3288–3295.

[22] B.J. Hering, et al., Single-donor, marginal-dose islet transplantation in patients with type 1 diabetes, JAMA 293 (7) (2005) 830–835.

15. New advanced therapy medicinal products

[23] D.E. Sutherland, et al., Islet autotransplant outcomes after total pancreatectomy: a contrast to islet allograft outcomes, Transplantation 86 (12) (2008) 1799–1802.

[24] L. Badet, et al., Expectations and strategies regarding islet transplantation: metabolic data from the GRAGIL 2 trial, Transplantation 84 (1) (2007) 89–96.

[25] M.R. Rickels, et al., Islet cell hormonal responses to hypoglycemia after human islet transplantation for type 1 diabetes, Diabetes 54 (11) (2005) 3205–3211.

[26] M.R. Rickels, et al., Glycemic thresholds for activation of counterregulatory hormone and symptom responses in islet transplant recipients, J. Clin. Endocrinol. Metab. 92 (3) (2007) 873–879.

[27] A. Gangemi, et al., Islet transplantation for brittle type 1 diabetes: the UIC protocol, Am. J. Transplant. 8 (6) (2008) 1250–1261.

[28] F.B. Barton, et al., Improvement in outcomes of clinical islet transplantation: 1999–2010, Diabetes Care 35 (7) (2012) 1436–1445.

[29] G.L. Warnock, et al., A multi-year analysis of islet transplantation compared with intensive medical therapy on progression of complications in type 1 diabetes, Transplantation 86 (12) (2008) 1762–1766.

[30] T. Tharavanij, et al., Improved long-term health related quality of life after islet transplantation, Transplantation 86 (9) (2008) 1161.

[31] clinicaltrials, Pancreatic Islets and Parathyroid Gland Co-transplantation for Treatment of Type 1 Diabetes (PARADIGM), 2020. https://clinicaltrials.gov/ct2/show/NCT03977662.

[32] J.L. Argo, et al., Pancreatic resection with islet cell autotransplant for the treatment of severe chronic pancreatitis, Am. Surg. 74 (6) (2008) 530–537.

[33] T. Anazawa, et al., Human islet isolation for autologous transplantation: comparison of yield and function using SERVA/Nordmark versus Roche enzymes, Am. J. Transplant. 9 (10) (2009) 2383–2391.

[34] M.R. Rickels, et al., Improvement in β-cell secretory capacity after human islet transplantation according to the CIT07 protocol, Diabetes 62 (8) (2013) 2890–2897.

[35] B. Chandravanshi, R.R. Bhonde, Shielding engineered islets with mesenchymal stem cells enhance survival under hypoxia, J. Cell. Biochem. 118 (9) (2017) 2672–2683.

[36] F. Djouad, et al., Immunosuppressive effect of mesenchymal stem cells favors tumor growth in allogeneic animals, Blood 102 (10) (2003) 3837–3844.

[37] X.-H. Wu, et al., Reversal of hyperglycemia in diabetic rats by portal vein transplantation of islet-like cells generated from bone marrow mesenchymal stem cells, World J. Gastroenterol. 13 (24) (2007) 3342.

[38] A. Mesples, et al., Early immunotherapy using autologous adult stem cells reversed the effect of anti-pancreatic islets in recently diagnosed type 1 diabetes mellitus: preliminary results, Med. Sci. Monit. 19 (2013) 852.

[39] U.G. Thakkar, et al., Insulin-secreting adipose-derived mesenchymal stromal cells with bone marrow–derived hematopoietic stem cells from autologous and allogenic sources for type 1 diabetes mellitus, Cytotherapy 17 (7) (2015) 940–947.

[40] S. Dave, et al., Novel therapy for insulin-dependent diabetes mellitus: infusion of in vitro-generated insulin-secreting cells, Clin. Exp. Med. 15 (1) (2015) 41–45.

[41] P.-O. Carlsson, et al., Preserved β-cell function in type 1 diabetes by mesenchymal stromal cells, Diabetes 64 (2) (2015) 587–592.

[42] J.C. Voltarelli, et al., Autologous nonmyeloablative hematopoietic stem cell transplantation in newly diagnosed type 1 diabetes mellitus, JAMA 297 (14) (2007) 1568–1576.

[43] W. Gu, et al., Diabetic ketoacidosis at diagnosis influences complete remission after treatment with hematopoietic stem cell transplantation in adolescents with type 1 diabetes, Diabetes Care 35 (7) (2012) 1413–1419.

[44] M.-G. Roncarolo, M. Battaglia, Regulatory T-cell immunotherapy for tolerance to self antigens and alloantigens in humans, Nat. Rev. Immunol. 7 (8) (2007) 585–598.

[45] Y. Zhao, et al., Human cord blood stem cell-modulated regulatory T lymphocytes reverse the autoimmune-caused type 1 diabetes in nonobese diabetic (NOD) mice, PLoS One 4 (1) (2009) e4226.

[46] Y. Zhao, et al., Reversal of type 1 diabetes via islet β cell regeneration following immune modulation by cord blood-derived multipotent stem cells, BMC Med. 10 (1) (2012) 1–11.

[47] N. Marek-Trzonkowska, et al., Administration of CD4+ CD25highCD127− regulatory T cells preserves β-cell function in type 1 diabetes in children, Diabetes Care 35 (9) (2012) 1817–1820.

[48] J.A. Bluestone, et al., Type 1 diabetes immunotherapy using polyclonal regulatory T cells, Sci. Transl. Med. 7 (315) (2015) 315ra189.

[49] L.P. De Marquesini, et al., IFN-γ and IL-10 islet-antigen-specific T cell responses in autoantibody-negative first-degree relatives of patients with type 1 diabetes, Diabetologia 53 (7) (2010) 1451–1460.

[50] M. Van Sandwijk, F. Bemelman, I. Ten Berge, Immunosuppressive drugs after solid organ transplantation, Neth. J. Med. 71 (6) (2013) 281–289.

[51] P. Soon-Shiong, et al., Insulin independence in a type 1 diabetic patient after encapsulated islet transplantation, Lancet (London, England) 343 (8903) (1994) 950.

[52] A. Murua, et al., Cell microencapsulation technology: towards clinical application, J. Control. Release 132 (2) (2008) 76–83.

[53] N. Dadheech, A.J. Shapiro, Human induced pluripotent stem cells in the curative treatment of diabetes and potential impediments ahead, in: Cell Biology and Translational Medicine, vol. 5, Springer, 2018, pp. 25–35.

[54] M. Cito, et al., The potential and challenges of alternative sources of β cells for the cure of type 1 diabetes, Endocr. Connect. 7 (3) (2018) R114–R125.

[55] J.R. Millman, F.W. Pagliuca, Autologous pluripotent stem cell–derived β-like cells for diabetes cellular therapy, Diabetes 66 (5) (2017) 1111–1120.

[56] E. Akinci, et al., Reprogramming of pancreatic exocrine cells towards a beta (β) cell character using Pdx1, Ngn3 and MafA, Biochem. J. 442 (3) (2012) 539–550.

[57] Q. Zhou, et al., In vivo reprogramming of adult pancreatic exocrine cells to β-cells, Nature 455 (7213) (2008) 627–632.

[58] X. Xiao, et al., Endogenous reprogramming of alpha cells into beta cells, induced by viral gene therapy, reverses autoimmune diabetes, Cell Stem Cell 22 (1) (2018) 78–90. e4.

[59] I.B. McInnes, G. Schett, The pathogenesis of rheumatoid arthritis, N. Engl. J. Med. 365 (23) (2011) 2205–2219.

[60] T. Bongartz, et al., Anti-TNF antibody therapy in rheumatoid arthritis and the risk of serious infections and malignancies: systematic review and meta-analysis of rare harmful effects in randomized controlled trials, JAMA 295 (19) (2006) 2275–2285.

[61] C. Salliot, et al., Infections during tumour necrosis factor-alpha blocker therapy for rheumatic diseases in daily practice: a systematic retrospective study of 709 patients, Rheumatology (Oxford) 46 (2) (2007) 327–334.

[62] C. Fournier, Where do T cells stand in rheumatoid arthritis? Joint Bone Spine 72 (6) (2005) 527–532.

[63] A. Farini, et al., Clinical applications of mesenchymal stem cells in chronic diseases, Stem Cells Int. 2014 (2014) 306573.

[64] Y.M. Pers, et al., Mesenchymal stem cells for the management of inflammation in osteoarthritis: state of the art and perspectives, Osteoarthr. Cartil. 23 (11) (2015) 2027–2035.

[65] S. Shadmanfar, et al., Intra-articular knee implantation of autologous bone marrow-derived mesenchymal stromal cells in rheumatoid arthritis patients with knee involvement: results of a randomized, triple-blind, placebo-controlled phase 1/2 clinical trial, Cytotherapy 20 (4) (2018) 499–506.

[66] L. Wang, et al., Human umbilical cord mesenchymal stem cell therapy for patients with active rheumatoid arthritis: safety and efficacy, Stem Cells Dev. 22 (24) (2013) 3192–3202.

[67] L. Wang, et al., Efficacy and safety of umbilical cord mesenchymal stem cell therapy for rheumatoid arthritis patients: a prospective phase I/II study, Drug Des. Devel. Ther. 13 (2019) 4331–4340.

[68] T.H. Shin, et al., Human umbilical cord blood-stem cells direct macrophage polarization and block inflammasome activation to alleviate rheumatoid arthritis, Cell Death Dis. 7 (12) (2016) e2524.

[69] J.M. Alvaro-Gracia, et al., Intravenous administration of expanded allogeneic adipose-derived mesenchymal stem cells in refractory rheumatoid arthritis (Cx611): results of a multicentre, dose escalation, randomised, single-blind, placebo-controlled phase Ib/IIa clinical trial, Ann. Rheum. Dis. 76 (1) (2017) 196–202.

[70] D.J. Joske, et al., Autologous bone-marrow transplantation for rheumatoid arthritis, Lancet 350 (9074) (1997) 337–338.

[71] R.K. Burt, et al., Treatment of autoimmune disease by intense immunosuppressive conditioning and autologous hematopoietic stem cell transplantation, Blood 92 (10) (1998) 3505–3514.

[72] R.K. Burt, et al., Autologous hematopoietic stem cell transplantation in refractory rheumatoid arthritis: sustained response in two of four patients, Arthritis Rheum. 42 (11) (1999) 2281–2285.

[73] R.M. Steinman, Dendritic cells: understanding immunogenicity, Eur. J. Immunol. 37 (Suppl. 1) (2007) S53–S60.

[74] S.S. Diebold, Determination of T-cell fate by dendritic cells, Immunol. Cell Biol. 86 (5) (2008) 389–397.

[75] G.M. Bell, et al., Autologous tolerogenic dendritic cells for rheumatoid and inflammatory arthritis, Ann. Rheum. Dis. 76 (1) (2017) 227–234.

[76] A. Nakajima, Application of cellular gene therapy for rheumatoid arthritis, Mod. Rheumatol. 16 (5) (2006) 269–275.

[77] A.A. Deviatkin, et al., Emerging concepts and challenges in rheumatoid arthritis gene therapy, Biomedicines 8 (1) (2020) 9.

[78] C.H. Evans, et al., Gene transfer to human joints: progress toward a gene therapy of arthritis, Proc. Natl. Acad. Sci. U. S. A. 102 (24) (2005) 8698–8703.

[79] P.A. Muraro, R. Martin, Immunological questions on hematopoietic stem cell transplantation for multiple sclerosis, Bone Marrow Transplant. 32 (Suppl. 1) (2003) S41–S44.

[80] E.M. Frohman, M.K. Racke, C.S. Raine, Multiple sclerosis—the plaque and its pathogenesis, N. Engl. J. Med. 354 (9) (2006) 942–955.

[81] J.W. Prineas, et al., Multiple sclerosis: remyelination of nascent lesions, Ann. Neurol. 33 (2) (1993) 137–151.

[82] P. Patrikios, et al., Remyelination is extensive in a subset of multiple sclerosis patients, Brain 129 (Pt 12) (2006) 3165–3172.

[83] I.D. Duncan, A.B. Radcliff, Inherited and acquired disorders of myelin: the underlying myelin pathology, Exp. Neurol. 283 (Pt B) (2016) 452–475.

[84] A. Uccelli, A. Laroni, M.S. Freedman, Mesenchymal stem cells for the treatment of multiple sclerosis and other neurological diseases, Lancet Neurol. 10 (7) (2011) 649–656.

[85] N. Payne, et al., The prospect of stem cells as multi-faceted purveyors of immune modulation, repair and regeneration in multiple sclerosis, Curr. Stem Cell Res. Ther. 6 (1) (2011) 50–62.

[86] E. Zappia, et al., Mesenchymal stem cells ameliorate experimental autoimmune encephalomyelitis inducing T-cell anergy, Blood 106 (5) (2005) 1755–1761.

[87] J. Zhang, et al., Bone marrow stromal cells reduce axonal loss in experimental autoimmune encephalomyelitis mice, J. Neurosci. Res. 84 (3) (2006) 587–595.

[88] L. Bai, et al., Human bone marrow-derived mesenchymal stem cells induce Th2-polarized immune response and promote endogenous repair in animal models of multiple sclerosis, Glia 57 (11) (2009) 1192–1203.

[89] B. Yamout, et al., Bone marrow mesenchymal stem cell transplantation in patients with multiple sclerosis: a pilot study, J. Neuroimmunol. 227 (1–2) (2010) 185–189.

[90] D. Karussis, et al., Safety and immunological effects of mesenchymal stem cell transplantation in patients with multiple sclerosis and amyotrophic lateral sclerosis, Arch. Neurol. 67 (10) (2010) 1187–1194.

[91] M. Mohyeddin Bonab, et al., Does mesenchymal stem cell therapy help multiple sclerosis patients? Report of a pilot study, Iran. J. Immunol. 4 (1) (2007) 50–57.

[92] M. Rabusin, et al., Long-term outcomes of hematopoietic stem cell transplantation for severe treatment-resistant autoimmune cytopenia in children, Biol. Blood Marrow Transplant. 19 (4) (2013) 666–669.

[93] J.L. Shevchenko, et al., Autologous hematopoietic stem cell transplantation with reduced-intensity conditioning in multiple sclerosis, Exp. Hematol. 40 (11) (2012) 892–898.

[94] M.C. Pasquini, et al., Transplantation for autoimmune diseases in north and South America: a report of the Center for International Blood and Marrow Transplant Research, Biol. Blood Marrow Transplant. 18 (10) (2012) 1471–1478.

[95] G.L. Mancardi, et al., Autologous haematopoietic stem cell transplantation with an intermediate intensity conditioning regimen in multiple sclerosis: the Italian multi-centre experience, Mult. Scler. 18 (6) (2012) 835–842.

[96] E. Carreras, et al., CD34+ selected autologous peripheral blood stem cell transplantation for multiple sclerosis: report of toxicity and treatment results at one year of follow-up in 15 patients, Haematologica 88 (3) (2003) 306–314.

[97] J. Liang, et al., Allogeneic mesenchymal stem cells transplantation in treatment of multiple sclerosis, Mult. Scler. 15 (5) (2009) 644–646.

[98] J.F. Li, et al., The potential of human umbilical cord-derived mesenchymal stem cells as a novel cellular therapy for multiple sclerosis, Cell Transplant. 23 (Suppl. 1) (2014) S113–S122.

[99] G. Shroff, Transplantation of human embryonic stem cells in patients with multiple sclerosis and Lyme disease, Am. J. Case Rep. 17 (2016) 944–949.

[100] A. Alikhan, et al., Vitiligo: a comprehensive overview part I. Introduction, epidemiology, quality of life, diagnosis, differential diagnosis, associations, histopathology, etiology, and work-up, J. Am. Acad. Dermatol. 65 (3) (2011) 473–491.

[101] S.A. Birlea, et al., Trends in regenerative medicine: repigmentation in vitiligo through melanocyte stem cell mobilization, Med. Res. Rev. 37 (4) (2017) 907–935.

[102] N. van Geel, et al., A review of non-cultured epidermal cellular grafting in vitiligo, J. Cutan. Aesthet. Surg. 4 (1) (2011) 17–22.

[103] S. Vertuani, A. Owczarczyk-Saczonek, The use of adipose-derived stem cells in selected skin diseases (vitiligo, alopecia, and nonhealing wounds), Int. J. Mol. Sci. 2017 (2017) 4740709.

[104] J.H. Lee, D.E. Fisher, Melanocyte stem cells as potential therapeutics in skin disorders, Expert. Opin. Biol. Ther. 14 (11) (2014) 1569–1579.

[105] Y. Gauthier, L. Benzekri, Non-cultured epidermal suspension in vitiligo: from laboratory to clinic, Indian J. Dermatol. Venereol. Leprol. 78 (1) (2012) 59–63.

[106] S. Zokaei, et al., Cultured epidermal melanocyte transplantation in vitiligo: a review article, Iran. J. Public Health 48 (3) (2019) 388–399.

[107] I. Majid, Grafting in vitiligo: how to get better results and how to avoid complications, J. Cutan. Aesthet. Surg. 6 (2) (2013) 83–89.

[108] V. Cervelli, et al., Treatment of stable vitiligo by ReCell system, Stem Cells Int. 17 (4) (2009) 273–278.

[109] N. van Geel, et al., Double-blind placebo-controlled study of autologous transplanted epidermal cell suspensions for repigmenting vitiligo, Arch. Dermatol. 140 (10) (2004) 1203–1208.

[110] N. van Geel, et al., Long-term results of noncultured epidermal cellular grafting in vitiligo, halo naevi, piebaldism and naevus depigmentosus, Br. J. Dermatol. 163 (6) (2010) 1186–1193.

[111] R.H. Huggins, et al., Melanocyte-keratinocyte transplantation procedure in the treatment of vitiligo: the experience of an academic medical center in the United States, J. Am. Acad. Dermatol. 66 (5) (2012) 785–793.

[112] P. Toossi, et al., Non-cultured melanocyte-keratinocyte transplantation for the treatment of vitiligo: a clinical trial in an Iranian population, J. Eur. Acad. Dermatol. Venereol. 25 (10) (2011) 1182–1186.

[113] P. Fioramonti, et al., Autologous cultured melanocytes in vitiligo treatment comparison of two techniques to prepare the recipient site: erbium-doped yttrium aluminum garnet laser versus dermabrasion, Dermatol. Surg. 38 (5) (2012) 809–812.

[114] P.C. Eves, et al., Establishing a transport protocol for the delivery of melanocytes and keratinocytes for the treatment of vitiligo, Tissue Eng. Part C Methods 17 (4) (2011) 375–382.

[115] D. Singh, et al., Scleroderma: an insight into causes, pathogenesis and treatment strategies, Pathophysiology 26 (2) (2019) 103–114.

[116] O. Distler, A. Cozzio, Systemic sclerosis and localized scleroderma—current concepts and novel targets for therapy, Semin. Immunopathol. 38 (1) (2016) 87–95.

[117] S.D. Sule, F.M. Wigley, Treatment of scleroderma: an update, Expert Opin. Investig. Drugs 12 (3) (2003) 471–482.

[118] A. Tyndall, et al., Treatment of systemic sclerosis with autologous haemopoietic stem cell transplantation, Lancet 349 (9047) (1997) 254.

[119] L. Keyes-Elstein, et al., Safety and efficacy of HSCT for systemic sclerosis across clinical trials, Nat. Rev. Rheumatol. 16 (2020) 661.

[120] U.A. Walker, L.A. Saketkoo, O. Distler, Haematopoietic stem cell transplantation in systemic sclerosis, RMD Open 4 (1) (2018), e000533.

[121] K.M. Sullivan, et al., Review: hematopoietic stem cell transplantation for scleroderma: effective immunomodulatory therapy for patients with pulmonary involvement, Arthritis Rheumatol. 68 (10) (2016) 2361–2371.

[122] J.M. van Laar, et al., Autologous hematopoietic stem cell transplantation vs intravenous pulse cyclophosphamide in diffuse cutaneous systemic sclerosis: a randomized clinical trial, JAMA 311 (24) (2014) 2490–2498.

[123] A.L. Strong, et al., Fat grafting for the treatment of scleroderma, Plast. Reconstr. Surg. 144 (6) (2019) 1498–1507.

[124] A.T. Maria, et al., Adipose-derived mesenchymal stem cells in autoimmune disorders: state of the art and perspectives for systemic sclerosis, Clin. Rev. Allergy Immunol. 52 (2) (2017) 234–259.

[125] P. Guillaume-Jugnot, et al., Autologous adipose-derived stromal vascular fraction in patients with systemic sclerosis: 12-month follow-up, Rheumatology (Oxford) 55 (2) (2016) 301–306.

[126] N. Scuderi, et al., Human adipose-derived stromal cells for cell-based therapies in the treatment of systemic sclerosis, Cell Transplant. 22 (5) (2013) 779–795.

[127] M.F. Griffin, A. Almadori, P.E. Butler, Use of lipotransfer in scleroderma, Nat. Rev. Rheumatol. 37 (suppl_3) (2017) S33–S37.

[128] J. Yamagami, Recent advances in the understanding and treatment of pemphigus and pemphigoid, F1000Res 7 (2018).

15. New advanced therapy medicinal products

[129] K. Izumi, K. Bieber, R.J. Ludwig, Current clinical trials in pemphigus and pemphigoid, Front. Immunol. 10 (2019) 978.
[130] D. Didona, et al., Pemphigus: current and future therapeutic strategies, Front. Immunol. 10 (2019) 1418.
[131] C.T. Ellebrecht, A.S. Payne, Setting the target for pemphigus vulgaris therapy, JCI Insight 2 (5) (2017) e92021.
[132] A.V. Vanikar, et al., Hematopoietic stem cell transplantation in autoimmune diseases: the Ahmedabad experience, Transplant. Proc. 39 (3) (2007) 703–708.
[133] A.V. Vanikar, et al., Allogenic hematopoietic stem cell transplantation in pemphigus vulgaris: a single-center experience, Indian J. Dermatol. 57 (1) (2012) 9–11.
[134] A. Albaghdadi, Current and under development treatment modalities of psoriasis: a review, Endocr. Metab. Immune Disord. Drug Targets 17 (3) (2017) 189–199.
[135] W.B. Kim, D. Jerome, J. Yeung, Diagnosis and management of psoriasis, Can. Fam. Physician 63 (4) (2017) 278–285.
[136] A. Osmancevic, M. Ståhle, Treatment of psoriasis: before and now, Lakartidningen 114 (2017) 1–13.
[137] A. Owczarczyk-Saczonek, et al., Stem cells as potential candidates for psoriasis cell-replacement therapy, Int. J. Mol. Sci. 18 (10) (2017) 1–16.
[138] B.H. Kaffenberger, et al., Remission of psoriasis after allogeneic, but not autologous, hematopoietic stem-cell transplantation, J. Am. Acad. Dermatol. 68 (3) (2013) 489–492.
[139] M.M. De Jesus, et al., Autologous adipose-derived mesenchymal stromal cells for the treatment of psoriasis vulgaris and psoriatic arthritis: a case report, Cell Transplant. 25 (11) (2016) 2063–2069.
[140] S.G. Wang, et al., Successful treatment of plaque psoriasis with allogeneic gingival mesenchymal stem cells: a case study, 2020 (2020) 4617520.
[141] S. Yoosuf, G.K. Makharia, Evolving therapy for celiac disease, Front. Pediatr. 7 (2019) 193.
[142] A.C. Piscaglia, Intestinal stem cells and celiac disease, World J. Stem Cells 6 (2) (2014) 213–229.
[143] A. Moheb-Alian, et al., Mesenchymal stem cells as potential therapeutic approaches in celiac disease, Gastroenterol. Hepatol. Bed Bench 9 (Suppl. 1) (2016) S1–S7.
[144] A. Al-toma, et al., Autologous hematopoietic stem cell transplantation in refractory celiac disease with aberrant T cells, Blood 109 (5) (2007) 2243–2249.
[145] R. Ciccocioppo, et al., A refractory celiac patient successfully treated with mesenchymal stem cell infusions, Mayo Clin. Proc. 91 (6) (2016) 812–819.
[146] J.K. Ko, K.K. Auyeung, Inflammatory bowel disease: etiology, pathogenesis and current therapy, Curr. Pharm. Des. 20 (7) (2014) 1082–1096.
[147] B.P. Abraham, T. Ahmed, T. Ali, Inflammatory bowel disease: pathophysiology and current therapeutic approaches, Handb. Exp. Pharmacol. 239 (2017) 115–146.
[148] H. Nakase, Current status and future of inflammatory bowel disease treatment, Nihon Shokakibyo Gakkai Zasshi 116 (3) (2019) 185–192.
[149] C.L. Hvas, et al., Current, experimental, and future treatments in inflammatory bowel disease: a clinical review, Immunopharmacol. Immunotoxicol. 40 (6) (2018) 446–460.
[150] A. Kashyap, S.J. Forman, Autologous bone marrow transplantation for non-Hodgkin's lymphoma resulting in long-term remission of coincidental Crohn's disease, Br. J. Haematol. 103 (3) (1998) 651–652.
[151] M.A. Ruiz, et al., Hematopoietic stem cell transplantation for Crohn's disease: gaps, doubts and perspectives, World J. Stem Cells 10 (10) (2018) 134–137.
[152] C.K. Brierley, et al., Autologous haematopoietic stem cell transplantation for Crohn's disease: a retrospective survey of long-term outcomes from the European Society for Blood and Marrow Transplantation, J. Crohns Colitis 12 (9) (2018) 1097–1103.
[153] M. Ditschkowski, et al., Improvement of inflammatory bowel disease after allogeneic stem-cell transplantation, Transplantation 75 (10) (2003) 1745–1747.
[154] D. García-Olmo, et al., A phase I clinical trial of the treatment of Crohn's fistula by adipose mesenchymal stem cell transplantation, Dis. Colon Rectum 48 (7) (2005) 1416–1423.
[155] L.J. Scott, Darvadstrocel: a review in treatment-refractory complex perianal fistulas in Crohn's disease, BioDrugs 32 (6) (2018) 627–634.
[156] B. Verstockt, et al., New treatment options for inflammatory bowel diseases, J. Gastroenterol. 53 (5) (2018) 585–590.
[157] H. Shimizu, et al., Stem cell-based therapy for inflammatory bowel disease, Intest. Res. 17 (3) (2019) 311–316.

[158] M.C. Barnhoorn, et al., Long-term evaluation of allogeneic bone marrow-derived mesenchymal stromal cell therapy for Crohn's disease perianal fistulas, J. Crohns Colitis 14 (1) (2020) 64–70.

[159] X. Shi, Q. Chen, F. Wang, Mesenchymal stem cells for the treatment of ulcerative colitis: a systematic review and meta-analysis of experimental and clinical studies, Stem Cell Res. Ther. 10 (1) (2019) 266.

[160] G.A. Salem, G.B. Selby, Stem cell transplant in inflammatory bowel disease: a promising modality of treatment for a complicated disease course, Stem Cell Res. Ther. 4 (2017) 95.

[161] D. Zucchi, et al., One year in review 2019: systemic lupus erythematosus, Clin. Exp. Rheumatol. 37 (5) (2019) 715–722.

[162] A.A. Justiz Vaillant, et al., Systemic lupus erythematosus (SLE), in: StatPearls, StatPearls Publishing Copyright © 2020, StatPearls Publishing LLC, Treasure Island, FL, 2020.

[163] K. Ichinose, Unmet needs in systemic lupus erythematosus, Nihon Rinsho Meneki Gakkai Kaishi 40 (6) (2017) 396–407.

[164] R.J. Cheng, et al., Mesenchymal stem cells: allogeneic MSC may be immunosuppressive but autologous MSC are dysfunctional in lupus patients, Front. Cell Dev. Biol. 7 (2019) 285.

[165] J. Liang, et al., Allogenic mesenchymal stem cells transplantation in refractory systemic lupus erythematosus: a pilot clinical study, Ann. Rheum. Dis. 69 (8) (2010) 1423–1429.

[166] D. Wang, et al., Umbilical cord mesenchymal stem cell transplantation in active and refractory systemic lupus erythematosus: a multicenter clinical study, Arthritis Res. Ther. 16 (2) (2014) R79.

[167] N.L. de Silva, S.L. Seneviratne, Haemopoietic stem cell transplantation in systemic lupus erythematosus: a systematic review, Allergy Asthma Clin. Immunol. 15 (2019) 59.

[168] E. Shavit, A. Alavi, R.G. Sibbald, Vasculitis-what do we have to know? A review of literature, Int. J. Low Extrem. Wounds 17 (4) (2018) 218–226.

[169] C. Fiehn, A.D. Ho, H.M. Lorenz, Hematopoietic stem cell transplantation (HSCT) for primary systemic vasculitis and related diseases, Autoimmunity 41 (8) (2008) 648–653.

[170] L. Liao, Mesenchymal stem cell and hematopoietic stem cell transplantation for vasculitis, Vasc. Invest. Ther. 3 (2020) 88–93.

CHAPTER

16

Targeting autoimmune disorders through metal nanoformulation in overcoming the fences of conventional treatment approaches

Krishna Yadav[a], Madhulika Pradhan[b], Deependra Singh[a], and Manju Rawat Singh[a],*

[a]University Institute of Pharmacy, Pt. Ravishankar Shukla University, Raipur, Chhattisgarh, India [b]Rungta College of Pharmaceutical Sciences and Research, Bhilai, Chhattisgarh, India
*Corresponding author

Abstract

Nanomedicine is a rapidly developing area of medicine with promising applications in molecular nanotechnology for safe, effective, and precise drug delivery. To date, many inorganic and polymeric nanoparticles (NPs) with and without surface modifications have been produced for selective drug delivery. An autoimmune disorder is a self-destructive immune cell condition that affects various body tissues and organs. Poor penetration and nonspecific delivery of therapeutic constituents to the targeted cells, which contributes to insufficient therapeutic effectiveness, is one of the main obstacles in targeting therapy for autoimmune diseases. Metallic nanoparticles provide a number of scopes in biomedical applications including diagnosis, treatment, and immunotherapy. Metal nanoparticles (MeNPs) (gold, silver, etc.) may suppress the immune system, causing a strong reaction to threatening cells. They are useful for drug targeting because of their nanosize, nontoxic properties, charge, and ease of high surface functionalization—all of which make them good carriers for drug transportation. This chapter intends to examine numerous strategic methods by integrating material science and immunobioengineering expertise for the safe and efficient delivery of metal-based nanoparticles for the treatment of various autoimmune disorders. Furthermore, the toxicity and safety issues of these metallic NPs are systematically presented.

Keywords

Metallic-nanoparticle, Autoimmune disorders, Nanomedicines, Targeting, Autoimmunity

1 Introduction

Nanotechnology has been widely used in several fields of research for decades, including submolecular chemistry, physics, quantum mechanics, material science, and bioengineering. This multidisciplinary science combines biophysics, atomic research, medicines, tissue engineering, and genetic biology, among other areas. Nanotechnology has shown potential in several clinical fields, including endocrinology, immunology, oncology, cardiology, ophthalmology, and so on. It is also commonly used in advanced fields including brain and tumor cell targeting and gene delivery [1, 2]. The development of nanotechnology in biomedical and medical research contributes to positive progress in conventional drug delivery approaches. It has built a significant method, tools, and materials to enhance pharmaceutical applications. In the treatment of several diseases, transporting medicinal active compounds to the right site is a major obstacle [3]. Poor biodistribution, reduced adequacy, undesirable effects, and lack of selectivity are common problems associated with the conventional dosage form. Strategies, like controlling medication conveyance, can conceivably defeat these restrictions by transporting medication to the place of activity. Furthermore, the drug delivery systems protect against rapid debasement or leeway as well as improving drug concentration in target tissues [4]. A more consistent strategy in drug targeting is to aim at the cell or individual tissue using carriers that are independently engineered and connected to an active therapeutic. A more crucial and efficient approach that structures the premise of nanotechnology is reducing the scale of the delivery carrier and engineering its lanes for acceptable drug conveyance [5]. Nanoparticles (NPs) have tremendous potential as drug transporters, as shown by recent advances in nanotechnology (Fig. 1). Nanostructures with novel physicochemical and natural properties are created using size reduction strategies and advances. These methods transform nanostructures into usable materials for biomedical applications, gaining importance in the pharmaceutical sciences as a result. Furthermore, these techniques assist in the elimination of unfavorable side effects, improving the controlled release of medicaments, drug solvency and bioavailability, and the accomplishment of other delivery objectives. Nanotechnology

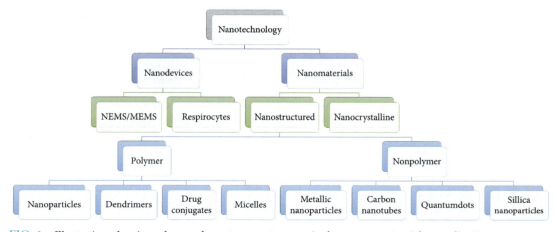

FIG. 1 Illustration of various classes of nanotransporters acquired awesome potential as medication transporters.

often improves the efficiency of active therapeutics in different dosage forms by allowing them to survive in nanoscales [6]. Nowadays, nanotechnology is seeking new applications in industries, researches, and medicine. Nanoparticles have been found to have distinct benefits in several biochemical, pathophysiological, and therapeutic applications. Nanoparticles may be rendered to evade immune system recognition or to directly restrain or upgrade immune responses. We also reviewed comprehensive perspectives on a nanoparticle in the treatment and targeting of medicine for different autoimmune disorders, focusing on possible theories on how particle physicochemical attributes may influence their interactions with immune cells to achieve alluring immunomodulation and escape unnecessary immunotoxicity.

The immune system protects us from native and external microorganisms such as microbes, viruses, and parasites that can affect the body in healthy people. However, in less population, this protection may be misdirected against the body's own tissues and cells, resulting in autoimmunity. Autoimmune disorders develop as a result of these occurrences. In normal situations, the immune response is controlled by the advanced system to ensure the host tissue is not attacked. Autoimmunity is characterized as a malfunction of the immune system in which antibodies (autoantibodies) and autoreactive immune cells invade the body's own tissues, resulting in immune system diseases [7]. According to the National Institute of Health (NIH), about 23.5 million Americans suffer from immune system dysfunction, and its prevalence is increasing. A total of 80–100 distinct autoimmune disorders have been identified by researchers [8]. All of these are long-lasting and potentially dangerous, with side effects varying over time. Autoimmune disorders are one of the top 10 causes of death for young women and people of all ages (up to 64 years of age). In 2003, the NIH funded $591 million for the research on autoimmune diseases, whereas the direct health care cost is $100 billion every year [9, 10].

Autoimmune diseases are physiological conditions that arise due to lack of self-resistance and immune obliteration of host tissues. Autoimmunity is caused by a variety of cellular and molecular events and reactions. The progression of autoimmune disorders is a highly dynamic mechanism in which the lymphocyte identification of self-antigens is intimately related to pathologic organ harm. Autoimmune disorders are complex characteristics of several loci controlling various facets of disease susceptibility [11]. Certain environmental influences, such as cigarette smoke, ultraviolet light, pathogens, and disease-causing agents, can interact with this genetic proclivity to initiate disease. Any immune system reaction is caused by a pathogen whose protein(s) shares auxiliary structural similarities with positions on the host's protein. As a result, antibodies induced against a pathogen can cross-react with a self-protein, forming autoantibodies, and the autoantigen in concern becomes a source of tenacious incitement [12, 13]. Even though the body includes a significant number of potentially autoreactive B and T cells, a range of factors function to create self-resistance during lymphocyte growth. This is particularly true for T cells that are not wiped out by self-epitopes. Autoantibodies form in animals when autoantigens are infused with adjuvants, signaling the production of autoreactive B cells in the healthy population (e.g., antithyroglobulin). When normal circulating T cells are activated by the required autoantigen (e.g. myelin critical protein) and interleukin-2, the involvement of autoreactive T cells in a healthy person is shown by the development of immune system lines of T cells [14].

The concept of autoimmunity was first proposed by Nobel Laureate Paul Ehrlich at the turn of the nineteenth century, and he called it "horror autotoxicus." His research led him to presume that the immune system is normally focused on responding to foreign materials and has an inbuilt tendency to avoid attacking self-tissues. When this mechanism is performed incorrectly, the immune system will attack self-tissues, resulting in autoimmune disease [15]. Ehrlich later redefined his hypothesis to perceive the probability of autoimmune tissue assaults but believed that certain inborn protection mechanisms would keep the immune reaction from becoming obsessive. The discovery of a material in the serum of a patient with paroxysmal cold hemoglobinuria that reacted to RBCs in 1904 put this theory to the test. Various diseases were related to allergic responses over the next several decades. The regulatory status of Ehrlich's theories, on the other hand, hindered understanding of these results. Immunology has devolved into a molecular science rather than a therapeutic one [16, 17]. The cutting-edge understanding of autoantibodies and immune system disorders started to propagate in the 1950s. Recently, it has been identified that autoimmune reactions are a critical component of the vertebrate immune system (also known as "natural autoimmunity"), which usually prevent disease production through the process of immunological tolerance to self-antigens [18].

Autoimmune disorders can be widely classified into systemic and organ-specific, contingent upon the foremost clinicopathologic character of each disorder. When the reaction is specifically directed toward antigens located only in certain organs, it is known as organ-specific, while when the reaction is directed toward antigens found in the body, it is classified as nonorgan specific. Many autoimmune diseases have been verified, and immune system components have been linked to the pathogenesis of a similar number of more persistent provocative conditions. Some autoimmune diseases affect a single organ (e.g., immune-mediated Hashimoto's thyroiditis), while others destroy several locations in a single organ system (e.g., immune-mediated vasculitis), while even others damage several organs through several processes (e.g., systemic lupus erythematosus [SLE]) [19, 20]. As a minimum, one autoimmune disorder has been recognized for almost every organ and tissue in the body. Although multiple autoimmune conditions target separate organs, diseases targeting a common location often have distinct clinical and pathological symptoms, more often owing to different antigenic boosts rather than anatomical and physiological variations among individuals. Other health disorders, including but not limited to atherosclerosis, amyotrophic lateral sclerosis, schizophrenia, infertility, and postmenopausal osteoporosis, may have an autoimmune component, according to thriving proof [21].

Treatment for autoimmune diseases normally entails addressing signs and monitoring the autoimmune mechanism while also attempting to maintain optimal immune function. Even though corticosteroids and other immunosuppressant medications do not function in all patients, they are nevertheless considered as front-line treatments. Furthermore, due to the activation of immunosuppression, these medications are attributed to severe adverse side effects [3]. Since these diseases affect the function of certain organs or tissues, remedial therapies may be needed to compensate for the tissues' reduced capacity as a result of autoimmune damage. Type 1 diabetics, for example, require long-term insulin substitution because their bodies refused to produce adequate insulin as a result of autoimmune destruction of pancreatic cells [22]. Similarly, patients with Addison's disease need regular pharmaceuticals to compensate for their failure to generate steroid hormones naturally [23]. Monoclonal antibodies, such as adalimumab, infliximab, and rituximab, have been incorporated with new therapeutic resources for coping with unsolicited inflammatory diseases in recent decades [24].

These drugs are examples of how a better understanding of the immune system and its regulatory mechanisms will lead to new therapies. However, such drugs are not uniformly convincing and should be used with caution due to the drawbacks of parenteral administration, a higher likelihood of diseases as a consequence of immunosuppression, a temporary effect, and a potential recurrence of disease if therapy is stopped for a prolonged period, as well as high prices. Nanomedicine approaches should be employed to resolve these problems to meet all future treatment targets. Nanotechnology has advantages over traditional medicine for autoimmune disorders, such as regulated and targeted delivery, fewer toxicities, and greater compatibility. Approaching autoimmune disorders at the nanoscale is a groundbreaking technology for solving many of the associated issues with various therapeutics for the management of autoimmune diseases. Therefore, this chapter focuses on metal nanoparticles (MeNPs) as nanomaterials in different autoimmune diseases in order to accomplish the therapeutic aim of various therapies available.

2 Nanotechnology and nanomaterials

Nanotechnology is a field of research that focuses on the mechanisms that take place at the subatomic level and how they function. Nanotechnology has evolved into an allied discipline that is commonly used in a variety of scientific fields. Nanotechnology is the analysis of materials for the building of ultra-tiny structures with measurements of 10^{-9}–10^{-7} m. Also, it is the study of materials, systems, nanoscale structures, and constituents that exhibit novel and alternate physical, synthetic, and biological properties. As a result, nanotechnology is described as the control of matter on a nuclear, subatomic, and supramolecular scale, as well as the design, development, characterization, and application of various nanoscale materials in various potential territories, primarily in the field of medicine [25]. This results in a self-contained division of nanostructures known as nanomedicine, which is mainly used for medicinal purposes. Nanomedicine includes the use of nanotechnology to enhance human health and prosperity. The European Science Foundation defines nanomedicine as "the science and invention of diagnosing, treating, and preventing disease and traumatic injury, of reducing pain, and of safeguarding and improving human health, using sub-atomic tools and sub-atomic learning of the human body" [26]. The utilization of nanotechnology in various clinical divisions has revolutionized the world of medicine, with nanoparticles being produced and used for therapeutics, diagnostics, and biomedical testing tools. Nanomaterials and nanoimaging devices, experimental therapeutics, drug conveyance methods, clinical and toxicological concerns are among the subdisciplines [27]. In the current scenario, an innovative method of nanomaterials is urgently needed for the diagnosis and treatment of a variety of diseases with significant assets, such as low affectability or precision, drug toxicities, and so on. These nanostructures are used as fluorescent materials and drug carriers with targeting antibodies, as well as being used as subatomic analysis instruments. Nanoparticulate materials, such as paramagnetic nanoparticles, nanoshells, quantum dots, and nanosomes, are currently being updated for analytical purposes. The nanoparticles-based delivery system provides various benefits [28] including:

✓ Expanded surface area
✓ Improved solvency

✓ An expanded rate of dissolution
✓ Diminished patient-to-persistent variability
✓ More rapid action of therapeutic activity
✓ Reduced dosing frequency
✓ Enhanced drug targeting and surface modifications
✓ Improve oral bioavailability
✓ Lessening poisonous quality of medications
✓ Augmentation in the stability of medication and formulation

As a significance of these advantages, the most efficient nanostructures are being upgraded, which can reform the drug manufacturing method and alter the scenario of pharmaceutical industries. Nanostructures have shown a guarantee of transporting a variety of molecules to desired locations in the body, based on their physicochemical properties. By focusing on nanomedicine, it is possible to improve the therapeutic index of drugs by increasing their viability and tolerance in the body [29]. Nanotechnology may also increase the bioavailability of water-insoluble drugs, protect therapeutic agents from physiological barriers, allow the development of new groups of bioactive macromolecules, and transport large payloads. Furthermore, combining imaging contrast agents within nanoparticles will allow for a drug delivery site that is exclusive to us, as well as testing the therapeutics' in vivo viability. Nanotechnology improves the protection profile of medications with elevated toxicity, and these nanoforms may be dynamically and passively coordinated to function specifically at the target tissue [30].

Nanoparticles are particles with a surrounding interfacial coating that is between 1 and 100 nm (nm) in dimension. The interfacial layer is an important component of nanoscale matter since it affects the bulk of its properties. Chemical and inorganic compounds, as well as ions, make up the interfacial base. Stabilizers, surface ligands, coatings, and passivating agents are all examples of organic molecules that coat inorganic nanoparticles. A nanoparticle is a miniature entity in nanotechnology that possesses many of the properties of its parent molecule as well as additional features. Because of a broad range of possible uses in optical, electronics, and biomedical sectors, nanoparticle exploration is currently a highly rational study area [27, 29]. Nanoparticles are a hot subject of research and they may serve as a connection between mass materials and nuclear or atomic structures. Nanoparticles demonstrate an especially welcoming level, exhibiting novel properties with possible therapeutic applications. The enormous assorted applications of nanoparticles in biology and medicine are given as follows:

✓ Medical imaging
✓ Examining of DNA structure
✓ Fluorescent biological markers
✓ Detection of pathogens
✓ Site of proteins
✓ Tumor annihilation through warming (hyperthermia)
✓ Phagokinetic investigations
✓ Tissue bioengineering
✓ Malignant growth cell imaging
✓ Detachment and purging of cells and biological molecules

✓ Gene and drug targeting
✓ Treatment of cancerous cells

Because of their contrived adaptability and tunable properties (e.g., pH response, thermosensitivity), nanoparticles (NPs) are very appealing as drug delivery systems. Nanoparticles are typically in the 10–100 nm scale, which is almost identical to the size of human proteins. Nanoparticles hold exciting potential for improving cellular absorption, distribution, and targeting of metallodrugs, especially anticancer medications, making them more appealing and stable. The early detection of malignant cells, specific tumor biomarkers, as well as the enhancement of the effectiveness of associated medications, are all addressed through nanoparticle-based medicine conveyance approaches [31]. In addition, novel treatment modalities such as near-infrared thermal therapy for tumors via nanoshells and gene therapy are being developed. The capacity of nanomedicines in malignancy is subjected to passive targeting (because of the upgrade of the penetrability and maintenance retention impact advanced by angiogenic vessels), which can be improved by concentrating on specific cells (because of multifunctional nanomaterials that detour the natural hindrances and achieve tumor cells). Immunotherapy advancements have aided the production of several novel therapeutics, including nanoparticles, peptides and proteins, cellular treatments, and monoclonal antibodies. Progress in immunotherapy has steered the development of various promising therapeutics, including tiny molecules, peptides and proteins, cellular treatments, and monoclonal antibodies. Despite this abundance of new therapeutics, the viability of immunotherapy has been constrained by difficulties in targeted delivery and controlled drug release, that is, spatial and transient regulation on deliverance. Particulate carrier systems, especially nanoparticles, have been extensively studied in the fields of drug distribution and immunization, and are increasingly being investigated as vehicles for distributing immunotherapies [9]. Nonspecific take-up by phagocytic cells, pervasion by tissue (transport constraint), off-target biodistribution, nonspecific activation of immunity, and inadequate control over intracellular confinement are the issues that can be solved with a nanoparticle-based method. Nanoparticle-intervened drug conveyance could give various advantages, including control of transport kinetics and biodistribution, immunogenicity, the potential for site-directed delivery, tracking ability utilizing medical imaging, and multitherapeutic loading [32]. The usage of nanoparticles to target and deliver individual drugs decreases toxicity and unintended complications while also improving the clinical index of the administered drug. With the support of nanotechnology, it is now feasible to offer therapy at the atomic level, which could aid in the diagnosis and treatment of several diseases.

2.1 Classification of nanoparticles

To appropriately comprehend and appreciate the assorted variety of nanomaterial some types of classification systems are required. In recent times, the most typical method for categorizing nanomaterials is to distinguish them as per their dimensions [33]. Nanomaterials are classified as:

i. Zero-dimensional (0-D)
ii. One-dimensional (1-D)
iii. Two-dimensional (2-D)
iv. Three-dimensional (3-D)

16. Targeting autoimmune disorders

This categorization depends on the number of measurements of dimensions that are not limited to the nanoscale run (<100 nm). To begin with, zero-dimensional nanomaterials are products of which all measurements estimated on the nanoscale (any of measurement, or 0-D, are bigger than 100 nm). Nanodots are perhaps the most well-known depiction of zero-dimensional nanomaterials. This molecule may be crystalline, amorphous, or polycrystalline, made up of single or multiple chemical components, have various shapes and configurations exist separately, or fuse in a matrix, polymeric, metallic, or ceramic, and be made up of single or multiple chemical components. 1-D nanomaterials, on the other hand, vary from 0-D nanomaterials in that one of their measurements is below the nanoscale. Needle-like-molded nanomaterials are the product of this structure dimension differentiation. Nanorods, nanotubes, and nanowires are several instances of one-dimensional nanomaterials. This 1-D nanomaterial, as 0-D nanomaterials, may be amorphous, crystalline, or polycrystalline, chemically untainted or tainted, independent material or entrenched inside another medium and it could be ceramic, polymeric, or metallic. Nanomaterials of two dimensions that are not bound to nanoscale are classified as 2-D nanomaterials. The nanomaterials have a plate-like shape as a result of this method. Nanocoating, nanolayer, and nanofilms are also two-dimensional nanomaterials. These nanomaterials could be comprised of different chemical compositions by single or multilayer structures of amorphous or crystalline, retained on a substrate, coordinated in a covering matrix material, and framed with polymeric, ceramic, or metallic materials. Furthermore, materials that are not bound to the nanoscale in any dimension are considered 3-D nanomaterials, commonly known as bulk or mass nanomaterials. Three random dimensions of over 100 nm are used to characterize these products. Regardless of the existence of these optional measurements, these products are referred to as nanomaterials because they have a nanocrystalline structure or contain properties at the nanoscale in terms of nanocrystalline structure and may be constructed from a variety of nanosized crystal arrangements, most typically in different orientations. 3-D nanomaterials may contain dispersions of nanoparticles, a heap of nanowires and nanotubes, as well as multilayers when it comes to the appearance of characters at the nanoscale. Metal, polymeric, or ceramic materials may also be used to make three-dimensional nanomaterials and may be crystalline or amorphous composite materials. As a result of this dimension-based grouping approach, nanomaterials may be recognized and organized in three dimensions [34].

The nanoparticles are of various sizes, shapes, and structures. It could be spherical, round and hollow, tubular, funnel-shaped, hollow core, flat, spiral, and so forth, or irregular and contrast from 1 nm to 100 nm in size. The surface can be uniform or asymmetrical with surface varieties. Some nanoparticles are amorphous or crystalline with one or multicrystal solids either free or clustered. Based on the nature and composition of constructing elements nanoparticles can be classified into I. Organic, II. Inorganic and III. Carbon-based nanoparticles.

I. **Organic nanoparticles**: These nanoparticles are biodegradable, nontoxic, and vulnerable to electromagnetic and thermal radiation, such as light and heat. Apart from their traditional characteristics, such as structure, scale, surface morphology, and so on, the pharmaceutical carrying capability, durability, physicochemical properties, and conveyance potential of adsorbed or entrapped drugs define their area of usage and productivity. These distinguishing characteristics make them an excellent alternative for drug delivery. Organic nanoparticles are widely employed in the pharmaceutical

368

industry for medicine or medicinal entity delivery since they are efficient and can be infused on specific areas of the body, a process known as targeted medication conveyance. Liposomes, micelles, dendrimers, and ferritin are typically recognized as organic nanoparticles [35, 36].

II. **Inorganic nanoparticles:** These are nanosized particles that are not composed of carbon. Metal [iron (Fe), aluminum (Al), zinc (Zn), copper (Cu), lead (Pb), cobalt (Co), silver (Ag), gold (Au), and their oxide (Fe_2O_3, Al_2O_3, TiO_2, ZnO, etc.) based nanoparticles are commonly considered as inorganic nanoparticles [35, 37].

III. **Carbon-based nanoparticles:** The nanoparticles furnished totally of carbon are known as carbon-based nanoparticles. They can be categorized into graphene, fullerenes, carbon nanotubes (CNT), carbon black and carbon nanofibers, and occasionally activated charcoal in nanosize [35].

Herein, in this chapter, we have given an astonishing accentuation on metal and metal oxide-based nanoparticles and their trademark in the different viewpoints of targeting and drug delivery in terms of autoimmunity.

2.2 Metal-based nanoparticles

Metals have been used to produce various devices and firearms for animal chasing and agricultural procedures since ancient times. After that, people started to look at the different uses of metals in various areas, such as hardware, constructions, devices, coverings, automobiles, and eventually biology and medicine. Remarkably, only a few metals found in living organisms are particularly essential for the normal operation of the human body. Zinc, for example, plays an important role in a variety of biological processes, including normal development, metabolism, immunity, wound healing, and neurological and enzymatic responses [38]. Magnesium and calcium are necessary for the proper functioning of ATP (the body's primary supply of energy) during metabolism. Calcium is also needed for signal transmission, muscle function, bone regeneration, and cell wall synthesis [39]. Manganese is involved in several redox reactions in living organisms, including photosynthesis in plants [40]. Heme, which contains iron, is a cofactor in hemoglobin and is responsible for transporting oxygen in the blood in all vertebrates [41]. Iron can also be present in metalloproteins such as cytochrome P450, xanthine oxidase, and monooxygenase. Copper is used in hemocyanin, which transports oxygen in arthropods and mollusks' blood. Cobalt is the most important metal in the B12 vitamin, which its deficiency could lead to anemia. Furthermore, zinc, manganese, and copper are assumed to serve as cofactors in various superoxide dismutase enzymes, which improve the conversion of superoxide to hydrogen peroxide, a crucial signaling molecule in several biological processes [41]. Since the mid-1980s, scientists also made significant progress in learning how these various metals work in biological systems. Despite the fact that these metals/metal ions have extensive biological interactions in living organisms, they can exhibit higher levels of cytotoxicity when applied externally for diagnostic or therapeutic purposes. According to different sources, these metal nanoparticulate types (nanoparticles, nanospheres, nanorods, etc.) can be used for in vivo therapeutic applications owing to their remarkable and exceptional biological and physicochemical properties as compared to bulk forms of related metals [40].

The expression "metal nanoparticle" refers to nanosized metallic particles with dimensions (length, width, or thickness) between 1 and 100 nm. Faraday detected metallic nanoparticles in solution for the first time in 1857, and Mie provided a theoretical clarification of their coloring in 1908. Because of their unique properties, metal nanoparticles have been widely used in a variety of areas, including hardware, sensors, catalysis, coatings, materials, solar cells, food manufacturing, packaging skincare goods, and biomedical applications, according to a large body of literature. Because of their size (nanoscale array) similitudes, metal nanoparticles have been commonly used in bioscience and medicine because they are biocompatible and easily interact with proteins, receptors, and nucleic acids. Furthermore, after proper functionalization, metal nanoparticles are shown to be capable of binding drugs, nucleic acids, peptides, antibodies, proteins, and targeting agents for delivery of such biomolecules to the desired locations. Furthermore, several studies have shown that metal nanoparticles can be eliminated by urine and defecation, demonstrating their biodegradability. As a result, researchers have been exceedingly occupied with numerous research assignments for the development of alternative diagnostic and therapeutic nanomedicine strategies for the treatment of various disorders (e.g., diabetes, malignancy, ischemic ailments, and neurodegenerative disorders) by using metal nanoparticles for the past couple of decades [34, 42].

2.2.1 *Production of metallic NPs*

Two fundamental procedures are utilized to create nanoparticles: "top-down" and "bottom-up." The name "top-down" alludes here to the mechanical squashing of source material utilizing a milling procedure. It denotes mechanical-physical nanosized particle fabrication methods based on ideologies of microsystem technology. This methodology is applied in the production of ceramic and metallic nanomaterials. In the "bottom-up" system, structures are developed by chemical procedures. The choice of the particular procedure relies upon the chemical composition and the desired characteristics indicated for the nanoparticles. It involves precipitation reactions, sol–gel processes, and aerosol processes. Bottom-up strategies depend on the physicochemical attributes of subatomic or molecular self-association. This methodology produces preferred and more perplexing structures from molecules or atoms, with better-controlling sizes and shapes [34].

Different physical, chemical, and organic strategies are presently utilized for the fabrication of metallic NPs that ought to be preferably controllable in regards to size and shape, surface functionalization, desired morphologies, and maximum product yield with narrow formulation compositions. Defined production and response conditions are essential in acquiring such desired nanosize particles and other features. Particle size, shape, composition, and crystallinity can be controlled by temperature, change in pH, surface modifications, chemical composition, and process controls. Lack of solvent contamination, hazardous and perilous materials, and chemicals inside the fabricated thin films, and the consistency of nanoparticle distribution are the most significant benefits of physical approaches in contrast with chemical strategy. Generally, all of them (methods such as chemical, ultrasonic-assisted, electrochemical, photocatalytic, photoinduced, biochemical reduction, and irradiation approaches) have their very own limitations, which incorporate toxicity concern, cost-effective and laborious nature, and numerous other effects [34].

2.3 Characteristic of metal nanoparticles as a delivery system

Before characterizing precisely what a perfect nanoparticle-based medication delivery system is made of, determining how the body interacts with the exogenous particulate matter is needed. Nanoparticles can enter into the human body, through three principle routes, infusion, inhalation, and oral consumption. When they enter the systemic circulation, biological protein and particle interaction is the primary process occurring before distribution into different organs [43]. Absorption from the blood vessels enables the lymphatic system to additionally convey and wipe out the particles. This system has three fundamental abilities, two of which are related to drug conveyance. The first, fluid recuperation includes the exudation of fluids by the lymphatic network from blood vessels. The second, which involves immunity, is perhaps the most relevant to this subject. As the system recuperates overabundant fluid, it additionally grabs chemical and external cells from tissues. As the fluids are once again filtered into the blood, the lymph nodes recognize any outside matter going through [44]. If macrophages consider anything as nonself, they can engorge and remove it from the body. This is a major problem with nanoparticle-based drug delivery; however, particle size and surface quality may affect clearance, as discussed in the following subsections [45].

Metal-based nanomaterials, including (bulk) metals, are anticipated to introduce a major improvement to many areas of our lives, such as technology, bioscience, and industry [46]. This is because metal nanoparticles have a variety of properties that are incredibly useful or can be monitored for a variety of new logical examinations and a large range of mechanical and biomedical applications.

The key features exhibited by MNPs

- Great surface energies
- Enormous surface-area-to-volume proportion when contrasted with the mass counterparts;
- Plasmon excitation;
- A huge number of low-coordination spots, for example, edges and corners, having countless "slewing bonds" and subsequently specific and chemical features and the capacity to store overabundance electrons.
- The progress among molecular and metallic states giving particular electronic structure (regional density of states LDOS);
- Amplified amount of crimps;
- Diminutive extend ordering;
- Quantum captivity

Recently, the world has witnessed great advances in the utilization of metal nanoparticles in the investigation of biomolecular associations, creating bioassays and biomedical tools, and different other biomedical applications, for example, gene delivery therapeutics, immunodiagnostics, and drug delivery. The shape, size, morphology, electrical charge, surface science, vicinity, and different features of metal nanoparticles are exploited in different means in the biomedical fields [47]. In the accompanying, we have discussed a couple of points of interest in metal nanoparticles that are vital to different biomedical applications.

Features, which are known to be consistent for bulk materials, rely upon the shape, size, crystallinity, surface structure, and phase of the nanomaterials. In the metal nanoparticles, shape and size are the two central points that decide the greater part of their properties. For instance, two nanoparticles made of the equivalent (pure) gold can display uniquely different shading, electrical conductivity, and a melting temperature if one is bigger than the other or one is circular and the other is nonspherical in shape [40].

2.3.1 *Smaller size and great surface area-to-volume ratio*

A nanosystem is made up of tens to thousands of units with a diameter of less than 100 nm. A biological system's most desirable metric is the nanoscale. Proteins (5–50 nm), viruses (20–450 nm), and genomes (10–100 nm long and 2 nm wide) are among the organic substances with nanoscale measurements. As a result, nanosystems can collaborate at the subatomic level or gain access to previously unreachable regions of biosystems. In terms of biomedical uses, this size match is extremely important [48, 49]. One of the critical requirements of nanomedicine applications is the creation of a device small enough to bypass the vasculature and access the cells to perform the desired purpose. Particles will only leave vascular pores if they are less than 50 nm in diameter. Nanomaterials with a diameter greater than 100 nm cannot be internalized by cells [50].

Nanosystems are not merely pieces of mass materials; they have outstanding properties considering their limited scale. The size of a substance at the nanoscale is equal to the de Broglie wavelengths of the electrons, excitons, and phonons that spread through it. If the size of a substance is reduced to the nanoscale, the phonons, electrons, and electric fields in and around the nanoparticles are spatially imprisoned, and quantum impacts continue to command. For example, inferable from the electron control effect in a nanoparticle, transformation probabilities and quantum thresholds transform, modifying its spectral properties [51]. The nanomaterials have measurements that fall between the Newtonian and quantum size regimes. Thus, the electrical, optical, magnetic, thermal, and chemical properties of the nanomaterials are not quite the same as their nuclear, atomic, and bulk counterparts.

The matter has "more surface" and "less mass" at the nanoscale. The "surface-to-volume ratios" of nanosystems are immense. Another important aspect that affects the different properties of such a small structure is its size. Surface molecules are unsaturated in a synchronizing way. The exposed surface area of the matter is responsible for a variety of properties. The surface-to-volume proportion is robust to properties such as surface adsorption, particle–molecule or particle–atmosphere associations, catalysis, and chemical reactivities. Scaling down drugs or potentially nanoparticles increases solvency, drug packing, and drug-target interaction by increasing the proportion of surface territories to volume. Significant surface curvature and high surface energy can be the source of anomalies from consistent mass atomic organizations at the nanoscale. Minor structural disorientation in the nanocrystal structure will alter material properties significantly [52]. Therefore, the chemical and physical properties of matter are exclusive to the nanoscale. Researchers exploit these exceptional characteristics of nanosystems in different fields of their applications. The size range of different nanosystems their characteristics and brief applications are mentioned in Table 1.

TABLE 1 Various characteristics and brief applications of nanosystems.

Types of nanosystems	Size (nm)	Characteristics	Applications
Liposome	50–100	Phospholipid vesicles, biocompatible, versatile, good entrapment efficiency, offer easy	Long circulatory, offer passive and active delivery of gene, protein, peptide and various other
Polymeric micelles	10–100 nm	Block amphiphilic copolymer micelles, high drug entrapment, payload, biostability	Long circulatory, target specific active and passive drug delivery, the diagnostic value
Polymeric nanoparticles	10–1000	Biodegradable, biocompatible, offer complete drug protection	Excellent carrier for controlled and sustained delivery of drugs. Stealth and surface-modified nanoparticles can be used for active and passive delivery of bioactives
Dendrimer	<10	Highly branched, nearly monodisperse polymer system produced by controlled polymerization; three main parts core, branch, and surface	Long circulatory, controlled delivery of bioactives, targeted delivery of bioactives to macrophages, liver targeting
Metallic nanoparticles	<100	Gold and silver colloids, very small size resulting in high surface area available for functionalization, stable	Drug and gene delivery, highly sensitive diagnostic assays, thermal ablation, and radiotherapy enhancement
Carbon nanotubes	0.5–3 diameter and 20–1000 length	Third allotropic crystalline form of carbon sheets either single layer (single-walled nanotube, SWNT) or multiple layers (multiwalled nanotube, MWNT). These crystals have remarkable strength and unique electrical properties (conducting, semiconducting, or insulating)	Functionalization enhanced solubility, penetration to cell cytoplasm and nucleus, as carrier for gene delivery, peptide delivery
Nanocrystals Quantum dots	2–9.5	Semiconducting material synthesized with II–VI and III–V column element; Size between 10 and 100 Å; Bright fluorescence, narrow emission, Broad UV excitation, and high photostability	The long term multiple color imaging of liver cell; DNA hybridization, immunoassay; receptor-mediated endocytosis; labeling of breast cancer marker HeR 2 surface of cancer cells

2.3.2 *Shape and morphology reliance*

The corner- and brim-like arched areas are abundant in nanomaterials. Most unsaturated atoms in synch (dangling security) occur in corners and sides, rather than on plane surfaces. The properties of nanomaterials are deeply affected by such a large separation of under-composed atoms in a nanoparticle. This opens up the possibility of developing new material functionality. Rather than modifying the structure, one may radically alter the properties of a substance by altering its form, scale, and morphology (Fig. 2). The small differences in form and scale of metallic nanomaterials have been perceived to induce major changes in their properties.

In the biomedical field, the configuration of metal nanoparticles is extremely significant. Researchers have also shown how the form of nanoparticles, regardless of surface coating, determines the effectiveness of nanoparticles in cellular uptake (Fig. 2). They claimed that tumor cells picked up spherical gold nanoparticles more efficiently than rod-shaped gold nanoparticles [53]. Size-dependent absorption efficacy by cells was discovered in studies involving metal nanoparticles of various sizes. In addition to both the tinier and larger spheres in the size range of 10–100 nm, 50 nm spherical nanoparticles were taken up more magnificently by the cells [54]. When it came to rod-shaped gold nanoparticles, the low-dimension ratio (1:3) nanorods had a higher cellular take-up than the high-dimension ratio (1:5) ones. In the size range of 10–100 nm, however, spherical nanoparticles were more effectively internalized than rod-shaped nanoparticles. The difference in take-up activity between the rod and spherical-shaped metal nanoparticles may also be due to surface structure and chemistry [53].

Due to their interesting geometry, gold nanostars are outstanding drug delivery systems [55]. Nanostars have a large surface area where a large variety of drugs and actives can be stacked due to their perplexing forms. Newly, it was demonstrated that gold nanostars transformed the shape of the nucleus of a cell when fused into malignant cells. This mechanism allowed improved drug release thus posing less of a barrier to outside therapy [55]. Silver nanoparticles have been shown to have an antibacterial activity that is shape-based. For example, truncated silver nano triangles showed bactericidal properties at a far lower silver content than spherical ones. Silver nanospheres, on the other hand, had superior bactericidal properties to silver nanorods [56].

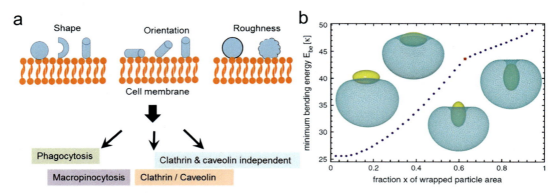

FIG. 2 Influences of particle shape, orientation, and surface roughness on the penetration of the cell membrane: (A) Depiction of the particle's cellular uptake and the endocytic route; and (B) orientation shift of the elliptical particle to reduce bending energy during the wrapping process; *Adopted from A. Yeste, M. Nadeau, E.J. Burns, H.L. Weiner, F.J. Quintana, Nanoparticle-mediated codelivery of myelin antigen and a tolerogenic small molecule suppresses experimental autoimmune encephalomyelitis, Proc. Natl. Acad. Sci. 109 (2012) 11270–11275. https://doi.org/10.1073/pnas.1120611109.*

2.3.3 *Biocompatibility, inertness, and simplicity of surface modifications*

Barely any nanoparticles satisfy every one of the prerequisites of nanomedicine applications. Nanosystems must meet several challenges/attributes in order to be considered for nanomedicine applications. On living organisms, a variety of biomedical applications can be carried out. As a result, several problems such as absorption, digestion, delivery, disposal, and biocompatibility of metal nanosystems should be addressed before they are used. Noble metals include gold, silver, platinum, copper, and palladium. Because each of these metals has a high oxidation potential, one would expect relative latency under normal environmental and biological conditions. At the nanoscale, though, the molecule surface is more receptive than the mass. Surface passivation of nanoparticles is accomplished by coating them with biocompatible materials such as silica and biomolecules [57]. Surface modernizers can render nanoparticles biocompatible while still ensuring their stability in a physiological setting. The cell state is enduring the dispersed gold nanoparticles all over [50].

Metal nanoparticles are linked to a variety of atoms and coating materials, allowing the chemistry and surface of particles to be customized. Metal nanoparticles attach to amines, disulfides, thiols, PEG, natural phosphates, and other molecules quickly. The surface conjugation of the functional groups is determined by the configuration of the metals and the reaction conditions. Sulfur-bearing functional groups, such as disulfides and thiols, for example, have a strong affinity for the gold surface. The selection of the coating materials relies upon the necessities or bigger objectives. For instance, analysts reported that connexion through CTAB-topping of gold nanorods on the exterior of gram-positive microorganisms was simpler than nucleic acid and peptide topping [58]. Biomolecules such as oligonucleotides, amino acids, peptides, proteins, and DNA have been coated on nanoparticles to give them a special bioactive interface that can interact with biological targets [59]. Antibodies, for example, have used the gold nanoparticle surface to achieve tumor-specific transport and cell membrane infiltration. The functionalization of gold nanoparticles with transferrin was shown to increase nanoparticle penetration into cells [60].

Protein or ligand-bound metal nanoparticles are used in label-free quantitative multiparameter biological analysis systems to determine the change in physical attributes caused by their interactions [61]. Metal nanoparticle-based label-free sensors have a cost-effective way to track well-known bimolecular activities in real-time [62]. A common surface modifier is PEG. Using ligand exchange reaction, PEG will easily take the place of the other surface atoms [63]. The addition of PEG to nanoparticles increased their stability and prevented salt-induced aggregation. PEG coatings have been used to greatly decrease the risk of metal nanoparticles interfering with the immune system [64].

Surface alterations of metal nanoparticles are also essential for the controlled release of the loaded therapeutic in addition to aiming at the target site or providing stabilization. For example, instead of thiols, glutathione was used on gold nanoparticle surfaces to monitor the release of drugs into the intracellular space [65]. The precise connection of the desired particles is allowed by bioconjugation responses at surface adsorbed layers [66]. For presenting multivalent functional multiplicity or multifunctionality onto metal particles, layer-by-layer addition of polyelectrolytes [67] was used. The advantages of nanoparticles are combined with new chemical and structural properties of the covering layers in certain structures. The multivalent linkage of small atoms to nanoparticles will result in a more powerful precise binding affinity. High-throughput drug development, diagnostics, and therapeutics may all benefit from the multivalent approach. Metal nanoparticles have a range of surface modification techniques that make them more compact, biocompatible, and capable of performing unique tasks in nanomedicine.

2.3.4 *Surface properties*

It has been observed that the size of nanoparticles affects the implementation of nanoparticle-based formulations; however, controlling surface qualities is another way to achieve the desired system. To create an optimal nanoparticle drug delivery system, a combination of appropriate targeting ligands, surface structure, flow, and reactivity is needed to avoid conglomeration, stabilization, and receptor binding, as well as pharmacological effects of the medication [51].

The clearance of the nanosystem from the body is the most important factor to consider. Since nanoparticles are detected by the lymphatic system, they are subject to the body's natural immune response to foreign substances. Because of greater binding to the blood component, the more hydrophobic a nanoparticle is, the more likely it is to be cleared [68]. Given how well hydrophobic nanoparticles are cleared, it seems safe to conclude that making their surfaces hydrophilic would lengthen their time in circulation. As a result, coating nanoparticles with surfactants or polymers, or making copolymers such as polyethylene glycol (PEG), reduces opsonization [69, 70]. Polyethylene glycol, polyethylene oxide (avoids splenic and hepatic localization), polysorbate 80, poloxamer, and poloxamine have all been shown to be important. PEG is a hydrophilic, moderately latent polymer that, when incorporated into the nanoparticle surface, prevents plasma proteins from binding to them (opsonization), preventing significant dose loss. PEGylated nanoparticles are also referred to as "stealth" nanoparticles because they do not opsonize and remain hidden by the reticuloendothelial system (RES) [71]. While clearance issues have been addressed by creating polymer complexes, aggregation remains a concern for tiny particles due to their large surface area. Nanoparticles, such as micelles, quantum dots, and dendrimers, are particularly susceptible to aggregation. To prevent particle aggregation and demand, a few methods have been used, including topping agents and changing the zeta potential (surface charges) [72]. The unique surface charge on the particles is important not only for their cellular interactions but also for their formulation stability (Fig. 3). In general, these methods and theories can be summarized as follows: particle size must be big enough to avoid outflow into blood vessels, but not too large to be vulnerable to macrophage leeway. The degree of accumulation and autonomy can be regulated by scheming the surface [73].

2.3.5 *Drug loading and release*

Nanoparticle surface features and sizes have been studied to improve bioavailability, decrease clearance, and increase stability. It is possible to bring drugs to tissues in the body that were histologically impossible to access by managing these characteristics. However, if the drug cannot be freed from the nanoparticle's matrix, this procedure would be meaningless. Desorption of the surface-bound or adsorbed product, medicate diffusion through the nanoparticle matrix erosion, and a combination of diffusion and erosion procedures, as well as swelling, temperature, pH, and drug solvency are all variables that affect medication release from nanoparticle-constructed formulations [16, 74].

The release of the drug can differ depending on the type of nanoparticle used. Depending on their structure, polymeric nanoparticles may be termed nanospheres or nanocapsules.

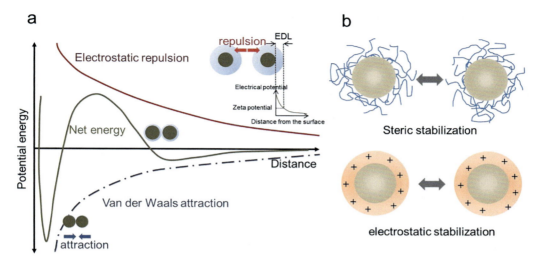

FIG. 3 Illustration showing the effect of surface charge on nanoparticles (A) potential energy between nanoparticles regulated by electrostatic repulsion and Van der Waals attraction, that can lead to particle agglomeration, and (B) the importance of steric and electrostatic to colloidal stability. *Adopted from S.-J. Seo, M. Chen, H. Wang, M.S. Kang, K.W. Leong, H.-W. Kim, Extra- and intra-cellular fate of nanocarriers under dynamic interactions with biology, Nano Today. 14 (2017) 84–99. https://doi.org/10.1016/j.nantod.2017.04.011.*

Nanospheres are homogeneous structures in which polymer chains coordinate like surfactants in the forming of micelles (phase-isolated from the bulk solution). Nanocapsules, on the other hand, are a heterogeneous structure in which the drug is stored inside a polymer reservoir (similar to a vesicle) [75].

The substance is activated by the disintegration of the lattice in nanospheres, which have a network like a grid where the medicine is mechanically and continuously scattered. With feebly bound medication to the large surface region of the nanoparticle, there is a short burst of medication release accompanied by a sustained release [76]. As nanocapsules are used, however, the release is regulated by pharmaceutical diffusion through the polymeric membrane, so drug diffusibility through the polymer is unquestionably a determining factor in its deliverability. If the polymer and the drug have some ionic reactions, they can form edifices that prevent the medication from being released from the capsule. Other ancillary agents, such as polyethylene oxide-propylene oxide (PEO-PPO), can be used to get around this. Given the increased release of drugs to target tissues, this would reduce the association between the capsule lattice and medication [77].

3 Targeting of metal nanoparticles for autoimmune conditions

Nowadays MeNPs are being expansively appraised as an appropriate carrier for therapy and diagnosis of autoimmune diseases. They are achieving a unique position in the area of drug delivery (as drug delivery carriers) and diagnosis due to their peerless properties such as minute size, higher surface area, competency for surface alteration, and great reactivity toward viable cells [78]. MeNPs that have been successfully employed for targeting autoimmune conditions include gold nanoparticles, silver nanoparticles, zinc oxide nanoparticles, magnetic nanoparticles, etc. However, the application of MeNPs for targeting autoimmune diseases is limited to diseases such as rheumatoid arthritis (RA), inflammatory bowel disease (IBD), psoriasis, multiple sclerosis (MS), myasthenia gravis, type 1 diabetes (T1D), etc. The application of metal nanoparticles for the treatment of various autoimmune conditions is presented in Table 2.

Nanomaterials have attracted a lot of attention and have become an interesting challenge for the advancement in nanotechnology in recent years since these materials have many phenomenal properties as compared to mass materials. Due to their excellent optical and electrical properties, magnetism, and other properties, a vast number of researchers are increasingly studying MeNPs. Metal nanoparticles have been widely used in bioengineering and material science, especially in medicine [79].

Metals of different kinds are present in all living organisms, which serve various biological functions. Since ancient times, metals and their ions have been used in a variety of biomedical applications. Advanced toxicological examinations, on the other hand, reveal various shortcomings of bulk materials in the drug (e.g., nonspecificity, poisonous content, and lower bioavailability). As a result, analysts have focused on developing nanoscale structures from these bulk metals and materials. Metal nanoparticles are commonly used in biomedical resolutions as biomolecule transporters (e.g., drugs, proteins, peptides, nucleic acid, antibodies, and aptamers). Aside from carrying biomolecules, metal nanoparticles have been commonly used as theranostic agents for several diseases (diabetes, cardiovascular conditions, cancer growth, neurodegenerative diseases, retinal disorders, microbial infections, etc.). Since there are several publications on metal nanoparticles throughout the inscription, this segment would focus solely on the progress of metal nanoparticles in immunological applications [47].

Metal nanoparticles are broadly utilized as carters for the conveyance of various therapeutic agents (e.g., antibodies, peptides, nucleic acids, chemotherapeutic medications) [46, 47]. Silver nanoparticles (AgNPs), gold nanoparticles (AuNPs), zinc, iron, titanium, and copper nanoparticles, for example, have extremely tunable optical properties. Furthermore, their surface can be easily functionalized either to conjugate with targeting agents and dynamic biomolecules through covalent bonding, electrostatic interactions, H-bonding, noncovalently, and other methods; or to stack multiple medications for improved therapeutic viability [80]. The primary goal of using a metal-nanoparticle-based drug delivery system (DDS) is to reduce therapeutic agent lethality while also improving their systemic transportation and therapeutic proficiency.

Metal nanoparticles (MeNPs) are used in a wide range of fields, including medicine, and almost everybody in developing countries is exposed to them (for diagnostic and therapeutic purposes). Ingestion, touching, inhalation, and infusion are also potential avenues for these nanoparticles to penetrate the bloodstream. Similar to any foreign matter, they may translocate to tissues and penetrate the innate immune mechanism, which acts as a nonspecific first line of protection against external threats to the host [81].

Metal-nanoparticle-focused medication conveyance is one of the new methodologies in the modern approach to the treatment of various ailments [82]. Proficient medication conveyance depends on two elements: (i) structure of nanocarriers for moderate and controlled release of medication; and (ii) capacity of the nanovehicles to deliver the medication entity to the

TABLE 2 Application of metal nanoparticles for treatment of various autoimmune disorders.

Autoimmune disease	Delivery carrier/metallic nanoparticle	Drug/therapeutic moiety used	Remark	Reference
Inflammatory bowels disease	peptide-gold nanoparticle (GNP)	Specific Peptide (P12)	Suppressed secretion of multiple pro-inflammatory chemokines and cytokines and decreased colonic inflammation in vivo	[120]
	ZnO-NP	Mesalazine	Enhanced therapeutic efficacy of 5-ASA in DSS-induced colitis model	[101]
Autoimmune encephalomyelitis	Gold nanoparticles	2-(1′H-indole-3′-carbonyl)-thiazole-4-carboxylic acid methyl ester (ITE) and myelin oligodendrocyte glycoprotein (MOG)35–55	NPs carrying ITE and MOG35–55 extended the FoxP3$^+$ Treg compartment and repressed the progress of experimental autoimmune encephalomyelitis (an experimental model of multiple sclerosis)	[121]
Rheumatoid arthritis	Silver nanoparticle	*Piper nigrum* extract	Silver nanoparticles stabilized with *Piper nigrum* extract (S-AgNPs) presented promising anti-arthritic activity by inhibiting TNF-α and suppressing certain proinflammatory cytokines	[122]
	Gum acacia (GA) stabilized Silver nanoparticle	Hesperidin (HP)	Reduced inflammatory cells influx and decreased inflammation in ankle joints tissues upon administration of HP loaded gum acacia (GA) stabilized silver nanoparticles	[123]
	PLGA-gold nanoparticles	Methotrexate	Enhanced therapeutic response as compared to free MTX therapy	[124]
	Hyaluronate-gold nanoparticles (HA-AuNP)	Tocilizumab (TCZ)	The enhanced therapeutic effect of HA-AuNP/TCZ complex	[125]
	RGD-attached gold (Au) half-shell nanoparticles (RGD peptide = Arginylglycylaspartic acid)	Methotrexate	Enhanced therapeutic efficacy with decreased dose and dose-dependent MTX side effects in the management of RA	[126]
	Gold nanoparticles (Nanogold)	Catalase	Enhanced antiangiogenic activities with subsequent minimization of macrophage infiltration and inflammation	[127]
Psoriasis	Gold and silver nanoparticle	*Cornus mas* extract	Significant decrease in CD68-positive macrophages and decreased production of IL-12 and TNF-α in psoriasis plaques	[128]

coveted destinations, saving the other healthy cells from their effects [83]. These prerequisites could be accomplished by utilizing two methodologies, known as active and passive targeting [84]. In active targeting, nanoparticles are conjugated with different dynamic ligands (e.g., sugars, peptides, recombinant proteins, antibodies, other miniature atoms) that are linked with particular cell surface receptors, and eventually drag the load to the chosen site and release the medication [143]. On the contrary, passive targeting is predominantly utilized for cancer therapies on account of the excellent pathophysiological acmes of tumor vessels with fissured vasculature. Essentially, these scattered veins in the tumor prompt an enhanced permeability and retention (EPR) impact that permits the nanoparticles to assemble more into the tumor [85]. The next discussion will focus on the advancement of nanoparticle-based DDS that can be used as a passive or active cancer therapeutic targeting device. Antibodies will determine the development of nanoparticle-based DDS that will function as either a passive or an active targeting system for cancer therapeutics.

Inflammation is the immune system's response to illness, injury, or infection in several pathological circumstances [86]. Using tiny organic molecules, scientists have developed a variety of antiinflammatory medicines. Despite this, researchers have recently discovered several nanoparticles that could have antiinflammatory effects in different animal models. For example, Uchiyama et al. developed an IgG-conjugated AuNPs (AuNP-IgG) device and demonstrated that intravenous infusion of AuNP-IgG did not cause hemolysis or hemorrhage in male Wistar rats, but rather smothered leukocyte adhesion to the postcapillary vessel wall, implying that AuNP-IgG has a potent antiinflammatory effect [87]. Rehman et al. found that Platinum NPs (PtNPs) had an antiinflammatory effect in the lipopolysaccharide-stimulated RAW264.7 cell line [88]. The findings revealed that PtNPs trigger a decrease in the lipopolysaccharide-induced formation of ROS, inhibit the phosphorylation of and Akt ERK1/2, and downregulate nuclear factor kappa-B (NF-kB), demonstrating PtNPs' potent antiinflammatory properties. The following sections go into several MeNPs that have been used to treat inflammatory diseases.

3.1 Gold nanoparticles

Gold is one of the biocompatible metals, with various beneficial properties against a variety of autoimmune diseases. AuNPs that have been meticulously designed have special characteristics such as being highly compliant with living systems, being very small, and having a wide range of shapes [89]. The US Food and Drug Administration (U.S. FDA) has also licensed AuNPs for the management of human RA. While the use of gold nanoparticles in the treatment of autoimmune diseases is still in its early stages, several studies have been conducted to target gold nanoparticles for drug delivery in autoimmune diseases such as IBD, RA, T1D, psoriasis, and others, which are addressed in the following portion of the chapter.

Hussein and Hanan generated naked gold nanoparticles (AuNPs) to test the therapeutic effect of two different doses of AuNPs in a dinitro-benzene sulfonic acid-induced colitis rat model. They found that when compared to the positive control group (dinitro-benzene sulfonic acid-colitis), the AuNPs treated group (for 72h) had improved kidney and liver functions, improved the renewing capacity of damaged colon tissues, suppressed inflammatory cytokine reaction, and decreased colonic myeloperoxidase and malondialdehyde production. Finally, they concluded that the newly discovered naked AuNPs are a promising and novel treatment for experimental colitis with no apparent drawbacks [90].

Using an experimental autoimmune encephalomyelitis model, Nosratabadi et al. attempted to fabricate a hyperforin (antiinflammatory compound) loaded gold nanoparticle (Hyp-GNP) for the treatment of MS. Following the administration of Hyp-GNP and hyperforin, a substantial decrease in the clinical incidence of EAE was found, as well as a reduction in the amount of inflammatory cell penetration in the spinal cord. Furthermore, as compared to other classes under study, Hyp-GNP substantially reduced disease-related cytokines, while significantly increasing antiinflammatory cytokines. Hyperforin and Hyp-GNP have also been shown to suppress Th1 and Th17 cell differentiation, while simultaneously promoting Treg and Th2 cell differentiation. Finally, they concluded that Hyp-GNP was substantially more successful than free hyperforin in the cases of EAE [91].

Gold nanoparticles have also been investigated for the treatment of RA, with promising findings. In this respect, Gul et al. explored the usage of gold nanoparticles in the treatment of RA. They investigated the immunomodulation potential of rutin and rutin-conjugated gold nanoparticles (R-AuNPs) in collagen-induced arthritis (CIA) model of rats by modulating iNOS and NF-kB expression. Rutin and R-AuNPs had antiarthritic effects in the CIA model of rats, as shown by a substantial decrease in the arthritic score and significant downregulation of NF-kB and iNOS expression in vivo. In summary, rutin and R-AuNPs were found to be potential therapeutic entities for the treatment of RA [92].

Furthermore, Leonaviien et al. demonstrated that AuNPs have therapeutic value in the treatment of RA. In a CIA rat model, the effect of AuNPs was investigated. They produced AuNPs with sizes ranging from 13 to 50 nm. In the CIA rat model, administration of 13-nm and 50-nm AuNPs decreased joint swelling by 49.7% (P0.002) and 45.03% (P0.01), respectively. Furthermore, the existence of a higher concentration of catalase in established AuNPs was confirmed to have an antioxidant effect (antioxidant enzyme). Overall, the results indicated that AuNPs may be used to treat RA [93].

Moving ahead, AuNPs have further proven themselves as a potential drug delivery cargo for efficient therapy of autoimmune Type 1 diabetes. In this regard, Shilo et al. fabricated insulin-coated gold nanoparticles (INS-GNPs) for prolonged and controlled regulation of glucose. They reported that intravenous as well as subcutaneous administration of INS-GNPs exhibited a decreased level of blood glucose for a duration of three times longer than free insulin in a mouse model of T1D. They further reported that linking insulin to GNPs quick degradation of insulin-by-insulin degrading enzymes, thereby providing controlled and prolonged therapeutic activity. Thus the newly fabricated INS-GNPs were reported to possess great potential to enhance patient compliance in T1D [94].

In this sequence, Selim et al. examined the effect of biologically fabricated gold nanoparticles (AuNPs) to manage hyperglycemic conditions in the T1D model of rats. A significant increase in the glucose level of diabetic control rats as compared to the normal control ($P < 0.001$) rats was reported. Furthermore, reduced kidney and liver function were observed in the diabetic treated and normal treated rats after the administration of AuNP. Conclusively, they suggested that AuNPs significantly enhanced antioxidant production in the T1D model of rats [95].

AuNPs have also shown promise as a delivery vehicle for the treatment of allergic, inflammatory skin disorders such as psoriasis. In this regard, Bessar et al. have created methotrexate (MTX) primed gold nanoparticles (AuNPs) for psoriasis therapy. To increase the solubility, durability, and biodistribution of MTX-loaded AuNPs, they functionalized them with sodium

3-mercapto-1-propane sulfonate (Au-3MPS). They conducted an ex vivo toxicological analysis in keratinocyte monolayers and discovered that Au-3MPS is not toxic. STEM images demonstrated that AuNPs were distributed correctly inside the cells. In vitro tests showed that MTX-Au-3MPS was more successful than MTX alone. Furthermore, MTX- Au-3MPS transmitted MTX to the epidermis and dermis at a higher pace than free MTX. Finally, they discovered that a newly formed MTX-Au-3MPS conjugate may be a safe, efficient, and nonirritating carrier for psoriasis topical therapy [96].

Sumbayev et al. examined the therapeutic ability of citrate-stabilized gold nanoparticles in the treatment of IL-1-dependent inflammatory conditions such as psoriasis. According to in vitro and in vivo studies, the fabricated AuNPs specifically downregulate cellular responses elicited by IL-1. They also reported that citrate-stabilized gold nanoparticles may be a promising new treatment option for psoriasis [97]. Both of the aforementioned study results suggest that AuNPs can produce medicines and cure autoimmune disorders.

3.2 Silver nanoparticles

Silver nanoparticles have been reported to possess potential immune-modulatory properties. AgNPs are readily internalized by immune system cells, can accumulate in peripheral lymphoid organs, and modify a variety of immune cell behavior indicators. Furthermore, silver nanoparticles' biocompatibility with living cells can explain why they are used to treat autoimmune diseases [96]. AgNPs used for the management of various autoimmune conditions have been elaborated in the following paragraph.

The use of AgNPs in the management of IBD has shown to be very successful. In this regard, Siczek et al. recently established and evaluated silver nanoparticle-loaded aqueous suspensions (NanoAg1 and NanoAg2) in a mouse model of ulcerative colitis (UC) and Crohn's disease (CD). They demonstrated antiinflammatory behavior in a semi-chronic inflammatory model caused by dextran sulfate sodium and 2,4,6-trinitrobenzene sulfonic acid administered into the colon (intracolonic) (i.c.). NanoAg1 and NanoAg2 (500 mg/dm^3, 100 μL/animal, i.c., once daily) reduced macroscopic, ulcer, and microscopic ratings, indicating substantial improvement of colitis in mouse models of colon inflammation. Furthermore, the fact that NanoAg1 has a weaker impact than NanoAg2 suggests that the form and diameter of silver nanoparticles affect the inflammatory properties. They also found that unlike NanoAg1, i.c. administration of formulation NanoAg2 changed the microbial flora of the colon by reducing the amount of *Escherichia coli* and *Clostridium perfringens* and growing the amount of *Lactobacillus* sp. In brief, the developed formulations (NanoAg1 and NanoAg2) have great promises for treating IBD since they effectively reduced the colon inflammation in UC and CD mouse models [98].

Nanocrystalline silver has also been investigated as a possible cure for autoimmune IBD. In this regard, Bhol et al. demonstrated that nanocrystalline silver (NPI 32101) has antiinflammatory properties in a rat model of ulcerative colitis. When opposed to the placebo and negative control classes, they observed that NPI 32101 at a dosage of 40 or 4 mg/kg (by intracolonic administration) greatly diminished colon inflammation. They also related NPI 32101 to sulfasalazine for antiinflammatory efficacy, finding that i.c. or oral administration of NPI 32101 greatly decreased UC in the rat model of the disease. They claimed that NPI 32101 inhibited MMP-9 expression as well as the expression of cytokines including IL-1, TNF-, and IL-12, proving the therapeutic value of nanocrystalline silver in the treatment of ulcerative colitis [99].

Apart from that, AgNPs have been used to deliver medications to people with psoriasis. In this background, David et al. developed AgNPs from polyphenol-rich fruit extract of the European blackberry and evaluated their antiinflammatory properties. They generated biocompatible AgNPs filled with European blackberry extract and evaluated their antiinflammatory ability on UVB-exposed HaCaT cells as well as in vivo potential on human psoriatic lesions and an acute inflammation model. Advanced AgNPs formulations are shown to have excellent antiinflammatory efficacy in vitro and in vivo [100].

Just a few studies have been performed on the fabrication of AgNPs to target autoimmune disorders, as shown earlier. However, efforts have been made to collect necessary evidence in order to show AgNPs' therapeutic capability for the successful treatment of autoimmune diseases.

3.3 Miscellaneous

Apart from gold and silver nanoparticles, other metal nanoparticles such as magnetic nanoparticles, titanium dioxide nanoparticles, and zinc oxide nanoparticles have also been used to target various autoimmune conditions. Although limited data exist, research findings demonstrating the therapeutic applicability of metal nanoparticles in autoimmune disorders have been elaborated in the following paragraph.

3.3.1 *Zinc oxide nanoparticles (ZnONPs)*

ZnONPs, are an innovative kind of economic and low-toxicity nanomaterial, tremendously employed in the area of drug delivery for delivery of antibacterial, anticancer, antioxidant, antiinflammatory, and antidiabetic agents. ZnONPs with a diameter of less than 100 nm is considered moderately biocompatible, making them a good carrier for promoting drug distribution. In addition, ZnONPs have been used to cure inflammatory disorders such as IBD. Li et al. documented the antiinflammatory ability of ZnO NPs in a dextran sulfate sodium (DSS)-induced ulcerative colitis model of mice by downregulating proinflammatory cytokines, IL-1 and TNF-α, and myeloperoxidase (MPO). They also found that combining ZnONPs with mesalazine (5-ASA) improved the therapeutic effectiveness of 5-ASA in DSS-induced colitis and restored improvements in DSS-unique mice's colonic microbiota, which 5-ASA could not [101].

3.3.2 *Titanium oxide nanoparticles (TiO2NPs)*

TiO2NPs have acquired a tremendous position for biological applications due to their exclusive biocompatible nature. The properties of TiO2NPs in relation to the immune system remain unclear. Sree Latha et al., on the other hand, found that TiO2NPs had immunomodulatory properties and may be used to treat autoimmune disorders [102]. However, only a few reports have shown that TiO2NPs may be used to administer medications to patients with autoimmune disorders. Arkhipova et al. investigated the association of blood serum with titanium oxide nanoparticles to see how it will remove the immune complex. The Laser correlation spectroscopy (LCS) technique was used to analyze the relationship of titanium oxide nanoparticles with the blood serum of patients with reported myasthenia. They used titanium oxide nanoparticles to incubate serum samples and then stabilized them with phosphoric acid, resulting in the production and precipitation of complexes including titanium oxide nanoparticles, serum globulins, and albumin. They discovered that when titanium dioxide nanoparticles were mixed with blood serum from myasthenia gravis patients, approximately 40% of circulating immune complexes were eliminated. Plasmapheresis is currently used to remove circulating blood immune complexes in patients with myasthenia gravis. However, the new process, which uses titanium oxide nanoparticles, maybe a successful treatment choice for myasthenia gravis [103].

3.3.3 *Superparamagnetic iron oxide nanoparticles (SPIONs) and ferromagnetic nanoparticles*

Superparamagnetism is acquired by nanoparticles that contain a solo magnetic domain. SPIONs have a broad variety of applications, including direct drug delivery, gene therapy, cancer tumor diagnosis, biomolecular isolation, tissue regeneration, and MRI imaging. SPIONs have also been used in siRNA distribution for the treatment of RA, in addition to the applications mentioned earlier. Duan et al. tested the effectiveness of a nanocarrier (polyethyleneimine [PEI]-superparamagnetic iron oxide nanoparticle [SPIONs]) for systemic transmission of therapeutic siRNA to experimental arthritic joints in this regard (arthritic rats). siRNA-loaded PEI-SPIOs displayed low cellular cytotoxicity, enhanced siRNA stability, increased macrophage absorption, and the capacity to silence particular genes in vitro. Joint macrophages and T cells quickly took up PEI-SPIONs-delivered siRNA, which collected effectively in inflamed joints. Briefly, PEI-functionalized SPIONs are effective carriers of systemic siRNA for the treatment of RA [104].

Zhang et al. fabricated magnetic nanoparticles to investigate the impact of the optimum size of magnetic nanoparticles (Fe3O4 nanoparticles) on RA targeting and photothermal therapy in a recent report. They created Fe3O4 nanoparticles of various sizes (70–350 nm) with similar surface properties. When irradiated with near-infrared light, the formed nanoparticles showed excellent biocompatibility as well as a higher temperature response. Furthermore, larger nanoparticles were more readily phagocytized than tiny nanoparticles during in vitro incubation with inflammatory cells, confirming size-dependent cellular internalization. Nonetheless, an in vivo experiment in the CIA model revealed that nanoparticles with a size of 220 nm had greater availability to inflamed joints and stronger therapeutic results when exposed to laser irradiation. Overall, they concluded that Fe3O4 nanoparticles may be used as a drug carrier for RA treatment [48].

3.3.4 *Copper-based nanoparticles*

Copper is an environmental bio component that plays a crucial part in the cell's physiology, as a cofactor or enzyme constituent, contributing to anti-oxidative processes or /detoxification of oxygen free radicals. Metallic copper (as a nutritional supplement) has been successfully used to combat autoimmune disorders such as RA for a long time [105].

In this sense, Lu et al. created the Cu7.2S4 nanoparticles (NPs) for the treatment of RA, which is focused on the premise that copper (Cu)-based nanomaterials could act as both photothermal therapy (PTT) agents and photosensitizers for photodynamic therapy (PDT). Cu can also promote chondrogenesis and osteogenesis. Furthermore, the Cu7.2S4 NPs produced have the potential to effectively kill pathogenic microorganisms such as *Staphylococcus aureus* and *Escherichia coli*, avoiding contamination during the intra-articular injection. Finally, they concluded that the combined PTT and PDT using multifunctional Cu7.2S4 NPs may be considered a novel and promising therapeutic option for RA [106].

4 Safety concern of metallic nanoparticles

The envisioned utilization of nanomaterials is expanding gradually in daily life from the family unit to human health. However, nothing is understood regarding the lethality of these NPs and their long-term impact on the welfare of living persons [107]. Regrettably, no strict regulatory standards or regulations exist or are being followed to evaluate the basic methodology and threat assessment methods for nanostructure toxicity calculation. Because of their limited scale, NPs are adept at penetrating within the body and can transcend biological barriers to access the body's cells and tissues [108, 109]. While the properties and toxicity dimensions of the bulk molecule from which nanomaterials are produced are certainly understood, there is a complete lack of evidence about how these materials' properties and toxicological composition alter at nanoscale measurements. Furthermore, deciding at what dosage and which size nanoscale materials experience differing toxic effects is problematic [110]. The overwhelming majority of published literature focuses on the planning, characterization, and widespread use of these nanocompounds in biomedicine. Only a few reports have looked at the toxicity and risk assessment of these NPs. Nanotoxicology is a topic that creates legitimate fear earlier rather than later, since the application of NPs to staff and end-users may have a lethal impact on their biological systems. In a nutshell, a fundamental question concerning the in vitro and in vivo toxicity of emerging nanomaterials, as well as recent progress on their safety, is discussed in the following paragraph [109].

When AgNPs (20 and 200 nm) and TiO2 NPs (21 nm) were applied to mouse testicular cells and human testicular embryonic carcinoma cells, the toxic quality of metal and metal oxide NPs of different sizes was expected. In comparison to TiO2-NPs, both sizes of AgNPs were found to be more cytostatic and cytotoxic. They have caused necrosis, apoptosis, and decreased proliferation in the dose and time-dependent ways. As compared to human testicular cells at the same dosage, all scaled AgNPs affected mouse testicular cells more prominently [111]. At an equal dosage, the toxicity of AgNPs (70 nm) and Ag ions against bacterial cells (*S. aureus* and *E. coli*), peripheral blood mononuclear cells (monocytes and T-lymphocytes), and human cells (human mesenchymal stem cells (hMSCs)) was studied. On monocytes, the cytotoxicity of Ag ions at doses greater than 1 ppm was studied in an expanding and concentration-dependent way, while AgNPs at doses greater than 30 ppm showed an expansion of cytotoxicity. T cell viability was affected when subjected to Ag ions at concentrations greater than 1.5 ppm, but no effect was shown when exposed to AgNPs. As opposed to AgNPs at the same concentration, Ag ions have a stronger lethal effect on bacterial cells [112]. The effects of AgNPs of different sizes (10, 20, 40, 60, and 80 nm) on yeast, bacteria, algae, and mammalian cells have been studied. As compared to larger particles, AgNPs of a smaller scale have caused more toxicity. The higher toxicity of smaller AgNPs may be attributed to more Ag release and therefore greater bioavailability of Ag, which can cause ROS to be generated in cells [113].

After 72 h of exposure, AuNPs (sizes 5 and 15 nm) were tested for toxicity in mouse fibroblast cell lines. The results revealed that 5 nm-sized AuNPs used at (concentration 50 m) were cytotoxic, but no substantial cytotoxicity was found when 15 nm AuNPs were used. It was estimated that AuNPs with a size of 4 nm will be active in cytoskeletal cell organization damage [50]. In PC12 rat pheochromocytoma cells, human umbilical vein endothelial cells, and neural progenitor cells, the toxicity of 4 nm-sized AuNPs was investigated at different doses and incubation times to explore parameters including morphology, functionality, and cell viability, cytoskeleton organization, and ROS formations. Because of the production of reactive oxygen species (ROS), a higher dose of AuNPs than 200 nm lowered cell viability. The effect of exposing cells to 10 nm on any of the cell parameters was not significant [114].

CuO NPs are shown to be cytotoxic to lung adenocarcinoma cells (A549 cells) and human bronchial epithelial cells in vitro (HBEC). CuO NPs have been shown to minimize cell viability, increase lactate dehydrogenase discharge, and increase IL-8 and ROS in a concentration-dependent manner [115]. In HBEC, the toxic impact of ZnO NPs at different concentrations (5–25 g/mL) was investigated to assess cell viability after 24 h of exposure [116]. Sub-acute lethality of ZnO NPs in rats has also been studied, with ZnO NPs being given at a concentration of 10 mg/kg body weight for 5 days. There was a small difference in the tissues of the rat, but no improvement in the exploratory activity of rats [38]. To explore acute toxicity, mice were given intraperitoneal infusions of TiO2 NPs at set doses of 2592, 1944, 1296, 972, 648, 324, and 0 mg/kg body weight [117]. Tremor, lack of appetite, passive activity, and torpidity were observed in the treated mice. MNPs such as cobalt oxide NPs [118] and Fe_2O_3 NPs have been analyzed for their lethality based on their structure, scale, and concentration.

After 48 h of exposure to SiO2 NPs of 15 or 46 nm duration, cell viability of human lung malignant growth cells was reduced at doses between 10 and 100 µg/mL [119]. Oral administration of SiO2 NPs (10–15 nm) resulted in significant changes in high- and low-density lipoproteins, triglycerides, mice egg albumin, cholesterol, total protein, and enzymatic operation. Aside from that, SiO2 NPs caused lethal results in mice kidney, testes, lung, and liver [119]. Depending on their form, scale, surface properties, and dosage, metal and metal oxide NPs, as well as quantum dots, may potentially be harmful to humans, microorganisms, and other living creatures. As a result, efforts should be made to develop healthy NPs for human gain.

5 Conclusion

The accessibility of metallic NPs has unlocked up new specialized applications in the therapeutic field. The distinct features of nanomaterials allow numerous precincts of human benefit including novel therapeutic agents, biosensors, antimicrobials, catalysis, electronics, and drug delivery. Metal NPs are currently being used in pharmaceutical sciences as a novel medication conveyance framework. Nanomaterials in medication conveyance may have dual functionality for analysis and therapeutics. Nanomedicines have discovered better approaches to treat life-threatening ailments. Though there are a few constraints, for example, functionalized drugs being conveyed by individual NPs are particularly restricted and their quantification is challenging. To accomplish the targeted medication conveyance system, conjugation of NPs with either a ligand or an antibody is vital. Nevertheless, the toxic impacts of metallic NPs must be considered before utilizing them for therapeutic purposes.

Acknowledgments

The authors would like to recognize DHR-ICMR project no. V.25011/286-HRD/2016-HR for financial assistance related to this study.

References

[1] H. Deng, Z. Zhang, The application of nanotechnology in immune checkpoint blockade for cancer treatment, J. Control. Release 290 (2018) 28–45, https://doi.org/10.1016/J.JCONREL.2018.09.026.

[2] R.N. AlKahtani, The implications and applications of nanotechnology in dentistry: a review, Saudi Dent. J. 30 (2018) 107–116, https://doi.org/10.1016/J.SDENTJ.2018.01.002.

[3] X. Feng, J. Liu, W. Xu, G. Li, J. Ding, Tackling autoimmunity with nanomedicines, Nanomedicine 15 (2020) 1585–1597, https://doi.org/10.2217/nnm-2020-0102.

[4] K. Yadav, N.S. Chauhan, S. Saraf, D. Singh, M.R. Singh, Challenges and need of delivery carriers for bioactives and biological agents: an introduction, in: Adv. Ave. Dev. Nov. Carriers Bioact. Biol. Agents, Elsevier, 2020, pp. 1–36, https://doi.org/10.1016/b978-0-12-819666-3.00001-8.

[5] Q. Muhammad, Y. Jang, S.H. Kang, J. Moon, W.J. Kim, H. Park, Modulation of immune responses with nanoparticles and reduction of their immunotoxicity, Biomater. Sci. 8 (2020) 1490–1501, https://doi.org/10.1039/C9BM01643K.

[6] R. Rezaei, M. Safaei, H.R. Mozaffari, H. Moradpoor, S. Karami, A. Golshah, B. Salimi, H. Karami, The role of nanomaterials in the treatment of diseases and their effects on the immune system, Open Access Maced. J. Med. Sci. 7 (2019) 1884–1890, https://doi.org/10.3889/oamjms.2019.486.

[7] G.R.G. Monif, The myth of autoimmunity, Med. Hypotheses 121 (2018) 78–79, https://doi.org/10.1016/J.MEHY.2018.09.023.

[8] Autoimmune Disease Statistics—AARDA, 2019. https://www.aarda.org/news-information/statistics/. accessed December 9, 2018.

[9] D.L. Hirsch, P. Ponda, Antigen-based immunotherapy for autoimmune disease: current status, ImmunoTargets Ther. 4 (2015) 1–11, https://doi.org/10.2147/ITT.S49656.

[10] A. Scanlin, Autoimmune diseases: the growing impact, BioSupply Trends Quarterl. (2014) 44–47.

[11] B. Antiochos, A. Rosen, Mechanisms of Autoimmunity, Clin. Immunol. (2019) 677. 684.e1. https://doi.org/10.1016/B978-0-7020-6896-6.00050-8.

[12] C.C. Denardin, G.E. Hirsch, R.F. da Rocha, M. Vizzotto, A.T. Henriques, J.C.F. Moreira, F.T.C.R. Guma, T. Emanuelli, Antioxidant capacity and bioactive compounds of four Brazilian native fruits, J. Food Drug Anal. 23 (2015) 387–398, https://doi.org/10.1016/j.jfda.2015.01.006.

[13] M.D. Rosenblum, K.A. Remedios, A.K. Abbas, Mechanisms of human autoimmunity, J. Clin. Invest. 125 (2015) 2228–2233, https://doi.org/10.1172/JCI78088.

[14] B. Zitti, Y.T. Bryceson, Natural killer cells in inflammation and autoimmunity, Cytokine Growth Factor Rev. 42 (2018) 37–46, https://doi.org/10.1016/J.CYTOGFR.2018.08.001.

[15] F. Bray, J. Ferlay, I. Soerjomataram, R.L. Siegel, L.A. Torre, A. Jemal, Global cancer statistics 2018: GLOBOCAN estimates of incidence and mortality worldwide for 36 cancers in 185 countries, CA Cancer J. Clin. 68 (2018) 394–424, https://doi.org/10.3322/caac.21492.

[16] N.R. Rose, I.R. Mackay, The Autoimmune Diseases, sixth ed., Academic Press, 2019, https://doi.org/10.1016/C2016-0-00383-2.

[17] A.B. Poletaev, L.P. Churilov, Y.I. Stroev, M.M. Agapov, Immunophysiology versus immunopathology: natural autoimmunity in human health and disease, Pathophysiology 19 (2012) 221–231, https://doi.org/10.1016/J.PATHOPHYS.2012.07.003.

[18] D. Zheng, T. Liwinski, E. Elinav, Interaction between microbiota and immunity in health and disease, Cell Res. 30 (2020) 492–506, https://doi.org/10.1038/s41422-020-0332-7.

[19] N.R. Rose, Human Organ-Specific Autoimmune Disease, Ref. Modul. Biomed. Sci. (2014), https://doi.org/10.1016/B978-0-12-801238-3.00124-0.

[20] M. Zeher, G. Szegedi, Types of autoimmune disorders. Classification, Orv. Hetil. 148 (2007) 21–24, https://doi.org/10.1556/OH.2007.28030.

[21] B. Bolon, Cellular and molecular mechanisms of autoimmune disease, Toxicol. Pathol. 40 (2012) 216–229, https://doi.org/10.1177/0192623311428481.

[22] A.L. McCall, L.S. Farhy, Treating type 1 diabetes: from strategies for insulin delivery to dual hormonal control, Minerva Endocrinol. 38 (2013) 145–163. http://www.ncbi.nlm.nih.gov/pubmed/23732369. (Accessed 10 December 2018).

[23] A. Hellesen, E. Bratland, E.S. Husebye, Autoimmune Addison's disease—an update on pathogenesis, Ann. Endocrinol. (Paris). 79 (2018) 157–163, https://doi.org/10.1016/J.ANDO.2018.03.008.

[24] A.F.U.H. Saeed, R. Wang, S. Ling, S. Wang, Antibody engineering for pursuing a healthier future, Front. Microbiol. 8 (2017) 495, https://doi.org/10.3389/fmicb.2017.00495.

[25] S.M. Moghimi, A.C. Hunter, J.C. Murray, Nanomedicine: current status and future prospects, FASEB J. 19 (2005) 311–330, https://doi.org/10.1096/fj.04-2747rev.

[26] T.J. Webster, Nanomedicine: what's in a definition? Int. J. Nanomedicine 1 (2006) 115–116, https://doi.org/10.2147/nano.2006.1.2.115.

[27] S.M. Bhagyaraj, O.S. Oluwafemi, N. Kalarikkal, S. Thomas, Characterization of Nanomaterials: Advances and Key Technologies, 2018, https://doi.org/10.1016/C2016-0-01721-7.

[28] K. Maroof, F. Zafar, H. Ali, S. Naveed, S. Tanwir, Scope of nanotechnology in drug delivery, J. Bioequiv. Availab. 08 (2015), https://doi.org/10.4172/jbb.1000257.

[29] Y. Li, X. Li, F. Zhou, A. Doughty, A.R. Hoover, R.E. Nordquist, W.R. Chen, Nanotechnology-based photoimmunological therapies for cancer, Cancer Lett. 442 (2019) 429–438, https://doi.org/10.1016/J.CANLET.2018.10.044.

[30] J.M. Blander, The many ways tissue phagocytes respond to dying cells, Immunol. Rev. 277 (2017) 158–173, https://doi.org/10.1111/imr.12537.

[31] S. Soares, J. Sousa, A. Pais, C. Vitorino, Nanomedicine: principles, properties, and regulatory issues, Front. Chem. 6 (2018), https://doi.org/10.3389/FCHEM.2018.00360.

[32] J. Mathew, J. Joy, S.C. George, Potential applications of nanotechnology in transportation: a review, J. King Saud Univ. - Sci. 31 (2019) 586–594, https://doi.org/10.1016/j.jksus.2018.03.015.

[33] V.N.S.K. Varma, P.V. Maheshwari, M. Navya, S.C. Reddy, H.G. Shivakumar, D.V. Gowda, Calcipotriol delivery into the skin as emulgel for effective permeation, Saudi Pharm. J. 22 (2014) 591–599, https://doi.org/10.1016/j.jsps.2014.02.007.

[34] S. Thota, D.C. Crans, Metal Nanoparticles: Synthesis and Applications in Pharmaceutical Sciences, 2018th ed., WILEY Blackwell, 2018, https://doi.org/10.1002/9783527807093.

[35] M.E. Grigore, Organic and inorganic Nano-Systems used in Cancer treatment abstract Nano-Systems in Cancer treatment, J. Med. Res. Heal. Educ. 1 (2017) 1–8. http://www.imedpub.com/articles/organic-and-inorganic-nanosystems-used-in-cancer-treatment.php?aid=18226. accessed December 16, 2018.

[36] A. Ficai, A.M. Grumezescu, Nanostructures for Cancer Therapy, 2017, https://doi.org/10.1016/c2015-0-04166-1.

[37] Z.P. Xu, Q.H. Zeng, G.Q. Lu, A.B. Yu, Inorganic nanoparticles as carriers for efficient cellular delivery, Chem. Eng. Sci. 61 (2006) 1027–1040, https://doi.org/10.1016/J.CES.2005.06.019.

[38] I. Ben Slama, Sub-acute Oral toxicity of zinc oxide nanoparticles in male rats, J. Nanomed. Nanotechnol. 06 (2015) 1–6, https://doi.org/10.4172/2157-7439.1000284.

[39] P. Hemon, Y. Renaudineau, M. Debant, N. Le Goux, S. Mukherjee, W. Brooks, O. Mignen, Calcium signaling: from normal B cell development to tolerance breakdown and autoimmunity, Clin. Rev. Allergy Immunol. 53 (2017) 141–165, https://doi.org/10.1007/s12016-017-8607-6.

[40] A.M. Grumezescu, Surface Chemistry of Nanobiomaterials: Applications of Nanobiomaterials Volume 3, Elsevier Science, 2016, https://doi.org/10.1016/C2015-0-00378-1.

[41] J. Anastassopoulou, T. Theophanides, The Role of Metal Ions in Biological Systems and Medicine, in: Bioinorg, Chem, Springer Netherlands, Dordrecht, 1995, pp. 209–218, https://doi.org/10.1007/978-94-011-0255-1_17.

[42] A. Bera, H. Belhaj, Application of nanotechnology by means of nanoparticles and nanodispersions in oil recovery - a comprehensive review, J. Nat. Gas Sci. Eng. 34 (2016) 1284–1309, https://doi.org/10.1016/J.JNGSE.2016.08.023.

[43] Q. Mu, G. Jiang, L. Chen, H. Zhou, D. Fourches, A. Tropsha, B. Yan, Chemical basis of interactions between engineered nanoparticles and biological systems, Chem. Rev. 114 (2014) 7740–7781, https://doi.org/10.1021/cr400295a.

[44] H.S. Park, S.H. Nam, J. Kim, H.S. Shin, Y.D. Suh, K.S. Hong, Clear-cut observation of clearance of sustainable upconverting nanoparticles from lymphatic system of small living mice, Sci. Rep. 6 (2016) 27407, https://doi.org/10.1038/srep27407.

[45] E.B. Thorp, C. Boada, C. Jarbath, X. Luo, Nanoparticle platforms for antigen-specific immune tolerance, Front. Immunol. 11 (2020) 945, https://doi.org/10.3389/fimmu.2020.00945.

[46] A.P. Ramos, M.A.E. Cruz, C.B. Tovani, P. Ciancaglini, Biomedical applications of nanotechnology, Biophys. Rev. 9 (2017) 79–89, https://doi.org/10.1007/s12551-016-0246-2.

[47] M.P. Nikolova, M.S. Chavali, Metal oxide nanoparticles as biomedical materials, Biomimetics (Basel, Switz.) 5 (2020) 27, https://doi.org/10.3390/biomimetics5020027.

[48] S. Zhang, L. Wu, J. Cao, K. Wang, Y. Ge, W. Ma, X. Qi, S. Shen, Effect of magnetic nanoparticles size on rheumatoid arthritis targeting and photothermal therapy, Colloids Surf. B: Biointerfaces 170 (2018) 224–232, https://doi.org/10.1016/j.colsurfb.2018.06.016.

[49] D.D. Verma, S. Verma, G. Blume, A. Fahr, Particle size of liposomes influences dermal delivery of substances into skin, Int. J. Pharm. 258 (2003) 141–151, https://doi.org/10.1016/S0378-5173(03)00183-2.

[50] R. Coradeghini, S. Gioria, C.P. García, P. Nativo, F. Franchini, D. Gilliland, J. Ponti, F. Rossi, Size-dependent toxicity and cell interaction mechanisms of gold nanoparticles on mouse fibroblasts, Toxicol. Lett. 217 (2013) 205–216, https://doi.org/10.1016/j.toxlet.2012.11.022.

[51] C. Bantz, O. Koshkina, T. Lang, H.-J. Galla, C.J. Kirkpatrick, R.H. Stauber, M. Maskos, The surface properties of nanoparticles determine the agglomeration state and the size of the particles under physiological conditions, Beilstein J. Nanotechnol. 5 (2014) 1774–1786, https://doi.org/10.3762/bjnano.5.188.

[52] D.R. Baer, M.H. Engelhard, G.E. Johnson, J. Laskin, J. Lai, K. Mueller, P. Munusamy, S. Thevuthasan, H. Wang, N. Washton, A. Elder, B.L. Baisch, A. Karakoti, S.V.N.T. Kuchibhtla, D. Moon, Surface characterization of nanomaterials and nanoparticles: important needs and challenging opportunities, J. Vac. Sci. Technol. A 31 (2013) 50820, https://doi.org/10.1116/1.4818423.

[53] B.D. Chithrani, A.A. Ghazani, W.C.W. Chan, Determining the size and shape dependence of gold nanoparticle uptake into mammalian cells, Nano Lett. 6 (2006) 662–668, https://doi.org/10.1021/nl052396o.

[54] B.D. Chithrani, W.C.W. Chan, Elucidating the mechanism of cellular uptake and removal of protein-coated gold nanoparticles of different sizes and shapes, Nano Lett. 7 (2007) 1542–1550, https://doi.org/10.1021/nl070363y.

[55] A.M. Fales, H. Yuan, T. Vo-Dinh, Silica-coated gold Nanostars for combined surface-enhanced Raman scattering (SERS) detection and singlet-oxygen generation: a potential Nanoplatform for Theranostics, Langmuir 27 (2011) 12186–12190, https://doi.org/10.1021/la202602q.

[56] S. Pal, Y.K. Tak, J.M. Song, Does the antibacterial activity of silver nanoparticles depend on the shape of the nanoparticle? A study of the gram-negative bacterium Escherichia coli, Appl. Environ. Microbiol. 73 (2007) 1712–1720, https://doi.org/10.1128/AEM.02218-06.

[57] R.A. Sperling, W.J. Parak, Surface modification, functionalization and bioconjugation of colloidal inorganic nanoparticles, Philos. Trans. R. Soc. A Math. Phys. Eng. Sci. 368 (2010) 1333–1383, https://doi.org/10.1098/rsta.2009.0273.

[58] V. Berry, A. Gole, S. Kundu, C.J. Murphy, R.F. Saraf, Deposition of CTAB-terminated Nanorods on Bacteria to form highly conducting hybrid systems, J. Am. Chem. Soc. 127 (2005) 17600–17601, https://doi.org/10.1021/ja056428l.

[59] G. Han, P. Ghosh, V.M. Rotello, Functionalized gold nanoparticles for drug delivery, Nanomedicine 2 (2007) 113–123, https://doi.org/10.2217/17435889.2.1.113.

[60] C.H.J. Choi, C.A. Alabi, P. Webster, M.E. Davis, Mechanism of active targeting in solid tumors with transferrin-containing gold nanoparticles, Proc. Natl. Acad. Sci. 107 (2010) 1235–1240, https://doi.org/10.1073/pnas.0914140107.

[61] S.K. Dondapati, T.K. Sau, C. Hrelescu, T.A. Klar, F.D. Stefani, J. Feldmann, Label-free biosensing based on single gold Nanostars as Plasmonic transducers, ACS Nano 4 (2010) 6318–6322, https://doi.org/10.1021/nn100760f.

[62] W. Li, L. Zhang, J. Zhou, H. Wu, Well-designed metal nanostructured arrays for label-free plasmonic biosensing, J. Mater. Chem. C 3 (2015) 6479–6492, https://doi.org/10.1039/C5TC00553A.

[63] A.C. Templeton, W.P. Wuelfing, R.W. Murray, Monolayer-protected cluster molecules, Acc. Chem. Res. 33 (2000) 27–36, https://doi.org/10.1021/ar9602664.

[64] S.E. McNeil, Nanotechnology for the biologist, J. Leukoc. Biol. 78 (2005) 585–594, https://doi.org/10.1189/jlb.0205074.

[65] R. Hong, G. Han, J.M. Fernández, B. Kim, N.S. Forbes, V.M. Rotello, Glutathione-mediated delivery and release using monolayer protected nanoparticle carriers, J. Am. Chem. Soc. 128 (2006) 1078–1079, https://doi.org/10.1021/ja056726i.

[66] R.A. Sperling, T. Pellegrino, J.K. Li, W.H. Chang, W.J. Parak, Electrophoretic separation of nanoparticles with a discrete number of functional groups, Adv. Funct. Mater. 16 (2006) 943–948, https://doi.org/10.1002/adfm.200500589.

[67] A.S. Angelatos, K. Katagiri, F. Caruso, Bioinspired colloidal systems vialayer-by-layer assembly, Soft Matter 2 (2006) 18–23, https://doi.org/10.1039/B511930H.

[68] L. Kou, J. Sun, Y. Zhai, Z. He, The endocytosis and intracellular fate of nanomedicines: implication for rational design, Asian J. Pharm. Sci. 8 (2013) 1–10, https://doi.org/10.1016/J.AJPS.2013.07.001.

[69] L. Araujo, R. Löbenberg, J. Kreuter, Influence of the surfactant concentration on the body distribution of nanoparticles, J. Drug Target. 6 (1999) 373–385, https://doi.org/10.3109/10611869908996844.

[70] V. Labhasetwar, C. Song, W. Humphrey, R. Shebuski, R.J. Levy, Arterial uptake of biodegradable nanoparticles: effect of surface modifications, J. Pharm. Sci. 87 (1998) 1229–1234, https://doi.org/10.1021/js980021f.

[71] P.K. Angra, S.A.A. Rizvi, C.W. Oettinger, M.J. D'Souza, Novel approach for preparing nontoxic stealth microspheres for drug delivery, Eur. J. Chem. 2 (2011) 125–129, https://doi.org/10.5155/eurjchem.2.2.125-129.394.

[72] D. Li, R.B. Kaner, Shape and aggregation control of nanoparticles: not shaken, not stirred, J. Am. Chem. Soc. 128 (2006) 968–975, https://doi.org/10.1021/JA056609N.

[73] E.A. Sykes, Q. Dai, C.D. Sarsons, J. Chen, J.V. Rocheleau, D.M. Hwang, G. Zheng, D.T. Cramb, K.D. Rinker, W.C.W. Chan, Tailoring nanoparticle designs to target cancer based on tumor pathophysiology, Proc. Natl. Acad. Sci. 113 (2016) E1142–E1151, https://doi.org/10.1073/pnas.1521265113.

[74] S. Mura, J. Nicolas, P. Couvreur, Stimuli-responsive nanocarriers for drug delivery, Nat. Mater. 12 (2013) 991–1003, https://doi.org/10.1038/nmat3776.

[75] C.E. Mora-Huertas, H. Fessi, A. Elaissari, Polymer-based nanocapsules for drug delivery, Int. J. Pharm. 385 (2010) 113–142, https://doi.org/10.1016/j.ijpharm.2009.10.018.

[76] J.H. Lee, Y. Yeo, Controlled drug release from pharmaceutical nanocarriers, Chem. Eng. Sci. 125 (2015) 75–84, https://doi.org/10.1016/j.ces.2014.08.046.

[77] P. Calvo, C. Remuñan-López, J.L. Vila-Jato, M.J. Alonso, Chitosan and chitosan/ethylene oxide-propylene oxide block copolymer nanoparticles as novel carriers for proteins and vaccines, Pharm. Res. 14 (1997) 1431–1436. http://www.ncbi.nlm.nih.gov/pubmed/9358557. (Accessed 16 December 2018).

[78] M. Pradhan, A. Alexander, M.R. Singh, D. Singh, S. Saraf, S. Saraf, Ajazuddin, understanding the prospective of nano-formulations towards the treatment of psoriasis, Biomed. Pharmacother. 107 (2018) 447–463, https://doi.org/10.1016/j.biopha.2018.07.156.

[79] T.O. McDonald, M. Siccardi, D. Moss, N. Liptrott, M. Giardiello, S. Rannard, A. Owen, The application of nanotechnology todrug delivery in medicine, Nano (2015) 173–223, https://doi.org/10.1016/B978-0-444-62747-6.00007-5.

[80] S.P. Boulos, T.A. Davis, J.A. Yang, S.E. Lohse, A.M. Alkilany, L.A. Holland, C.J. Murphy, Nanoparticle–protein interactions: a thermodynamic and kinetic study of the adsorption of bovine serum albumin to gold nanoparticle surfaces, Langmuir 29 (2013) 14984–14996, https://doi.org/10.1021/la402920f.

[81] Z.-R. Shi, G.-Z. Tan, Z. Meng, M. Yu, K.-W. Li, J. Yin, K.-H. Wei, Y.-J. Luo, S.-Q. Jia, S.-J. Zhang, J. Wu, X.-B. Mi, L. Wang, Association of anti-acidic ribosomal protein P0 and anti-galectin 3 antibodies with the development of skin lesions in systemic lupus erythematosus, Arthritis Rheumatol. (Hoboken, N.J.) 67 (2015) 193–203, https://doi.org/10.1002/art.38891.

[82] W.H. De Jong, P.J.A. Borm, Drug delivery and nanoparticles: applications and hazards, Int. J. Nanomedicine 3 (2008) 133–149, https://doi.org/10.2147/ijn.s596.

[83] K. Cho, X. Wang, S. Nie, Z. Chen, D.M. Shin, Therapeutic nanoparticles for drug delivery in cancer, Clin. Cancer Res. 14 (2008) 1310–1316, https://doi.org/10.1158/1078-0432.CCR-07-1441.

[84] V.P. Torchilin, Passive and active drug targeting: drug delivery to tumors as an example, Handb. Exp. Pharmacol. (2010) 3–53, https://doi.org/10.1007/978-3-642-00477-3_1.

[85] F. Danhier, O. Feron, V. Préat, To exploit the tumor microenvironment: passive and active tumor targeting of nanocarriers for anti-cancer drug delivery, J. Control. Release 148 (2010) 135–146, https://doi.org/10.1016/j.jconrel.2010.08.027.

[86] E. Ricciotti, G.A. FitzGerald, Prostaglandins and inflammation, Arterioscler. Thromb. Vasc. Biol. 31 (2011) 986–1000, https://doi.org/10.1161/ATVBAHA.110.207449.

[87] M.K. Uchiyama, D.K. Deda, S.F. de Paula Rodrigues, C.C. Drewes, S.M. Bolonheis, P.K. Kiyohara, S.P. de Toledo, W. Colli, K. Araki, S.H.P. Farsky, *In vivo* and In vitro toxicity and anti-inflammatory properties of gold

nanoparticle bioconjugates to the vascular system, Toxicol. Sci. 142 (2014) 497–507, https://doi.org/10.1093/toxsci/kfu202.

[88] M.U. Rehman, Y. Yoshihisa, Y. Miyamoto, T. Shimizu, The anti-inflammatory effects of platinum nanoparticles on the lipopolysaccharide-induced inflammatory response in RAW 264.7 macrophages, Inflamm. Res. 61 (2012) 1177–1185, https://doi.org/10.1007/s00011-012-0512-0.

[89] B. Ahmad, N. Hafeez, S. Bashir, A. Rauf, Mujeeb-ur-Rehman, Phytofabricated gold nanoparticles and their biomedical applications, Biomed. Pharmacother. 89 (2017) 414–425, https://doi.org/10.1016/j.biopha.2017.02.058.

[90] R.M. Hussein, H. Saleh, Promising therapeutic effect of gold nanoparticles against dinitrobenzene sulfonic acid-induced colitis in rats, Nanomedicine 13 (2018), https://doi.org/10.2217/nnm-2018-0009.nnm-2018-0009.

[91] R. Nosratabadi, M. Rastin, M. Sankian, D. Haghmorad, M. Mahmoudi, Hyperforin-loaded gold nanoparticle alleviates experimental autoimmune encephalomyelitis by suppressing Th1 and Th17 cells and upregulating regulatory T cells, nanomedicine nanotechnology, Biol. Med. 12 (2016) 1961–1971, https://doi.org/10.1016/j.nano.2016.04.001.

[92] A. Gul, B. Kunwar, M. Mazhar, S. Faizi, D. Ahmed, M.R. Shah, S.U. Simjee, Rutin and rutin-conjugated gold nanoparticles ameliorate collagen-induced arthritis in rats through inhibition of NF-κB and iNOS activation, Int. Immunopharmacol. 59 (2018) 310–317, https://doi.org/10.1016/j.intimp.2018.04.017.

[93] L. Leonavičiene, G. Kirdaite, R. Bradunaite, D. Vaitkiene, A. Vasiliauskas, D. Zabulyte, A. Ramanavičiene, A. Ramanavičius, T. Ašmenavičius, Z. Mackiewcz, Effect of gold nanoparticles in the treatment of established collagen arthritis in rats, Med. 48 (2012) 91–101, https://doi.org/10.3390/medicina48020016.

[94] M. Shilo, P. Berenstein, T. Dreifuss, Y. Nash, G. Goldsmith, G. Kazimirsky, M. Motiei, D. Frenkel, C. Brodie, R. Popovtzer, Insulin-coated gold nanoparticles as a new concept for personalized and adjustable glucose regulation, Nanoscale 7 (2015) 20489–20496, https://doi.org/10.1039/c5nr04881h.

[95] M.E. Selim, A.A. Hendi, E. Alfallaj, The possible counteractive effect of gold nanoparticles against streptozotocin-induced type 1 diabetes in young male albino rats, Pak. J. Pharm. Sci. 29 (2016) 823–836. http://www.ncbi.nlm.nih.gov/pubmed/27166528. (Accessed 16 December 2018).

[96] H. Bessar, I. Venditti, L. Benassi, C. Vaschieri, P. Azzoni, G. Pellacani, C. Magnoni, E. Botti, V. Casagrande, M. Federici, A. Costanzo, L. Fontana, G. Testa, F.F. Mostafa, S.A. Ibrahim, M.V. Russo, I. Fratoddi, Functionalized gold nanoparticles for topical delivery of methotrexate for the possible treatment of psoriasis, Colloids Surf., B 141 (2016) 141–147, https://doi.org/10.1016/j.colsurfb.2016.01.021.

[97] V.V. Sumbayev, I.M. Yasinska, C.P. Garcia, D. Gilliland, G.S. Lall, B.F. Gibbs, D.R. Bonsall, L. Varani, F. Rossi, L. Calzolai, Gold nanoparticles downregulate interleukin-1β-induced pro-inflammatory responses, Small 9 (2013) 472–477, https://doi.org/10.1002/smll.201201528.

[98] K. Siczek, H. Zatorski, A. Chmielowiec-Korzeniowska, J. Pulit-Prociak, M. Śmiech, R. Kordek, L. Tymczyna, M. Banach, J. Fichna, Synthesis and evaluation of anti-inflammatory properties of silver nanoparticle suspensions in experimental colitis in mice, Chem. Biol. Drug Des. 89 (2017) 538–547, https://doi.org/10.1111/cbdd.12876.

[99] K.C. Bhol, P.J. Schechter, Effects of Nanocrystalline silver (NPI 32101) in a rat model of ulcerative colitis, Dig. Dis. Sci. 52 (2007) 2732–2742, https://doi.org/10.1007/s10620-006-9738-4.

[100] L. David, B. Moldovan, A. Vulcu, L. Olenic, M. Perde-Schrepler, E. Fischer-Fodor, A. Florea, M. Crisan, I. Chiorean, S. Clichici, G.A. Filip, Green synthesis, characterization and anti-inflammatory activity of silver nanoparticles using European black elderberry fruits extract, Colloids Surf., B 122 (2014) 767–777, https://doi.org/10.1016/j.colsurfb.2014.08.018.

[101] J. Li, H. Chen, B. Wang, C. Cai, X. Yang, Z. Chai, W. Feng, ZnO nanoparticles act as supportive therapy in DSS-induced ulcerative colitis in mice by maintaining gut homeostasis and activating Nrf2 signaling, Sci. Rep. 7 (2017) 43126, https://doi.org/10.1038/srep43126.

[102] T.S. Latha, M.C. Reddy, P.V.R. Durbaka, S.V. Muthukonda, D. Lomada, Immunomodulatory properties of titanium dioxide nanostructural materials, Indian J. Pharmacol. 49 (2017) 458–464, https://doi.org/10.4103/ijp.IJP_536_16.

[103] E. Arkhipova, I. Alchinova, A. Sanadze, L. Goldenberg, M. Karganov, Interaction of titanium dioxide nanoparticles and blood serum of patients with bronchial asthma and Myasthenia Gravis, Am. J. Clin. Exp. Med. 3 (2015) 128, https://doi.org/10.11648/j.ajcem.20150303.20.

16. Targeting autoimmune disorders

[104] J. Duan, J. Dong, T. Zhang, Z. Su, J. Ding, Y. Zhang, X. Mao, Polyethyleneimine-functionalized iron oxide nanoparticles for systemic siRNA delivery in experimental arthritis, Nanomedicine 9 (2014) 789–801, https://doi.org/10.2217/nnm.13.217.

[105] J.S. Smolen, G. Steiner, Therapeutic strategies for rheumatoid arthritis, Nat. Rev. Drug Discov. 2 (2003) 473–488, https://doi.org/10.1038/nrd1109.

[106] Y. Lu, L. Li, Z. Lin, L. Wang, L. Lin, M. Li, Y. Zhang, Q. Yin, Q. Li, H. Xia, A new treatment modality for rheumatoid arthritis: combined photothermal and photodynamic therapy using $Cu_{7.2}S_4$ nanoparticles, Adv. Healthc. Mater. 7 (2018), https://doi.org/10.1002/adhm.201800013, 1800013.

[107] K.L. Aillon, Y. Xie, N. El-Gendy, C.J. Berkland, M.L. Forrest, Effects of nanomaterial physicochemical properties on in vivo toxicity, Adv. Drug Deliv. Rev. 61 (2009) 457–466, https://doi.org/10.1016/j.addr.2009.03.010.

[108] M. Ahamed, M. Javed Akhtar, S. Kumar, M. Khan, J. Ahmad, S.A. Alrokayan, Zinc oxide nanoparticles selectively induce apoptosis in human cancer cells through reactive oxygen species, Int. J. Nanomedicine 7 (2012) 845, https://doi.org/10.2147/IJN.S29129.

[109] D. Singh, S. Singh, J. Sahu, S. Srivastava, M.R. Singh, Ceramic nanoparticles: Recompense, cellular uptake and toxicity concerns, Artif. Cells, Nanomedicine, Biotechnol. 44 (2016) 401–409, https://doi.org/10.3109/21691401.2014.955106.

[110] S. Sharifi, S. Behzadi, S. Laurent, M.L. Forrest, P. Stroeve, M. Mahmoudi, Toxicity of nanomaterials, Chem. Soc. Rev. 41 (2012) 2323–2343, https://doi.org/10.1039/c1cs15188f.

[111] N. Asare, C. Instanes, W.J. Sandberg, M. Refsnes, P. Schwarze, M. Kruszewski, G. Brunborg, Cytotoxic and genotoxic effects of silver nanoparticles in testicular cells, Toxicology 291 (2012) 65–72, https://doi.org/10.1016/j.tox.2011.10.022.

[112] C. Greulich, D. Braun, A. Peetsch, J. Diendorf, B. Siebers, M. Epple, M. Köller, The toxic effect of silver ions and silver nanoparticles towards bacteria and human cells occurs in the same concentration range, RSC Adv. 2 (2012) 6981, https://doi.org/10.1039/c2ra20684f.

[113] A. Ivask, I. Kurvet, K. Kasemets, I. Blinova, V. Aruoja, S. Suppi, H. Vija, A. Käkinen, T. Titma, M. Heinlaan, M. Visnapuu, D. Koller, V. Kisand, A. Kahru, Size-dependent toxicity of silver nanoparticles to Bacteria, yeast, algae, crustaceans and mammalian cells in vitro, PLoS One 9 (2014), https://doi.org/10.1371/journal.pone.0102108, e102108.

[114] S.J. Soenen, B. Manshian, J.M. Montenegro, F. Amin, B. Meermann, T. Thiron, M. Cornelissen, F. Vanhaecke, S. Doak, W.J. Parak, S. De Smedt, K. Braeckmans, Cytotoxic effects of gold nanoparticles: a multiparametric study, ACS Nano 6 (2012) 5767–5783, https://doi.org/10.1021/nn301714n.

[115] X. Jing, J.H. Park, T.M. Peters, P.S. Thorne, Toxicity of copper oxide nanoparticles in lung epithelial cells exposed at the air-liquid interface compared with in vivo assessment, Toxicol. in Vitro 29 (2015) 502–511, https://doi.org/10.1016/j.tiv.2014.12.023.

[116] B.C. Heng, X. Zhao, S. Xiong, K. Woei Ng, F. Yin-Chiang Boey, J. Say-Chye Loo, Toxicity of zinc oxide (ZnO) nanoparticles on human bronchial epithelial cells (BEAS-2B) is accentuated by oxidative stress, Food Chem. Toxicol. 48 (2010) 1762–1766, https://doi.org/10.1016/j.fct.2010.04.023.

[117] J. Chen, X. Dong, J. Zhao, G. Tang, *In vivo* acute toxicity of titanium dioxide nanoparticles to mice after intraperitoneal injection, J. Appl. Toxicol. 29 (2009) 330–337, https://doi.org/10.1002/jat.1414.

[118] W.-S. Cho, K. Dart, D.J. Nowakowska, X. Zheng, K. Donaldson, S.E. Howie, Adjuvanticity and toxicity of cobalt oxide nanoparticles as an alternative vaccine adjuvant, Nanomedicine 7 (2012) 1495–1505, https://doi.org/10.2217/nnm.12.35.

[119] R. Hassankhani, M. Esmaeillou, A.A. Tehrani, K. Nasirzadeh, F. Khadir, H. Maadi, In vivo toxicity of orally administered silicon dioxide nanoparticles in healthy adult mice, Environ. Sci. Pollut. Res. 22 (2015) 1127–1132, https://doi.org/10.1007/s11356-014-3413-7.

[120] H. Yang, L. Kozicky, A. Saferali, S.-Y. Fung, N. Afacan, B. Cai, R. Falsafi, E. Gill, M. Liu, T.R. Kollmann, R.E.W. Hancock, L.M. Sly, S.E. Turvey, Endosomal pH modulation by peptide-gold nanoparticle hybrids enables potent anti-inflammatory activity in phagocytic immune cells, Biomaterials 111 (2016) 90–102, https://doi.org/10.1016/j.biomaterials.2016.09.032.

[121] A. Yeste, M. Nadeau, E.J. Burns, H.L. Weiner, F.J. Quintana, Nanoparticle-mediated codelivery of myelin antigen and a tolerogenic small molecule suppresses experimental autoimmune encephalomyelitis, Proc. Natl. Acad. Sci. 109 (2012) 11270–11275, https://doi.org/10.1073/pnas.1120611109.

[122] A. Mani, C. Vasanthi, V. Gopal, D. Chellathai, Role of phyto-stabilised silver nanoparticles in suppressing adjuvant induced arthritis in rats, Int. Immunopharmacol. 41 (2016) 17–23, https://doi.org/10.1016/j.intimp.2016.10.013.

[123] K. Rao, S. Aziz, T. Roome, A. Razzak, B. Sikandar, K.S. Jamali, M. Imran, T. Jabri, M.R. Shah, Gum acacia stabilized silver nanoparticles based nano-cargo for enhanced anti-arthritic potentials of hesperidin in adjuvant induced arthritic rats, Artif. Cells, Nanomedicine, Biotechnol. (2018) 1–11, https://doi.org/10.1080/21691401.2018.1431653.

[124] H.J. Kim, S.-M. Lee, K.-H. Park, C.H. Mun, Y.-B. Park, K.-H. Yoo, Drug-loaded gold/iron/gold plasmonic nanoparticles for magnetic targeted chemo-photothermal treatment of rheumatoid arthritis, Biomaterials 61 (2015) 95–102, https://doi.org/10.1016/j.biomaterials.2015.05.018.

[125] H. Lee, M.-Y. Lee, S.H. Bhang, B.-S. Kim, Y.S. Kim, J.H. Ju, K.S. Kim, S.K. Hahn, Hyaluronate–gold nanoparticle/tocilizumab complex for the treatment of rheumatoid arthritis, ACS Nano 8 (2014) 4790–4798, https://doi.org/10.1021/nn500685h.

[126] S.-M. Lee, H.J. Kim, Y.-J. Ha, Y.N. Park, S.-K. Lee, Y.-B. Park, K.-H. Yoo, Targeted chemo-Photothermal treatments of rheumatoid arthritis using gold half-Shell multifunctional nanoparticles, ACS Nano 7 (2013) 50–57, https://doi.org/10.1021/nn301215q.

[127] F. Ba Fakih, A. Shanti, C. Stefanini, S. Lee, Optimization of gold nanoparticles for efficient delivery of catalase to macrophages for alleviating inflammation, ACS Appl. Nano Mater. 3 (2020) 9510–9519, https://doi.org/10.1021/acsanm.0c02234.

[128] D. Crisan, K. Scharffetter-Kochanek, M. Crisan, S. Schatz, A. Hainzl, L. Olenic, A. Filip, L.A. Schneider, A. Sindrilaru, Topical silver and gold nanoparticles complexed with *Cornus mas* suppress inflammation in human psoriasis plaques by inhibiting NF-κB activity, Exp. Dermatol. 27 (2018) 1166–1169, https://doi.org/10.1111/exd.13707.

CHAPTER

17

Immunomodulatory effects of parasites on autoimmunity

Amir Abdoli[a,b], Alireza Badirzadeh[c], Nazanin Mojtabavi[d,e], Ahmadreza Meamar[c], and Reza Falak[d,e,]*

[a]Zoonosis Research Center, Jahrom University of Medical Sciences, Jahrom, Iran [b]Department of Parasitology and Mycology, Jahrom University of Medical Sciences, Jahrom, Iran [c]Department of Parasitology and Mycology, School of Medicine, Iran University of Medical Sciences, Tehran, Iran [d]Department of Immunology, School of Medicine, Iran University of Medical Sciences, Tehran, Iran [e]Immunology Research Center, Iran University of Medical Sciences, Tehran, Iran *Corresponding author

Abstract

Some helminthic and protozoan infections become chronic with mild symptoms; however, they can gradually affect the immune system and skew its balance toward antiinflammatory conditions. Noticeably, infection with helminths is usually related to reduced cellular immune responses and a shift of T-cell responses to two types of T helper. An inverse association was also found between the prevalence of autoimmune diseases and helminthic infections which suggests that "helminthic therapy" might be beneficial in patients with autoimmune diseases. Helminthic therapy can mitigate the intensity of inflammatory responses and improve the clinical symptoms of autoimmune diseases with minor side effects. However, some intracellular protozoan infections will skew the immune responses toward T helper 1 type and may trigger the development of autoimmune disease. In this chapter, we will mainly focus on this idea and will discuss the possible mechanisms and also the challenges behind them. The main idea in helminthic therapy is the application of some parasites and their products as immunomodulatory agents for the development of new drugs and novel optimistic therapeutic agents for the treatment of autoimmune disease.

Keywords

Helminthic therapy, Autoimmunity, Immunomodulation, Excretory/secretory products, Cytokine balance, T helper, Th1/Th2 ratio, *Leishmania*, *Toxoplasma*

Translational Autoimmunity, Vol. 2
https://doi.org/10.1016/B978-0-12-824390-9.00005-0

Copyright © 2022 Elsevier Inc. All rights reserved.

1 Introduction

Helminth infections are among the most prevalent chronic infectious diseases in under-developed or developing nations [1, 2]. Soil transmitted helminths (STHs) (ascariasis, hook-worm, and trichuriasis), schistosomiasis, and enterobiasis are the most prevalent helminth infections worldwide (Table 1) [2, 3]. Typically, the majority of helminth infections (especially STHs) have minor clinical symptoms, hence, if the infection is left untreated, the infection usually becomes chronic and remains for a long period [4]. Interestingly, these chronic infections regulate the immune responses toward antiinflammatory conditions and autoimmunity diseases [5]. Epidemiological investigations reveal an inverse association between the prevalence of autoimmune diseases and helminth infections [6], whereas a high prevalence of autoimmunity was reported in nations with high sanitation status with low exposure to helminth infections [6–8]. In animal models, helminth infections or helminth-driven excretory/secretory products (ESPs) can protect the host against severe autoimmune diseases [9, 10]. Human clinical trials have shown the beneficial roles of "helminthic therapy" in patients with autoimmune diseases [11], while helminthic therapy mitigated the intensity of inflammatory responses and improved the clinical symptoms of autoimmune diseases with minor side effects [11–13].

TABLE 1 Worldwide prevalence of the most common human helminth infections.

Helminth species	Disease or condition in humans	Estimate prevalence worldwide	Habitat of adult worm in humans
Nematodes			
Ascaris lumbricoides and *A. suum*	Ascariasis	804 million	Small intestine
Trichuris trichiura	Trichuriasis	477 million	Large intestine
Enterobius vermicularis	Enterobiasis (Oxyuriasis)	>200 million	
Toxocara canis	Visceral or ocular larva migrans	Unknown	N/A
Necator americanus	Necatoriasis	472 million	Small intestine
Ancylostoma duodenale	Ancylostomiasis		
Ancylostoma ceylanicum			
Strongyloides stercoralis	Strongyloidiasis	30–100 million	
Wuchereria bancrofti	Lymphatic filariasis	44 million	Lymphatic vessels
Brugia malayi or *Brugia timori*			
Onchocerca volvulus	Onchocerciasis (river blindness)	17 million	Subcutaneous tissue
Trichinella spiralis	Trichinellosis	0.066 million	Small intestine

TABLE 1 Worldwide prevalence of the most common human helminth infections—cont'd

Helminth species	Disease or condition in humans	Estimate prevalence worldwide	Habitat of adult worm in humans
Trematodes			
Schistosoma mansoni	Intestinal schistosomiasis	206 million	Mesenteric veins
Schistosoma haematobium	Urogenital schistosomiasis		Venous plexus of urinary bladder
Schistosoma japonicum	Intestinal schistosomiasis		Mesenteric veins
Fasciola hepatica	Fascioliasis	80 million	Bile ducts
Clonorchis sinensis	Clonorchiasis		Bile ducts and gall bladder
Opisthorchis spp.	Opisthorchiasis		
Paragonimus spp.	Paragonimiasis		Lungs
Cestodes			
Echinococcus granulosus	Hydatid disease	0.8 million	N/A
Echinococcus multilocularis	Alveolar echinococcosis	0.019 million	N/A
Cysticercus cellulosae (Taenia solium larva)	Cysticercosis and Neurocysticercosis	1 million	N/A
Taenia solium	Intestinal taeniasis	0.38 million	Small intestine

N/A, not applicable. There is no development of adult worms in humans.
Reproduced from ref. P. Gazzinelli-Guimaraes, T. Nutman, Helminth parasites and immune regulation [version 1; peer review: 2 approved], F1000Research. 7(1685) 2018. (Open access publication under a creative commons license).

2 Mechanism of action in helminth therapy

Contrary to the host immune response against the majority of intracellular pathogens (e.g., bacteria, fungi, viruses, and protozoa), the protective immune response against helminths is characterized by T helper type 2 (Th2) cells and their related antiinflammatory cytokines (e.g., IL-4, IL-5, IL-9, and IL-13), increase in the frequency of eosinophils, mast cells, basophils, and secretion of some immunoglobulin (Ig) isotypes including IgG1, IgG4, and IgE [14–16]. Furthermore, chronic helminth infections induce regulatory cells, such as regulatory T cells (Treg), B cells (Breg), and dendritic cells (DCreg), and consequently, these cells secret immunomodulatory cytokines such as IL-10 and transforming growth factor-β (TGF-β) (Fig. 1) [17–19]. These regulatory cells and their antiinflammatory cytokines play a pivotal role in the regulation of inflammatory reactions in autoimmune diseases [20].

Recent studies indicate that the gut microbiota has an important role in immune regulation by helminth infections [21]. Intestinal helminths can maintain the gastrointestinal (GI) microbiota to induce antiinflammatory responses [22]. In fact, there is a reciprocal link between

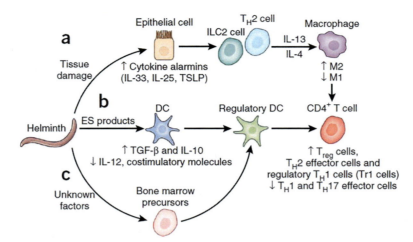

FIG. 1 Mechanisms of helminth-induced immune alteration. Helminth infection stimulates and activates various aspects of the type 2 immune response. (A) Tissue injury induced by helminths triggers the production of the cytokine alarmins (IL-25, IL-33, and the group 2 innate lymphoid cell (ILC2)), that trigger production of Th2 cytokines by the thymic stromal lymphopoietin (TSLP) cells and Th2 cells as well as by basophils and eosinophils. Macrophages exposure to the antiinflammatory cytokines IL-4 or IL-13 lead to suppression of the classical activation of macrophages (M1) and stimulate the expansion of the M2 phenotype. (B) Excretory/secretory (ES) antigens of helminths promote DC to produce the immunoregulatory cytokines, such as TGF-β and IL-10, and also silence DC synthesis of proinflammatory chemokines, cytokines, and costimulatory molecules. (C) Helminth infection promote regulatory DCs that are in favor for the generation of Treg cells. As well the Th1 and Th17 cells compromises during helminth infections. *Reproduced from the ref. P. Salgame, G.S. Yap, W.C. Gause, Effect of helminth-induced immunity on infections with microbial pathogens, Nat. Immunol. 14(11) (2013) 1118 with permission from Springer-Nature.*

GI microbiota and helminths, while helminths alter the GI microbiota composition and the helminths' colonization is influenced by the persistence of microbiota [23–25]. For instance, mice with *Heligmosomoides polygyrus* infection (an intestinal nematode of rodents) have higher colonization of *Lactobacillus* species, and this colonization is associated with enhancement of Treg cells [26]. Transferring of intestinal contents from *H. polygyrus* infected mice to uninfected mice with allergic airway inflammation led to immunomodulation of allergic reactivity [27]. Helminth therapy with human whipworm (*Trichuris trichiura*) in Macaques with idiopathic chronic diarrhea leads to modulation of GI microbiota, induction of Th2 responses, and clinical improvement [28]. In human studies, individuals with intestinal nematode infections (*Ascaris lumbricoides*, *T. trichiura*, and hookworms) had increased and decreased proportions of the families of Paraprevotellaceae and the genus *Bifidobacterium* in their feces, respectively, compared to noninfected individuals [29]. Antihelminth treatment led to decline in proportion of the order Clostridiales and increased the order of Bacteroidales in humans with GI helminth infections [30]. In patients with celiac disease, helminth therapy with *Necator americanus* enhanced the proportion of the Bacteroidetes phylum in patients compared to control individuals [31, 32]. Therefore, these data indicate the important role of microbiota in the regulation of immunity by helminth infections.

3 Application and protective roles of helminth therapy

It is well documented that the imbalance of type 1 and type 2 immunity can lead to autoimmune and allergic disorders [33]. While Th1/Th17 axis and their inflammatory cytokines mediated autoimmune disorders, immunopathogenesis of allergies are principally mediated by Th2 immune responses [34]. Although helminths induce a Th2 immune response, they can augment regulatory immune responses, which are characterized by expansion of Treg, Breg, and DCreg cells, as well as M2 type macrophages and immunoregulatory cytokines, IL-10 and TGF-β [17–19, 34] (Fig. 2).

Resolution of inflammation is an important therapeutic approach for autoimmune diseases and the immunosuppressive therapy have been used as the major treatment for these diseases [35, 36]. However, immunosuppressive agents have different side effects [37], such as cardiovascular toxicity [38] and increased risk of opportunistic infections [39–41]. Meanwhile, helminthic therapy is a novel and optimistic therapeutic option for the treatment of autoimmune diseases with minor side effects [42]. Till now, helminthic therapy has been

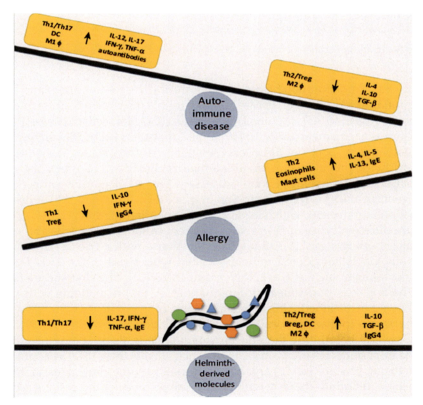

FIG. 2 Immune profiles of the autoimmune and allergic disorders in comparison to the long-term/tolerated immune response to helminth infection. *Reproduced from the ref. J. Kahl, N. Brattig, E. Liebau, The untapped Pharmacopeic potential of Helminths, Trends Parasitol. 34(10) (2018) 828–42 with permission from Elsevier.*

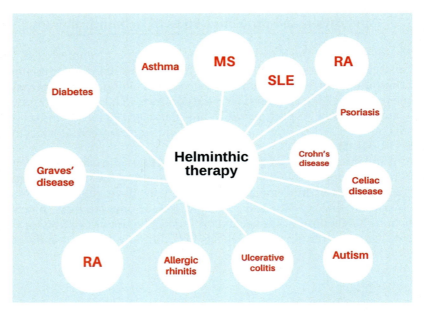

FIG. 3 A snapshot on the application of helminthic therapy in autoimmunity diseases.

used for treatment or amelioration of such autoimmune diseases in human and animal models, including inflammatory bowel disease (IBD) (Crohn's disease and ulcerative colitis) [43], multiple sclerosis (MS) [44, 45], rheumatoid arthritis (RA) [46], celiac disease [47], psoriasis [48], systemic lupus erythematosus (SLE) [49], type 1 diabetes (T1D) [50], allergic rhinitis [51], asthma [52], and autism spectrum disorders (ASD) [53, 54] (Fig. 3).

IBD is a worldwide prevalent chronic inflammatory disorder that affects the gastrointestinal (GI) tract. IBD mainly includes Crohn's disease (CD) and ulcerative colitis (UC) [55]. The typical pathogenesis of IBD is a dysregulation in mucosal immunity at the epithelial barriers and tight-junction impairment, which leads to mucosal inflammation [12, 56]. Although both CD and UC are different types of IBD, rather different inflammatory cells and cytokines are involved in their pathogenesis. A Th2-mediated response with a rise of IL-5 and IL-13 play a role in UC, the CD is considered to be associated with a rise in the Th1/Th17 and their inflammatory cytokines, such as IL-12, IFN-γ, and IL-23 [12]. The first successful small trial of helminth therapy was performed by Summers et al. [57] in patients with CD and UC. The results showed a sustained clinical improvement of the patients who received repeated doses of *Trichuris suis* (pig whipworm) via oral inoculation of the helminth ova (2500 ova). Subsequently, several helminthic therapies in small-scale trials are being used by *N. americanus* or *T. suis* in patients with UC and CD. As such, *T. suis* ova (TSO) was prepared under good manufacturing practice (GMP) and has been used in some clinical tests [58]. In patients with celiac disease, helminth therapy with *N. americanus* revealed no serious adverse events [47, 59, 60]. In one clinical trial, the patients successfully completed low-dose gluten challenge after helminth therapy [59]. The helminth therapy led to increase in production of IL-5 and IL-10 in duodenal biopsies after exposure to gluten antigen [60].

MS is one of the major neurological diseases that affect vision, coordination, and mobility, which ultimately may lead to paralysis [61]. Inflammatory reactions that are mediated by Th1/Th17 cells lead to neuron demyelination both in MS and experimental autoimmune encephalomyelitis (EAE), which is an animal model of the disease [61]. Regarding MS patients, results of the first clinical study published in 2007 by Correale and Farez [44] monitored 12 parasites-infected patients and 12 noninfected patients. They showed fewer numbers of exacerbations, which is found in infected patients than in noninfected counterparts. Immunological findings revealed a significant decrease in IL-12 and IFN-γ and an increase in TGF-β and IL-10 of parasite-infected patients [44]. Interestingly, monitoring of the same patients after antiparasitic treatment demonstrated increased numbers of exacerbations alongside a decrease in antiinflammatory mediators such as IL-10- and TGF-β-secreting cells [62]. Helminth therapy with T. suis has shown increases in serum IL-4 and IL-10 and a decrease in disease index with no serious adverse events of the helminth infection [63].

Autism spectrum disorder (ASD) is a developmental disorder linked to genetic background and immunological disorders. ASD affects communication and behavior. Helminth therapy is also proposed for the treatment and prevention of ASD [64, 65]. Two recent studies evaluated the experiences of individuals who had self-treating with helminths [66, 67]. Cheng et al. estimated that about 6000 and 7000 individuals had self-treating with the helminths worldwide [66]. Interview with five physicians who monitored more than 700 self-treating individuals with helminths revealed that helminth therapy can be efficacious to treat a wide range of autoimmune conditions, allergies, and various neuropsychiatric disorders (NPDs), such as anxiety disorders and major depressive disorder [67]. Interestingly, about 57% of the self-treating patients have autism and the majority of these patients responded favorably to therapy with T. suis and H. diminuta. Side effects of helminth infections, such as gastrointestinal pains, were only reported in 1% of pediatric patients with H. diminuta, although antihelminthic treatment resolved these symptoms. Nevertheless, helminth therapy did not affect the social-communication traits of autistic individuals [67]. The results of a recent randomized trial of T. suis versus placebo in adult individuals with ASD revealed that helminth therapy had only minimal and nonserious side effects, but no significant changes were found in the social-communication traits [68]. Nevertheless, fecal microbiota transfer therapy has shown some improvement in gastrointestinal and autism related symptoms [69, 70]. It should be noted that abnormal gastrointestinal symptoms alongside microbiota perturbations are found to be associated with ASD [71, 72].

Reduced risk of atopy and asthma have been reported among school-age children with STHs and Schistosoma infections [73–76]. For example, it was observed that children with Schistosoma infection were significantly less prone to allergy as measured by skin prick test (SPT) reactivity to house dust mite allergens [77]. An interesting study among Gabonese schoolchildren has shown that long-term treatment and follow-up of STHs increases allergen skin-test reactivity up to 30 months after treatment [78], while another study among the schoolchildren in Ecuador did not show the raise of atopy during 12 months after the treatment [79]. Helminthic therapy with TSO revealed no therapeutic effect for patients with allergic rhinitis [80].

Although helminthic therapy in animal models of RA, T1D, and SLE (Table 4) has shown reduced inflammatory conditions and alleviation in the severity of diseases, clinical trials in this regard are ongoing and their results have not been published until now.

4 Current challenges in helminth therapy

It is important to note that some helminths are also associated with allergic reactions and autoimmunity disorders and rheumatic syndromes [112–114]. For instance, *Toxocara canis* [115, 116] and *Anisakis simplex* [117] infections were reported to be associated with allergic and hypersensitivity reactions. Hence, helminthic therapy should be performed with helminths that induced immunoregulation without hypersensitivity reactions.

Another important challenge of helminthic therapy is the domestication of helminths. While some helminths that are used in helminthic therapy require human hosts (e.g., *N. americanus* or *T. trichiura*), humans are the accidental host of some other helminths (e.g., *H. diminuta* or *T. suis*) [118]. Hence, the use of helminths that do not have domesticated and established clinical problems is desirable for helminthic therapy.

Safe and costly production of some widely used therapeutic helminths, such as *T. suis*, is not available at the moment. For instance, the production of TSO requires pigs as reservoir hosts; in this condition, isolation of TSO from porcine feces requires specific settings to eliminate potential pathogens. Hence, safe and costly production of TSO has not been available so far [66, 118].

In recent studies, helminth-derived compounds have been used for helminth therapy in animal models instead of live worm [118]. These recombinant components may be faced with several technical challenges, including diminished biological activity due to limitations of current expression systems [118, 119].

5 Animal models for helminth therapy

Various animal models of helminth infection have been developed for the assessment of immune responses in the context of autoimmune disorders [118], for instance, EAE and NOD mouse models are used as models of multiple sclerosis and type 1 diabetes for research purposes (Table 2). Moreover, multiple helminths and their compounds have been identified which possess desirable immunoregulatory effects (Table 3).

Animal models of IBD show that helminth or helminth-derived antigens can ameliorate IBD symptoms (Table 4). For instance, it is observed that *S. mansoni* infection attenuates trinitrobenzene sulfonic acid (TNBS)-induced colitis in mice by the expansion of Th2 and their antiinflammatory cytokines, IL-4 and IL-10, and suppression of IFN-γ production [81, 82]. Recombinant antigens from *A. simplex* attenuates dextran sodium sulfate (DSS)-induced colitis by induction of Treg cells and increase of IL-10 secretion [89].

Several helminths have been used for helminth therapy in the animal model of multiple sclerosis, which is known as experimental autoimmune encephalomyelitis (EAE) (Table 4). In this regard, *S. mansoni* infection significantly delayed the development of EAE symptoms through the decrease of proinflammatory cytokine and increase in IL-4 production [94, 95]. *S. japonicum* infection reduced spinal cords inflammation and demyelination by a Th2 mediated mechanism, such as suppression of IFN-γ and high-level production of IL-4 [98]. *T. spiralis* [96] and *Fasciola hepatica* [97] induced immunoregulation in EAE model by mechanisms related to the Th2 immunity.

Rheumatoid arthritis (RA) is another autoimmune disease that affects the synovium of the joints and lead to erosive injury to joint cartilage and bone [46]. In an animal model of RA,

TABLE 2 Animal models used in helminth therapy.

Human CIAD	CIADs	Animal models
Multiple sclerosis	AI	EAE
Cohn's disease	AI	TNBS- or DNBS-induced colitis
Ulcerative colitis	AI	DSS- or oxazolone-induced colitis
	–	Idiopathic chronic diarrhea (macaques)
IBD-like	AT	T cell transfer model of chronic colitis
	KO	Mdr1a-spontaneous colitis
Type 1 diabetes	IM	NOD mice model
	AI	Cyp-accelerated diabetes in NOD mice
	AI	STZ-induced diabetes
Rheumatoid arthritis	AI	Collagen-, CFA- or zymosan-induced arthritis
	AT	K/BxN-induced arthritis
	IM	MRL/MpJ polyarthritis model (also model for SLE)
Multiple sclerosis	AI	Experimental autoimmune encephalomyelitis
Dermal allergies	AI	DFNB-induced contact hypersensitivity
	AI	OVA-atopic eczema
Respiratory allergies	AI	LPS- or CXCL8-induced pulmonary neutrophil model
	AI	OVA- or Derp1-induced allergic airways inflammation
Other allergies	AI	Ocular allergic inflammation
	AI	Food allergy
	AI	OVA-induced delayed-hypersensitivity
Obesity	HFD	High-fat diet-induced obesity

Abbreviations: *AI*, adjuvant-induced model, a model of disease in animals induced by some chemical substance; *AT*, adoptive transfer model, disease induction mediated by transfer of immune cells or antibodies between wild-type and specific animal strains; *CFA*, Freund's complete adjuvant; *CIADs*, chronic inflammatory-associated diseases; *CXCL8*, interleukin 8; *Cyp*, cyclophosphamide; *Derp1*, peptidase 1 from house dust mites; *DFNB*, dinitrofluorobenzene; *DNBS*, dinitrobenzene sulfonic acid; *DSS*, dextran sodium; *EAE*, Experimental Autoimmune Encephalomyelitis; *HFD*, high-fat diet-induced model; *IM*, inbred murine model; *K/BxN*, mice expressing both the T cell receptor transgene KRN and the MHC class II molecule A(g7); *KO*, gene knock-out model; *LPS*, lipopolysaccharide; *Mdr1a* mice, mice lacking key multidrug-resistance genes; *MRL*, Murphy Roths large; *NOD* mice, non-obese diabetic mice; *OVA*, ovalbumin; *SLE*, systematic lupus erythematosus; *STZ*, streptozotocin; *TNBS*, trinitrobenzene sulfonic acid. *Reproduced with some modification from the ref. K. Sobotková, W. Parker, J. Levá, J. Růžková, J. Lukeš, K. Jirků Pomajbíková, Helminth therapy—from the parasite perspective, Trends Parasitol. 35(7) (2019) 501–15 with permission from Elsevier.*

helminth therapy with *S. mansoni* and *S. japonicum* showed attenuation of disease intensity through increased secretion of IL-4 and IL-10 [103, 104] and decreased levels of inflammatory cytokines, namely IL-17, TNF-α, and IFN-γ [103], and autoantibodies [26]. Collectively, results of a recent meta-analysis regarding the animal model of RA revealed that helminthic therapy significantly reduced arthritis score and IFN-γ, but increased IL-10 levels [26].

17. Immunomodulatory effects of parasites on autoimmunity

TABLE 3 Summary of helminths, their life stages, and compounds used in helminth therapy.

Helminths	Life stages used in HT	Helminth form tested in HT		Specific compounds[a]	In vivo/in vitro models
		Live worms	HDeCs		
Trematoda					
Fasciola hepatica	Adult	✓	Ag[b]/ESPs	Proteins	Allergies, MS, RA, T1D in vitro cell culture
Schistosoma japonicum	Adult	–	–	Proteins, killed eggs	IBD, MS, RA in vitro cell culture
	Eggs		Ag		
Schistosoma mansoni	Adult	✓	Ag/ESPs	Proteins, glycan, glycoprotein, killed eggs	Allergies, IBD, MS, RA, T1D, obesity in vitro cell culture
	Larvae		Ag		
	Eggs		Ag		
Clonorchis sinensis	Adult	–	Ag	Protein	Allergies, IBD in vitro cell culture
Cestoda					
Hymenolepis diminuta	Adult	✓	Ag/ESPs	Helminth-influenced cells [c]	IBD, RA in vitro cell culture
	Larvae		–		
Taenia taeniiformis	Larvae	✓	ESPs	–	In vitro cell culture
Taenia crassiceps	Larvae	✓	Ag/ESPs	Helminth-influenced cells	MS, RA, T1D in vitro cell culture
Taenia solium	Adult	✓	–	Protein	IBD in vitro cell culture
	Larvae		Ag		
Echinococcus granulosus	Larvae	–	Ag	Protein	IBD in vitro cell culture
Echinococcus multilocularis	Larvae	–	ESPs	Protoscolexes compound, *alveococcus* vesicles	In vitro cell culture
Nematoda					
Spirurida					
Acantocheilonema vitae	Adult	–	–	Protein, glycoprotein	Allergies, IBD, RA in vitro cell culture
	L4 larvae				
Brugia malayi	Adult	–	Ag	Proteins, peptide	Allergies, IBD, RA, T1D in vitro cell culture
	Larvae		Ag/ESPs		
Dirofilaria immitis	Adult	✓	ESPs	Protein	T1D in vitro cell culture

404

TABLE 3 Summary of helminths, their life stages, and compounds used in helminth therapy—cont'd

		Helminth form tested in HT			
Helminths	Life stages used in HT	Live worms	HDeCs	Specific compounds[a]	In vivo/in vitro models
Litostomoides sigmoidalis	Adult	✓	Ag	–	T1D
	L3 larvae		–		
Onchocerca volvulus	Adult	–	–	Protein	In vitro cell culture
	L4 larvae				
Wuchereria bancrofti	Adult	–	–	Protein	T1D
Strongylida					
Ancylostoma caninum	Adult	–	ESPs	Peptide	Allergies, IBD in vitro cell culture
Ancylostoma ceylanicum	Adult	–	Ag/ESPs	Peptide	Allergies, IBD in vitro cell culture
Heligmosomoides polygyrus	Adult	✓	Ag/ESPs	Helminth-influenced cells, protein	Allergies, IBD, RA, T1D, obesity in vitro cell culture
	L3 larvae		–		
Haemonchus contortus	Adult	–	–	Glycoprotein	In vitro cell culture
	L3 larvae		Ag		
Necator americanus	L3 larvae	✓	–	–	Allergies, CED, IBD in vitro cell culture
Nippostrongylus brasiliensis	Adult	✓	ESPs	Protein	Allergies, RA, obesity in vitro cell culture
	L3 larvae		–		
Oxyurida					
Enterobius vermicularis	Adult	✓	–	–	MS
Syphacia obveolata		✓	–		RA
Rhabditida					
Strongyloides stercoralis	Adult	✓	–	–	Allergies, MS
Strongyloides venezuelensis	Adult	✓	–	–	T1D
	L3 larvae		ESPs		
Ascaridida					
Anisakis simplex	L3 larvae	–	ESPs	Glycoprotein	Allergies, IBD in vitro cell culture
Ascaris lumbricoides	Adult	✓	–	Protein	Allergies, IBD, MS

Continued

17. Immunomodulatory effects of parasites on autoimmunity

TABLE 3   Summary of helminths, their life stages, and compounds used in helminth therapy—cont'd

| Helminths | Life stages used in HT | Helminth form tested in HT | | | | In vivo/in vitro models |
		Live worms	HDeCs	Specific compounds[a]		
Ascaris suum	Adult	–	Ag	Protein helminth-influenced cells		RA in vitro cell culture
	Eggs		Ag			
Toxocara canis	Adult	–	Ag/ESPs	–		In vitro cell culture
Enoplida						
Trichinella pseudospiralis	Adults	✓	–	–		MS
Trichinella spiralis	Adults	✓	–	Protein, killed larvae, helminth-influenced cells		Allergies, IBD, MS, RA, T1D, in vitro cell culture
	Larvae					
Trichuris muris	Eggs	✓	–	–		IBD in vitro cell culture
Trichuris trichiura	Adults	✓	–	–		IBD, MS
Trichuris suis	Adults	✓	ESPs	Lipid		Allergies, IBD, MS in vitro cell culture

[a] *Specific compound: a particular antigenic substance that was either isolated from a worm or ESPs, or its recombinant or synthesized form. This category comprises several types of biomolecule.*

[b] *Ag: crude antigen from the helminth's stage, soluble extract from a part of, or the whole, helminth's stage (synonyms: stage extract, crude extract, crude soluble antigen, whole antigen, soluble stage proteins). This category also includes HMW Ag (high-molecular-weight fraction of an antigen, usually >50 kDa), crude antigen from laminated layer of hydatid cyst, pseudocoelomic fluids, or hydatid fluids.*

[c] *Helminth-influenced cells: T or B lymphocytes adopted from animals that are colonized by the helminth.*

Abbreviations used in this table: *CED*, celiac disease; *ESPs*, excretory/secretory products, material released by a part of, or the whole, helminth's stage; *HDeCs*, helminth-derived compounds; *HT*, helminth therapy; *IBD*, inflammatory bowel disease; *MS*, multiple sclerosis; *RA*, rheumatoid arthritis; *T1D*, type-1 diabetes; *TSO*, *Trichuris suis* ova.

Reproduced with some modification from the ref K. Sobotková, W. Parker, J. Levá, J. Růžková, J. Lukeš, K. Jirků Pomajbíková, Helminth therapy—from the parasite perspective, Trends Parasitol. 35(7) (2019) 501–15 with permission from Elsevier.

Type 1 diabetes (T1D) is a common autoimmune disease worldwide. Helminthic therapy in animal models of T1D ameliorated Th1-mediated immunity, conversely, helminths augment antiinflammatory Th2-mediated responses. As such, helminth therapy prevents disease progression and pancreas damage [50, 99–102] (Table 4).

Helminth therapy has been developed for the treatment of atopy and allergic hypersensitivity in animal models [120, 121]. In mice with airway hyperresponsiveness, helminth infections diminished numbers of eosinophils in bronchoalveolar lavage fluid (BALF) of the infected mice [108]. *S. japonicum* infection reduced eosinophilia and mucus production as well as IL-4, IL-5, and allergen-specific IgE levels [110]. In a food allergy model, *H. polygyrus* infection protected against production of peanut-specific IgE and symptoms of anaphylaxis in an IL-10–dependent manner [111] (Table 4).

TABLE 4 Helminth therapy in animal models of autoimmune diseases.

Disease	Inflammatory bowel disease		
Animal model	Helminth	Outcomes	References
Trinitrobenzene sulfonic acid (TNBS)	Schistosoma mansoni	Helminth infection attenuates TNBS-induced colitis via Th2 polarization. Mediated through increases in IL-4 and IL-10 and decreases in IFNγ	[81, 82]
TNBS	Heligmosomoides polygyrus	Helminth infection attenuates TNBS-induced colonic injury and inflammation via Th2 polarization. Mediated through increases in IL-4 and IL-13	[83]
TNBS	Schistosoma cercariae	Both infections with helminth and immunization with recombinant P28GST attenuates TNBS-induced colitis. Mediated through Th2 polarization and modulation of eosinophil recruitment	[84]
TNBS	Schistosoma japonicum	Ova infection prevents TNBS-induced colitis via Th2 polarization. Mediated through increases in IL-4, IL-5, and IL-10 and decreases in IFNγ	[85–87]
Dextran sodium sulfate (DSS)	S. mansoni	Helminth infection attenuates DSS-induced colitis. Egg injections are ineffective. Mediated through macrophage trafficking	[88]
DSS	Anisakis simplex	Therapeutic treatment with recombinant rAs-migration inhibitory factor protein attenuates DSS-induced colitis. Thought to be mediated through regulatory T cell (Treg) expansion and increases in IL-10	[89]
DSS	Acanthocheilonema viteae	Therapeutic treatment with recombinant cystatin protein attenuates DSS-induced colitis. Thought to be mediated via targeting and modulation of macrophages	[90]
Dinitrobenzene sulfonic acid (DNBS)	Trichinella spiralis	Helminth infection reduced severity of DNBS-induced colonic damage. Mediated through increases in IL-4 and IL-13 and a decrease in IFNγ	[91]
DNBS	Hymenolepis diminuta	Helminth infection in WT and IL-22$^{-/-}$ mice attenuates DNBS-induced colitis. An increase in the number of mucus-containing goblet cells in the small intestine was observed in WT but not IL-22$^{-/-}$ mice	[92]
Nonsteroidal antiinflammatory drugs (NSAIDs)	Trichuris muris	Helminth infection in Nod2$^{-/-}$ mice restored SI goblet cell numbers/morphology and decreased IFNγ-secreting CD8$^+$ T cells in the intestine	[30]
T cell transfer model of colitis (TCT)	H. polygyrus	Helminth infection in Rag mice attenuates TCT-induced colitis. Mediated through decreases in IL-12 and IFNγ and increases in IL-13 and Treg	[93]
TCT	H. polygyrus	Helminth infection in Rag mice attenuates TCT-induced colitis. Mediated through altered dendritic cell (DC) function in the mucosa	[85]

Continued

17. Immunomodulatory effects of parasites on autoimmunity

TABLE 4 Helminth therapy in animal models of autoimmune diseases—cont'd

Disease	Inflammatory bowel disease		
Animal model	**Helminth**	**Outcomes**	**References**
Dinitrobenzene sulfonic acid (DNBS)	Trichinella spiralis	Helminth infection reduced the severity of DNBS-induced colonic damage. Mediated through increases in IL-4 and IL-13 and a decrease in IFNγ	[91]
DNBS	Hymenolepis diminuta	Helminth infection in WT and IL-22$^{-/-}$ mice attenuates DNBS-induced colitis. An increase in the number of mucus-containing goblet cells in the small intestine was observed in WT but not IL-22$^{-/-}$ mice	[92]
Nonsteroidal antiinflammatory drugs (NSAIDs)	Trichuris muris	Helminth infection in Nod2$^{-/-}$ mice restored SI goblet cell numbers/morphology and decreased IFNγ-secreting CD8$^+$ T cells in the intestine	[30]
T cell transfer model of colitis (TCT)	H. polygyrus	Helminth infection in Rag mice attenuates TCT-induced colitis. Mediated through decreases in IL-12 and IFNγ and increases in IL-13 and Treg	[93]
TCT	H. polygyrus	Helminth infection in Rag mice attenuates TCT-induced colitis. Mediated through altered dendritic cell (DC) function in the mucosa	[85]
Dinitrobenzene sulfonic acid (DNBS)	Trichinella spiralis	Helminth infection reduced the severity of DNBS-induced colonic damage. Mediated through increases in IL-4 and IL-13 and a decrease in IFNγ	[91]
DNBS	Hymenolepis diminuta	Helminth infection in WT and IL-22$^{-/-}$ mice attenuates DNBS-induced colitis. An increase in the number of mucus-containing goblet cells in the small intestine was observed in WT but not IL-22$^{-/-}$ mice	[92]
Nonsteroidal antiinflammatory drugs (NSAIDs)	Trichuris muris	Helminth infection in Nod2$^{-/-}$ mice restored SI goblet cell numbers/morphology and decreased IFNγ-secreting CD8$^+$ T cells in the intestine	[30]
T cell transfer model of colitis (TCT)	H. polygyrus	Helminth infection in Rag mice attenuates TCT-induced colitis. Mediated through decreases in IL-12 and IFNγ and increases in IL-13 and Treg	[93]
TCT	H. polygyrus	Helminth infection in Rag mice attenuates TCT-induced colitis. Mediated through altered dendritic cell (DC) function in the mucosa	[85]
Dinitrobenzene sulfonic acid (DNBS)	Trichinella spiralis	Helminth infection reduced the severity of DNBS-induced colonic damage. Mediated through increases in IL-4 and IL-13 and a decrease in IFNγ	[91]
DNBS	Hymenolepis diminuta	Helminth infection in WT and IL-22$^{-/-}$ mice attenuates DNBS-induced colitis. An increase in the number of mucus-containing goblet cells in the small intestine was observed in WT but not IL-22$^{-/-}$ mice	[92]
Nonsteroidal antiinflammatory drugs (NSAIDs)	Trichuris muris	Helminth infection in Nod2$^{-/-}$ mice restored SI goblet cell numbers/morphology and decreased IFNγ-secreting CD8$^+$ T cells in the intestine	[30]

TABLE 4 Helminth therapy in animal models of autoimmune diseases—cont'd

Disease	Inflammatory bowel disease		
Animal model	**Helminth**	**Outcomes**	**References**
T cell transfer model of colitis (TCT)	*H. polygyrus*	Helminth infection in Rag mice attenuates TCT-induced colitis. Mediated through decreases in IL-12 and IFNγ and increases in IL-13 and Treg	[93]
TCT	*H. polygyrus*	Helminth infection in Rag mice attenuates TCT-induced colitis. Mediated through altered dendritic cell (DC) function in the mucosa	[85]
Dinitrobenzene sulfonic acid (DNBS)	*Trichinella spiralis*	Helminth infection reduced the severity of DNBS-induced colonic damage. Mediated through increases in IL-4 and IL-13 and a decrease in IFNγ	[91]
DNBS	*Hymenolepis diminuta*	Helminth infection in WT and IL-22$^{-/-}$ mice attenuates DNBS-induced colitis. An increase in the number of mucus-containing goblet cells in the small intestine was observed in WT but not IL-22$^{-/-}$ mice	[92]
Nonsteroidal antiinflammatory drugs (NSAIDs)	*Trichuris muris*	Helminth infection in Nod2$^{-/-}$ mice restored SI goblet cell numbers/morphology and decreased IFNγ-secreting CD8^{+} T cells in the intestine	[30]
T cell transfer model of colitis (TCT)	*H. polygyrus*	Helminth infection in Rag mice attenuates TCT-induced colitis. Mediated through decreases in IL-12 and IFNγ and increases in IL-13 and Treg	[93]
TCT	*H. polygyrus*	Helminth infection in Rag mice attenuates TCT-induced colitis. Mediated through altered dendritic cell (DC) function in the mucosa	[85]
Dinitrobenzene sulfonic acid (DNBS)	*Trichinella spiralis*	Helminth infection reduced the severity of DNBS-induced colonic damage. Mediated through increases in IL-4 and IL-13 and a decrease in IFNγ	[91]
DNBS	*Hymenolepis diminuta*	Helminth infection in WT and IL-22$^{-/-}$ mice attenuates DNBS-induced colitis. An increase in the number of mucus-containing goblet cells in the small intestine was observed in WT but not IL-22$^{-/-}$ mice	[92]
Nonsteroidal antiinflammatory drugs (NSAIDs)	*Trichuris muris*	Helminth infection in Nod2$^{-/-}$ mice restored SI goblet cell numbers/morphology and decreased IFNγ-secreting CD8^{+} T cells in the intestine	[30]
T cell transfer model of colitis (TCT)	*H. polygyrus*	Helminth infection in Rag mice attenuates TCT-induced colitis. Mediated through decreases in IL-12 and IFNγ and increases in IL-13 and Treg	[93]
TCT	*H. polygyrus*	Helminth infection in Rag mice attenuates TCT-induced colitis. Mediated through altered dendritic cell (DC) function in the mucosa	[85]
Dinitrobenzene sulfonic acid (DNBS)	*Trichinella spiralis*	Helminth infection reduced the severity of DNBS-induced colonic damage. Mediated through increases in IL-4 and IL-13 and a decrease in IFNγ	[91]

Continued

17. Immunomodulatory effects of parasites on autoimmunity

TABLE 4 Helminth therapy in animal models of autoimmune diseases—cont'd

Disease	**Inflammatory bowel disease**		
Animal model	**Helminth**	**Outcomes**	**References**
DNBS	*Hymenolepis diminuta*	Helminth infection in WT and IL-22$^{-/-}$ mice attenuates DNBS-induced colitis. An increase in the number of mucus-containing goblet cells in the small intestine was observed in WT but not IL-22$^{-/-}$ mice	[92]
Nonsteroidal antiinflammatory drugs (NSAIDs)	*Trichuris muris*	Helminth infection in Nod2$^{-/-}$ mice restored SI goblet cell numbers/morphology and decreased IFNγ-secreting CD8$^+$ T cells in the intestine	[30]
T cell transfer model of colitis (TCT)	*H. polygyrus*	Helminth infection in Rag mice attenuates TCT-induced colitis. Mediated through decreases in IL-12 and IFNγ and increases in IL-13 and Treg	[93]
TCT	*H. polygyrus*	Helminth infection in Rag mice attenuates TCT-induced colitis. Mediated through altered dendritic cell (DC) function in the mucosa	[85]
Dinitrobenzene sulfonic acid (DNBS)	*Trichinella spiralis*	Helminth infection reduced the severity of DNBS-induced colonic damage. Mediated through increases in IL-4 and IL-13 and a decrease in IFNγ	[91]
DNBS	*Hymenolepis diminuta*	Helminth infection in WT and IL-22$^{-/-}$ mice attenuates DNBS-induced colitis. An increase in the number of mucus-containing goblet cells in the small intestine was observed in WT but not IL-22$^{-/-}$ mice	[92]
Disease	**Multiple Sclerosis**		
Experimental autoimmune encephalomyelitis (EAE)	*S. mansoni*	Helminth infection attenuated the clinical course of EAE. Therapeutic exposure significantly delayed the development of symptoms. Mediated through an increase of IL-4 and decrease of proinflammatory cytokines	[94, 95]
EAE	*T. spiralis*	Helminth infection maintained Th2 immunity after EAE induction. Transfer of T cells from infected mice to EAE immunized mice amelioration disease and protected from disease	[96]
EAE	*Fasciola hepatica*	Helminth infection attenuated the clinical course of EAE. Mediated through migration interference of DCs, macrophages eosinophils, neutrophils, and CD4$^+$ T cells	[97]
EAE	*S. japonicum*	Helminth infection reduced inflammation and demyelination in spinal cords. Mediated through a Th2-biased microenvironment of low IFNγ and high IL-4 production in the spleen and CNS	[98]

TABLE 4 Helminth therapy in animal models of autoimmune diseases—cont'd

Disease		Inflammatory bowel disease	
Animal model	**Helminth**	**Outcomes**	**References**
Disease		**Type 1 diabetes**	
Nonobese diabetic (NOD)	S. mansoni	Helminth infection or ova injection prevented disease if administered before the onset of pancreatic infiltration (<4 weeks of age). Mediated through a Th2-biased environment of increased IL-4, IL-5, IL-10, and IL-13	[99, 100]
NOD	H. polygyrus	Helminth infection protects animals from disease for <35 weeks. Thought to be mediated through Th2 skewing and modulation of IL-4 and IL-13 expression. Mechanism independent of IL-10 and CD4$^+$/CD25$^+$ T cells	[50, 101]
NOD	T. spiralis	Helminth infection protected animals from disease for <37 weeks. Thought to be mediated by increases in CD4$^+$ cells and decreases in CD8$^+$ and NK cells in the pancreas. Th2 skewing noted	[50]
Diabetic retinopathy	Ancylostoma caninum	Transgenic mice expressing neutrophil inhibitory factor (NIF) are protected from diabetic retinopathy. NIF did not compromise normal immune surveillance but did result in large amounts of superoxide	[102]
Nonobese diabetic (NOD)	S. mansoni	Helminth infection or ova injection prevented disease if administered before the onset of pancreatic infiltration (<4 weeks of age). Mediated through a Th2-biased environment of increased IL-4, IL-5, IL-10, and IL-13	[99, 100]
NOD	H. polygyrus	Helminth infection protects animals from disease for <35 weeks. Thought to be mediated through Th2 skewing and modulation of IL-4 and IL-13 expression. Mechanism independent of IL-10 and CD4$^+$/CD25$^+$ T cells	[50, 101]
Disease		**Rheumatoid arthritis**	
Collagen-induced arthritis (CIA)	S. mansoni	Helminth infection attenuates disease through decreases in IFNγ, TNFα, and IL-17 and increases in IL-4 and IL-10	[103]
CIA	S. japonicum	Helminth infection attenuates disease incidence and severity. Protection was infection stage-dependent through decreases in IFNγ and autoantibodies and increases in IL-4 and IL-10	[104]

Continued

17. Immunomodulatory effects of parasites on autoimmunity

TABLE 4   Helminth therapy in animal models of autoimmune diseases—cont'd

Disease	Inflammatory bowel disease		
Animal model	Helminth	Outcomes	References
CIA	*A. viteae*	Prophylactic and therapeutic admiration of an excretory/secretory (ES)-62 analog attenuates disease through the decrease in inflammasome activity and IL-1β at the disease site	[105]
MRL/lpr Mouse Strain	*H. polygyrus*	Helminth infection attenuates the incidence and severity of spontaneous disease through increases in IL-4 and IgG1 and decreases in lymphocyte infiltration at the disease site	[106]
Collagen-induced arthritis (CIA)	*S. mansoni*	Helminth infection attenuates disease through decreases in IFNγ, TNFα, and IL-17 and increases in IL-4 and IL-10	[103]
CIA	*S. japonicum*	Helminth infection attenuates disease incidence and severity. Protection was infection stage-dependent. Mediated through decreases in IFNγ and autoantibodies and increases in IL-4 and IL-10	[104]
CIA	*A. viteae*	Prophylactic and therapeutic admiration of an excretory/secretory (ES)-62 analog attenuates disease through the decrease in inflammasome activity and IL-1β at the disease site	[105]
MRL/lpr Mouse Strain	*H. polygyrus*	Helminth infection attenuates the incidence and severity of spontaneous disease through increases in IL-4 and IgG1 and decreases in lymphocyte infiltration at the disease site	[106]
Collagen-induced arthritis (CIA)	*S. mansoni*	Helminth infection attenuates disease through decreases in IFNγ, TNFα, and IL-17 and increases in IL-4 and IL-10	[103]
Disease	Systemic lupus erythematosus		
MRL/Lpr	*A. viteae*	Therapeutic administration of ES-62 analogs attenuates the incidence and severity of the disease. Mediated by reducing MyD88 and IL-6 in kidney infiltrating macrophages	[107]
Disease	Hypersensitivity and allergic reactions		
OVA (ovalbumin)-induced airway hyperresponsiveness (AHR)	*H. polygyrus*	Reduced numbers of total cells and eosinophils were detected in bronchoalveolar lavage fluid (BALF) of infected mice. mesenteric lymph node cells (MLNC) from infected animals contained increased numbers of CD4$^+$CD25$^+$Foxp3$^+$ T cells, higher TGF-β expression, and produced strong IL-10 responses to parasite antigen.	[108]
OVA-induced AHR	*Strongyloides venezuelensis*	Infection reduced AHR 48h after challenge	[109]

TABLE 4 Helminth therapy in animal models of autoimmune diseases—cont'd

Disease		Inflammatory bowel disease	
Animal model	Helminth	Outcomes	References
OVA-induced AHR	S. japonicum	Infection reduced mucus production, eosinophilia, IL-4, and IL-5, and allergen-specific IgE levels. Protection was also elicited through adoptive transfer of dendritic cells (DCs) from infected animals	[110]
Food allergy	H. polygyrus	Infection protected against production of peanut-specific IgE and symptoms of anaphylaxis in an IL-10–dependent manner.	[111]

Reproduced with some modifications from T.B. Smallwood, P.R. Giacomin, A. Loukas, J.P. Mulvenna, R.J. Clark, J.J. Miles, Helminth immunomodulation in autoimmune disease, Front. Immunol. 8 (2017) 453. (Open access publication under a creative common license).

6 Immunomodulatory roles of parasites on inflammatory or autoimmune diseases

Although the potential link between distinct bacterial and viral infectious diseases and inflammatory or autoimmunity diseases is well documented, it seems that the role of infection with various parasites has been vastly neglected. According to the literature, it is believed that parasites have a complicated immunomodulatory effect in the human host [122] and might be involved in the evolution of autoimmunity [123].

Parasite antigens play vital roles in immune dysregulation through interaction with the host immune system, which can finally lead to various spectrum of autoimmune disorders [124]. Those infections in line with host genetic background or endocrine disorders could be considered as a possible route for autoimmunity development [122, 125].

Some studies show the correlation of autoimmunity disorders with parasitic infections. *Trypanosoma cruzi*, the causative agent of Chagas disease, can directly activate various autoimmunity pathways and lead to severe cardiomyopathy following the development of autoreactive antibodies as well as cytotoxic T cells and consequently affect different organs especially the heart and nervous system [126–128]. In some long-standing severe infections such as malaria, the development of anemia due to complement-mediated hemolytic conditions is associated with the development of various autoantibodies against different proteins and enzymes [129]. *Toxoplasma* infection can trigger a high level of specific antibodies. Moreover, anti-*Toxoplasma* antibody titer is higher in autoimmune diseases [130]. In onchocerciasis (river blindness), the development of autoantibodies plays a destructive function against the patients' inner retina antigens [131].

Infecting parasites may modify host proteins' structure to be perceived as an extrinsic or a neoantigen, capable of stimulating autoimmune responses [122, 125]. Although autoimmunity due to a parasitic infection was vastly reported, little is known about its exact mechanisms and pathogenesis [129, 132]. Autoantibodies raised against nuclear antigens in Schistosoma, malaria, and trematode infections are similar to human anti-DNA antibodies found in patients with SLE [133, 134]. Generally, autoimmunity-related clinical manifestations can happen in chronic parasitic infections [128].

17. Immunomodulatory effects of parasites on autoimmunity

7 Leishmaniasis and autoimmune disorders

Leishmaniasis is a spectrum of vector-borne tropical parasitic infection, which is caused by different species of genus *Leishmania*. The main cellular environment around these intracellular parasites is mononuclear phagocytes such as macrophages and dendritic cells (DCs) [135, 136]. This infection has several major clinical manifestations including cutaneous, visceral, and mucocutaneous lesions, depending on the distinct *Leishmania* species, the host may develop localized or disseminated forms of the infection. Nowadays, leishmaniasis is endemic among approximately 100 countries, with an annual incidence of 1.2 million and 0.4 million cases of cutaneous (CL) and visceral leishmaniasis (VL), respectively [135, 137].

Leishmania has a dimorphic life cycle with distinct stages including flagellated promastigote form in sand fly, as its intermediate insect vector and amastigote stage in mononuclear phagocytic cells of mammalian hosts. Amastigote form lives in phagolysosomal compartments of the macrophages [138]. Pathogenesis of leishmaniasis is due to complex interactions between parasite antigens and the host's immune system [139].

The similarity between host and *Leishmania* antigens has been reported in some studies and points out the possibility of the development of high titer lupus-related antinuclear antibodies in VL and CL patients. So that, patients demonstrate different autoimmune manifestations, such as cutaneous vasculitis and arthralgia. Moreover, some laboratory findings, such as hypergammaglobulinemia, cryoglobulinemia, decreased CH50 level, and development of antinuclear antibodies are commonly observed [140, 141].

In brief, distinct autoantibodies against nuclear antigens, such as Sm, SS-A, SS-B, RNP, native DNA, as well as non-nuclear antigens, such as smooth muscle, cyclic citrullinated peptide (CCP), myeloperoxidase (MPO), cardiolipin, b2-glycoprotein, hemoglobin, and actin might be detectable [141–145].

Similar to many other autoimmune diseases, the mechanism of development of autoantibodies in leishmaniasis is not clear yet. Argov et al. suggested that either polyclonal activation of lymphocytes or molecular mimicry between distinct *leishmania* antigens and extractable ribonucleoproteins may play role in the induction of autoantibodies against the nuclear antigens [145]. Molecular mimicry induces not only an antibody-related humoral response but also a cellular cytotoxic T cell response as well, which leads to various tissues damages [145, 146].

General laboratory findings in VL patients are pancytopenia and hypergammaglobulinemia, which resemble various autoimmune features [141, 144, 147]. By applying antiglobulin Coombs' test and immunofluorescence techniques, IgG antibodies against cell surface components of erythrocytes, platelets and neutrophils were reported in these patients [147]. VL is a well-known mimicker of autoimmune diseases such as SLE [148]. The SLE is a disease with a thousand faces was specified by several features such as thrombocytopenia, skin lesions, nephritis, positive ANAs, and anticardiolipin [148]. In some cases, after treating the leishmaniasis, ANAs vanished and SLE symptoms were completely treated [146].

In leishmaniasis, different organs such as the kidney and skin may be involved. Following renal involvement, glomerulonephritis, kidney fibrosis, and hypertrophy, nephrotic syndrome and acute interstitial nephritis may occur [146, 149]. In one study, *Leishmania* parasites were observed in renal tissue [146, 150]. In another experiment, the search for the parasite in the patient's kidney was negative [151]. In some studies, renal biopsies elucidated evidence of the precipitation of immunoglobulins, complement, and fibrinogen as well as the presence of *Leishmania* antigens, without direct evidence of leishmanial parasite in the tissue [149, 152]. Furthermore, in the sera of VL patients, distinct immune complexes, capable of directly stimulating monocytes/macrophages and consequently the production of various proinflammatory and antiinflammatory cytokines including GM-CSF, IL-6, IL-10, and IL-1RA were detected. These immune complexes affect the progression and outcome of leishmaniasis via the induction of inflammatory cytokines [150].

8 *Toxoplasmosis* and autoimmune disorders

Toxoplasmosis is a zoonotic disease with a significant public health concern, caused by the ubiquitous obligatory intracellular parasite *Toxoplasma gondii* [153, 154]. *T. gondii* belongs to apicomplexan parasites capable of invading nucleated cells in almost all warm-blooded animals and humans, while felines (cats) are regarded as its primary host [155]. Toxoplasmosis is usually due to ingestion of contaminated food or water with oocysts shed by cats, or through consuming raw animal meat containing cysts and rarely across the placenta, from infected mother to her fetus. It is assumed that almost one-third of any population has experienced this parasitic infection [154].

Nowadays, toxoplasmosis is considered an emerging chronic opportunistic infection in immunocompromised individuals [156]. Combination of potent cell-mediated (Th1) and humoral immune responses may put an end to toxoplasmosis, however, its possible role in autoimmunity has been studied scarcely [157, 158].

Innate immune response and production of inflammatory cytokines are the initial events in the immunity to toxoplasmosis [157, 159]. Meanwhile, resistance to toxoplasmosis mainly relies on cell-mediated immune response through activation of specific Th1 lymphocytes and production of IL-12 and IFN-γ [157].

Following infection, *Toxoplasma* tachyzoites, as the active form of the parasite stimulate neutrophils, which consequently produce IL-12 and TNF-α, leading to a strong Th1 response [157]. Neutrophil extracellular traps (NETs) effectively contribute to *Toxoplasma* entrapment and its clearance and could be involved in autoimmunity as well [160, 161].

It seems that toxoplasmosis is linked with various autoimmune disorders. Percutaneous injection of the tachyzoites into the rats' footpad induced a localized inflammatory arthritic process such as rheumatoid arthritis with iridocyclitis and triggered immune response against ocular and also articular antigens [162].

However, some animal studies show that toxoplasmosis has protective effects against autoimmunity and is capable of preventing the development of autoimmune renal disorders and lupus-like syndrome of NZBW mice and potentially prolong their life. Moreover, the parasite downregulates the induction of IFN-γ and IL-10 cytokines and anti-HSP70 autoantibody titer and stops the progression of glomerulonephritis in NZBW mice [163]. Furthermore, in patients with autoimmune T1D, the anti-*Toxoplasma* antibody titer is lower than healthy controls [164].

However, most of the studies show a positive correlation between anti-*Toxoplasma* antibodies with various autoimmune disorders including rheumatoid arthritis (RA), polymyositis, Crohn's disease, thyroid diseases, Wegener's granulomatosis, antiphospholipid syndrome (APS), and autoimmune bullous diseases [165–171].

In addition, a higher prevalence of anti-*Toxoplasma* IgG was identified in patients with SLE, APS, cryoglobulinemia, vasculitides associated with antineutrophil cytoplasmic autoantibodies (ANCA), autoimmune thyroid diseases, and systemic sclerosis (SSc) [130, 172–174].

Toxoplasmosis is possibly associated with RA, especially in older patients [165, 166]. *T. gondii* can develop spontaneous RA in IL-1Ra-deficient mice [175]. IL-1 is a crucial cytokine in immune responses against the infection and IL-1Ra is considered as a negative regulator of IL-1 signaling because it competes with IL-1α and IL-1β in binding to IL-1 receptors. Therefore, IL-1Ra defects could potentially cause severe autoimmune manifestations. The severity of arthritis was also linked with cell-mediated response through Th1 polarization accompanied by Th17 response in mice [175, 176]. In a study in Brazil, a remarkable relation was reported between atopic syndrome and negative serology to *Toxoplasma* infection. This experiment indicates that the immunomodulation triggered by *Toxoplasma* may play a protective role in the expansion of distinct allergic diseases [177]. Altogether, various studies have found associations between Toxoplasmosis and induction of specific autoantibodies, which results in autoimmune conditions.

9 Conclusion

In conclusion, helminthic therapy of patients with autoimmune diseases, including administration of distinct types of manageable parasites or their excretory/secretory products can shift immune response toward Th2 and improve the clinical symptoms and the inflammatory condition of the patients. Inversely, some intracellular protozoa such as *Leishmania* and *Toxoplasma* can skew the immune response toward Th1 and play role in the development of autoimmunity due to molecular mimicry of some mammalian and parasite antigens. Parasites' immunosuppressive excretory/secretory products can boost tolerance in the host immune system and based on the mentioned molecular structure similarities with mammalian antigens have the authority to evade the host humoral and cellular immune system mechanisms and survive and even induce hypersensitivity reactions. Currently, several immunoparasitology studies have focused on these ideas and try to find, characterize and synthetize recombinant forms of parasite-derived immunomodulatory agents to apply as novel medications for the treatment of autoimmune disease in the future.

References

[1] P.J. Hotez, M. Alvarado, M.-G. Basáñez, I. Bolliger, R. Bourne, M. Boussinesq, et al., The global burden of disease study 2010: interpretation and implications for the neglected tropical diseases, PLoS Negl. Trop. Dis. 8 (7) (2014), e2865.

[2] P.M. Jourdan, P.H. Lamberton, A. Fenwick, D.G. Addiss, Soil-transmitted helminth infections, Lancet 391 (10117) (2018) 252–265.

[3] P. Gazzinelli-Guimaraes, T. Nutman, Helminth parasites and immune regulation [version 1; peer review: 2 approved], F1000Research 7 (1685) (2018).

[4] P.J. Hotez, P.J. Brindley, J.M. Bethony, C.H. King, E.J. Pearce, J. Jacobson, Helminth infections: the great neglected tropical diseases, J. Clin. Invest. 118 (4) (2008) 1311–1321.

[5] N.L. Harris, L. Pn, Recent advances in Type-2-cell-mediated immunity: insights from helminth infection, Immunity 47 (6) (2017) 1024–1036.

[6] L.J. Wammes, H. Mpairwe, A.M. Elliott, M. Yazdanbakhsh, Helminth therapy or elimination: epidemiological, immunological, and clinical considerations, Lancet Infect. Dis. 14 (11) (2014) 1150–1162.

[7] A.E. Wiria, Y. Djuardi, T. Supali, E. Sartono, M. Yazdanbakhsh (Eds.), Helminth infection in populations undergoing epidemiological transition: a friend or foe? Semin. Immunopathol. (2012). Springer.

[8] H. Okada, C. Kuhn, H. Feillet, J.F. Bach, The 'hygiene hypothesis' for autoimmune and allergic diseases: an update, Clin. Exp. Immunol. 160 (1) (2010) 1–9.

[9] J.P. Hewitson, J.R. Grainger, R.M. Maizels, Helminth immunoregulation: the role of parasite secreted proteins in modulating host immunity, Mol. Biochem. Parasitol. 167 (1) (2009) 1–11.

[10] W. Harnett, Secretory products of helminth parasites as immunomodulators, Mol. Biochem. Parasitol. 195 (2) (2014) 130–136.

[11] J. Fleming, J. Weinstock, Clinical trials of helminth therapy in autoimmune diseases: rationale and findings, Parasite Immunol. 37 (6) (2015) 277–292.

[12] T.B. Smallwood, P.R. Giacomin, A. Loukas, J.P. Mulvenna, R.J. Clark, J.J. Miles, Helminth immunomodulation in autoimmune disease, Front. Immunol. 8 (453) (2017).

[13] D.E. Elliott, J.V. Weinstock, Nematodes and human therapeutic trials for inflammatory disease, Parasite Immunol. 39 (5) (2017), e12407.

[14] R.M. Anthony, L.I. Rutitzky, J.F. Urban Jr., M.J. Stadecker, W.C. Gause, Protective immune mechanisms in helminth infection, Nat. Rev. Immunol. 7 (12) (2007) 975.

[15] J.E. Allen, R.M. Maizels, Diversity and dialogue in immunity to helminths, Nat. Rev. Immunol. 11 (6) (2011) 375.

[16] A. Abdoli, M. Pirestani, Are pregnant women with chronic helminth infections more susceptible to congenital infections? Front. Immunol. 5 (53) (2014).

[17] C.M. Finlay, K.P. Walsh, K.H. Mills, Induction of regulatory cells by helminth parasites: exploitation for the treatment of inflammatory diseases, Immunol. Rev. 259 (1) (2014) 206–230.

[18] B. Everts, H.H. Smits, C.H. Hokke, M. Yazdanbakhsh, Helminths and dendritic cells: sensing and regulating via pattern recognition receptors, Th2 and Treg responses, Eur. J. Immunol. 40 (6) (2010) 1525–1537.

[19] S. Babu, T.B. Nutman, 31 - Immune responses to helminth infection, in: R.R. Rich, T.A. Fleisher, W.T. Shearer, H.W. Schroeder, A.J. Frew, C.M. Weyand (Eds.), Clinical Immunology (Fifth Edition), Content Repository Only, London, 2019. 437–47.e1.

[20] S. Sakaguchi, T. Yamaguchi, T. Nomura, M. Ono, Regulatory T cells and immune tolerance, Cell 133 (5) (2008) 775–787.

[21] F. Varyani, J.O. Fleming, R. Maizels, Helminths in the gastrointestinal tract as modulators of immunity and pathology, Am. J. Physiol. Gastrointest. Liver Physiol. (2017).

[22] T.P. Brosschot, L.A. Reynolds, The impact of a helminth-modified microbiome on host immunity, Mucosal Immunol. 11 (2018) 1039–1046.

[23] L.A. Reynolds, B.B. Finlay, R.M. Maizels, Cohabitation in the intestine: interactions among helminth parasites, bacterial microbiota, and host immunity, J. Immunol. 195 (9) (2015) 4059–4066.

[24] A. Rapin, N.L. Harris, Helminth–bacterial interactions: cause and consequence, Trend Immunol. (2018).

[25] A. Hoerauf, Microflora, helminths, and the immune system—who controls whom? N. Engl. J. Med. 363 (15) (2010) 1476–1478.

[26] L.A. Reynolds, K.A. Smith, K.J. Filbey, Y. Harcus, J.P. Hewitson, S.A. Redpath, et al., Commensal-pathogen interactions in the intestinal tract, Gut Microbes 5 (4) (2014) 522–532.

[27] M. Zaiss Mario, A. Rapin, L. Lebon, K. Dubey Lalit, I. Mosconi, K. Sarter, et al., The intestinal microbiota contributes to the ability of helminths to modulate allergic inflammation, Immunity 43 (5) (2015) 998–1010.

[28] M.J. Broadhurst, A. Ardeshir, B. Kanwar, J. Mirpuri, U.M. Gundra, J.M. Leung, et al., Therapeutic helminth infection of macaques with idiopathic chronic diarrhea alters the inflammatory signature and mucosal microbiota of the colon, PLoS Pathog. 8 (11) (2012), e1003000.

[29] S.C. Lee, M. San Tang, Y.A. Lim, S.H. Choy, Z.D. Kurtz, L.M. Cox, et al., Helminth colonization is associated with increased diversity of the gut microbiota, PLoS Negl. Trop. Dis. 8 (5) (2014), e2880.

[30] D. Ramanan, R. Bowcutt, S.C. Lee, M. San Tang, Z.D. Kurtz, Y. Ding, et al., Helminth infection promotes colonization resistance via type 2 immunity, Science 352 (6285) (2016) 608–612.

[31] C. Cantacessi, P. Giacomin, J. Croese, M. Zakrzewski, J. Sotillo, L. McCann, et al., Impact of experimental hookworm infection on the human gut microbiota, J. Infect. Dis. 210 (9) (2014) 1431–1434.

[32] P. Giacomin, M. Zakrzewski, T.P. Jenkins, X. Su, R. Al-Hallaf, J. Croese, et al., Changes in duodenal tissue-associated microbiota following hookworm infection and consecutive gluten challenges in humans with coeliac disease, Sci. Rep. 6 (2016) 36797.

[33] M. Veldhoen, The role of T helper subsets in autoimmunity and allergy, Curr. Opin. Immunol. 21 (6) (2009) 606–611.

[34] J. Kahl, N. Brattig, E. Liebau, The untapped pharmacopeic potential of helminths, Trends Parasitol. 34 (10) (2018) 828–842.

[35] G. Rogler, Resolution of inflammation in inflammatory bowel disease, Lancet Gastroenterol. Hepatol. 2 (7) (2017) 521–530.

[36] C.D. Buckley, D.W. Gilroy, C.N. Serhan, B. Stockinger, P.P. Tak, The resolution of inflammation, Nat. Rev. Immunol. 13 (1) (2013) 59–66.

[37] J.M. Smith, T.L. Nemeth, R.A. McDonald, Current immunosuppressive agents: efficacy, side effects, and utilization, Pediatr. Clin. N. Am. 50 (6) (2003) 1283–1300.

[38] L.W. Miller, Cardiovascular toxicities of immunosuppressive agents, Am. J. Transplant. 2 (9) (2002) 807–818.

[39] S. Husain, N. Singh, The impact of novel immunosuppressive agents on infections in organ transplant recipients and the interactions of these agents with antimicrobials, Clin. Infect. Dis. 35 (1) (2002) 53–61.

[40] K. Orlicka, E. Barnes, E.L. Culver, Prevention of infection caused by immunosuppressive drugs in gastroenterology, Ther. Adv. Chronic. Dis. 4 (4) (2013) 167–185.

[41] J.A. Fishman, Opportunistic infections—coming to the limits of immunosuppression? Cold Spring Harb. Perspect. Med. 3 (10) (2013).

[42] S.M. Ryan, R.M. Eichenberger, R. Ruscher, P.R. Giacomin, A. Loukas, Harnessing helminth-driven immunoregulation in the search for novel therapeutic modalities, PLoS Pathog. 16 (5) (2020), e1008508.

[43] A. Abdoli, Therapeutic potential of helminths and helminth-derived antigens for resolution of inflammation in inflammatory bowel disease, Arch. Med. Res. (2019).

[44] J. Correale, M. Farez, Association between parasite infection and immune responses in multiple sclerosis, Ann. Neurol. 61 (2) (2007) 97–108.

[45] J.O. Fleming, Helminth therapy and multiple sclerosis, Int. J. Parasitol. 43 (3) (2013) 259–274.

[46] K. Langdon, J. Phie, C.B. Thapa, E. Biros, A. Loukas, N. Haleagrahara, Helminth-based therapies for rheumatoid arthritis: a systematic review and meta-analysis, Int. Immunopharmacol. 66 (2019) 366–372.

[47] A.J. Daveson, D.M. Jones, S. Gaze, H. McSorley, A. Clouston, A. Pascoe, et al., Effect of hookworm infection on wheat challenge in celiac disease – a randomised double-blinded placebo controlled trial, PLoS One 6 (3) (2011), e17366.

[48] O. Atochina, D. Harn, Prevention of psoriasis-like lesions development in fsn/fsn mice by helminth glycans, Exp. Dermatol. 15 (6) (2006) 461–468.

[49] A. Olia, C. Shimokawa, T. Imai, K. Suzue, H. Hisaeda, Suppression of systemic lupus erythematosus in NZBWF1 mice infected with Hymenolepis microstoma, Parasitol. Int. 76 (2020) 102057.

[50] K.A. Saunders, T. Raine, A. Cooke, C.E. Lawrence, Inhibition of autoimmune type 1 diabetes by gastrointestinal helminth infection, Infect. Immun. 75 (1) (2007) 397–407.

[51] A.M. Croft, P. Bager, S.K. Garg, Helminth therapy (worms) for allergic rhinitis, Cochrane Database Syst. Rev. 4 (2012).

[52] S. Navarro, D.A. Pickering, I.B. Ferreira, L. Jones, S. Ryan, S. Troy, et al., Hookworm recombinant protein promotes regulatory T cell responses that suppress experimental asthma, Sci. Transl. Med. 8 (362) (2016). 362ra143-362ra143.

[53] A. Abdoli, A.H. Mirzaian, Potential application of helminth therapy for resolution of neuroinflammation in neuropsychiatric disorders, Metab. Brain Dis. 35 (1) (2020) 95–110.

[54] E. Hollander, G. Uzunova, B.P. Taylor, R. Noone, E. Racine, E. Doernberg, et al., Randomized crossover feasibility trial of helminthic Trichuris suis ova versus placebo for repetitive behaviors in adult autism spectrum disorder, World J. Biol. Psychiatry 21 (4) (2020) 291–299.

[55] D.C. Baumgart, S.R. Carding, Inflammatory bowel disease: cause and immunobiology, Lancet 369 (9573) (2007) 1627–1640.

[56] B. Khor, A. Gardet, R.J. Xavier, Genetics and pathogenesis of inflammatory bowel disease, Nature 474 (7351) (2011) 307.

[57] R.W. Summers, D.E. Elliott, K. Qadir, J.F. Urban Jr., R. Thompson, J.V. Weinstock, Trichuris suis seems to be safe and possibly effective in the treatment of inflammatory bowel disease, Am. J. Gastroenterol. 98 (9) (2003) 2034.

[58] J.V. Weinstock, D.E. Elliott, Translatability of helminth therapy in inflammatory bowel diseases, Int. J. Parasitol. 43 (3) (2013) 245–251.

[59] J. Croese, P. Giacomin, S. Navarro, A. Clouston, L. McCann, A. Dougall, et al., Experimental hookworm infection and gluten microchallenge promote tolerance in celiac disease, J. Allergy Clin. Immunol. 135 (2) (2015). 508–16. e5.

[60] H.J. McSorley, S. Gaze, J. Daveson, D. Jones, R.P. Anderson, A. Clouston, et al., Suppression of inflammatory immune responses in celiac disease by experimental hookworm infection, PLoS One 6 (9) (2011), e24092.

[61] D.S. Reich, C.F. Lucchinetti, P.A. Calabresi, Multiple sclerosis, N. Engl. J. Med. 378 (2) (2018) 169–180.

[62] J. Correale, M.F. Farez, The impact of parasite infections on the course of multiple sclerosis, J. Neuroimmunol. 233 (1) (2011) 6–11.

[63] J.O. Fleming, A. Isaak, J.E. Lee, C.C. Luzzio, M.D. Carrithers, T.D. Cook, et al., Probiotic helminth administration in relapsing–remitting multiple sclerosis: a phase 1 study, Mult. Scler. J. 17 (6) (2011) 743–754.

[64] D. Siniscalco, N. Antonucci, Possible use of Trichuris suis ova in autism spectrum disorders therapy, Med. Hypotheses 81 (1) (2013) 1–4.

[65] C. Arroyo-López, Helminth therapy for autism under gut-brain axis-hypothesis, Med. Hypotheses 125 (2019) 110–118.

[66] A.M. Cheng, D. Jaint, S. Thomas, J. Wilson, W. Parker, Overcoming evolutionary mismatch by self-treatment with helminths: current practices and experience, J. Evol. Med. 3 (2015) 1–22.

[67] J. Liu, R. Morey, J. Wilson, W. Parker, Practices and outcomes of self-treatment with helminths based on physicians' observations, J. Helminthol. 91 (3) (2017) 267–277.

[68] E. Hollander, G. Uzunova, B.P. Taylor, R. Noone, E. Racine, E. Doernberg, et al., Randomized crossover feasibility trial of helminthic Trichuris suis ova versus placebo for repetitive behaviors in adult autism spectrum disorder, World J. Biol. Psychiatry. (2018) 1–9.

[69] D.-W. Kang, J.B. Adams, A.C. Gregory, T. Borody, L. Chittick, A. Fasano, et al., Microbiota transfer therapy alters gut ecosystem and improves gastrointestinal and autism symptoms: an open-label study, Microbiome 5 (1) (2017) 10.

[70] D.-W. Kang, J.B. Adams, D.M. Coleman, E.L. Pollard, J. Maldonado, S. McDonough-Means, et al., Long-term benefit of microbiota transfer therapy on autism symptoms and gut microbiota, Sci. Rep. 9 (1) (2019) 5821.

[71] F. Strati, D. Cavalieri, D. Albanese, C. De Felice, C. Donati, J. Hayek, et al., New evidences on the altered gut microbiota in autism spectrum disorders, Microbiome 5 (1) (2017) 24.

[72] J.S. Son, L.J. Zheng, L.M. Rowehl, X. Tian, Y. Zhang, W. Zhu, et al., Comparison of fecal microbiota in children with autism spectrum disorders and neurotypical siblings in the simons simplex collection, PLoS One 10 (10) (2015), e0137725.

[73] M.I. Araujo, A.A. Lopes, M. Medeiros, Á.A. Cruz, L. Sousa-Atta, D. Solé, et al., Inverse association between skin response to aeroallergens and *Schistosoma mansoni* infection, Int. Arch. Allergy Immunol. 123 (2) (2000) 145–148.

[74] P.J. Cooper, M.E. Chico, L.C. Rodrigues, M. Ordonez, D. Strachan, G.E. Griffin, et al., Reduced risk of atopy among school-age children infected with geohelminth parasites in a rural area of the tropics, J. Allergy Clin. Immunol. 111 (5) (2003) 995–1000.

[75] E.V. Ponte, D. Rasella, C. Souza-Machado, R. Stelmach, M.L. Barreto, A.A. Cruz, Reduced asthma morbidity in endemic areas for helminth infections: a longitudinal ecological study in Brazil, J. Asthma 51 (10) (2014) 1022–1027.

[76] J. Feary, J. Britton, J. Leonardi-Bee, Atopy and current intestinal parasite infection: a systematic review and meta-analysis, Allergy 66 (4) (2011) 569–578.

[77] A.H. van den Biggelaar, R. van Ree, L.C. Rodrigues, B. Lell, A.M. Deelder, P.G. Kremsner, et al., Decreased atopy in children infected with Schistosoma haematobium: a role for parasite-induced interleukin-10, Lancet 356 (9243) (2000) 1723–1727.

[78] A.H.J. van den Biggelaar, L.C. Rodrigues, R. van Ree, J.S. van der Zee, Y.C.M. Hoeksma-Kruize, J.H.M. Souverijn, et al., Long-term treatment of intestinal helminths increases mite skin-test reactivity in Gabonese schoolchildren, J. Infect. Dis. 189 (5) (2004) 892–900.

[79] P.J. Cooper, M.E. Chico, M.G. Vaca, A.-L. Moncayo, J.M. Bland, E. Mafla, et al., Effect of albendazole treatments on the prevalence of atopy in children living in communities endemic for geohelminth parasites: a cluster-randomised trial, Lancet 367 (9522) (2006) 1598–1603.

[80] P. Bager, J. Arnved, S. Rønborg, J. Wohlfahrt, L.K. Poulsen, T. Westergaard, et al., Trichuris suis ova therapy for allergic rhinitis: A randomized, double-blind, placebo-controlled clinical trial, J. Allergy Clin. Immunol. 125 (1) (2010). 123–30.e3.

[81] D.E. Elliott, J. Li, A. Blum, A. Metwali, K. Qadir, J.F. Urban Jr., et al., Exposure to schistosome eggs protects mice from TNBS-induced colitis, Am. J. Physiol. Gastrointest. Liver Physiol. 43 (2003) 293–299.

[82] T. Moreels, R. Nieuwendijk, J. De Man, D. Winter, A. Herman, E. Van Marck, et al., Concurrent infection with Schistosoma mansoni attenuates inflammation induced changes in colonic morphology, cytokine levels, and smooth muscle contractility of trinitrobenzene sulphonic acid induced colitis in rats, Gut 53 (1) (2004) 99–107.

[83] T.L. Sutton, A. Zhao, K.B. Madden, J.E. Elfrey, B.A. Tuft, C.A. Sullivan, et al., Anti-inflammatory mechanisms of enteric Heligmosomoides polygyrus infection against trinitrobenzene sulfonic acid-induced colitis in a murine model, Infect. Immun. 76 (10) (2008) 4772–4782.

[84] V. Driss, M. El Nady, M. Delbeke, C. Rousseaux, C. Dubuquoy, A. Sarazin, et al., The schistosome glutathione S-transferase P28GST, a unique helminth protein, prevents intestinal inflammation in experimental colitis through a Th2-type response with mucosal eosinophils, Mucosal Immunol. 9 (2) (2016) 322.

[85] Y. Zhao, S. Zhang, L. Jiang, J. Jiang, H. Liu, Preventive effects of Schistosoma japonicum ova on trinitrobenzenesulfonic acid-induced colitis and bacterial translocation in mice, J. Gastroenterol. Hepatol. 24 (11) (2009) 1775–1780.

[86] M. H-m, L. W-q, L. J-h, Y.-l. Cheng, L. Y-l, Schistosoma japonicum eggs modulate the activity of CD4+ CD25+ Tregs and prevent development of colitis in mice, Exp. Parasitol. 116 (4) (2007) 385–389.

[87] C.-M. Xia, Y. Zhao, L. Jiang, J. Jiang, S.-C. Zhang, Schistosoma japonicum ova maintains epithelial barrier function during experimental colitis, World J. Gastroenterol. 17 (43) (2011) 4810.

[88] P. Smith, N.E. Mangan, C.M. Walsh, R.E. Fallon, A.N. McKenzie, N. van Rooijen, et al., Infection with a helminth parasite prevents experimental colitis via a macrophage-mediated mechanism, J. Immunol. 178 (7) (2007) 4557–4566.

[89] M. Cho, C. Lee, H. Yu, Amelioration of intestinal colitis by macrophage migration inhibitory factor isolated from intestinal parasites through Toll-like receptor 2, Parasite Immunol. 33 (5) (2011) 265–275.

[90] C. Schnoeller, S. Rausch, S. Pillai, A. Avagyan, B.M. Wittig, C. Loddenkemper, et al., A helminth immunomodulator reduces allergic and inflammatory responses by induction of IL-10-producing macrophages, J. Immunol. 180 (6) (2008) 4265–4272.

[91] W. Khan, P. Blennerhasset, A. Varghese, S. Chowdhury, P. Omsted, Y. Deng, et al., Intestinal nematode infection ameliorates experimental colitis in mice, Infect. Immun. 70 (11) (2002) 5931–5937.

[92] J.L. Reyes, M.R. Fernando, F. Lopes, G. Leung, N.L. Mancini, C.E. Matisz, et al., IL-22 restrains tapeworm-mediated protection against experimental colitis via regulation of IL-25 expression, PLoS Pathog. 12 (4) (2016), e1005481.

[93] D.E. Elliott, T. Setiawan, A. Metwali, A. Blum, J.F. Urban Jr., J.V. Weinstock, Heligmosomoides polygyrus inhibits established colitis in IL-10-deficient mice, Eur. J. Immunol. 34 (10) (2004) 2690–2698.

[94] D. Sewell, Z. Qing, E. Reinke, D. Elliot, J. Weinstock, M. Sandor, et al., Immunomodulation of experimental autoimmune encephalomyelitis by helminth ova immunization, Int. Immunol. 15 (1) (2003) 59–69.

[95] A.C. La Flamme, K. Ruddenklau, B.T. Bäckström, Schistosomiasis decreases central nervous system inflammation and alters the progression of experimental autoimmune encephalomyelitis, Infect. Immun. 71 (9) (2003) 4996–5004.

[96] A. Gruden-Movsesijan, N. Ilic, M. Mostarica-Stojkovic, S. StosiC-Grujicic, M. Milic, SOFRONIC-MILOSAVLJEVIC L., Mechanisms of modulation of experimental autoimmune encephalomyelitis by chronic Trichinella spiralis infection in dark Agouti rats, Parasite Immunol. 32 (6) (2010) 450–459.

[97] K.P. Walsh, M.T. Brady, C.M. Finlay, L. Boon, K.H. Mills, Infection with a helminth parasite attenuates autoimmunity through TGF-β-mediated suppression of Th17 and Th1 responses, J. Immunol. 183 (3) (2009) 1577–1586.

[98] X. Zheng, X. Hu, G. Zhou, Z. Lu, W. Qiu, J. Bao, et al., Soluble egg antigen from Schistosoma japonicum modulates the progression of chronic progressive experimental autoimmune encephalomyelitis via Th2-shift response, J. Neuroimmunol. 194 (1–2) (2008) 107–114.

[99] A. Cooke, P. Tonks, F.M. Jones, H. O'SHEA, P. Hutchings, A.J. Fulford, Infection with Schistosoma mansoni prevents insulin dependent diabetes mellitus in non-obese diabetic mice, Parasite Immunol. 21 (4) (1999) 169–176.

[100] P. Zaccone, Z. Fehérvári, F.M. Jones, S. Sidobre, M. Kronenberg, D.W. Dunne, et al., Schistosoma mansoni antigens modulate the activity of the innate immune response and prevent onset of type 1 diabetes, Eur. J. Immunol. 33 (5) (2003) 1439–1449.

[101] Q. Liu, K. Sundar, P.K. Mishra, G. Mousavi, Z. Liu, A. Gaydo, et al., Helminth infection can reduce insulitis and type 1 diabetes through CD25-and IL-10-independent mechanisms, Infect. Immun. 77 (12) (2009) 5347–5358.

[102] A.A. Veenstra, J. Tang, T.S. Kern, Antagonism of CD11b with neutrophil inhibitory factor (NIF) inhibits vascular lesions in diabetic retinopathy, PLoS One 8 (10) (2013), e78405.

[103] Y. Osada, S. Shimizu, T. Kumagai, S. Yamada, T. Kanazawa, Schistosoma mansoni infection reduces severity of collagen-induced arthritis via down-regulation of pro-inflammatory mediators, Int. J. Parasitol. 39 (4) (2009) 457–464.

[104] Y. He, J. Li, W. Zhuang, L. Yin, C. Chen, J. Li, et al., The inhibitory effect against collagen-induced arthritis by Schistosoma japonicum infection is infection stage-dependent, BMC Immunol. 11 (1) (2010) 28.

[105] J. Rzepecka, M.A. Pineda, L. Al-Riyami, D.T. Rodgers, J.K. Huggan, F.E. Lumb, et al., Prophylactic and therapeutic treatment with a synthetic analogue of a parasitic worm product prevents experimental arthritis and inhibits IL-1β production via NRF2-mediated counter-regulation of the inflammasome, J. Autoimmun. 60 (2015) 59–73.

[106] M.C. Salinas-Carmona, G. De la Cruz-Galicia, I. Pérez-Rivera, J.M. Solís-Soto, J.C. Segoviano-Ramirez, A.V. Vázquez, et al., Spontaneous arthritis in MRL/lpr mice is aggravated by Staphylococcus aureus and ameliorated by Nippostrongylus brasiliensis infections, Autoimmunity 42 (1) (2009) 25–32.

[107] D. Rodgers, M. Pineda, C. Suckling, W. Harnett, M. Harnett, Drug-like analogues of the parasitic worm-derived immunomodulator ES-62 are therapeutic in the MRL/Lpr model of systemic lupus erythematosus, Lupus 24 (13) (2015) 1437–1442.

[108] M.S. Wilson, M.D. Taylor, A. Balic, C.A.M. Finney, J.R. Lamb, R.M. Maizels, Suppression of allergic airway inflammation by helminth-induced regulatory T cells, J. Exp. Med. 202 (9) (2005) 1199–1212.

[109] D. Negrao-Corrêa, M.R. Silveira, C.M. Borges, D.G. Souza, M.M. Teixeira, Changes in pulmonary function and parasite burden in rats infected with Strongyloides venezuelensis concomitant with induction of allergic airway inflammation, Infect. Immun. 71 (5) (2003) 2607–2614.

[110] P. LIU, LI J, YANG X, SHEN Y, ZHU Y, WANG S, et al., Helminth infection inhibits airway allergic reaction and dendritic cells are involved in the modulation process, Parasite Immunol. 32 (1) (2010) 57–66.

[111] M.E.H. Bashir, P. Andersen, I.J. Fuss, H.N. Shi, C. Nagler-Anderson, An enteric helminth infection protects against an allergic response to dietary antigen, J. Immunol. 169 (6) (2002) 3284–3292.

[112] D.M. McKay, Not all parasites are protective, Parasite Immunol. 37 (6) (2015) 324–332.

[113] A. Abdoli, H.M. Ardakani, Helminth infections and immunosenescence: the friend of my enemy, Exp. Gerontol. 133 (2020) 110852.

[114] S.L. Peng, Rheumatic manifestations of parasitic diseases, Semin. Arthritis Rheum. 31 (4) (2002) 228–247.

[115] P.J. Cooper, Toxocara canis infection: an important and neglected environmental risk factor for asthma? Clin Exp Allergy 38 (4) (2008) 551–553.

[116] I. Mohammadzadeh, S. Darvish, S.M. Riahi, S.A. Moghaddam, M. Pournasrollah, M. Mohammadnia-Afrozi, et al., Exposure to Toxocara spp. and Ascaris lumbricoides infections and risk of allergic rhinitis in children, Allergy, Asthma Clin. Immunol. 16 (1) (2020) 69.

[117] M.T. Audicana, M.W. Kennedy, Anisakis simplex: from obscure infectious worm to inducer of immune hypersensitivity, Clin. Microbiol. Rev. 21 (2) (2008) 360–379.

[118] K. Sobotková, W. Parker, J. Levá, J. Růžková, J. Lukeš, P.K. Jirků, Helminth therapy – from the parasite perspective, Trends Parasitol. 35 (7) (2019) 501–515.

[119] L. Nascimento Santos, L.G. Carvalho Pacheco, C. Silva Pinheiro, N.M. Alcantara-Neves, Recombinant proteins of helminths with immunoregulatory properties and their possible therapeutic use, Acta Trop. 166 (2017) 202–211.

[120] H. Evans, E. Mitre, Worms as therapeutic agents for allergy and asthma: understanding why benefits in animal studies have not translated into clinical success, J. Allergy Clin. Immunol. 135 (2) (2015) 343–353.

[121] R.M. Maizels, Regulation of immunity and allergy by helminth parasites, Allergy 75 (3) (2020) 524–534.

17. Immunomodulatory effects of parasites on autoimmunity

[122] G. Zandman-Goddard, Y. Shoenfeld, Parasitic infection and autoimmunity, Lupus 18 (13) (2009) 1144–1148.
[123] M. Abu-Shakra, Y. Shoenfeld, Chronic infections and autoimmunity, Immunol. Ser. 55 (1991) 285.
[124] E. van Riet, F.C. Hartgers, M. Yazdanbakhsh, Chronic helminth infections induce immunomodulation: consequences and mechanisms, Immunobiology 212 (6) (2007) 475–490.
[125] M. Abu-Shakra, D. Buskila, Y. Shoenfeld, Molecular mimicry between host and pathogen: examples from parasites and implication, Immunol. Lett. 67 (2) (1999) 147–152.
[126] D.F. Nunes, G. PMdM, C. de Mesquita Andrade, C. ACJd, E. Chiari, G. LMdC, Troponin T autoantibodies correlate with chronic cardiomyopathy in human C hagas disease, Tropical Med. Int. Health 18 (10) (2013) 1180–1192.
[127] A.R. Teixeira, M.M. Hecht, M.C. Guimaro, A.O. Sousa, N. Nitz, Pathogenesis of chagas' disease: parasite persistence and autoimmunity, Clin. Microbiol. Rev. 24 (3) (2011) 592–630.
[128] R. Tarleton, L. Zhang, Chagas disease etiology: autoimmunity or parasite persistence? Parasitol. Today 15 (3) (1999) 94–99.
[129] J. Rivera-Correa, A. Rodriguez, Autoimmune Anemia in Malaria, Trends Parasitol. 36 (2) (2020) 91–97.
[130] Y. Shapira, N. Agmon-Levin, C. Selmi, J. Petríková, O. Barzilai, M. Ram, et al., Prevalence of anti-toxoplasma antibodies in patients with autoimmune diseases, J. Autoimmun. 39 (1) (2012) 112–116.
[131] C.-C. Chan, R.B. Nussenblatt, M.K. Kim, A.G. Palestine, K. Awadzi, E.A. Ottesen, Immunopathology of ocular onchocerciasis: 2. Anti-retinal autoantibodies in serum and ocular fluids, Ophthalmology 94 (4) (1987) 439–443.
[132] K. Ritter, R. Thomssen, A. Kuhlencord, W. Bommer, Prolonged haemolytic anaemia in malaria and autoantibodies against triosephosphate isomerase, Lancet 342 (8883) (1993) 1333–1334.
[133] Y. Shoenfeld, J. Rauch, H. Massicotte, S.K. Datta, J. André-Schwartz, B.D. Stollar, et al., Polyspecificity of monoclonal lupus autoantibodies produced by human-human hybridomas, N. Engl. J. Med. 308 (8) (1983) 414–420.
[134] G. Bendixen, T. Hadidi, R. Manthorpe, H. Permin, J. Struckmann, A. Wiik, et al., Antibodies against nuclear components in schistosomiasis: results compared to values in patients with rheumatoid arthritis, systemic lupus erythematosus, and osteoarthrosis, Allergy 39 (2) (1984) 107–113.
[135] S.M. Muxel, J.I. Aoki, J.C.R. Fernandes, M.F. Laranjeira-Silva, R.A. Zampieri, S.M. Acuña, et al., Arginine and polyamines fate in Leishmania infection, Front. Microbiol. 8 (2017) 2682.
[136] S. Santos-Pereira, F.O. Cardoso, K.S. Calabrese, T. Zaverucha do Valle, Leishmania amazonensis resistance in murine macrophages: Analysis of possible mechanisms, Plos One 14 (12) (2019), e0226837.
[137] J. Alvar, I.D. Vélez, C. Bern, M. Herrero, P. Desjeux, J. Cano, et al., Leishmaniasis worldwide and global estimates of its incidence, PLoS One 7 (5) (2012), e35671.
[138] U.A. Wenzel, Bank E, C. Florian, S. Förster, N. Zimara, J. Steinacker, et al., Leishmania major parasite stage-dependent host cell invasion and immune evasion, FASEB J. 26 (1) (2012) 29–39.
[139] P. Kaye, P. Scott, Leishmaniasis: complexity at the host–pathogen interface, Nat. Rev. Microbiol. 9 (8) (2011) 604–615.
[140] P.V. Voulgari, G. Pappas, E. Liberopoulos, M. Elisaf, F. Skopouli, A. Drosos, Visceral leishmaniasis resembling systemic lupus erythematosus, Ann. Rheum. Dis. 63 (10) (2004) 1348–1349.
[141] E. Liberopoulos, A. Kei, F. Apostolou, M. Elisaf, Autoimmune manifestations in patients with visceral leishmaniasis, J. Microbiol. Immunol. Infect. 46 (4) (2013) 302–305.
[142] E. Ahlin, A. Elshafei, M. Nur, S.H. El Safi, R. Johan, G. Elghazali, Anti-citrullinated peptide antibodies and rheumatoid factor in Sudanese patients with Leishmania donovani infection, Rev. Bras. Reumatol. 51 (6) (2011) 579e86.
[143] K.P. Makaritsis, N.K. Gatselis, M. Ioannou, E. Petinaki, G.N. Dalekos, Polyclonal hypergammaglobulinemia and high smooth-muscle autoantibody titers with specificity against filamentous actin: consider visceral leishmaniasis, not just autoimmune hepatitis, Int. J. Infect. Dis. 13 (4) (2009) e60–e157.
[144] K.-L. Koster, H.-J. Laws, A. Troeger, R. Meisel, A. Borkhardt, P.T. Oommen, Visceral leishmaniasis as a possible reason for pancytopenia, Front. Pediatr. 3 (2015) 59.
[145] S. Argov, C. Jaffe, M. Krupp, H. Slor, Y. Shoenfeld, Autoantibody production by patients infected with Leishmania, Clin. Exp. Immunol. 76 (2) (1989) 190.
[146] B. Granel, J. Serratrice, L. Swiader, F. Gambarelli, L. Daniel, C. Fossat, et al., Crossing of antinuclear antibodies and anti-leishmania antibodies, Lupus 9 (7) (2000) 548–550.
[147] S. Pollack, A. Nagler, D. Liberman, I. Oren, G. Alroy, R. Katz, et al., Immunological studies of pancytopenia in visceral leishmaniasis, Isr. J. Med. Sci. 24 (2) (1988) 70.

[148] F. Chasset, C. Richez, T. Martin, A. Belot, A.-S. Korganow, L. Arnaud, Rare diseases that mimic systemic lupus erythematosus (lupus mimickers), Joint Bone Spine. 86 (2) (2019) 165–171.

[149] P. Desjeux, F. Santoro, D. Afchain, M. Loyens, A. Capron, Circulating immune complexes and anti-IgG antibodies in mucocutaneous leishmaniasis, Am. J. Trop. Med. Hyg. 29 (2) (1980) 195–198.

[150] A.I. Elshafie, E. Åhlin, L. Mathsson, G. ElGhazali, J. Rönnelid, Circulating immune complexes (IC) and IC-induced levels of GM-CSF are increased in Sudanese patients with acute visceral Leishmania donovani infection undergoing sodium stibogluconate treatment: implications for disease pathogenesis, J. Immunol. 178 (8) (2007) 5383–5389.

[151] J.M. Romero, C.L. López, M. Mayol, P. Roig, J.R. Gómez, J.F. Quilez, Renal and urinary tract leishmaniasis. A disease to keep in mind, Actas Urol. Esp. 19 (10) (1995) 789–794.

[152] C. Mary, G. Ange, S. Dunan, D. Lamouroux, M. Quilici, Characterization of a circulating antigen involved in immune complexes in visceral leishmaniasis patients, Am. J. Trop. Med. Hyg. 49 (4) (1993) 492–501.

[153] M. Mareze, B. AdN, B. APD, F. Pinto-Ferreira, A.C. Miura, M. FDC, et al., Socioeconomic vulnerability associated to Toxoplasma gondii exposure in southern Brazil, PloS One 14 (2) (2019), s.

[154] S.-H. Lee, K.-B. Chu, H.-J. Kang, F.-S. Quan, Virus-like particles containing multiple antigenic proteins of toxoplasma gondii induce memory T cell and B cell responses, PLoS One 14 (8) (2019), e0220865.

[155] D. Fisch, B. Clough, E.-M. Frickel, Human immunity to toxoplasma gondii, PLoS Pathog. 15 (12) (2019), e1008097.

[156] Z.-D. Wang, H.-H. Liu, Z.-X. Ma, H.-Y. Ma, Z.-Y. Li, Z.-B. Yang, et al., *Toxoplasma gondii* infection in immuno-compromised patients: a systematic review and meta-analysis, Front. Microbiol. 8 (2017) 389.

[157] S.K. Bliss, A.J. Marshall, Y. Zhang, E.Y. Denkers, Human polymorphonuclear leukocytes produce IL-12, TNF-α, and the chemokines macrophage-inflammatory protein-1α and-1β in response to toxoplasma gondii antigens, J. Immunol. 162 (12) (1999) 7369–7375.

[158] E.Y. Denkers, R.T. Gazzinelli, S. Hieny, P. Caspar, A. Sher, Bone marrow macrophages process exogenous toxoplasma gondii polypeptides for recognition by parasite-specific cytolytic T lymphocytes, J. Immunol. 150 (2) (1993) 517–526.

[159] L. Meda, S. Gasperini, M. Ceska, M.A. Cassatella, Modulation of proinflammatory cytokine release from human polymorphonuclear leukocytes by gamma interferon, Cell. Immunol. 157 (2) (1994) 448–461.

[160] L.C. Lacerda, J.L. Dos Santos, A.B. Wardini, A.N. da Silva, A.G. Santos, H.P.S. Freire, et al., Toxoplasma gondii induces extracellular traps release in cat neutrophils, Exp. Parasitol. 207 (2019) 107770.

[161] D.S. Abi Abdallah, C. Lin, C.J. Ball, M.R. King, G.E. Duhamel, E.Y. Denkers, Toxoplasma gondii triggers release of human and mouse neutrophil extracellular traps, Infect. Immun. 80 (2) (2012) 768–777.

[162] M. Romero-piffiguer, M.E. Ferro, C.M. Riera, Potentiation of autoimmune response in rats infected with toxoplasma gondii. Effect of the infection route, Jpn. J. Med. Sci. Biol. 40 (5–6) (1987) 175–185.

[163] M. Chen, F. Aosai, K. Norose, H.S. Mun, H. Ishikura, S. Hirose, et al., Toxoplasma gondii infection inhibits the development of lupus-like syndrome in autoimmune (New Zealand black× New Zealand white) F1 mice, Int. Immunol. 16 (7) (2004) 937–946.

[164] I. Krause, J.M. Anaya, A. Fraser, O. Barzilai, M. Ram, V. Abad, et al., Anti-infectious antibodies and autoimmune-associated autoantibodies in patients with type I diabetes mellitus and their close family members, Ann. N. Y. Acad. Sci. 1173 (1) (2009) 633–639.

[165] S. Fischer, N. Agmon-Levin, Y. Shapira, B.-S.P. Katz, E. Graell, R. Cervera, et al., Toxoplasma gondii: bystander or cofactor in rheumatoid arthritis, Immunol. Res. 56 (2–3) (2013) 287–292.

[166] Z. Hosseininejad, M. Sharif, S. Sarvi, A. Amouei, S.A. Hosseini, T.N. Chegeni, et al., Toxoplasmosis seroprevalence in rheumatoid arthritis patients: a systematic review and meta-analysis, PLoS Negl. Trop. Dis. 12 (6) (2018), e0006545.

[167] E. Adams, G. Hafez, M. Carnes, J. Wiesner, F. Graziano, The development of polymyositis in a patient with toxoplasmosis: clinical and pathologic findings and review of literature, Clin. Exp. Rheumatol. 2 (3) (1984) 205.

[168] E.E. Wasserman, K. Nelson, N.R. Rose, C. Rhode, J.P. Pillion, E. Seaberg, et al., Infection and thyroid autoimmunity: a seroepidemiologic study of TPOaAb, Autoimmunity 42 (5) (2009) 439–446.

[169] M. Lidar, N. Lipschitz, P. Langevitz, O. Barzilai, M. Ram, B.S. Porat-Katz, et al., Infectious serologies and autoantibodies in Wegener's granulomatosis and other vasculitides: novel associations disclosed using the rad BioPlex 2200, Ann. N. Y. Acad. Sci. 1173 (1) (2009) 649–657.

[170] L. Sagi, S. Baum, N. Agmon-Levin, Y. Sherer, B.S.P. Katz, O. Barzilai, et al., Autoimmune bullous diseases: the spectrum of infectious agent antibodies and review of the literature, Autoimmun. Rev. 10 (9) (2011) 527–535.

17. Immunomodulatory effects of parasites on autoimmunity

[171] H. Zinger, Y. Sherer, G. Goddard, Y. Berkun, O. Barzilai, N. Agmon-Levin, et al., Common infectious agents prevalence in antiphospholipid syndrome, Lupus 18 (13) (2009) 1149–1153.

[172] R. Tozzoli, O. Barzilai, M. Ram, D. Villalta, N. Bizzaro, Y. Sherer, et al., Infections and autoimmune thyroid diseases: parallel detection of antibodies against pathogens with proteomic technology, Autoimmun. Rev. 8 (2) (2008) 112–115.

[173] Y. Berkun, G. Zandman-Goddard, O. Barzilai, M. Boaz, Y. Sherer, B. Larida, et al., Infectious antibodies in systemic lupus erythematosus patients, Lupus 18 (13) (2009) 1129–1135.

[174] D. Zamir, M. Amar, G. Groisman, P. Weiner (Eds.), Toxoplasma infection in systemic lupus erythematosus mimicking lupus cerebritis, Mayo Clin. Proc. (1999). Elsevier.

[175] T. Washino, M. Moroda, Y. Iwakura, F. Aosai, Toxoplasma gondii infection inhibits Th17-mediated spontaneous development of arthritis in interleukin-1 receptor antagonist-deficient mice, Infect. Immun. 80 (4) (2012) 1437–1444.

[176] K. Hirota, M. Hashimoto, H. Yoshitomi, S. Tanaka, T. Nomura, T. Yamaguchi, et al., T cell self-reactivity forms a cytokine milieu for spontaneous development of IL-17+ Th cells that cause autoimmune arthritis, J. Exp. Med. 204 (1) (2007) 41–47.

[177] J.F. Fernandes, E.A. Taketomi, J.R. Mineo, D.O. Miranda, R. Alves, R.O. Resende, et al., Antibody and cytokine responses to house dust mite allergens and toxoplasma gondii antigens in atopic and non-atopic Brazilian subjects, Clin. Immunol. 136 (1) (2010) 148–156.

CHAPTER

18

Prediction of autoimmune diseases: From bench to bedside

Álvaro J. Vivas[a,b] *and Gabriel J. Tobón*[b,*]

[a]Universidad Icesi, Facultad de Ciencias de la Salud, Calle 18 No. 122 -135, Cali, Colombia

[b]Universidad Icesi, CIRAT: Centro de Investigación en Reumatología, Autoinmunidad y Medicina Traslacional, Cali, Colombia

*Corresponding author

Abstract

Autoimmune diseases (AIDs) include an increasingly prevalent group of disorders. If diagnosed at a later stage, AIDs can be associated with significant morbidity and mortality and subsequently lead to incalculable economic and intangible losses. Fortunately, there are detectable factors that can arise years before the onset of clinical manifestations, which are referred to as biomarkers. This chapter describes how the rise of new technologies has promoted great advances in the identification of novel biomarkers for the prediction of AIDs, including systemic lupus erythematosus (SLE), rheumatoid arthritis (RA), Sjögren's syndrome (SS), and type 1 diabetes (T1D). Preventive approaches, their outcomes, and ongoing clinical trials are also discussed.

Keywords

Systemic lupus erythematosus, Sjögren's syndrome, Type 1 diabetes, Rheumatoid arthritis, Biomarker, Prediction, Prevention

1 Introduction

Autoimmune diseases (AIDs) include a heterogeneous group of disorders characterized by a dysregulation of the immune system resulting in the loss of tolerance to self-antigens, cells, tissues, or organs, leading to excessive inflammation and tissue damage. Although many of these diseases are rare, they affect about 5% of the global population [1], and their frequency has significantly increased over the last 30 years due to different environmental factors such as diet, pollution exposure, infection, and stress load, among others [2]. AIDs are chronic and often disabling, which can lead to considerable health care costs and other intangible losses [3–5]. Hence, prediction and risk assessment for autoimmune diseases and preventing the disease development is a necessary but challenging task; however, recent findings promise future breakthroughs. In the remaining part of the chapter, we use the term "prediction" to describe the capability of a parameter to diagnose diseases at early stages.

AIDs are believed to progress sequentially through phases of initiation, propagation, and resolution (Fig. 1). The first phase is a result of genetic predisposition and environmental triggers; the second phase is characterized by cytokine production, epitope spreading, and imbalances in adaptive and innate immunity; and the third phase involves the induction and activation of regulatory mechanisms [6]. In general, genetic polymorphisms, especially those located in regulatory regions of genes related to self-antigen presentation (e.g., HLA) and regulation of the immune response, induce a variable predisposition to autoimmunity. Environmental factors, such as infections, UV radiation, trauma, or certain chemical substances, trigger autoimmune reactions that would eventually result in the manifestation of disease [7–9]. These reactions may leave detectable traces, such as the production of antibodies, changes in complement components, chemokines, cytokines, or other molecules. Molecules that are associated with the intensity of a disease or other pathophysiological state are referred to as biomarkers [10] (Fig. 2). The study of risk factor genes and biomarkers (cytokines and antibodies) is a cornerstone for the prediction of AIDs, as we will discuss here.

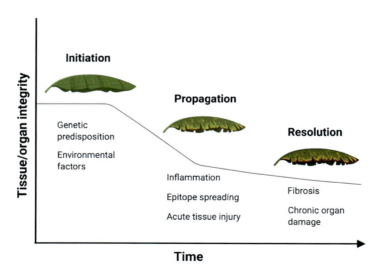

FIG. 1 Phases of autoimmune diseases. In this metaphoric image, the ants represent the immune system cells and the leaves constitute organ/tissue integrity. In normal conditions, certain ant species have a symbiotic relationship with plants (e.g., myrmecophytes). However, in autoimmune diseases (AIDs), the immune system starts to recognize self-antigens as foreign, initiating and amplifying an immune response. Later, once chronic damage is established, disease activity tends to decrease with fewer inflammatory cell-infiltrating tissues.

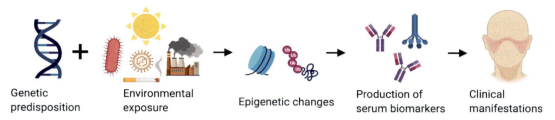

FIG. 2 Pathogenesis of autoimmune diseases. HLA and non-HLA SNPs or mutations predispose individuals to develop the disease. Environmental exposure to UV radiation, pollution or other agents, as well as infections, induce aberrant immunological phenomena (pathogenic or not) that can be detected years before the onset of clinical manifestations. Technological advances have allowed earlier detection of these changes, expanding the possibility of early intervention.

2 Using genetics to estimate the risk of developing AIDs

With the advent of next-generation sequencing, an unimaginable amount of information suddenly became available, the majority of which had unknown significance or was impossible to interpret. However, advances in computational biology have changed this picture, leading to encouraging results across a broad spectrum of AIDs.

2.1 Type 1 diabetes (T1D)

During the last decade, genetic studies, typically in the form of genome-wide association studies (GWASs), have identified more than 50 distinct genetic signals that impact predisposition to T1D [11, 12]. These studies have determined that about 50% of the heritability of T1D is attributed to human leukocyte antigen (HLA) alleles, and the remainder to several non-HLA loci [13]. Efforts have been made to develop Genetic Risk Scores (GRS), which summarize risk-associated variations by aggregating information from multiple single nucleotide polymorphisms (SNPs), to predict T1D diagnoses. One of the first research groups to do so were Aly et al. [14] who studied participants who were siblings of patients with T1D in the Diabetes Autoimmunity Study in the Young (DAISY) cohort. It was found that individuals who shared both haplotypes for DR3/DR3-DQ8 had a much higher risk of developing islet autoimmunity than those who only shared one haplotype (islet autoimmunity by age 15, 85% vs 20%, and T1D diagnosis by age 12, 55% vs 7%). Years later, other researchers determined that measuring non-HLA genetic risk could provide additional predictive power. Steck et al. [15] defined a genetic risk stratum for the DAISY cohort in which PTPN22 and UBASH3A were also included as risk factors. This genetic risk stratum significantly improved prediction of the general population of children with a risk of diabetes by age 15 for those subjects in the high-risk group (45%), compared with children of all other genotypes (3%). In addition, the positive predictive value for diabetes was slightly better with this genetic risk stratum than with HLA-DR3/4 alone (17.4 vs 6.4), while the negative predictive value was similar (98.6 vs 99.2). Sensitivity was decreased (42% vs 75%), while specificity was increased (95% vs 74%).

Recently, two independently developed GRSs [16, 17] were combined into a single GRS that included 41 HLA and non-HLA SNPs [18]. This merged GRS was tested in the T1D in the Environmental Determinants of Diabetes in the Young (TEDDY) study, a multicenter prospective cohort study that followed thousands of children with high T1D-risk HLA genotypes from birth by using the development of islet autoantibodies and T1D as outcomes indicative of disease progression [19]. This GRS could effectively predict T1D to a significantly higher degree: individuals with a score >14.4 had an 11% cumulative risk of developing multiple islet autoantibodies by age 6, compared with those with a lower score, who had a risk of 4.1%. The cumulative risk for developing diabetes by age 10 was 7.6% in children with a score of >14.4, compared with 2.7% in children with a score of ≤14.4. Experts generally consider this a successful risk stratification [11].

2.2 Systemic lupus erythematosus (SLE)

A study conducted by Chen et al. [20] used three European and two Chinese GWASs to investigate the performance of GRS in predicting the susceptibility to and severity of SLE. It was found that within the European population and across the Chinese and European populations, a genetic score incorporating linkage disequilibrium pruned-SNPs (at $R^2 = 0.2$) with modest (P <1e-05) evidence for association with disease predicted SLE with area under the receiver operating characteristic curve (AUC) of ≥0.64. In general, a higher GRS was associated with a greater risk of developing the disease, higher disease severity, and earlier disease onset, all independent of sex.

In a similar study, Almlöf et al. [21] used machine learning based on random forests to design a SNP genotype classifier to predict the risk of SLE and previously unknown genes and genetic variants that conferred the risk of SLE. Researchers used genotype data generated on the "Immunochip" (Illumina) platform from 1160 patients with SLE and 2711 controls. The random forest classifier yielded a probability that each given sample originated from a patient with SLE. This probability value was used to calculate the AUC as a measure of prediction accuracy. The AUC for the random forest prediction was 0.74, with a sensitivity of around 76% and a specificity of approximately 85%. In addition, the random forest algorithm was used to calculate "importance scores," which described to what extent a gene or region conferred risk for SLE based on the classification performance of the SNPs in the gene region. More than 40 genes were identified as high-risk factors for SLE progression, including three genes that were not previously described to be associated with the disease (*ZNF804A*, *ANK3*, and *DOCK3*). Compared to the regular single-SNP association analysis, the random forest method identified additional risk genes for SLE based on the same data from the Immunochip dataset.

2.3 Rheumatoid arthritis (RA)

There is an urgent need to identify reliable diagnostic biomarkers to detect early stages of RA. Different methods have been used to identify potential markers. One novel modeling approach was developed by Scott et al. [22], who combined odds ratios for 15 four-digit/10 two-digit HLA-DRB1 alleles, 31 SNPs, and male smoking status in males. This model was applied in seropositive cases and controls with HLA-DRB1 tissue data available from two large multi-center cohorts of European ancestry: the Wellcome Trust Case Control Consortium (WTCCC) and UK RA Genetics Group Consortium (UKRAGG). These cohorts added more than 4000 RA cases and 3000 controls, even after considering the inclusion criteria. This model was able to identify individuals with clinically relevant increased risks for seropositive RA; the AUCs calculated for discriminating between ACPA-positive RA and controls were 0.837 and 0.857 for each cohort, respectively, using this HLA-SNP-Smoking model. This model identified 7.53% and 3.75% of ACPA-positive male patients, respectively, to have ORs for seropositive RA >20 (lifetime risk >22%). In addition, researchers identified that individuals with higher HLA-derived ORs developed RA at a younger age. Conversely, smoking, either presently or in the past, was associated with later onset RA with a median time to onset 7–12 years later compared to never-smokers. Authors considered that although their approach significantly improved the discriminatory abilities of existing models at that time, it remained unsuitable for population screening, as only a minority of patients demonstrated significantly increased lifetime risks for RA. Nevertheless, they stated that if it was used to target groups with a priori increased risks, such as first-degree relatives of RA patients, then a greater proportion of high-risk individuals could be identified.

Other groups have combined GWAS with experimental studies. For example, in a study conducted by Shervington et al. [23], primary normal human fibroblast-like synoviocytes (HFLS) and phenotype rheumatic HFLS-RA cells were used to identify differentially expressed genes using microarrays. Seventy-four genes were identified as having differential expression, which were then mapped against an RA inflammatory pathway, shortlisting candidate genes. *HSPA6, MMP1, MMP13,* and *TNFSF10* gene expression profiles were suggested to be potential diagnostic biomarkers, since they had the highest expression in HFLS-RA compared to HFLS. Furthermore, the cytokine IL-7 was found to be significantly more expressed (2.4×10^3-fold) in HFLS-RA cells compared with normal synoviocytes. Moreover, Zhang et al. [24] conducted a study that aimed to identify potential biomarkers for differential diagnosis between RA and osteoarthritis (OA) through genome-wide gene expression profiling analysis. Researchers obtained and profiled three genome-wide transcriptomic datasets of synovial tissues from RA and OA cohorts, including GSE55235, GSE55457, and GSE55584 datasets. It was found that IL7R+STAT1 had promising diagnostic ability to differentiate between these two diseases; more importantly, it was considered that these markers could be used to predict disease occurrence, considering their key role in the pathogenesis of these diseases. To our knowledge, there are no reviews of IL-7 or its receptor being evaluated as predictors of RA diagnosis in previously healthy patients. The closest report is from Goëb et al. [25], in which it was found that low IL-7 levels predicted RA progression in patients with very early inflammatory joint symptoms.

2.4 Sjögren's syndrome (SS)

There are fewer genetic association studies available for SS compared with other AIDs in terms of disease prediction. However, recent large-scale studies have been conducted in SS patients identifying that the human leukocyte antigen (HLA) class 2 molecules convey the largest heritable predisposition to SS [26]. A meta analysis identified the DRB1*0301, DQA1*0501, DQB1*0201, and DRB1*03 alleles as risk factors for SS [27]. Another study found HLA-DQ1/HLA-DQ2 heterozygous patients have increased anti-Ro and anti-La production [28].

The most significant genetic association with SS outside of the HLA region is in the interferon-regulatory factor 5 (IRF5) locus [29]. This group of transcription factors regulates and controls the expression of target genes. They act with Toll-like receptors (TLRs) and type 1 interferons to express proinflammatory cytokines. SS patients have demonstrated elevated expression of IRF5, which may be partly explained by the fact that the transcription factor ZBTB3 has increased binding to the IRF5 promoter [30], although the current evidence is limited. Another strong genetic association described is found in the gene encoding IL12a. IL-12 activates STAT4, a signaling event crucial for CD4$^+$ Th1 cell differentiation [31]. SS patients with the *IL12A* rs485497 polymorphism have increased IL-12p70 levels, which associate with disease activity. Compared with healthy controls, SS patients have significantly higher IL-12p70 levels [32].

Some genetic associations have only been discovered in specific populations. For example, the general transcription factor IIi (GTF2i) has been described as the gene with the most strong association with SS in a Northern Han Chinese population. Nevertheless, this association was not observed in European SS patients [33]. Thus, further studies are needed to explore the significance of these findings. It is also necessary to evaluate genetic associations in different populations.

3 Epigenetics to predict AIDs

3.1 T1D

Post translational modifications (PTMs) in T1D may result in neoepitopes that can be recognized with the subsequent development of pathogenic autoantibodies. One such example is antibodies specific to oxidative PTM-insulin (oxPTM-INS-Ab), which are present in around 84% of individuals with newly diagnosed T1D [34]. A longitudinal study developed by Strollo et al. [35] included serum samples from the ABIS study (a prospective population-based follow-up study, which included 17,055 unselected children born between October 1, 1997, and October 1, 1999, in southeast Sweden) [36]. The authors tested 51 samples from the 23 children in the cohort that developed T1D; these samples were obtained longitudinally before diagnosis at three different times (at ages of 5, 7, and 11). As controls, samples from 63 matched children were used, including 64 samples from 32 autoantibody-positive children who did not develop T1D, and 31 samples from autoantibody-negative children who did not develop to T1D (both after median follow-ups of 10.8 years). Autoantibody-positivity was defined as at least one positive islet antibody marker (insulin autoantibodies (IAA), glutamic acid decarboxylase antibodies (GADA), islet tyrosine phosphatase 2 antibodies (IA-2A), and zinc transporter 8 antibodies (ZnT8)). Researchers found that oxPTM-INS autoreactivity was present before T1D diagnosis in over 90% of T1D patients; oxPTM-INS-Abs were able to discriminate between children who progressed to T1D and those who did not, regardless of their islet autoantibody status. In addition, oxPTM-INS-Ab identified over 80% of individuals with the disease, including more than 30% of patients who were negative for the IAA.

On the other hand, it has been reported that insulin-producing beta cells are the only cells in the body with a significant amount of unmethylated *INS* DNA; thus, when these cells are destroyed, serum levels of unmethylated insulin are increased [37, 38]. Simmons et al. hypothesized that unmethylated insulin DNA could be an adjunctive marker of beta-cell death and progression to T1D in individuals at risk for diabetes [39]. Hence, researchers measured the unmethylated *INS* ratio (unmethylated over methylated INS DNA), as well as the four aforementioned islet autoantibodies, in 57 patients by electrochemiluminescence (ECL) assays and radioimmunoassays longitudinally for 24 months before diagnosis. Interestingly, no significant associations were found between the level of unmethylated *INS* ratio and islet autoantibodies at baseline; however, at different times (18, 12, 6, and 2 months), sera were positive for different antibodies, with IAA and IA-2A being positive 0–2 months before diagnosis. Only IAA levels were significantly associated with the unmethylated *INS* ratio over time. In addition, a larger increase in this ratio was associated with an earlier age of T1D onset, suggesting that beta-cell death occurs more quickly in younger participants.

3.2 SLE

SLE is a polygenic and widely heterogeneous disease, known to have a strong genetic component with a 2–5% concordance in dizygotic twins, and a 30%–40% concordance in monozygotic twins [40]. Accordingly, there is still a high percentage attributed to environmental factors, many of which induce epigenetic changes that can be detected before the onset of clinical manifestations [41].

DNA methylation changes have been widely described in SLE patients. Lupus patients have also been reported to have abnormal DNA demethylation in peripheral blood mononuclear cells (PBMCs), CD4$^+$ T cells, B cells, neutrophils, and in interferon-related genes (e.g., IFI44L, IFIT1, and STAT1) [42, 43]. Of these, T cells are the best understood, in which the promoters of *CD11a*, *CD40L*, *CD70*, *PRF1* and other genes are demethylated, contributing to the pathogenesis of the SLE [44].

Considering the above-mentioned data, specific DNA methylation states of particular genes have been proposed as biomarkers that can predict SLE. The presence of significant hypomethylation status in CpG Site 1 (Chr1: 79085222) and Site 2 (Chr1: 79085250; cg06872964) within the promoter region of *IFI44L* (IFN-induced protein 44-like) has been identified as a biomarker for SLE diagnosis with good diagnostic performance (93% sensitivity, 96% specificity) [45]. These results were validated in a Chinese cohort consisting of 529 patients with SLE, 569 healthy controls, 429 patients with RA, and 199 patients with primary Sjögren's syndrome. In addition, this biomarker was also validated in a European cohort consisting of 615 patients with SLE and 781 healthy controls. In both cohorts, these epigenetic changes were only found in SLE patients [45].

Other methylation-sensitive genes have also been described to be potential SLE biomarkers. Zhang et al. ingeniously developed a novel approach to measure the methylation status of *CD11a* and *CD70* promoter sequences by combining the standard method of bisulfite conversion of methylated CpG pairs with high-throughput oligonucleotide microarray-based technology. This allowed a rapid quantification of methylation levels of the *CD70* and *CD11a* promoters in bisulfite-treated DNA samples, detecting significantly lower methylation levels in SLE patients CD4$^+$ T cells compared with healthy controls [46].

On the other hand, microRNAs (miRNAs) might also represent future biomarkers for detecting SLE. In a meta analysis conducted by Zheng et al. [47] that included 17 studies of different miRNAs, the overall performance of total mixed miRNAs was moderate in discriminating SLE patients from healthy controls, with a combined area under the ROC curve (AUC) of 0.8797, 71% pooled sensitivity, and 81% pooled specificity. In addition, authors examined individual miRNAs among the total miRNA library, and found that miRNA21 was repeatedly used in individual studies; its diagnostic performance was essentially equivalent to the miRNA pool, with an AUC value of 0.828, a pooled sensitivity of 68%, and a pooled specificity of 77% [47].

3.3 RA

DNA methylation also plays an important role in RA. However, trials evaluating its application are mostly oriented towards therapeutic response in a specific treatment. To our knowledge, no reports are analyzing differential DNA methylation in predicting RA diagnosis. Conversely, citrullination is a deeply studied epigenetic change in RA patients, and it plays a critical role in RA pathogenesis. Anticitrullinated protein antibodies (ACPA) are one result of this post-translational modification and are described to predict the development of RA, as discussed later in this chapter.

One category of epigenetic changes that has a key role in many AIDs and that has not been mentioned in this chapter is histone modifications. Histone modifications status can be very unstable, as it can be easily altered by the environment and drug treatment, which may be why they are seldom suggested as biomarkers for diagnosis.

3.4 SS

SS patients exhibit differential expression of miRNAs, with associated (depending on the miRNA) dry eyes, parotid swelling, overactivation of B and T cells, and neuropathy [48, 49]. Pauley et al. investigated miR-146a in SS patients and in SS-prone C57BL/6.NOD-*Aec1Aec2* mouse model to elucidate its involvement in SS pathogenesis. Expression of miR-146a was examined in the PBMCs of 25 SS patients and 10 healthy controls, as well as in PBMCs, salivary glands, and lacrimal glands of the SS-prone mice. miR-146a expression was increased in SS patients compared to healthy controls and that SS mice had elevated miR-146a expression in salivary glands and PBMCs. In the latter, miR-146a was increased 3.7-fold at 8 weeks, and 30-fold at 20 weeks. Considering this, alterations in miRNA expression in humans may be present even before disease onset in target tissues, and that expression in PBMCs could serve as a biomarker in SS-prone individuals [50]. Years later, Jiang et al. [51] evaluated the value of miR-146a and miR-4484 in the diagnosis of anti-Ro-positive SS. 70 SS patients and 60 healthy controls were selected for the study. Quantitative polymerase chain reaction (qPCR) was used to detect serum expression of these two miRNAs in both groups, finding that their expression was upregulated in SS patients. Statistical analysis revealed that the sensitivity and specificity for both miRNAs combined in the diagnosis of SS were 91.43% and 86.36%, respectively.

Considering the above factors, differential miRNA expression may be detected in SS patients years before diagnosis, which could be a promising biomarker performance. Trials evaluating miRNAs for the prediction of SS in humans are still required.

4 Using antibodies and serum biomarkers to predict AIDs

Autoantibodies and antinuclear antibodies (ANA) serve as key diagnostic and classification criteria for many AIDs. Some of them are described as pathogenic, while others are believed to be protective or to ameliorate disease progression [52]. Moreover, many of these antibodies are detected years before a patient presents with clinical manifestations. Therefore, they have been made to use these molecules to predict AIDs.

4.1 T1D

As in other AIDs, T1D has a preclinical stage in which autoantibodies are produced. In general, when beta-cell destruction reaches a point at which insulin production becomes insufficient, clinical manifestations are observed. Different autoantibodies with prediction potential have been identified for T1D, including islet cell antibodies (ICA), IAA, GADA, IA-2A, and ZnT8. It has been postulated that after seroconversion of any two of these five autoantibodies, individuals will almost always develop T1D given sufficient time [53]. Progression to T1D in children with a single of these autoantibodies is estimated in 10% within 10 years, and for more than two autoantibodies, it increases by 11% each year, reaching >70% in the following 10 years [53–55]. The rate of progression depends on additional factors, such as age, genotype, sex, and fitness.

However, it is important to consider that some autoantibodies may be present only during limited periods. For example, IAA and GADA are most frequently detected as the first autoantibodies in children, but disappear in 25% and 10% of cases in children at clinical onset, respectively [56]. Nevertheless, these two have low predictive accuracy when used as a single test, while IA-2A has a highly specific association with T1D progression [53]. Therefore, the use of multiple biomarkers may be necessary due to the heterogeneity of the disease. Also, first-degree relatives of patients diagnosed with T1D or those having high-risk HLA genotypes, are highly recommended to be screened for these autoantibodies to estimate the risk of T1D development [56].

Another proposed biomarker is the ratio of proinsulin to C-peptide that when elevated, indicates beta-cell endoplasmic reticulum (ER) dysfunction [57]. Some authors have proposed that this ratio may be an effective screening tool to identify multiple autoantibody-positive individuals with high diabetes risk [58–60]. Nevertheless, multiple factors may generate variation in this measurement between assays, negatively influencing the consistency of this marker during the follow-up examination [58, 61]. In an attempt to improve this variability, Van Dalem et al. [62] developed a trefoil-type-time resolved fluorescence immunoassay (TT-TRFIA) for simultaneous measurement of C-peptide and proinsulin. The diagnostic performance of this immunoassay to predict progression to T1D within 2 years in first-degree relatives of 49 patients with high autoantibody-inferred risk (IA-2A$^+$ or ZnT8$^+$ plus $\geq$1 other autoantibody) was tested. The authors of this study found that this ratio had an AUC of 0.68, a sensitivity of 70%, and a specificity of 77%, in predicting impending diabetes, equal to the gold standard, hyperglycemic clamp test and oral glucose tolerance test, although the former is a noninvasive test.

Omics technologies have allowed large-scale profiling of protein expression and gene expression changes in T1D patients relative to disease-free controls [56]. However, very few studies using omics to predict T1D have been developed. Genome-wide transcriptome analysis of blood RNA samples from 28 autoantibody-positive children found that type I interferon-related transcriptomic signatures were already detectable up to two years before the detection of T1D-associated autoantibodies [63].

4.2 SLE

Arbuckle et al. [64] conducted a retrospective study of 130 former military SLE patients whose sera were available from the USA Department of Defense Serum Repository. They detected that in 115 of the 130 patients (88%), at least one autoantibody for SLE was present up to 9 years before diagnosis (mean 3.3 years). ANA, anti-Ro, and anti-La antibodies were the earliest autoantibodies to appear (mean 3.4 years), while others such as anti-Sm and anti-U1RNP antibodies appeared just months before diagnosis. The most common autoantibodies were ANA (78%), anti-dsDNA (55%), anti-Ro (47%), and anti-La (34%). Using the same database, McClain et al. [65] found that 24/130 (18.5%) patients were positive for IgG and/or IgM anticardiolipin antibodies (aCL) before the SLE diagnosis. Individuals produced aCL from as early as 7.6 years before SLE diagnosis to within a month of SLE diagnosis (median 3.2 years). The presence of aCL also predicted a more severe clinical outcome including renal disease, central nervous system disease, and clotting events. Interestingly, antiphospholipid (aPL)-positive SLE patients evaluated throughout the study met a significantly higher number of ACR SLE criteria (mean 6.1) than the other lupus patients analyzed (4.9; P <0.001). Moreover, when the patients who were positive for IgG aCL were analyzed separately, this difference became even more pronounced (6.5 vs 4.8 criteria; P <0.001). In addition, aCL positive patients presented with SLE at a younger age than aCL- patients (mean, 27.1 and 31.6 years of age, respectively).

One of the challenges in using antibodies as predictors of disease is that, together with ANA, they are detectable in up to 20% [52] of apparently healthy individuals, and there is even higher prevalence in first-degree relatives of SLE patients [66]. However, many of these normal patients exhibit dysregulation in the immune system [67, 68]. Therefore, efforts have been made to develop more sensitive and precise methods to predict future SLE. Researchers have begun to explore new alternatives, such as the use of cell-bound complement activation products (CB-CAPs) as predictors of SLE and potential future disease progression. Recently, a product called AVISE CTD test, which is a test that combines autoantibody, Erythrocyte-bound C4d (EC4d), B-cell bound C4d (BC4d), and platelet-bound C4d (PC4d), was developed [69]. A retrospective longitudinal observational study conducted by Liang et al. [70] examined patients from a single rheumatic individual without a confirmed SLE diagnosis, and who had undergone AVISE CTD testing as part of their routine clinical care over 2 years. The AVISE test was ordered for all patients within this time frame who had inflammatory arthritis, undifferentiated connective tissue disease, or other diagnoses with symptoms or features that suggested a possible SLE diagnosis. dsDNA indirect fluorescent antibody (IFA) status (crithidia), antibody titers (ELISA), and ACPA antibody titers (ELISA) were collected as part of the AVISE testing panel. The study cohort consisted of 117 patients; of these, the diagnoses in 2 years indicated that 16/20 (80%) were positive for disease, compared with 28/97 (28.9%) of patients with a nonpositive test. In contrast, the diagnosis of SLE was confirmed in 3 out of 4 patients with a positive dsDNA IFA (75%) at baseline, versus 20/113 (17.7%) without a positive dsDNA IFA test.

Furthermore, to evaluate this test's performance compared to traditional biomarkers of SLE (dsDNA, C3, C4, and ANA), all of these biomarkers were also evaluated at the beginning of the study ($t = 0$) and 2 years later ($t = 2$). It was found that elevated dsDNA, low C3, and low C4 demonstrated high specificity (>90%), but poor sensitivity (<20%) for predicting a diagnosis of SLE at $t = 2$. Conversely, ANA positivity at $t = 0$ had good sensitivity (87%) but low specificity (39%). AVISE positivity demonstrated a specificity of 93%, a sensitivity of 57%, PPV of 65%, and NPV of 90%. Using logistic regression, only AVISE positivity was significantly associated with a confirmed diagnosis of SLE at $t = 2$, with an OR of 10.7 (95% CI 2.6–44.9, $P = 0.001$) [70].

4.3 RA

The presence of autoantibodies is a distinctive feature of RA. The two autoantibodies most commonly used in clinical practice are rheumatoid factor (RF) and ACPA, which are generally used for the classification/diagnosis of this disorder. These antibodies may be associated with greater disease activity (only RF) [71], higher radiographic progression [71, 72], lower chances of disease remission, and higher probability of disease recurrence [73], suggesting a pathogenic role. More importantly, they can be present years before the onset of clinical manifestations and are also associated with a higher risk of developing RA [74, 75].

For instance, in a prospective cohort study [74], blood samples drawn from 12,698 white Danish individuals from the general population (aged 20–100 years old) without RA at study entry (1981–1983) were used to perform RF tests. Then, in the years 2009–2010, plasma from 9712 of these patients was drawn to measure RF levels again. Participants diagnosed clinically with RA during the study were identified by means of the national Danish Patient Registry, requiring only a single inpatient or outpatient hospital diagnosis. Researchers found that during the 181,654 person-years of follow-up, 183 participants developed RA. The median time from the provision of the sample to development of RA was 15 years for those with RF levels of <25 IU/mL, 12 years for those with RF levels of 25–50 UI/mL, 7 years for 50.1–100 IU/mL, and 7 years for >100 IU/mL. The cumulative incidence of RA increased with increasing RF, with up to 26-fold higher long-term risk of developing RA and up to 32% 10-year absolute risk of developing RA. In addition, high RF levels were associated with the development of other AIDs (SS, SLE, and systemic sclerosis).

Likewise, the appearance of RF in serum is sequential leading up to diagnosis: first IgM RF appears, then IgA RF, and finally IgG RF [75]. This was reported in a study that evaluated stored samples from 73 military cases with seropositive RA before RA diagnosis (mean 2.9 samples per case; sample collected at a mean of 6.6 years before diagnosis). Samples were tested for RF isotypes and ACPA. It was also found that ACPA positivity at any point prediagnosis had a sensitivity of 69.6% for future seropositive RA, with a specificity of 100% compared to controls. Prediagnosis positivity for ACPA and/or >2 RF isotypes (IgM, IgG, IgA) had an overall sensitivity of 74% and specificity of 98.6% for future seropositive RA compared with matched military controls.

Anticarbamylated protein (anti-CarP) antibodies are also useful in predicting RA. In an observational prospective cohort study conducted by Shi et al. [76] sera were drawn from 340 arthralgia patients who did not have clinical signs of arthritis, but who were positive for IgM RF and/or ACPA. Of the patients with arthralgia, 111 were RF-positive/ACPA-negative, and 229 were ACPA-positive. Patients were observed for the development of RA (based on the 2010 American College of Rheumatology/European League Against Rheumatism classification criteria) during a median follow-up period of 36 months. It was found that Anti-CarP antibodies were present in the sera of 30% of patients. 120 patients developed RA after a median of 12 months. The presence of anti-CarP antibodies was associated with the development of RA in the entire arthralgia cohort after correction for RF and ACPA status (hazard ratio 1.56 [95% confidence interval 1.06–2.29], $P < 0.023$), as well as in the ACPA2 antibody-positive subgroup (odds ratio 2.231 [95% confidence interval 1.31–3.79], $P < 0.003$). However, whether anti-CarP antibodies may predict the development of RA in arthralgia patients who were negative for ACPA and RF could not be addressed due to the nature of the cohort (Tables 1 and 2).

18. Prediction of autoimmune diseases: From bench to bedside

TABLE 1   Predictive value and associations of biomarkers of some systemic autoimmune diseases.

Autoimmune disease	Biomarker	Predictive value	Time from first detection to diagnosis (years)	Associations
SLE	ds-DNA, C3, C4 (together)	Se: <20% Sp: >90%	Up to 9.2 (mean 2.7)	Higher disease activity, renal involvement, hematological involvement [77–79]
	ANAs	Se: 87% Sp: 39%	Mean 9.2	Immune dysregulation
	AVISE test	Se: 57% Sp: 93%	N/A	Rheumatoid Arthritis, UCTD, higher SLICC
	Anti-Ro	Se: 47% Sp: N/A	Mean 9.4	Congenital heart block, Sjögren's syndrome
	Anti-La	Se: 34% Sp: N/A	Mean 8.1	Sjögren's syndrome
	IgM aCL and IgG aCL	N/A	Up to 7.6 (median 3.2)	White, male, concomitant APS, earlier disease onset, more severe disease course, thrombocytopenia. Hemolytic anemia
	ds-DNA	Se: 55% Sp: N/A	Mean 9.3	Higher disease activity, renal involvement, hematological involvement [77–79]
RA	RF	Se: 74% Sp:98.6%	Up to 15 (mean 6.6)	Disease activity, Radiographic progression, less remission, disease recurrence, lymphoma [80], presence of other AIDs
	ACPA	Se: 69.6% Sp: 90%–100%	Up to 10 (mean 6.6)	Radiographic progression, less remission, disease recurrence
	anti-CarP	Se: 30% Sp: N/A	N/A	Presence of RF and ACPA
SS	ANAs	OR 7.4	Up to 20 (median 4.3–5.1)	Immune dysregulation
	Anti-Ro	OR 30	Up to 20 (median 4.3–5.1)	Disease activity, glandular and extraglandular manifestations
	Anti-La	OR 34	Up to 16.1 (median 3.5)	Disease activity, glandular and extraglandular manifestations

APS: antiphospholipid syndrome, *N/A*: not available, *Se*: sensitivity, *Sp*: specificity.
SLICC: Systemic Lupus International Collaborating Clinics.
P.D. All table references are included in the References section of the Manuscript.

Álvaro J. Vivas and Gabriel J. Tobón

TABLE 2 Predictive value and associations of biomarkers of some organ-specific autoimmune diseases.

Autoimmune disease	Biomarker	Predictive value	Time from first detection to diagnosis (years)	Associations
Type 1 diabetes	TT-TRFIA for simultaneous measurement of C peptide and insulin	Se: 70% Sp: 77%	2	Not determined
	ICA, IAA, GADA, IA-2A	Progression: 10% at 1 year with a single of these autoantibodies >70% in the following 10 years or more than two autoantibodies	Up to 10 years	Faster disease progression (for IA-2A and ZnT8 positive) [81]
Primary biliar cholangitis (PBC)	Antimitochondrial antibodies (AMAs)	N/A	Mean 8.7–9	Chronic hepatitis, liver fibrosis, lymphoid aggregates within portal areas [82]
	ANAs (multiple nuclear dot and nuclear membrane/ rim like patterns)	N/A	N/A	Progressive form of the disease [83]
Neonatal hyperthyroidism	TSH level <0.9 mIU/L between days 3 and 7 of life [84]	Se: 78% Sp: 99%	N/A	Intellectual dysfunction, heart failure
Hashimoto's thyroiditis	Antithyroidal peroxidase (TPO) titers over 17 IU/ mL [85]	Se: 90% Sp: 75%	N/A	Asthma, rheumatoid arthritis, type 1 diabetes, celiac disease [86]

It is important to remember that both ACPA and RF are usually tested for only one isotype (IgG and IgM, respectively). Interestingly, it has been described that testing for multiple autoantibody subtypes increases diagnostic power and potential of predicting AIDs. Sieghart et al. tested for IgM, IgG, and IgA isotypes of RF, ACPA, and RA33 antibodies in 290 patients with RA, 261 disease controls, and 100 healthy subjects. Investigators found that about one third of seronegative patients generated antibodies known to be highly associated with RA, including IgA isotypes of RF and ACPA [87]. Diagnostic performance for each isotype is described in Table 3 and illustrated in Fig. 3. Similarly, Brink et al. evaluated different RF and ACPA isotypes to predict RA. RF-IgA was significantly more prevalent than the most frequent ACPA subtypes in samples collected ≥15 years before the onset of symptoms. The frequency of RF-positivity of the IgA, IgG, and IgM isotypes in all samples from pre-symptomatic individuals was 25%, 18%, and 26%, respectively; positivity after the onset of disease was

TABLE 3 Diagnostic performance and discriminatory capacity of RF, ACPA and RA33 isotypes for the diagnosis of rheumatoid arthritis (RA).

Biomarker	Diagnostic performance	Area under the curve (AUC)	Positive predictive value (PPV)
IgA-RF	Se: 50.7% Sp: 98%	0.775	95.4%
IgG-RF	Se: 14.4% Sp: 98%	0.643	85.4%
IgM-RF	Se: 64.8% Sp: 92%	0.785	86.8%
IgA-ACPA	Se: 34.1% Sp: 99%	0.742	96.5%
IgG-ACPA	Se: 57.9% Sp: 99%	0.754	97.9%
IgM-ACPA	Se: 28.6% Sp: 95%	0.67	82.3%
IgA-RA33	Se: 6% Sp: 98%	0.55	63.1%
IgG-RA33	Se: 6.2% Sp: 98%	0.608	71.6%
IgM-RA33	Se: 17.7% Sp: 98%	0.481	84.2%

Adapted from D. Sieghart, A. Platzer, P. Studenic, F. Alasti, M. Grundhuber, S. Swiniarski, et al, Determination of autoantibody isotypes increases the sensitivity of serodiagnostics in rheumatoid arthritis, Front. Immunol. 9(APR) (2018).

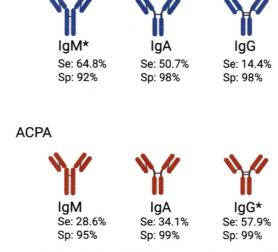

FIG. 3 Diagnostic performance of different RF and ACPA isotypes for RA. In generally, IgM and IgG are evaluated when performing RF and ACPA tests, respectively. However, other subtypes of these autoantibodies also demonstrate acceptable diagnostic performance. Individuals may be positive for only one isotype; therefore, including a panel evaluating IgM, IgA, and IgG for RF and ACPA may increase sensitivity and specificity for the diagnosis of RA.

significantly increased (65%, 57%, and 79%, respectively). Biomarkers with the highest odds ratios for RA development in pre-symptomatic individuals were CCP2 (OR: 20.26), IgM-RF (OR: 11.08), and IgA-RF (OR: 9.07). Additional results are listed in Tables 4 and 5.

The performance of these three biomarkers together in predicting RA development has also been evaluated in a cohort of early arthritis patients. When comparing the presence of one, two, or three of these biomarkers to patients with zero autoantibodies, the odds ratio (OR) of having a positive RA diagnosis increased from 3.8 (95% CI: 2.9–5.0), to 20.9 (95% CI: 12.7–34.3), and to 112.2 (95% CI: 52.4–240.5), respectively [91, 92].

TABLE 4 Diagnostic accuracy of determined ACPAs, anti-CCP2 antibodies, anti-CarP antibodies, and RF isotypes for RA development in presymptomatic individuals.[a]

Biomarker	Diagnostic performance (95% CI)	Odds ratio for RA development in presymptomatic individuals (95% CI)
CCP-2	Se: 29.6% (26.08–33.39)	20.6 (10.58–38.3)
CEP-1	Se: 23.9% (20.64–27.51)	4.75 (3.14–7.2)
Filaggrin	Se: 21.8% (18.72–25.39)	9.39 (5.33–16.55)
Fibß$_{36-52}$	Se: 22.5 (19.36–26.1)	3.98 (2.66–5.95)
Vim$_{60-75}$	Se: 9.49 (7.38–12.15)	1.93 (1.18–3.14)
CarP	Se: 13.78 (10.81–17.43)	5.83 (2.08–16.36)
IgA-RF	Se: 24.75 (21.46–28.37)	9.07 (5.5–14.96)
IgG-RF	Se: 17.56 (14.72–20.83)	5.89 (3.53–9.82)
IgM-RF	Se: 26.09 (22.73–29.76)	11.08 (6.64–18.5)

[a] Adapted from M. Brink, et al., Rheumatoid factor isotypes in relation to antibodies against citrullinated peptides and carbamylated proteins before the onset of rheumatoid arthritis, Arthritis Res. Ther. 18(1) (2016) 1–11, https://doi.org/10.1186/s13075-016-0940-2.

TABLE 5 Cytokines/chemokines detected by multiplex assays for the prediction of SLE and RA.

Cytokine/chemokine	AID predicted	Association	Median time before disease onset (years)	Odds ratio (95% CI)
Interferon- γ inducible protein-10	SLE	interferon α concentrations, ANAs, anti-Ro, anti-Jo-1	8.9	N/A
MCP-1 [88]	SLE	Inverse correlation with ANAs, anti-Ro, anti-La	8.9	N/A
IL-1RA, IL-12, GM-CSF, IFN-y [89, 90]	RA	ACPA and/or RF positivity	3.3–5	4.7 (2.12–10.4)
IL-4 [89, 90]	RA	ACPA and/or RF positivity	3.3–5	4.3 (1.94–9.7)
Eotaxin [89]	RA	ACPA and/or RF positivity	3.3	5.8 (2.7–12.62)
IL-17 [89]	RA	Significantly high levels before disease, lowering after disease onset	3.3	N/A

4.4 SS

Autoantibodies are also highly characteristic of Sjögren's syndrome (SS). Patients with high titers of anti-Ro and anti-La tend to have higher disease activity, extraglandular manifestations and lymphoma [93, 94]. Similar to the aforementioned AIDs, it has also been shown that individuals that present with autoantibodies will develop SS in the following months to years.

Theander et al. [95] conducted a retrospective study that evaluated ANA, anti-Ro, anti-La, and RF from 117 patients with primary SS from whom serum samples had been obtained before diagnosis and saved in biobanks. In addition, 117 control subjects (with one serum sample each) were randomly selected from the same biobank from which the patient samples were obtained. The controls were matched for sex and age at the time of acquisition of the respective patient's earliest serum sample. It was found that 75% of the patients were positive for at least one of the autoantibodies detected pre-diagnosis. ANA was present in 64% of the patients, RF in 53%, and anti-Ro 60, anti Ro 52, and anti-La in 51%, 41%, and 20%, respectively. The predictive value for developing primary SS was highest for anti-La (OR 34), followed by anti-Ro 60 (OR 30), ANAs (OR 7.4), and RF (OR 4.1). An OR could not be calculated for anti-Ro 52, as none of the controls were positive for this autoantibody. There were no significant correlations between the levels of these autoantibodies and time from sampling to diagnosis. However, ANA, RF, and antibodies against Ro were detected in samples obtained as early as 19–20 years (median 4.3–5.1) before diagnosis. In addition, it is important to highlight the fact that patients diagnosed as having primary SS earlier than the age of 40 had a significantly higher prevalence of prediagnostic autoantibodies with higher titers.

Furthermore, other biomarkers have also been described to increase the risk of developing SS. A longitudinal study conducted by Shiboski et al. [96] included all participants in the Sjögren's International Collaborative Clinical Alliance (SICCA) registry who were found to have any objective measures of salivary hypofunction, dry eye, focal lymphocytic sialadenitis in minor salivary gland biopsy, or anti-Ro antibodies. Patients were recalled over a 2–3-year interval after their baseline examinations to repeat all clinical examinations and specimen collections. 771 patients returned for a follow-up visit; researchers found that individuals with hypergammaglobulinemia, defined as IgG >1445 mg/dL at study entry, were four times more likely to progress to SS than those with lower values. Likewise, patients with hypocomplementemia, defined as C4 <16 mg/dL at study entry, were 6 times more likely to progress to SS than those without this phenotype.

5 Perspectives

5.1 Multiplex assay technologies (MAS)

In recent years, multiplex assay technologies (MAS) such as addressable laser bead immunoassays and line immunoassays have been developed. These allow for the detection of up to 100 different autoantibodies in a single assay. Therefore, they could provide a broad antibody profile that may lead to previously unappreciated associations [52]. Additionally, although the ANA indirect immunofluorescence (IIF) test is considered the gold standard for the classification of some AIDs, some evidence suggests that follow-up testing algorithms might be inverted, wherein MAS detect antibodies to disease-specific autoantibody targets is a more cost-effective approach. Samples that have negative MAS results might then be tested by ANA IIF assays to determine whether antibodies to targets not included in the MAS are also detected [97–100]. In addition, the extra antibodies tested in the MAS could provide physicians additional information about prognosis, risk of a flare-up, or specific clinical manifestations. Experts consider that adding algorithmic analysis to MAS, called MAAA (Multiplex assay technologies with algorithmic analysis), could significantly increase its sensibility and sensitivity, and even be useful in predicting AIDs [52, 97].

There are still challenges to consider in predicting AIDs [52]. For example, if a healthy patient is found to have a high risk of developing an AID, the physician may be obliged to advise the patient of the test result and its clinical implications, which could be considered unethical if taking into account the consequent anxiety associated with the possibility of developing chronic and even life-threatening disease. This may also have implications for employment prospects, and healthcare insurance policy rates, and eligibility. Hence, strict policies protecting the patients' rights should be implemented.

6 Prevention

6.1 T1D

T1D is one of the few AIDs in which multiple prevention trials have been completed, some of which have used dietary intervention. For example, the BABYDIET, TRIGR, and FINDIA studies have analyzed the avoidance of certain proteins, such as bovine insulin and gluten that have been postulated to cause T1D. The BABYDIET study did not find significant differences after modulating gluten exposure [101]. The TRIGR study found no difference with bovine milk protein avoidance in autoantibody development or T1D progression [102]. However, the FINDIA study observed a significant reduction in autoantibody positivity in individuals after bovine insulin avoidance (FINDIA formula) compared to ordinary cow's milk [103].

Other authors have proposed a different approach. In T1D-susceptible patients identified by genetic studies, cellular stressors could lead to a release of B cell antigens to which immune tolerance has not been achieved [104]. Hence, it was hypothesized that B cell-rest, achieved by administration of insulin, could protect B cells [105]. In other studies in which this was tested in NOD mice, both parenteral and oral insulin administration prevented or delayed the onset of T1D [106, 107]. Later, the Diabetes Prevention Trial-Type 1 (DPT-1) evaluated this intervention in humans. Subcutaneous [108] and oral [109] insulin were provided to first- and second-degree relatives of T1D patients; none of the interventions prevented the development of the disease. Nevertheless, in an ad hoc analysis of the subgroup of high-islet cell autoantibody-positive patients, a projected delay of 4.8 years in the disease onset was observed [109].

Another evaluated intervention was the induced tolerance to GAD65, which is a diabetes antigen. Trials in which GAD65 was administrated to spontaneously diabetic nonobese mice prevented autoimmune beta-cell destruction [110, 111]. This motivated researchers to investigate the effect of this intervention in T1D patients. In line with this, a double-blind placebo-controlled clinical trial evaluated nondiabetic children aged 4–17.9, with GADA and at least one of IA-2A or ZnT8. These patients were randomly given GAD or placebo, and cumulative incidence of T1D onset over a 5-year follow-up was determined. GAD did not affect progression to T1D [112].

Some recently evaluated interventions are abatacept and teplizumab. The former selectively blocks CD28-mediated T cell costimulation, interfering with T cell activation, proliferation, and survival [113]. This drug has been described to have good efficacy in conserving beta-cell function in patients recently diagnosed with T1D, but only transiently [114]. Currently, on-going trials are examining the effect of abatacept in preventing progression to clinical T1D in Stage 1 and 2 patients with islet autoantibodies (Clinicaltrials.gov, NCT03929601, and NCT01773707). Another trial is evaluating whether intervention with abatacept will prevent or delay the development of abnormal glucose tolerance in at-risk autoantibody positive non-diabetic relatives of patients with T1D (Clinicaltrials.gov, NCT01773707). Teplizumab is a hu-manized monoclonal antibody against CD3 on T cells; in one of the first trials evaluating this drug it failed to meet primary endpoints (insulin use of less than 0.5 unit/kg/day and HbA1c of less than 6.5% at 1 year) [115]. However, another study found that it preserved C-peptide secretion by 30%, and after 2 years, individuals maintained residual insulin production [116]. Later, in a recent phase II randomized, placebo-controlled, double-blind trial involving rel-atives of patients with T1D who did not have diabetes but were at high risk for developing disease, it was found that teplizumab almost doubled the median time to the diagnosis of T1D compared to the placebo group (48.4 months vs 24.4 months). In addition, 43% of the partic-ipants who received teplizumab were diagnosed with T1D, compared to 72% of those who received the placebo.

Similarly, otelixizumab, a chimeric monoclonal antibody that targets the ε-chain of the CD3 T-lymphocyte surface receptor, has been shown to have beneficial effects on beta-cell function, although at the cost of significant side effects. At low doses, studies have postulated that it is not effective on beta-cell preservation [117]. Lastly, rituximab, an anti-CD20 monoclonal antibody, showed some efficacy in beta-cell function preservation, but only for a short time [44, 118].

6.2 SLE

Different authors have confirmed that vitamin D supplementation in SLE patients in-creased regulatory T cells, decreased effector Th1 and Th17 cells [119], and lowered the dis-ease activity score [120]. Additionally, it has been reported that anti-C1q, anti-dsDNA, and disease activity may be aggravated by vitamin D insufficiency [121, 122].

These findings motivated experts to investigate whether this vitamin could affect the prevention of SLE. Costenbader et al. assessed vitamin D intake in SLE incident cases via semiquantitative food frequency questionnaires among a cohort of more than 180,000 women followed from 1980 to 2002. The relationship between vitamin D intake and incidence SLE was examined, but no association was found [123]. Similarly, Young et al. measured 25-hydroxy vitamin D levels in 436 individuals who had a relative with SLE, but did not have SLE them-selves. Fifty-six of these individuals developed SLE after a follow-up of 6.3 years. Mean base-line vitamin D levels and vitamin D supplementation were not different between those who did and did not develop SLE, although these results were not statistically significant ($P = 0.42$ and $P = 0.65$, respectively). Vitamin D deficiency was greater in those who developed the disease compared with those who did not progress to SLE (46 vs 33%, $P = 0.05$). Further stud-ies are needed to evaluated this intervention [124].

6.3 RA

Dietary interventions have been evaluated in the treatment of RA [125], one of the most studied of which is the Mediterranean diet. A recent systematic review evaluating the effects of this diet in the treatment and prevention of RA found that it reduces pain, decreases RA score as assessed by health questionnaire, and reduces the 28 joint-count disease activity score (DAS28). Nevertheless, the authors concluded that there is insufficient evidence to support widespread recommendation of this diet for the prevention of RA [126].

Another lifestyle intervention studied for the prevention of RA is smoking cessation. In a recent trial, smoking cessation and RA risk were investigated in two cohorts of more than 230,000 women, in which 1528 incident cases of RA were identified. Among the seropositive RA patients, those who were current smokers had a hazard ratio for RA of 1.67 (1.38–2.01) compared to never-smokers (1.0). Likewise, compared to never-smokers, a slightly elevated risk for seropositive RA was still detectable among past smokers, even 30 years after smoking cessation. Additionally, in women who quit smoking and had not smoked for >30 years, the risk of seropositive RA was reduced by 37% (HR 0.63, 95% IC 0.44–0.9) compared to women who quit smoking for 0 to <5 years. Considering this, the authors concluded that sustained smoking cessation may reduce the risk of seropositive RA [127].

A retrospective cohort study conducted by Chodick et al. [128] used computerized medical databases of a large health organization to identify diagnosed RA cases among adults who began statin therapy between 1998 and 2007. Compliance with statins was assessed by calculating the mean proportion of follow-up days covered (PDC) with statins with all study participants. The crude incidence density rate of RA among noncompliant patients (PDC <20%) was 51% higher (3.98 per 1000 person-years) compared to highly compliant patients who took statins for at least 80% of the follow-up period. These findings motivated other researchers to evaluate if atorvastatin could halt RA development in persons at risk of this disease with the STAPRA (Statins to Prevent Rheumatoid Arthritis) trial, which is still ongoing.

In the PRIARI (Prevention of RA by Rituximab) study [129], individuals positive for both ACPA and RF, but without arthritis, were included in a randomized, double-blind, placebo-controlled study to receive a single infusion of 1000 mg of rituximab or placebo. Forty-one individuals received rituximab and 40 individuals received placebo and they were followed up for a mean of 29 (0–54) months. The risk of developing arthritis in the placebo group was 40%, which was decreased by 55% in the rituximab group (HR 0.45, 95% CI 0.154–1322) (not statistically significant). In addition, rituximab treatment caused a delay in arthritis development of 12 months compared with placebo treatment, at the point at which 25% of the subjects had developed arthritis ($P < 0.001$). Further studies with larger sample sizes evaluating this monoclonal antibody for the prevention of RA are needed.

Glucocorticoids have also been tested for the prevention of RA. In a study conducted by Bos et al. [130], 83 patients with arthralgia positive for ACPA or IgM RF were randomly allocated to groups given intramuscular injections of 100 mg dexamethasone or placebo for 6 weeks. Although patients treated with dexamethasone had reduced antibody levels after 1 month (ACPA 222% and IgM-RF 214%), arthritis development in both groups was similar (20% vs 21%) during a median follow-up of 26 months. Hence, it is important to consider that surrogate markers may not always be a reliable indicator of clinical outcomes.

Various additional trials are currently ongoing testing other agents such as hydroxychloroquine (Clinicaltrials.gov, NCT02603146) (StopRA), abatacept (IRSCTNregistry, IRSCTN46017566) (APIPPRA), and glucocorticoids (Clinicaltrialsregister.eu, 2014–004472-35) (TREAT EARLIER) to prevent or delay the development of RA. The use of new technologies, and further understanding of the pathophysiology of this disease, will provide better

18. Prediction of autoimmune diseases: From bench to bedside

TABLE 6 Recently completed or ongoing trials for the prevention of Type 1 diabetes and rheumatoid arthritis.

Pathology	Intervention	Trial name	Identifier	Estimated study completion date
RA	Abatacept	ARIAA (arthritis prevention in the preclinical phase of rheumatoid arthritis with abatacept)	NCT02778906	December 2019
	Abatacept	APIPPRA (abatacept reversing subclinical inflammation as measured by MRI in ACPA positive arthralgia)	ISRCTN46017566	July 2021
	Hydroxychloroquine	StopRA (strategy to prevent the onset of clinically apparent rheumatoid arthritis)	NCT02603146	November 2023
	Methylprednisolone	TREAT EARLIER (treat early arthralgia to reverse or limit impending exacerbation to rheumatoid arthritis)	2014–004472-35	Not available
	Atorvastatin	STAPRA (statins to prevent rheumatoid arthritis)	2013–005524-42	Not available
T1D	Abatacept	CTLA4-Ig for prevention of abnormal glucose tolerance and diabetes in relatives at risk for Type 1 Diabetes	NCT01773707	November 2021
	Rituximab and abatacept	Rituximab and abatacept for prevention or reversal of type 1 diabetes	NCT03929601	July 2026
	MAS-1 adjuvanted insulin B-chain	MER3101 (MAS-1 adjuvanted antigen-specific immunotherapeuthic for prevention and treatment of type 1 diabetes)	NCT3624062	April 2022
	Hydroxychloroquine	Hydroxychloroquine in individuals at risk for type 1 diabetes mellitus (TN-22)	NCT03428945	August 2024
	Oral insulin	GPPAD-POinT (global platform of autoimmune diabetes—primary oral insulin trial)	NCT03364868	January 2025

opportunities to hopefully achieve RA prevention in the near future. A summary containing ongoing prevention trials of the former AIDs can be found in Table 6.

7 Conclusion

Genetic and epigenetic studies have facilitated great advances in the understanding and prediction of various AIDs. Multiomic technology has the potential to unveil novel aspects of these pathologies, and to identify new substances and approaches to diagnose and predict their progression. Further observational and experimental studies are imperative to achieve this goal. Furthermore, biomarkers have the potential not only to predict the development of a disease but also the extent and severity of a disease, bringing clinicians' valuable information in terms of additional intervention options.

References

[1] N. Dragin, R. Le Panse, S. Berrih-Aknin, Prédisposition aux pathologies auto-immmunes, Medecine/Sciences 33 (2) (2017) 169–175.

[2] A. Lerner, P. Jeremias, T. Matthias, The world incidence and prevalence of autoimmune diseases is increasing, Int. J. Celiac. Dis. 3 (4) (2015) 151–155.

[3] E.E. Carter, S.G. Barr, A.E. Clarke, The global burden of SLE: prevalence, health disparities and socioeconomic impact, Nat. Rev. Rheumatol. 12 (10) (2016 Oct) 605–620.

[4] S.M.M. Verstappen, Rheumatoid arthritis and work: the impact of rheumatoid arthritis on absenteeism and presenteeism, Best Pract. Res. Clin. Rheumatol. 29 (3) (2015 Jun) 495–511.

[5] V. Foos, N. Varol, B.H. Curtis, K.S. Boye, D. Grant, J.L. Palmer, et al., Economic impact of severe and non-severe hypoglycemia in patients with type 1 and type 2 diabetes in the United States, J. Med. Econ. 18 (6) (2015 Jun) 420–432.

[6] M.D. Rosenblum, K.A. Remedios, A.K. Abbas, Mechanisms of human autoimmunity, J. Clin. Invest. 125 (6) (2015) 2228–2233.

[7] J.C. Knight, Regulatory polymorphisms underlying complex disease traits, J. Mol. Med. (Berl.) 83 (2) (2005) 97–109.

[8] M. Alvaro-Benito, E. Morrison, M. Wieczorek, J. Sticht, C. Freund, Human leukocyte antigen-DM polymorphisms in autoimmune diseases, Open Biol. 6 (8) (2016).

[9] F.W. Miller, Environmental agents and autoimmune diseases, Adv. Exp. Med. Biol. 711 (2011) 61–81.

[10] G. Shi, Z. Zhang, Q. Li, New biomarkers in autoimmune disease, J Immunol Res 2017 (2017) 1–2.

[11] M.S. Udler, M.I. McCarthy, J.C. Florez, A. Mahajan, Genetic risk scores for diabetes diagnosis and precision medicine, Endocr. Rev. 40 (6) (2019) 1500–1520.

[12] S. Onengut-Gumuscu, W.-M. Chen, O. Burren, N.J. Cooper, A.R. Quinlan, J.C. Mychaleckyj, et al., Fine mapping of type 1 diabetes susceptibility loci and evidence for colocalization of causal variants with lymphoid gene enhancers, Nat. Genet. 47 (4) (2015 Apr) 381–386.

[13] M.J. Redondo, R.A. Oram, A.K. Steck, Genetic risk scores for type 1 diabetes prediction and diagnosis, Curr. Diab. Rep. 17 (129) (2017) 1–10.

[14] T.A. Aly, A. Ide, M.M. Jahromi, J.M. Barker, M.S. Fernando, S.R. Babu, et al., Extreme genetic risk for type 1A diabetes, Proc. Natl. Acad. Sci. U. S. A. 103 (38) (2006 Sep) 14074–14079.

[15] A.K. Steck, F. Dong, R. Wong, A. Fouts, E. Liu, J. Romanos, et al., Improving prediction of type 1 diabetes by testing non-HLA genetic variants in addition to HLA markers, Pediatr. Diabetes 15 (5) (2014 Aug) 355–362.

[16] C. Winkler, J. Krumsiek, F. Buettner, C. Angermüller, E.Z. Giannopoulou, F.J. Theis, et al., Feature ranking of type 1 diabetes susceptibility genes improves prediction of type 1 diabetes, Diabetologia 57 (12) (2014 Dec) 2521–2529.

[17] R.A. Oram, K. Patel, A. Hill, B. Shields, T.J. McDonald, A. Jones, et al., A type 1 diabetes genetic risk score can aid discrimination between type 1 and type 2 diabetes in Young adults, Diabetes Care 39 (3) (2016 Mar) 337–344.

[18] E. Bonifacio, A. Beyerlein, M. Hippich, C. Winkler, K. Vehik, M.N. Weedon, et al., Genetic scores to stratify risk of developing multiple islet autoantibodies and type 1 diabetes: a prospective study in children, PLoS Med. 15 (4) (2018 Apr), e1002548.

[19] M. Rewers, J.X. She, A.G. Ziegler, O.G. Simell, Å. Lernmark, W.A. Hagopian, et al., The environmental determinants of diabetes in the young (TEDDY) study, Ann. N. Y. Acad. Sci. 1150 (2008) 1–13.

[20] L. Chen, Y. Wang, L. Liu, A. Bielowka, R. Ahmed, H. Zhang, et al., Genome-wide assessment of genetic risk for systemic lupus erythematosus and disease severity, Hum. Mol. Genet. 44 (0) (2020).

[21] J.C. Almlöf, A. Alexsson, J. Imgenberg-Kreuz, L. Sylwan, C. Bäcklin, D. Leonard, et al., Novel risk genes for systemic lupus erythematosus predicted by random forest classification, Sci. Rep. 7 (1) (2017) 1–11.

18. Prediction of autoimmune diseases: From bench to bedside

[22] I.C. Scott, S.D. Seegobin, S. Steer, R. Tan, P. Forabosco, A. Hinks, et al., Predicting the risk of rheumatoid arthritis and its age of onset through modelling genetic risk variants with smoking, PLoS Genet. 9 (9) (2013).

[23] L. Shervington, A. Darekar, M. Shaikh, R. Mathews, A. Shervington, Identifying reliable diagnostic/predictive biomarkers for rheumatoid arthritis, Biomark. Insights 13 (2018).

[24] R. Zhang, X. Yang, J. Wang, L. Han, A. Yang, J. Zhang, et al., Identification of potential biomarkers for differential diagnosis between rheumatoid arthritis and osteoarthritis via integrative genome-wide gene expression profiling analysis, Mol. Med. Rep. 19 (1) (2019) 30–40.

[25] V. Goëb, P. Aegerter, R. Parmar, P. Fardellone, O. Vittecoq, P.G. Conaghan, et al., Progression to rheumatoid arthritis in early inflammatory arthritis is associated with low IL-7 serum levels, Ann. Rheum. Dis. 72 (6) (2013 Jun) 1032–1036.

[26] T.R. Reksten, C.J. Lessard, K.L. Sivils, Genetics in Sjögren's syndrome, Rheum. Dis. Clin. N. Am. 42 (3) (2016) 435–447.

[27] P. Cruz-Tapias, A. Rojas-Villarraga, S. Maier-Moore, J.M. Anaya, HLA and Sjögren's syndrome susceptibility. A meta-analysis of worldwide studies, Autoimmun. Rev. [Internet] 11 (4) (2012) 281–287. Available from: https://doi.org/10.1016/j.autrev.2011.10.002.

[28] J.B. Harley, M. Reichlin, F.C. Arnett, E.L. Alexander, W.B. Bias, T.T. Provost, Gene interaction at HLA-DQ enhances autoantibody production in primary Sjögren's syndrome, Science 232 (4754) (1986 May) 1145–1147.

[29] C.J. Lessard, H. Li, I. Adrianto, J.A. Ice, A. Rasmussen, K.M. Grundahl, et al., Variants at multiple loci implicated in both innate and adaptive immune responses are associated with Sjögren's syndrome, Nat. Genet. 45 (11) (2013 Nov) 1284–1292.

[30] L.C. Kottyan, E.E. Zoller, J. Bene, X. Lu, J.A. Kelly, A.M. Rupert, et al., The IRF5-TNPO3 association with systemic lupus erythematosus has two components that other autoimmune disorders variably share, Hum. Mol. Genet. 24 (2) (2015 Jan) 582–596.

[31] J. Anaya, J.C. Sarmiento-monroy, Síndrome de Sjögren. Second Edi, Universidad del Rosario, Bogotá, 2017.

[32] O. Fogel, E. Rivière, R. Seror, G. Nocturne, S. Boudaoud, B. Ly, et al., Role of the IL-12/IL-35 balance in patients with Sjögren's syndrome, J. Allergy Clin. Immunol. 142 (1) (2018) 258. 268.e5.

[33] Y. Li, K. Zhang, H. Chen, F. Sun, J. Xu, Z. Wu, et al., A genome-wide association study in Han Chinese identifies a susceptibility locus for primary Sjögren's syndrome at 7q11.23, Nat. Genet. 45 (11) (2013 Nov) 1361–1365.

[34] R. Strollo, C. Vinci, M.H. Arshad, D. Perrett, C. Tiberti, F. Chiarelli, et al., Antibodies to post-translationally modified insulin in type 1 diabetes, Diabetologia 58 (12) (2015 Dec) 2851–2860.

[35] R. Strollo, C. Vinci, N. Napoli, P. Pozzilli, J. Ludvigsson, A. Nissim, Antibodies to post-translationally modified insulin as a novel biomarker for prediction of type 1 diabetes in children, Diabetologia 60 (8) (2017) 1467–1474.

[36] J. Ludvigsson, M. Ludvigsson, A. Sepa, Screening for prediabetes in the general child population: maternal attitude to participation, Pediatr. Diabetes 2 (4) (2001 Dec) 170–174.

[37] A. Kuroda, T.A. Rauch, I. Todorov, H.T. Ku, I.H. Al-Abdullah, F. Kandeel, et al., Insulin gene expression is regulated by DNA methylation, PLoS One 4 (9) (2009 Sep), e6953.

[38] M.I. Husseiny, A. Kaye, E. Zebadua, F. Kandeel, K. Ferreri, Tissue-specific methylation of human insulin gene and PCR assay for monitoring beta cell death, PLoS One 9 (4) (2014).

[39] K.M. Simmons, A. Fouts, L. Pyle, J. Clark, F. Dong, L. Yu, et al., Unmethylated insulin as an adjunctive marker of beta cell death and progression to type 1 diabetes in participants at risk of diabetes, Int. J. Mol. Sci. 20 (16) (2019).

[40] J.J. Connolly, H. Hakonarson, Role of cytokines in systemic lupus erythematosus: recent progress from GWAS and sequencing, J. Biomed. Biotechnol. 2012 (2012) 798924.

[41] Y. Zhan, Y. Guo, Q. Lu, Aberrant epigenetic regulation in the pathogenesis of systemic lupus erythematosus and its implication in precision medicine, Cytogenet. Genome Res. 149 (3) (2016) 141–155.

[42] H. Wu, J. Liao, Q. Li, M. Yang, M. Zhao, Q. Lu, Epigenetics as biomarkers in autoimmune diseases, Clin. Immunol. [internet] 196 (2018) 34–39. Available from https://doi.org/10.1016/j.clim.2018.03.011.

[43] S.H. Chen, Q.L. Lv, L. Hu, M.J. Peng, G.H. Wang, B. Sun, DNA methylation alterations in the pathogenesis of lupus, Clin. Exp. Immunol. 187 (2) (2017) 185–192.

[44] M. Jeffries, A. Sawalha, Epigenetics in systemic lupus erythematosus: leading the way for specific therapeutic agents, Int. J. Clin. Rheumtol. 6 (4) (2011) 423–439.

[45] M. Zhao, Y. Zhou, B. Zhu, M. Wan, T. Jiang, Q. Tan, et al., IFI44L promoter methylation as a blood biomarker for systemic lupus erythematosus, Ann. Rheum. Dis. 75 (11) (2016 Nov) 1998–2006.

[46] X. Zhang, D. Zhou, M. Zhao, Y. Luo, P. Zhang, Z. Lu, et al., A proof-of-principle demonstration of a novel microarray-based method for quantifying DNA methylation levels, Mol. Biotechnol. 46 (3) (2010) 243–249.

[47] X. Zheng, Y. Zhang, P. Yue, L. Liu, C. Wang, K. Zhou, et al., Diagnostic significance of circulating miRNAs in systemic lupus erythematosus, PLoS One 14 (6) (2019) 1–19.

[48] M. Reale, C. D'Angelo, E. Costantini, M. Laus, A. Moretti, A. Croce, MicroRNA in Sjögren's syndrome: their potential roles in pathogenesis and diagnosis, J Immunol Res 2018 (2018).

[49] Y.J. Kim, Y. Yeon, W.J. Lee, Y.U. Shin, H. Cho, Y.K. Sung, et al., Comparison of microRNA expression in tears of normal subjects and Sjögren's syndrome patients, Investig. Ophthalmol. Vis. Sci. 60 (14) (2019) 4889–4895.

[50] K.M. Pauley, C.M. Stewart, A.E. Gauna, C. Dupre, R. Kuklani, A.L. Chan, et al., Altered miR-146a expression in Sjögren's syndrome and its functional role in innate immunity, Eur. J. Immunol. 41 (7) (2013) 2029–2039.

[51] C.-R. Jiang, H.-L. Li, The value of MiR-146a and MiR-4484 expressions in the diagnosis of anti-SSA antibody positive Sjögren's syndrome and the correlations with prognosis, Eur. Rev. Med. Pharmacol. Sci. 22 (15) (2018 Aug) 4800–4805.

[52] M.Y. Choi, M.J. Fritzler, Autoantibodies in SLE: prediction and the p value matrix, Lupus 28 (11) (2019) 1285–1293.

[53] A.G. Ziegler, M. Rewers, O. Simell, T. Simell, J. Lempainen, A. Steck, et al., Seroconversion to multiple islet autoantibodies and risk of progression to diabetes in children, JAMA 309 (23) (2013 Jun) 2473–2479.

[54] E. Bonifacio, Predicting type 1 diabetes using biomarkers, Diabetes Care 38 (6) (2015 Jun) 989–996.

[55] P.J. Bingley, Clinical applications of diabetes antibody testing, J. Clin. Endocrinol. Metab. 95 (1) (2010 Jan) 25–33.

[56] L. Yi, A.C. Swensen, W.J. Qian, Serum biomarkers for diagnosis and prediction of type 1 diabetes, Transl. Res. 201 (2018) 13–25.

[57] E.K. Sims, Z. Chaudhry, R. Watkins, F. Syed, J. Blum, F. Ouyang, et al., Elevations in the fasting serum proinsulin-to-C-peptide ratio precede the onset of type 1 diabetes, Diabetes Care 39 (9) (2016) 1519–1526.

[58] I. Truyen, P. De Pauw, P.N. Jørgensen, C. Van Schravendijk, O. Ubani, K. Decochez, et al., Proinsulin levels and the proinsulin:c-peptide ratio complement autoantibody measurement for predicting type 1 diabetes, Diabetologia 48 (11) (2005 Nov) 2322–2329.

[59] M.E. Røder, M. Knip, S.G. Hartling, J. Karjalainen, H.K. Akerblom, C. Binder, Disproportionately elevated proinsulin levels precede the onset of insulin-dependent diabetes mellitus in siblings with low first phase insulin responses. The childhood diabetes in Finland study group, J. Clin. Endocrinol. Metab. 79 (6) (1994 Dec) 1570–1575.

[60] R.A. Watkins, C. Evans-Molina, J.K. Terrell, K.H. Day, L. Guindon, I.A. Restrepo, et al., Proinsulin and heat shock protein 90 as biomarkers of beta-cell stress in the early period after onset of type 1 diabetes, Transl. Res. 168 (2016). 96–106.e1.

[61] P.E.M. De Pauw, I. Vermeulen, O.C. Ubani, I. Truyen, E.M.F. Vekens, F.T. van Genderen, et al., Simultaneous measurement of plasma concentrations of proinsulin and C-peptide and their ratio with a trefoil-type time-resolved fluorescence immunoassay, Clin. Chem. 54 (12) (2008 Dec) 1990–1998.

[62] A. Van Dalem, S. Demeester, E.V. Balti, B. Keymeulen, P. Gillard, B. Lapauw, et al., Prediction of impending type 1 diabetes through automated dual-label measurement of proinsulin: C-peptide ratio, PLoS One 11 (12) (2016) 1–14.

[63] H. Kallionpää, L.L. Elo, E. Laajala, J. Mykkänen, I. Ricaño-Ponce, M. Vaarma, et al., Innate immune activity is detected prior to seroconversion in children with HLA-conferred type 1 diabetes susceptibility, Diabetes 63 (7) (2014) 2402–2414.

[64] M.R. Arbuckle, M.T. McClain, M.V. Rubertone, R.H. Scofield, G.J. Dennis, J.A. James, et al., Development of autoantibodies before the clinical onset of systemic lupus erythematosus, N. Engl. J. Med. 349 (16) (2003 Oct) 1526–1533.

[65] M.T. McClain, M.R. Arbuckle, L.D. Heinlen, G.J. Dennis, J. Roebuck, M.V. Rubertone, et al., The prevalence, onset, and clinical significance of antiphospholipid antibodies prior to diagnosis of systemic lupus erythematosus, Arthritis Rheum. 50 (4) (2004) 1226–1232.

[66] D.S. Pisetsky, Antinuclear antibody testing - misunderstood or misbegotten? Nat. Rev. Rheumatol. 13 (8) (2017 Aug) 495–502.

[67] T. Aberle, R.L. Bourn, M.E. Munroe, H. Chen, V.C. Roberts, J.M. Guthridge, et al., Clinical and serologic features in patients with incomplete lupus classification versus systemic lupus erythematosus patients and controls, Arthritis Care Res. (Hoboken) 69 (12) (2017 Dec) 1780–1788.

18. Prediction of autoimmune diseases: From bench to bedside

[68] S. Slight-Webb, R. Lu, L.L. Ritterhouse, M.E. Munroe, H.T. Maecker, C.G. Fathman, et al., Autoantibody-positive healthy individuals display unique immune profiles that may regulate autoimmunity, Arthritis Rheumatol. (Hoboken, NJ) 68 (10) (2016) 2492–2502.

[69] J. Mossell, J.A. Goldman, D. Barken, R.V. Alexander, The Avise lupus test and cell-bound complement activation products aid the diagnosis of systemic lupus erythematosus, Open Rheumatol. J. 10 (1) (2016) 71–80.

[70] E. Liang, M. Taylor, M. McMahon, Utility of the AVISE connective tissue disease test in predicting lupus diagnosis and progression, Lupus Sci. Med. 7 (1) (2020) 1–7.

[71] D. Aletaha, F. Alasti, J.S. Smolen, Rheumatoid factor determines structural progression of rheumatoid arthritis dependent and independent of disease activity, Ann. Rheum. Dis. 72 (6) (2013) 875–880.

[72] A. Gupta, R. Kaushik, R.M. Kaushik, M. Saini, R. Kakkar, Association of anti-cyclic citrullinated peptide antibodies with clinical and radiological disease severity in rheumatoid arthritis, Curr. Rheumatol. Rev. 10 (2) (2014) 136–143.

[73] S. Bugatti, A. Manzo, C. Montecucco, R. Caporali, The clinical value of autoantibodies in rheumatoid arthritis, Front. Med. 5 (December) (2018) 1–10.

[74] S.F. Nielsen, S.E. Bojesen, P. Schnohr, B.G. Nordestgaard, Elevated rheumatoid factor and long term risk of rheumatoid arthritis: a prospective cohort study, BMJ 345 (7878) (2012) 1–9.

[75] K.D. Deane, C.I. O'Donnell, W. Hueber, D.S. Majka, A.A. Lazar, L.A. Derber, et al., The number of elevated cytokines and chemokines in preclinical seropositive rheumatoid arthritis predicts time to diagnosis in an age-dependent manner, Arthritis Rheum. 62 (11) (2010 Nov) 3161–3172.

[76] J. Shi, L.A. Van De Stadt, E.W.N. Levarht, T.W.J. Huizinga, R.E.M. Toes, L.A. Trouw, et al., Anti-carbamylated protein antibodies are present in arthralgia patients and predict the development of rheumatoid arthritis, Arthritis Rheum. 65 (4) (2013) 911–915.

[77] E. Mummert, et al., The clinical utility of anti-double-stranded DNA antibodies and the challenges of their determination, J. Immunol. Methods 459 (2018) 11–19. https://doi.org/10.1016/j.jim.2018.05.014.

[78] V.V. Vasilev, et al., Autoantibodies against C3b-functional consequences and disease relevance, Front. Immunol. 10 (2019) 64. https://doi.org/10.3389/fimmu.2019.00064.

[79] J.H. Jung, et al., Thrombocytopenia in systemic lupus erythematosus, Medicine 95 (6) (2016) 1–7. https://doi.org/10.1097/MD.0000000000002818.

[80] G. Nocturne, et al., Rheumatoid factor and disease activity are independent predictors of lymphoma in primary Sjögren's syndrome, Arthritis Rheumatol. 68 (4) (2016) 977–985. https://doi.org/10.1002/art.39518.

[81] F.K. Gorus, et al., Screening for insulinoma antigen 2 and zinc transporter 8 autoantibodies: a cost-effective and age-independent strategy to identify rapid progressors to clinical onset among relatives of type 1 diabetic patients, Clin. Exp. Immunol. 171 (1) (2013) 82–90. https://doi.org/10.1111/j.1365-2249.2012.04675.x.

[82] H.C. Mitchison, et al., Positive antimitochondrial antibody but normal alkaline phosphatase: is this primary biliary cirrhosis? Hepatology (Baltimore, Md.) 6 (6) (1986) 1279–1284. https://doi.org/10.1002/hep.1840060609.

[83] M. Milkiewicz, et al., Predicting and preventing autoimmunity: the case of anti-mitochondrial antibodies, Autoimmun. Highlights 3 (3) (2012) 105–112. https://doi.org/10.1007/s13317-012-0038-z.

[84] T.G.A. Strieder, et al., Prediction of progression to overt hypothyroidism or hyperthyroidism in female relatives of patients with autoimmune thyroid disease using the thyroid events Amsterdam (THEA) score, Arch. Internal Med. 168 (15) (2008) 1657–1663. https://doi.org/10.1001/archinte.168.15.1657.

[85] B. Bromińska, et al., Anti-thyroidal peroxidase antibodies are associated with thyrotropin levels in hypothyroid patients and in euthyroid individuals, Ann. Agric. Environ. Med. 24 (3) (2017) 431–434. https://doi.org/10.5604/12321966.1232090.

[86] E. Fröhlich, R. Wahl, Thyroid autoimmunity: role of anti-thyroid antibodies in thyroid and extra-thyroidal diseases, Front. Immunol. 8 (May) (2017). https://doi.org/10.3389/fimmu.2017.00521.

[87] D. Sieghart, A. Platzer, P. Studenic, F. Alasti, M. Grundhuber, S. Swiniarski, et al., Determination of autoantibody isotypes increases the sensitivity of serodiagnostics in rheumatoid arthritis, Front. Immunol. 9 (APR) (2018).

[88] C. Eriksson, S. Rantapää-Dahlqvist, Cytokines in relation to autoantibodies before onset of symptoms for systemic lupus erythematosus, Lupus 23 (7) (2014) 691–696. https://doi.org/10.1177/0961203314523869.

[89] H. Kokkonen, et al., Up-regulation of cytokines and chemokines predates the onset of rheumatoid arthritis, Arthritis Rheum. 62 (2) (2010) 383–391. https://doi.org/10.1002/art.27186.

[90] K.T. Jørgensen, et al., Cytokines, autoantibodies and viral antibodies in premorbid and postdiagnostic sera from patients with rheumatoid arthritis: case-control study nested in a cohort of Norwegian blood donors, Ann Rheum Dis 67 (6) (2008) 860–866. https://doi.org/10.1136/ard.2007.073825.

[91] M.K. Verheul, S. Bohringer, M.A.M. van Delft, J.D. Jones, W.F.C. Rigby, R.W. Gan, et al., Triple positivity for anti-citrullinated protein autoantibodies, rheumatoid factor, and anti-carbamylated protein antibodies conferring high specificity for rheumatoid arthritis: implications for very early identification of at-risk individuals, Arthritis Rheumatol. (Hoboken, NJ) 70 (11) (2018) 1721–1731.

[92] N. Lingampalli, J. Sokolove, L.J. Lahey, J.D. Edison, W.R. Gilliland, V.M. Holers, et al., Combination of anti-citrullinated protein antibodies and rheumatoid factor is associated with increased systemic inflammatory mediators and more rapid progression from preclinical to clinical rheumatoid arthritis, Clin. Immunol. 195 (2018 Oct) 119–126.

[93] S. Fragkioudaki, C.P. Mavragani, H.M. Moutsopoulos, Predicting the risk for lymphoma development in Sjögren's syndrome: an easy tool for clinical use, Medicine (Baltimore) 95 (25) (2016 Jun), e3766.

[94] P. Brito-Zeron, N. Acar-Denizli, W.-F. Ng, M. Zeher, A. Rasmussen, T. Mandl, et al., How immunological profile drives clinical phenotype of primary Sjögren's syndrome at diagnosis: analysis of 10,500 patients (Sjögren Big Data Project), Clin. Exp. Rheumatol. 36 (Suppl 1(3)) (2018) 102–112.

[95] E. Theander, R. Jonsson, B. Sjöström, K. Brokstad, P. Olsson, G. Henriksson, Prediction of Sjögren's syndrome years before diagnosis and identification of patients with early onset and severe disease course by autoantibody profiling, Arthritis Rheumatol. 67 (9) (2015) 2427–2436.

[96] C.H. Shiboski, A.N. Baer, S.C. Shiboski, M. Lam, S. Challacombe, H.E. Lanfranchi, et al., Natural history and predictors of progression to Sjögren's syndrome among participants of the Sjögren's international collaborative clinical Alliance registry, Arthritis Care Res. (Hoboken) 70 (2) (2018 Feb) 284–294.

[97] M.J. Fritzler, L. Martinez-Prat, M.Y. Choi, M. Mahler, The utilization of autoantibodies in approaches to precision health, Front. Immunol. 9 (NOV) (2018) 1–7.

[98] D. Perez, B. Gilburd, D. Azoulay, O. Shovman, N. Bizzaro, Y. Shoenfeld, Antinuclear antibodies: is the indirect immunofluorescence still the gold standard or should be replaced by solid phase assays? Autoimmun. Rev. 17 (6) (2018 Jun) 548–552.

[99] N. Bizzaro, I. Brusca, G. Previtali, M.G. Alessio, M. Daves, S. Platzgummer, et al., The association of solid-phase assays to immunofluorescence increases the diagnostic accuracy for ANA screening in patients with autoimmune rheumatic diseases, Autoimmun. Rev. 17 (6) (2018 Jun) 541–547.

[100] P.L. Meroni, M.O. Borghi, Diagnostic laboratory tests for systemic autoimmune rheumatic diseases: unmet needs towards harmonization, Clin. Chem. Lab. Med. 56 (10) (2018 Sep) 1743–1748.

[101] S. Hummel, M. Pflüger, M. Hummel, E. Bonifacio, A.-G. Ziegler, Primary dietary intervention study to reduce the risk of islet autoimmunity in children at increased risk for type 1 diabetes: the BABYDIET study, Diabetes Care 34 (6) (2011 Jun) 1301–1305.

[102] M. Knip, H.K. Åkerblom, D. Becker, H.-M. Dosch, J. Dupre, W. Fraser, et al., Hydrolyzed infant formula and early β-cell autoimmunity: a randomized clinical trial, JAMA 311 (22) (2014 Jun) 2279–2287.

[103] O. Vaarala, J. Ilonen, T. Ruohtula, J. Pesola, S.M. Virtanen, T. Härkönen, et al., Removal of bovine insulin from Cow's Milk formula and early initiation of Beta-cell autoimmunity in the FINDIA pilot study, Arch. Pediatr. Adolesc. Med. 166 (7) (2012 Jul) 608–614.

[104] C.M. Dayan, M. Korah, D. Tatovic, B.N. Bundy, K.C. Herold, Changing the landscape for type 1 diabetes: the first step to prevention, Lancet [Internet] 394 (10205) (2019) 1286–1296. Available from https://doi.org/10.1016/S0140-6736(19)32127-0.

[105] S.C. Shah, J.I. Malone, N.E. Simpson, A randomized trial of intensive insulin therapy in newly diagnosed insulin-dependent diabetes mellitus, N. Engl. J. Med. 320 (9) (1989) 550–554.

[106] M.A. Atkinson, N.K. Maclaren, R. Luchetta, Insulitis and diabetes in NOD mice reduced by prophylactic insulin therapy, Diabetes 39 (8) (1990 Aug) 933–937.

[107] R.J. Keller, G.S. Eisenbarth, R.A. Jackson, Insulin prophylaxis in individuals at high risk of type I diabetes, Lancet (London, England) 341 (8850) (1993) 927–928.

[108] Diabetes Prevention Trial- -Type 1 Diabetes Study Group, Effects of insulin in relatives of patients with type 1 diabetes mellitus, N. Engl. J. Med. 346 (22) (2002) 1685–1691.

[109] J.S. Skyler, J.P. Krischer, J. Wolfsdorf, C. Cowie, J.P. Palmer, C. Greenbaum, et al., Effects of oral insulin in relatives of patients with type 1 diabetes: the diabetes prevention trial-type 1, Diabetes Care 28 (5) (2005 May) 1068–1076.

[110] R. Tisch, R.S. Liblau, X.D. Yang, P. Liblau, H.O. McDevitt, Induction of GAD65-specific regulatory T-cells inhibits ongoing autoimmune diabetes in nonobese diabetic mice, Diabetes 47 (6) (1998 Jun) 894–899.

18. Prediction of autoimmune diseases: From bench to bedside

[111] J. Tian, M. Clare-Salzler, A. Herschenfeld, B. Middleton, D. Newman, R. Mueller, et al., Modulating autoimmune responses to GAD inhibits disease progression and prolongs islet graft survival in diabetes-prone mice, Nat. Med. 2 (12) (1996 Dec) 1348–1353.

[112] H. Elding Larsson, M. Lundgren, B. Jonsdottir, D. Cuthbertson, J. Krischer, Safety and efficacy of autoantigen-specific therapy with 2 doses of alum-formulated glutamate decarboxylase in children with multiple islet autoantibodies and risk for type 1 diabetes: a randomized clinical trial, Pediatr. Diabetes 19 (3) (2018) 410–419.

[113] O. Rachid, A. Osman, R. Abdi, Y. Haik, CTLA4-Ig (abatacept): a promising investigational drug for use in type 1 diabetes, Expert Opin. Investig. Drugs [Internet] 29 (3) (2020) 221–236. Available from https://doi.org/10.1080/13543784.2020.1727885.

[114] T. Orban, B. Bundy, D.J. Becker, L.A. DiMeglio, S.E. Gitelman, R. Goland, et al., Co-stimulation modulation with abatacept in patients with recent-onset type 1 diabetes: a randomised, double-blind, placebo-controlled trial, Lancet (London, England) 378 (9789) (2011) 412–419.

[115] N. Sherry, W. Hagopian, J. Ludvigsson, S.M. Jain, J. Wahlen, R.J.J. Ferry, et al., Teplizumab for treatment of type 1 diabetes (Protégé study): 1-year results from a randomised, placebo-controlled trial, Lancet (London, England) 378 (9790) (2011) 487–497.

[116] W. Hagopian, R.J.J. Ferry, N. Sherry, D. Carlin, E. Bonvini, S. Johnson, et al., Teplizumab preserves C-peptide in recent-onset type 1 diabetes: two-year results from the randomized, placebo-controlled Protégé trial, Diabetes 62 (11) (2013 Nov) 3901–3908.

[117] C. Guglielmi, S.R. Williams, R. Del Toro, P. Pozzilli, Efficacy and safety of otelixizumab use in new-onset type 1 diabetes mellitus, Expert. Opin. Biol. Ther. 16 (6) (2016 Jun) 841–846.

[118] D.J. Becker, S.E. Gitelman, R. Goland, P.A. Gottlieb, J.B. Marks, P.F. Mcgee, et al., Rituximab, B-Lymphocyte Depletion, and Preservation of Beta-Cell Function, 2009.

[119] B. Terrier, N. Derian, Y. Schoindre, W. Chaara, G. Geri, N. Zahr, et al., Restoration of regulatory and effector T cell balance and B cell homeostasis in systemic lupus erythematosus patients through vitamin D supplementation, Arthritis Res. Ther. 14 (5) (2012 Oct) R221.

[120] G. Ruiz-Irastorza, S. Gordo, N. Olivares, M.-V. Egurbide, C. Aguirre, Changes in vitamin D levels in patients with systemic lupus erythematosus: effects on fatigue, disease activity, and damage, Arthritis Care Res. (Hoboken) 62 (8) (2010 Aug) 1160–1165.

[121] C.C. Mok, D.J. Birmingham, L.Y. Ho, L.A. Hebert, H. Song, B.H. Rovin, Vitamin D deficiency as marker for disease activity and damage in systemic lupus erythematosus: a comparison with anti-dsDNA and anti-C1q, Lupus 21 (1) (2012) 36–42.

[122] Y. Schoindre, M. Jallouli, M.L. Tanguy, P. Ghillani, L. Galicier, O. Aumaître, et al., Lower vitamin D levels are associated with higher systemic lupus erythematosus activity, but not predictive of disease flare-up, Lupus Sci. Med. 1 (1) (2014) 1–8.

[123] K.H. Costenbader, D. Feskanich, M. Holmes, E.W. Karlson, E. Benito-Garcia, Vitamin D intake and risks of systemic lupus erythematosus and rheumatoid arthritis in women, Ann. Rheum. Dis. 67 (4) (2008) 530–535.

[124] K.A. Young, M.E. Munroe, J.M. Guthridge, D.L. Kamen, T.B. Niewold, G.S. Gilkeson, et al., Combined role of vitamin D status and CYP24A1 in the transition to systemic lupus erythematosus, Ann. Rheum. Dis. 76 (1) (2017 Jan) 153–158.

[125] K. Hagen, M. Byfuglien, L. Falzon, S. Olsen, G. Smedslung, Dietary Interventions for Rheumatoid Arthritis, Cochrane Library, 2009.

[126] C. Forsyth, M. Kouvari, N.M. D'Cunha, E.N. Georgousopoulou, D.B. Panagiotakos, D.D. Mellor, et al., The effects of the Mediterranean diet on rheumatoid arthritis prevention and treatment: a systematic review of human prospective studies, Rheumatol. Int. 38 (5) (2018 May) 737–747.

[127] X. Liu, S.K. Tedeschi, M. Barbhaiya, C.L. Leatherwood, C.B. Speyer, B. Lu, et al., Impact and timing of smoking cessation on reducing risk of rheumatoid arthritis among women in the nurses' health studies, Arthritis Care Res. 71 (7) (2019) 914–924.

[128] G. Chodick, H. Amital, Y. Shalem, E. Kokia, A.D. Heymann, A. Porath, et al., Persistence with statins and onset of rheumatoid arthritis: a population-based cohort study, PLoS Med. 7 (9) (2010) 1–13.

[129] D.M. Gerlag, M. Safy, K.I. Maijer, M.W. Tang, S.W. Tas, M.J.F. Starmans-Kool, et al., Effects of B-cell directed therapy on the preclinical stage of rheumatoid arthritis: the PRAIRI study, Ann. Rheum. Dis. 78 (2) (2019 Feb) 179–185.

[130] W.H. Bos, B.A.C. Dijkmans, M. Boers, R.J. Van De Stadt, D. Van Schaardenburg, Effect of dexamethasone on autoantibody levels and arthritis development in patients with arthralgia: a randomised trial, Ann. Rheum. Dis. 69 (3) (2010) 571–574.

Index

Note: Page numbers followed by *f* indicate figures and *t* indicate tables.

A

Abatacept, 231–234
Absent in melanoma 2 (AIM2), 150–151
Activation and/or survival signals, 28
ActivinA/nodal signaling, 139
Acute coronary syndrome (ACS), 300–301
Acute inflammation, 116
Acute-phase proteins (APPs), 86
Adalimumab (ADA), 210, 211–212*t*, 214–215*t*, 217–218*t*, 220*t*, 222–223*t*, 225–226*t*, 228*t*, 230*t*, 232*t*
Adaptive immunity, 86–87, 194–195
Adipose tissue, 332
Adult-onset Still's disease (AOSD), 90
Advanced therapy medicinal products (ATMPs)
    biologic origin, 320
    treatment, 321, 321*f*
    types of products, 320
Adverse effects (AEs), 97–99, 98*t*
Aging
    accumulation of errors, 195–196
    age and sex differences, 196–197
    cancer development, 199
    clinical presentation, 196–197
    epidemiological data related, 196–197, 197–199*t*
    history, 195–196
    process, 120–121
    thymus involution, 196
Akkermansia muciniphila, 283
AkT-mTOR-SMAD3 pathway, 63
ANCA-associated vasculitis (AAV), 90
Animal models, 402–406, 403–413*t*
Ankylosing spondylitis (AS), 60, 90–91, 155, 159–160, 303
Anti-AchR antibodies, 91
Antibody-dependent cellular cytotoxicity (ADCC), 308–309
Anti-CD20 mAb (rituximab), 40, 44–45
Anti-CD52mAb (alemtuzumab), 45–46
Anticitrullinated peptide antibody (ACPA), 118, 159, 432
Anticyclic citrullinated peptide (anti-CCP) antibodies, 44, 275, 303
Antidrug antibodies (ADAs), 206
Antigen-presenting cells (APCs), 4–6, 57
Antiinflammatory cytokines, 119
Antiinflammatory treatments, 307–308

Anti-mitotic reagents, 180
Antinuclear antibodies (ANA), 432
Antineutrophil cytoplasmic autoantibodies (ANCA), 68–69, 416
Antiphospholipid syndrome (APS), 415
Antismooth muscle antibody titres, 68–69
Anti-TNF-α agents
    certolizumab pegol, 213
    etanercept, 213–216
    golimumab, 213
    inflammatory diseases, 207
    infliximab, 207–210, 208–209*t*
    therapies, 118
Apremilast, 45
A proliferation inducing ligand (APRIL), 181–182
Artificial thymic organoids (ATOs), 142
ASCERTAIN trial, 97–98
Atacicept, 185
Atherosclerosis, 162–163
Atopic dermatitis (AD), 13–14
Autism spectrum disorder (ASD), 401
Autoantibodies, 363, 432
Autoimmune bullous diseases, 415
Autoimmune cardiac diseases
    myocarditis, 21–22
    rheumatic heart diseases (RHD), 21
Autoimmune digestive disorders
    celiac disease (CeD), 345–347
    inflammatory bowel disease (IBD), 347–350
Autoimmune diseases (AIDs). *See also* Chronotherapy; Clock; Clock-controlled pathway; Inflammatory cytokine inhibition (ICI); Systemic lupus erythematosus (SLE)
    chronic and systemic inflammatory disorders, 155
    description, 150
    heterogeneous group of disorders, 425–426
    and leishmaniasis, 414–415
    NLRP3/IL-1β axis, 154–155
    pathogenesis, 425–426, 427*f*
    phases, 425–426, 426*f*
    psoriasis, 20–21
    and toxoplasmosis, 415–416
    type I cytokines, 19–20
Autoimmune diseases-induced atherosclerosis, 162–163
Autoimmune lymphoproliferative syndrome (ALPS), 61

452　　Index

Autoimmune neurological disorder, 44
Autoimmune polyendocrine syndrome-1 (APS-1), 137–138
Autoimmune polyendocrinopathy-candidiasis-ectodermal dystrophy (APECED), 137–138
Autoimmune regulator, 137
Autoimmune-related uveitic disorders, 91
Autoimmune skin disorders
　pemphigus, 343
　psoriasis, 343–345
　systemic sclerosis (SSc), 339–343
　vitiligo, 339, 340t
Autoimmune thyroid diseases (AITD), 283–284
　bile acid metabolism, 274
　etiology, 274
　immune-mediated mechanisms, 273
　Lactobacillus species, 275
　specific pathogen-free rats, 274
Autoimmunity malignancies, 38
"Autoimmunity Theory of Aging", 196
Autologous hematopoietic stem cell transplantation, 187

B

Bacillus Calmette-Guérin (BCG) disease, 68
Bacteria-derived LPS, 154
B-cell activation factor from the TNF superfamily (BAFF), 183–184
B-cell depletion, 185
B-cell maturation antigen (BCMA), 181–182
B cells into antibody-producing cells (BSF-2), 86
Behçet's syndrome (BS), 91
Belatacept, 234
Biomarker, 426, 429, 431
Blood–brain barrier (BBB), 24
Body composition and metabolic health
　immune profiles and inflammatory status, 244
　metabolic syndrome (MetS), 245–246
　overweight and obesity, 244–245
Body mass index (BMI), 244
Bortezomib, 185–186
Brain and Muscle ARNT-like 1 (BMAL1), 163
B regulatory cell (Breg cells). *See also* In vivo maintenance/expansion
　defined, 38
　expansion of, 46
　functional properties, 39–40, 39f
　granzyme B (GrB), 42
　IL-10 producing, 40–41
　IL-35 producing, 41
　receptor-mediated inhibitory mechanisms, 42–43
　TGF-β producing, 41–42
Brodalumab, 224
Bystander suppression, 5–6

C

Cancer
　description, 308
　immune system involvement, 308–309
　inflammatory pathways, 308–309, 309f
　precision medicine, 309–310
CAR-BCMA T cells, 185–186
Carbohydrates, 249–250
Carbon-based nanoparticles (CNT), 369
Cardiovascular disease (CVD)
　atherosclerotic plaque formation and progression, 300–301, 301f
　cholesterol-lowering statins, 303
　inflammatory pathways, 302
　mortality and morbidity, 300–301
　musculoskeletal diseases, 303
　risk assessment and prognosis, 303
CARMIL2 deficiency, 69
CAR T-cell therapies, 310
Caspase 8-dependent alternative inflammasome activation pathway, 154
Caspase 1 inhibitors, 150–151, 167
Castleman's disease, 84
CD19+ CD5+ CD1dhi B cells, 38
CD19 expression, 185
CD20 expression, 183, 185–186
CD25 deficiency, 68
CD122 deficiency, 68–69
CD138 expression, 181–182
Celiac disease (CeD), 345–347
Cell adhesion molecules (CAMs), 117
Cell-based therapies, 320
Cell therapy, 6–7, 136, 322–336, 339, 343–350, 352
Central nervous system (CNS), 24
Certolizumab pegol inhibitors, 125, 213
Chimeric antigen receptor (CAR), 298–299
Chloride intracellular channels (CLICs), 153–154
Chronic inflammation, 116, 120–121
Chronic lymphocytic thyroiditis, 274
Chronotherapy
　berberine, 168
　caspase 1 inhibitors, 167
　CCR2/CCL2 axis, 168
　defined, 168
　IL-1 blockade, 167
　NLRP3 inhibitors, 166–167
Ciliary neurotrophic factor (CNTF), 85
Circadian immunity, defined, 163
Circadian rhythms, 163
Clock
　alteration, 163–165
　macrophages harbor, 163
　structure, 163, 164f

Clock-controlled pathway, 165–166
Collaborative Islet Transplant Registry (CITR), 323
Collagen-induced arthritis (CIA), 26, 39–40, 284
Combined ATMPs (cATMPs), 320
Common lymphoid progenitor (CLP) cells, 15–16, 56–57
Common variable immunodeficiency (CVID), 65, 66t
Complement-dependent cytotoxicity (CDC), 308–309
Congenital deficiencies, 137–138
Copper-based nanoparticles, 384–385
Cord blood-derived HSCs (CB-HSCs), 142
Cortical thymic epithelial cells (cTECs), 137
Corticoids, 180
Corticosteroids, 2–3
C-reactive protein (CRP), 302
Crohn's disease (CD), 22–23, 91, 415
Cryopyrin-associated periodic syndrome (CAPS), 151, 155
C-type lectin receptors (CLRs), 150–151
Cultured melanocyte transplantation, 339
Cyclic GMP-AMP synthase (cGAS), 150–151
Cysteine-rich domains (CRDs), 122
Cytokines, 4. *See also* Inflammatory cytokine inhibition (ICI)
  balance, 399–400
  immune responses, 206
Cytoplasmic nucleotide-binding, 150–151
Cytotoxic T-lymphocyte-associated antigen-4 (CTLA-4), 206, 310

D

Damage-associated molecular patterns (DAMPs), 150–151
Danish National Birth Cohort, 244–245
Definitive endoderm cells (DEs), 139
Delayed-type hypersensitivity (DTH), 38
Dendritic cells (DCs), 332
DEP domain containing mTOR interacting protein (DEPTOR), 159–160
Depression
  antiinflammatory treatments, 307–308
  description, 306
  epidemiological research, 306
  inflammation, 306–307, 307f
Diabetes Autoimmunity Study in the Young (DAISY) cohort, 427
Diabetes mellitus
  genome-wide association studies (GWAS), 299
  immune system and inflammatory factors, 299–300
  immunomodulatory therapies, 300
  rheumatoid arthritis (RA), 25–26
  type 1 diabetes (T1D), 24–25
  type 2 diabetes (T2D), 25
  uncontrolled hyperglycemia, 299

Dietary patterns
  defined, 246
  Mediterranean diet, 247–249
  western diet, 246–247
DiGeorge syndrome, 137–138
Directed differentiation protocols, 138–141, 143f
Disease Activity Score of 28 joints (DAS-28), 285
Disease-modifying anti-rheumatic drugs (DMARDs), 3, 94, 276
Disease pathology, 19
DOCK8 deficiency, 67–68
Double-negative T (DNT) cells, 61
Dysbiosis. *See also* Autoimmune thyroid diseases (AITD); Rheumatoid arthritis (RA); Sjögren's syndrome (SS); Systemic lupus erythematosus (SLE)
  autoimmunity development, 273
  etiology, 272
  germ-free nonobese diabetic (NOD) mice, 272
  HbA1c, 273
  impaired epithelial barrier function, 271–272, 271f
  mechanisms, 271–272
  and mucosal immune system, 273
  prediabetic children, 272

E

Edmonton protocol, 322–323
Effector functions, 27–28
Effector T cells, 57
Endothelial nitric oxide synthase (eNOS), 116–117
Enhanced permeability and retention (EPR), 378–380
Epidemiologists, 194
Erythrocyte sedimentation rate (ESR), 309–310
Etanercept, 213–216
European bone marrow transplantation (EBMT) database, 352
European league against rheumatism (EULAR) database, 352
Excretory/secretory products (ESPs), 396, 407–413t
Expanded Disability Status Scale (EDSS) score, 44, 91, 336
Experimental autoimmune encephalitis (EAE) model, 38–40, 44, 401–402
Extracellular signal-regulated kinases (ERK), 121
Extracellular signals, 150–151
Extra virgin olive oil (EVOO), 248–249

F

Fas ligand (FasL), 40
Ferromagnetic nanoparticles, 384
Fibroblast-like synoviocytes (FLS), 25–26
First-degree relatives (FDRs), 325
Flavin-dependent monooxygenase (FMO3) enzyme, 284

454   Index

Follicular regulatory T cells (fTreg), 60
FoxP3⁺ γδT cells, 60
FoxP3, 431 amino acid-long protein, 58

G

Galphaq (Gαq), 38
Gastrointestinal perforations, 99
General transcription factor IIi (GTF2i), 430
Gene therapy, 6, 326, 332–333
Gene therapy medicinal products (GTMPs), 320
Genetic Risk Scores (GRS), 427
Genome-wide association studies (GWASs), 65, 427
Giant cell arteritis (GCA), 90
Glial fibrillary acidic protein (GFAP), 93
Glucocorticoid-induced TNFR-related ligand (GITRL)
    expression, 40
Glucocorticoid therapy, 2–3
Gold nanoparticles (AuNPs), 378, 380–382
Golimumab, 213
Graft-*versus*-host disease, 84
Granulocyte-macrophage colony-stimulating factor
    (GM-CSF), 16–17, 87
Granulomatosis with polyangiitis (GPA), 90
Granzyme B (GrB) cells, 42
Graves' disease (GD), 61, 273
Graves' ophthalmopathy (GO), 91
Guselkumab, 227

H

Hashimoto's thyroiditis (HT), 61, 273–274
Hassell's corpuscles, 137
Helminthic therapy. *See also* Animal models
    antihelminth treatment, 397–398
    application of, 399–400, 400*f*
    atopy and allergic hypersensitivity, 406
    challenges, 402
    epidemiological investigations, 396
    immune profiles, 399, 399*f*
    immune regulation, 397–398
    immunosuppressive agents, 399–400
    intracellular pathogens, 397
    prevalence of, 396, 396–397*t*
    underdeveloped or developing nations, 396
Hematopoietic stem cells (HSCs), 137
Hematopoietic stem cell transplantation (HSCT), 6–7,
    67, 332
Henoch-Schönlein purpura (HSP), 90
Heparan sulfate proteoglycans (HSPG), 181–182
High-mobility group box-1 (HMGB1) levels, 93
High-sensitivity C-reactive protein (hs-CRP), 250
Homeostasis, 18–19
Homeostatic model assessment-B cell function
    (HOMA-B), 285
"Horror autotoxicus", 363–364

hPSC-derived anterior foregut endoderm, 139
Human embryonic stem cells (hESC), 138
Human fibroblast-like synoviocytes (HFLS), 429
Human-induced pluripotent stem cells (hiPSC), 138
Human leukocyte antigen (HLA) alleles, 427
Human pluripotent stem cells (hPSC), 138
Human thymus development and function, 137,
    142–144
Human umbilical cord blood-derived MSCs (hUCB-
    MSCs), 332
Humoral immunity, 183–184, 184*f*
Hypothalamus-pituitary-adrenal (HPA) axis, 89

I

Idiopathic thrombocytopenic purpura (ITP), 4–5
Idiopathic uveitis, 91
IκBKβ deficiency, 68
ILC 1, 15–16
ILC 2, 16
ILC 3, 16–17, 17*t*
ILC populations, 28
IL-6 trans-presentation, 86
IL-6 trans-signaling, 85–86
IL-23/IL-17A pathway, 20–21
Immune checkpoint blockade (ICB) treatment, 310
Immune checkpoint inhibitors (ICIs), 206
    abatacept, 231–234
    antagonists, 231
    belatacept, 234
    CTLA-4 genes, 231
Immune deficiency, 68
Immune dysregulation polyendocrinopathy
    enteropathy X-linked (IPEX) syndrome, 56, 65–67
Immune-mediated Hashimoto's thyroiditis, 364
Immune system dysfunction, 296
Immunoglobulins (Ig), 3–4, 206
"Immunological Theory of Aging", 195–196
Immunometabolism, 7
Immunomodulation, 300, 397–398, 416
Immunoregulators, 26–27
Immunosenescence
    immune cells, 296–297, 297*f*
    and inflammatory pathways, 298
    senescent cells, 296
    senolytic therapies, 298–299
    T and B cells, 296
Immunosuppressant indoleamine dioxygenase (IDO1),
    308
Immunotherapy, 3–4
Inborn errors, Treg dysfunction
    CARMIL2 deficiency, 69
    CD25 deficiency, 68
    CD122 deficiency, 68–69
    DOCK8 deficiency, 67–68

IκBKβ deficiency, 68
  mutations, 67
Inducible nitric oxide synthase (iNOS) expression, 116–117
Inducible Treg (iTreg) cells, 4
Inflammaging/immunosenescence, 194–195
Inflammatory bowel disease (IBD), 13–14, 22–23, 70–71, 91, 118, 161, 347–350, 400
Inflammatory cytokine inhibition
  anti-TNF-α (*see* Anti-TNF-α agents)
  interleukin-6 (IL-6) (*see* Interleukin-6 (IL-6))
  interleukin-17 (*see* Interleukin-17 (IL-17))
  interleukin-23 (*see* Interleukin-23 (IL-23))
Inflammatory pathways, 298
Inflammatory skin disease, 44
Infliximab, 207–210, 208–209t
Inhaled/topical corticosteroids, 2–3
Innate effector cells, 119
Innate immune system, 150–151, 194–196
Innate lymphoid cells (ILCs). *See also* Autoimmune cardiac diseases; Autoimmune diseases; Diabetes; Immunoregulators; Inflammatory bowel disease (IBD); Systemic lupus erythematosus (SLE)
  and adaptive immunity, 13–14
  characteristics of, 15
  disease pathology, 19
  features, 13–14
  groups of, 15
  homeostasis, 18–19
  ILC 1 (*see* ILC 1)
  ILC 2 (*see* ILC 2)
  ILC 3 (*see* ILC 3)
  lymphoid and nonlymphoid tissues, 13–14, 18
  protective immune functions, 18, 19f
  roles, 13–14
Innate/natural immunity, 194–195
Inorganic nanoparticles, 369
Intercellular adhesion molecule 1 (ICAM-1), 117
Interferon regulatory factor 3 (IRF3), 123
Interleukin-6 (IL-6)
  and acute-phase proteins, 92–93, 93t
  adverse effects (AEs), 97–99, 98t
  cell types, 84, 84t
  drug interactions, warnings, and immunogenicity, 101
  efficacy, 95–97
  factors, 84
  four-helix protein, 83–84
  hepcidin production, 92–93
  host defense mechanism, 86–87
  on lymphoid cells, 88, 89t
  mild elevations, 95, 95f
  off-label use, 101–103
  physiological and nonphysiological stimuli, 84, 85t
  pleyotropic effects, 86, 87f
  sarilumab, 219

signaling, 85–86, 86f
  sirukumab, 219–221
  targeting levels, 94, 94t
  T cell differentiation, 87–88, 88f
  tocilizumab, 216
  urinary, 93
Interleukin-17 (IL-17)
  brodalumab, 224
  ixekizumab, 224
  secukinumab, 221
Interleukin-23 (IL-23)
  guselkumab, 227
  risankizumab, 227–231
  tildrakizumab, 227
  ustekinumab, 227
International Union of Immunological Societies (IUIS), 15
Intestinal microbiota, 270
Intestinal pathobionts, 278
Intraarticular (IA) injection, 332
Intracellular staining protocol (CD4$^+$ CD25$^+$ FoxP3$^+$), 62–63
Intrauterine fetal growth retardation (IUGR), 119–120
Invariant natural killer T cells (iNKT), 60
In vitro coculture systems, 142–144
In vivo maintenance/expansion, anti-CD20 mAb (rituximab), 44–45
Islet transplantation, 322–323
Ixekizumab, 224

J

JAK/STAT signaling, 28
Janus kinases (JAKs), 3–4, 85
Joint inflammation, 25–26
Juvenile idiopathic arthritis (JIA), 90, 159

K

Kawasaki disease (KD), 71, 90
Killer cell lectin-like receptor 1 (KLRG1) expression, 298

L

Leishmaniasis, 414–415
Leucine-rich repeat (LRR), 150–151
Leukemia inhibitory factor (LIF), 85
Lipopolysaccharide-responsive and beige-like anchor protein (LRBA), 65
Local tissue homeostasis, 63
Low carbohydrate diet (LCD), 249
Lymphocyte activation gene-3 (LAG-3), 61

M

Macronutrients
  carbohydrates, 249–250
  omega-3 polyunsaturated fatty acids, 251–252
  protein, 250–251

Macrophage colony-stimulating factor (M-CSF), 87
Macrophages, 25–26
Magnetic associated cell sorter (MACS), 63
Major histocompatibility complexes (MHC), 137
Matrix metallopeptidase (MMP)-9 activity, 119
Maximum lifespan, 193–194
Mediterranean diet, 245–249
Medullary thymic epithelial cells (mTECs), 137
Memory plasmocytes, 181
Mental health conditions. *See* Depression
Mesenchymal stem cells (MSCs), 324
Mesenchymal stromal cell therapy, 6–7
Metabolic syndrome (MetS), 245–246
Metacarpophalangeal (MCP) joints, 333
Metal-based nanoparticles
  biocompatibility, inertness and surface
    modifications, 375–376
  biological processes, 369
  characteristics, 371–377
  drug loading and release, 376–377
  drug delivery system (DDS), 378
  in vivo therapeutic applications, 369
  production of, 370
  safety concern, 385–386
  shape and morphology reliance, 373–374, 374f
  size (nanoscale array), 370
  smaller size and great surface area-to-volume ratio,
    372
  surface properties, 376
MHC Class I expression, 309
Microbiota
  autoimmune diseases development, 271–272
  determinants, 274
  duodenal mucosa biopsies, 273
  HT patients, 274–275
  human health and disease, 278
  intestinal, 270
  manipulation and probiotic application, 7
  oxidative phosphorylation and glycan metabolism
    pathways, 277
  prediabetic children, 272
  primary SS patients, 279
  Th17 lymphocytes, 275–276
Micronutrients
  autoimmune disorders, 252
  selenium (Se), 253–254
  sodium, 254
  vitamin D, 252–253
miR-155 inhibitor, 160
Mitochondrial antiviral signaling protein (MAVS), 123
Mitogen-activated protein kinase (MAPK), 85
Monoclonal antibodies (mAbs), 92–93, 99–100, 206,
    364–365
Mononuclear phagocytes, 116

mTOR pathway, 298
Multimorbidity, 310–311
Multiple sclerosis (MS), 13–14, 24, 44–46, 71, 91, 401
  cell therapy, 333–336
  central nervous system (CNS), 333
  ongoing clinical trials, 337–338t
Multiplex assay technologies (MAS), 440–441
Multiplex assay technologies with algorithmic analysis
    (MAAA), 440–441
Muromonab, 4–5
Musculoskeletal conditions
  immune system involvement, 304–305, 304f
  morbidity and disability, 303
  precision medicine, 305–306
Myocarditis, 21–22

N
NADPH oxidase (NOX) family, 117
Nanomedicines, 367, 386
Nanoparticles (NPs), 362–363, 362f, 366
  chemical and inorganic compounds, 366
  classification, 367–369
  metal-based (*see* Metal-based nanoparticles)
  particulate carrier systems, 367
Nanotechnology
  clinical fields, 362–363
  and nanomaterials, 365–377
National Institute of Health (NIH), 363
Natural autoimmunity, 363–364
Natural/innate immunity, 194–195
Neuromyelitis optica spectrum disorder (NMOSD), 219
Neuropsychiatric disorders (NPDs), 401
Neutropenia, 99
Neutrophil extracellular traps (NETs), 151–153, 158,
    298, 415
Niches, 181
Nicotinamide adenine dinucleotide phosphate
    (NADPH), 117
Nitric oxide (NO) synthesis, 116–117
NK cell depletion, 24
NLRP3 inflammasome
  activation, 153–154, 155–157t
  and autoimmune diseases (*see* Autoimmune
    diseases)
  pathway, 121
  priming, 151–153
  structure and function, 151, 152f
Non-B/non-T (NBNT) cells, 16
Noncultured epidermal suspension transplant, 339
Noninfectious endogenous danger molecules, 150–151
Non-nutrient dietary factors, 254–255
Nonrelevant pathways and cell functions, 2
Non-ST wave-elevated myocardial infarction
    (NSTEM1), 300–301

Index

457

Nordic diet, 245–246
Nucleotide-binding domain (NOD), 150–151
nude phenotype, 137–138

O

OKT3 (Ortho Kung 3), 4–5
Oligomerization domain (NOD)-like receptors (NLR), 150–151
Omega-3 polyunsaturated fatty acids, 251–252
Oral tolerance, 6, 18–19
Organic nanoparticles, 368–369
Osteoarthritis (OA), 303
Overweight and obesity, 244–245
Oxidative PTM-insulin (oxPTM-INS-Ab), 430

P

Palindromic rheumatism (PR) severity, 248
Parasites, 413
Parvovirus B19 (B19V), 160
Pathogen-associated molecular patterns (PAMPs), 150–151
Pattern recognition receptors (PRRs), 150–151
Pemphigus
    cell therapy, 343
    ongoing clinical trials, 343, 344*t*
    pathogenic relevance, 343
Peripheral blood mononuclear cells (PBMCs), 38, 158
Peripheral clocks, 163
Peripheral neutrophilia, 86–87
Phagocytosis of crystals, 153
Pharmacodynamics, 99–101
Pharmacokinetics, 99–101, 100*t*
Pharmacological treatments, autoimmune diseases, 27–29
Phase II ANDANTE I and II trials, 102
Phase III SIRROUND trials, 101–102
Phosphatidylinositol-4, 5-biphosphate 3-kinase (PI3K), 85
Plant-based diets, 250–251
Plasmablasts, 180–181
Plasmacytoid dendritic cells (pDCs), 245
Plasma viscosity (PV), 309–310
Plasmocytes
    chemokines, 181
    effector cells, 182–183
    humoral immunity, 180–181
    low-affinity antibodies, 180–181
    targeting, 187–188, 188*t*
Plasmocyte-specific niches, 186–187
Platelet hyperreactivity, 121
Platinum NPs (PtNPs), 380
Pluripotent stem cells. *See* Human pluripotent stem cells (hPSC)
Polyarteritis nodosa (PAN), 90

Polyarticular JIA (PJIA), 90
Polymyalgia rheumatica (PMR), 90
Polymyositis, 415
Positive and negative selection, 137, 142–144
Post-translational modifications (PTMs), 123–124, 153, 430
Precision medicine, 296, 305–306. *See also* Immunosenescence; Musculoskeletal conditions
Preeclampsia, 120
Pregnancy, 119–120
Preligand-binding assembly domain (PLAD), 122
Primary Sjögren's syndrome, 60
Probiotics
    autoimmune diabetes, 280–283, 281–282*t*
    autoimmune diseases, 279–280
    autoimmune thyroid diseases, 283–284
    rheumatoid arthritis (RA), 284–285
    Sjögren's syndrome (SS), 286–287
    systemic lupus erythematous (SLE), 285–286
Programmed cell death 1 (PD-1), 206
Programmed cell death-ligand 1 (PD-L1), 40, 206
Proinflammatory cytokines, 302
Promote *vs.* mitigate autoimmune disease, 255, 255*f*
Promyelocytic leukemia zinc finger protein (PLZF), 60
Prostacyclin, 116–117
Prostaglandin E (PGE2), 116–117
Prostaglandin F2α (PGF2 α), 116–117
Prostaglandin PGI2, 116–117
Protective/adaptive immunity, 194–195
Protein, 250–251
Protein inhibitors of activated STATs (PIAS), 85
Protein methylation, 123–124
Psoralen plus ultraviolet A (PUVA), 339
Psoriasis, 13–14, 20–21, 44–45, 117–118
    cell therapy, 343–345
    immune-mediated chronic systemic inflammatory disease, 343
    ongoing clinical trials, 343, 346*t*
Psoriasis Area and Severity Index (PASI), 246–247
Psoriatic arthritis (PsA), 44–45, 90–91, 159, 244–245, 303
P2X purinoceptor 7 (P2rx7), 153
Pyrin domain-containing protein 3 (NLRP3). *See* NLRP3 inflammasome

Q

Quantitative polymerase chain reaction (qPCR), 432

R

Rapamycin (mTOR) protein kinase, 63
Reactive arthritis (ReA), 90–91
Reactive oxygen species (ROS), 153
Reaggregated thymic organotypic cultures (RTOCs), 142
Receptor activator of NF-κβ ligand (RANKL), 88

Receptor-binding, 121–123
Receptor-mediated inhibitory mechanisms, 42–43
Regulatory T cells (Treg cells)
  in bone marrow, 56–57
  canonical markers, 58
  CD4$^+$ CD25^{high} cells, 58
  cell surface markers, 56
  clinical implications, 72, 73–74t
  cytokines, 72
  developmental trajectory, 56–57, 57f
  discovery, 56
  dose-dependent, 75
  homeostasis, 324
  IL-2, 72
  intracellular and extracellular markers, 58, 59t
  pathogenesis, 72
  phenotype, 58, 59f
  randomized trials, 72
  surface receptors, 75
  transforming growth factor-β1(TGF-β1), 57
Remitting seronegative symmetrical synovitis with
    pitting edema (RS3PE) syndrome, 90
Respiratory burst, 195–196
Retinoic acid receptor-related orphan receptor-α
    (RORα), 16
Retinoic acid receptor-related orphan receptor γt
    (RORγt) expression, 63–64
Rheumatic heart diseases (RHD), 21
Rheumatoid arthritis (RA), 13–14, 25–26, 43–44, 60,
    69–70, 118–119, 155, 158–159, 402–403, 415, 428–429,
    432, 435–440, 436–439t, 438f, 443–444
  antibiotic administration, 275–276
  cell therapy, 326–332
  chronic inflammatory arthropathy, 326
  etiopathogenesis, 276–277
  fecal transplantation, 275–276
  gene therapy, 332–333
  joint inflammation, 275
  methotrexate-treated patients, 276
  ongoing clinical trials, 326, 334–335t
  oral administration, 276
  osteomicrobiology, 276–277
  probiotics, 284–285
  systemic autoimmune disease, 275
Rheumatoid factor (RF), 44
Risankizumab, 227–231

S

Sarcoidosis, 91
SARIL-RA-KAKEHASI phase III trial, 96
SARIL-RA-MOBILITY Part A phase II RCT, 96
SARIL-RA-TARGET phase III study, 96
Sarilumab, 219
Secukinumab, 221

Selenium (Se), 253–254
Selenomethionine (SeMet), 253–254
Senescence-associated secretory phenotype (SASP), 296
Senolytics, 298–299
Serum high-sensitivity C-reactive protein (hs-CRP), 285
Serum pathogenic IL-17 cells, 89
Severe combined immune deficiency (SCID), 68
Signal transducer and activator of transcription 3
    (STAT3), 85
Silver nanoparticles (AgNPs), 378, 382–383
"Silver Tsunami", 193–195
Single nucleotide polymorphisms (SNPs), 118
Sirukumab, 219–221
Sjögren's syndrome (SS), 90, 155, 160–161, 278–279,
    286–287, 429–430, 432, 440
Skin prick test (SPT), 401
SLE disease activity index (SLEDAI), 64
Sodium, 254
Soluble gp130 (sgp130Fc), 85–86
Soluble TNF-α (sTNF-α), 121–122
Somatic cell therapy medicinal products (SCTMPs), 320
Spondyloarthritis (SpA), 159–160
Stimulator of interferon genes (STING), 123
ST wave-elevated myocardial infarction (STEM1),
    300–301
Subcutaneous (SC) administration, 216
Superparamagnetic iron oxide nanoparticles (SPIONs),
    384
Suppressor of cytokine signaling (SOCS3) protein, 85
Surface staining protocol (CD4$^+$ CD25$^+$ CD127$^{-/low}$), 62
Synovial membrane (synovitis), 118–119
Systemic JIA (SJIA), 90
Systemic lupus erythematosus (SLE), 13–14, 23, 56, 60,
    64–65, 89, 155, 158, 277–278, 303, 428, 431, 433–434,
    442
  conventional immunosuppressive therapies, 350
  ongoing clinical trials, 350, 351t
  probiotics, 285–286
Systemic sclerosis (SSc), 43–44, 155, 160, 219
  cell therapy, 342–343
  heterogeneous autoimmune disease, 339
  ongoing clinical trials, 341t

T

T cells, 3–4, 27
T1D in the Environmental Determinants of Diabetes in
    the Young (TEDDY) study, 427–428
T helper 1 (Th1) cells, 118
T helper 3 (Th3) cells, 61
T helper 17 (Th17) cells, 4, 118
Therapeutic agents, 2
Thioredoxin-interacting protein (TXNIP), 154
Th1/Th2 ratio, 397
Thymic deficiencies, 137–138

Thymic epithelial cells (TECs). *See also* Human
 pluripotent stem cells (hPSC)
 chemokines, 136–137
 E-cadherin, 136–137
 human-based model systems, 136–137
 mouse models, 136–137
Thymic epithelial progenitor cells (TEPs)
 hPSC-derived, 141–142, 143*f*
 in vitro coculture systems, 139–144
Thymic nurse cells, 137
Thymus gland, 136
Thymus organogenesis, 136–137
Thyroid diseases, 415
Thyroid peroxidase antibodies (TPOAb), 253–254
Thyrotropin receptor (TSHR) expression, 91
Tildrakizumab, 227
Tissue-engineered products (TEPs), 320
Tissue engineering, 325–326
Tissue-resident Treg cells, 63–64
Titanium oxide nanoparticles (TiO2NPs), 383–384
TNF-α converting enzyme (TACE), 121–122
TNF-α inhibitors (TNFi) function, 124–125
TNF homology domain (THD), 122
Toll-like receptor adaptor molecule (TRIF), 123
Toll-like receptors (TLRs), 3–4, 38, 150–151
Toxoplasmosis, 415–416
Trafficking, 29
Transforming growth factor-β1(TGF-β1), 57, 397, 398*f*
Translational studies, 8
Tr1 cells, 61
T regulatory (Treg) cells, 3–4, 38
Trimethylamine N-oxide (TMAO), 302
Tuft cells, 137
Tumor necrosis factor (TNF), 15–16
Tumor necrosis factor alpha (TNF-α). *See also*
 Pregnancy; Psoriasis
 acute and chronic, 116
 cell adhesion molecules (CAMs), 117
 complex structure and receptor-binding, 121–123
 development and application, 125–127
 edema, 117
 foreign or damaging entity, 115–116
 leukocytes, 116
 nitric oxide (NO) synthesis, 116–117
 proinflammatory cytokine, 116
 RA, 118–119
Tumor necrosis factor alpha converting enzyme
 (TACE), 302
Tumor necrosis factor receptor 1 (TNFR1), 119
Tumor necrosis factor superfamily (TNFSF13), 181–182

Type I cytokines, 19–20
Type 1 diabetes mellitus (T1DM), 56, 65
Type 1 diabetes (T1D), 24–25, 161–162, 406, 427–428,
 430–431, 433, 441–442. *See also* Dysbiosis
 cell therapy, 322–325
 gene therapy, 326
 insulin-producing beta cells, 322
 ongoing clinical trials, 322, 327–331*t*
 tissue engineering, 325–326
Type 2 diabetes (T2D), 25
Type I interferons (IFN-I), 158

U

UK RA Genetics Group Consortium (UKRAGG),
 428–429
Ulcerative colitis (UC), 22–23
Umbilical cord blood (UCB), 63
Umbilical cord-derived MSCs (UC-MSCs), 326–332
Urokinase-type plasminogen activator receptor (uPAR),
 298–299
Ustekinumab, 227

V

Vaccination, 5–6
Vascular cell adhesion molecule 1 (VCAM-1), 117
Vascular endothelial growth factor (VEGF), 310
Vasculitis
 cell therapy, 352
 inflamed blood vessel, 352
 ongoing clinical trials, 352, 352*t*
Vegetarian diets, 250–251
Ventral anterior foregut endoderm (vAFE), 139
Visceral adipose tissue (VAT), 63
Vitamin D supplementation, 65, 252–253
Vitiligo
 cell therapy, 339
 human pigmentation disease, 339
 ongoing clinical trials, 340*t*
Vogt-Koyanagi-Harada syndrome, 91

W

"Wear and Tear Theory of Aging", 195–196
Wegener's granulomatosis, 415
Wellcome Trust Case Control Consortium (WTCCC),
 428–429
Western diet, 246–247

Z

Zinc oxide nanoparticles (ZnONPs), 383